# Emergency Patient Care for the EMT-A

# Contributors

David DeGroote, EMT-P
Director, Ambulance Service
Bloomington Hospital
Bloomington, Indiana

John Goll, EMT-P
EMS Educator, Ambulance Service
Wishard Memorial Hospital
Indianapolis, Indiana

Nancy McClure, RPT
Assistant Supervisor
Physical Therapy Department
Wishard Memorial Hospital
Indianapolis, Indiana

Paul J. Smith, EMT-P, MS
Director, Ambulance Service
Wishard Memorial Hospital
Indianapolis, Indiana

Paul W. Thorensen, Ph.D.
Assistant Professor of Clinical Psychology
Psychiatry Department
Indiana University School of Medicine
Indianapolis, Indiana

Gary E. Zeller, REMT-A
EMS Educator, Ambulance Service
Wishard Memorial Hospital
Indianapolis, Indiana

# Emergency Patient Care for the EMT-A

Janet M. Barber, R. N., M. S.
United States Air Force, N.C.
Wilford Hall USAF MEDICAL CENTER (AFSC)
Lackland Air Force Base, Texas

Peter A. Dillman, EMT-P, M. S.
Director of Education and Medical Quality Assurance
Wishard Memorial Hospital Ambulance Service
Indianapolis, Indiana

Reston Publishing Company, Inc.
*A Prentice Hall Company*
Reston, Virginia

*Respectfully dedicated to*
*the men and women of the*
*Wishard Memorial Hospital Ambulance Service*
*Indianapolis, Indiana*

The opinions or assertions in this book are those of the authors, and do not necessarily reflect those of the United States Air Force or the Department of Defense.

**Library of Congress Cataloging in Publication Data**

Barber, Janet Miller.
Emergency patient care for the EMT-A.

Includes index.
1. Emergency medicine. 2. Emergency medical technicians. I. Dillman, Peter. II. Title. [DNLM: 1. Ambulances. 2. Emergency medical services. 3. Transportation of patients. WX 215 B234e]
RC86.7.B36 616'.025 81-825
ISBN 0-8359-1671-5 AACR2


*A Prentice-Hall Company*
Reston, Virginia 22090



10 9 8 7 6 5 4 3 2 1

Printed in the United States of America

# Contents

# Preface

*Emergency Patient Care for the EMT-A* has been written in response to the learning needs of today's EMT. Its primary mission is to prepare the beginning student for certification as a basic EMT. The authors recognize that EMTs are curious and eager to know more than what is minimally required, and thus this text includes many opportunities for additional learning.

The EMT is a developing member in a dynamic career field and must know the definition, responsibilities, and legal risks of his role; in addition, he must appreciate associations with other team members within Emergency Medical Services. Historical developments and trends in practice have been included to explain the evolution of the EMT's role and to place it in perspective with other emergency care disciplines. Such understandings will assist in daily practice associations and will set the stage for continued growth within the career field.

The EMT must acquire a working knowledge of the "language of medicine" in order to communicate with peers and co-workers. Throughout the text, phonetic spellings are included, along with a Glossary at the end, so that EMTs will not only know what words *mean*, but will appreciate how they *sound* when pronounced properly. Anatomy and physiology have been thoroughly considered, since communications regarding descriptions of illness and injury inherently demand a working knowledge of associated terms that identify body parts or functions, or life processes.

Assessment skills are fundamental to the EMT's role. Extensive coverage of evaluation of illness or injury as well as suggestions on relating to the patient in distress are included. Particular attention has been paid to communications with children, the elderly, and blind, hearing-impaired, retarded, brain-damaged, and handicapped persons. A special chapter deals with individuals with behavioral disorders, and offers the EMT some suggestions for handling personal stressors in the work-related environment.

Unlike traditional EMT texts, this book recognizes that today's EMT must be knowledgeable regarding a wide range of medical problems in addition to traumatic injuries. Cardiovascular disease, respiratory distress, diabetes, alcoholism, and environmental illness have been included to ensure that the student will possess the knowledge and skills to deal with the broad range of problems that realistically comprise pre-hospital care.

The defined tasks of an EMT cannot be accomplished apart from the "tools of the trade." The EMT must be thoroughly familiar with the ambulance, its equipment and supplies, EMS radio and telemetric devices, and specialized rescue apparatus. Safe driving of an emergency vehicle is also imperative for successful patient transport, and this subject has been considered as well.

Initially the reader is introduced to the role of the EMT within today's EMS arena. Chapters dealing with assessment skills, techniques of basic life support, and shock management are followed by discussions of major pre-hospital problems. Emphasis has been placed on *presenting signs and symtoms* to encourage the EMT to follow a logical format in the assessment and management of the patient's problem *as it exists*—not as a suspected medical diagnosis. The content has been selected and organized to foster the development of a systematic and consistent framework for EMT problem-solving in the pre-hospital care environment.

A generous supply of illustrations, tables, and appendixes have been incorporated to amplify material throughout the textbook and to serve as a readily accessible reference source during daily practice. Considerable attention has been paid to incorporating the "why's" as well as the "how to's" of technical practice. The authors believe that understanding the rationale of action is of critical importance when circumstances demand on-the-spot modifications to standard EMT procedures.

In any career field, the basic textbook is only a beginning tool for acquiring knowledge and a skill base. It must be supplemented with other instructional modes in the classroom and with well-supervised field experience. The authors urge the EMT to become familiar with additional resource books, and to read EMT journals and relevant EMS publications regularly to encourage self-growth and continuing education.

*Emergency Patient Care* is more than a basic textbook of fundamentals for the EMT—it is a resource manual that will be of significant value in day-to-day problem-solving, and can be used to refine and expand knowledge and skills acquired as a product of actual patient care experiences.

Janet M. Barber
Peter A. Dillman

# Acknowledgments

We wish to express our appreciation to the library personnel of Wishard Memorial Hospital, Indianapolis, Indiana, who provided professional direction and research assistance throughout the time of preparation of this text; and to Debbie Faulk, who assisted in last-minute typing details.

Thanks also go to Tom Tilton, owner of the Reptile Kingdom Serpentarium in Nashville, Indiana, who permitted us the use of his reptiles; to David Fisher, Coordinator of Audiovisual Services, Welborn Baptist Hospital, Evansville, Indiana, who provided all the photographs for the chapter on extrication; and to Bob Biehn, Special Relations Coordinator, Wishard Memorial Hospital Ambulance Service, who provided selected photographs throughout the text.

A special thanks goes to all the EMTs and paramedics of Wishard Memorial Hospital Ambulance Service, who over the years have inspired me in my educational and writing endeavors; and to my educational colleagues in EMS, who have consistently provided encouragement in their own special ways.

Finally, I am personally indebted to my family and friends for their understanding of my social absences during the writing of this book; and to Connie and Ryan, for making me happy through it all.

Peter A. Dillman

# A Note to the Reader

Throughout this text, the abbreviated terms EMT, EMT-A, advanced EMT, and EMT-P have been used. For clarity, the following definitions for each term should be understood:

EMERGENCY MEDICAL TECHNICIAN (EMT) A general term used to denote all Emergency Medical Technicians.

EMERGENCY MEDICAL TECHNICIAN–AMBULANCE (EMT–A) Any person who has completed an EMT-A course, regardless of whether he functions in a prehospital or a hospital setting.

ADVANCED EMERGENCY MEDICAL TECHNICIAN (A–EMT) OR EMERGENCY MEDICAL TECHNICIAN–INTERMEDIATE (EMT–I) Any person who has completed a prescribed number of modules in the EMT-P course curriculum, which enables the individual to perform selected advanced life support skills such as airway maintenance (esophageal obturator airway insertion and intubation), intravenous techniques, and drug therapy.

EMERGENCY MEDICAL TECHNICIAN–PARAMEDIC (EMT–P) Any person who has completed the 15-module paramedic curriculum that has been adopted by the Department of Transportation (DOT), Department of Health and Human Resources (DHHR), and Department of Labor. Upon completion of the didactic, clinical, and field internship portions of the course, the EMT-P is trained to perform any of a number of advanced life suport skills and procedures such as intubation, defibrillation, intravenous techniques, drug therapy, and ECG monitoring.

It must be realized that all skills and procedures that may be performed by an EMT, EMT-A, advanced EMT or EMT-I, or EMT-P are to be performed under the authority or direction of a licensed physician.

Chapter 1

# Emergency Medical Services (EMS) History

Early written history has provided little information regarding the use of a transportation system for the sick or injured. Throughout early ages, however, it has always been known that specific treatments (mostly religious or herbal) were administered to those who required obvious medical attention. Some of the earliest records indicate that the Egyptians used definitive care techniques by splinting and dressing wounds. For the lack of quick transportation during these early ages, most injured or ill persons were carried to a designated healer or helper or treated at the site of the medical emergency.

It was not until the Napoleonic Wars that a system of service to the injured was realized. During these wars, a French surgeon general (Baron Dominique Jean Larrey) utilized a transportation system of light carriages for casualty transport. The medical crews operating these carriages were trained in controlling hemorrhage and splinting fractures. One of the first ambulance services was born on those battle fields, and the idea persisted throughout Europe and Asia.

The first ambulance service in the United States is believed to have been in the U.S. Army in 1865. No doubt this service was conceived and initiated to decrease mortality on the battle field, much like that during the Napoleonic Wars.

Many of the first ambulance services in American cities began as hospital-based operations. New York's Bellevue Hospital, Cincinnati's General Hospital, Wishard Memorial Hospital in Indianapolis and a few others all operated ambulance transportation systems in the late 1800s. (See Fig. 1-1.) Although the city population during these times was provided with an emergency transportation (ambulance) and protection (fire) service, it was not until the mid-1940s that communities away from cities recognized a need for local fire protection and first aid. In outlying communities the time factor of getting to an injured person or burning building was either too long from the city, or the city itself did not provide services

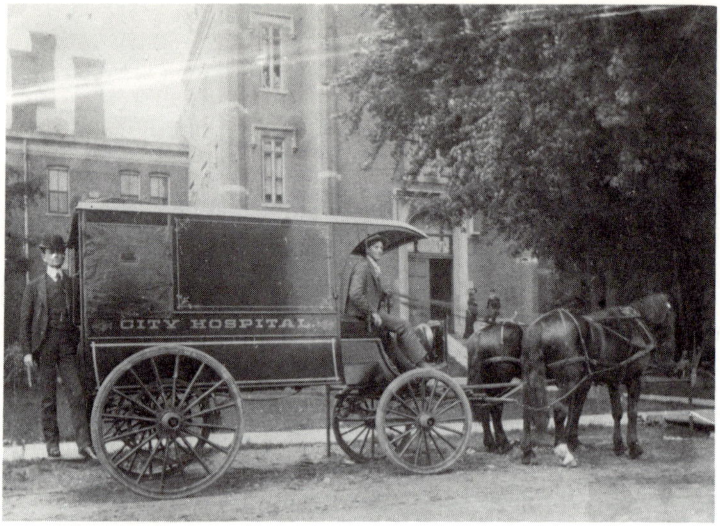


**Figure 1–1.** The horsedrawn ambulance was a common means of transportation in the late 1800s for the sick or injured. (*Courtesy of Wishard Memorial Hospital, Indianapolis, Indiana*)

to a community outside the city. Because of this situation, local community governments initiated volunteer services for first aid and fire protection, and usually both were housed under the same roof. In this way the volunteer fire departments were born.

Ambulance service in the ensuing years was a "pick 'em up and run" proposition. Little or no patient stabilization at the emergency scene was realized; let alone was there qualified medical personnel to definitively treat and care for the patient. As a matter of fact, one of the best qualifications for being behind the wheel of an ambulance was knowing well the city streets (hence the ambulance name, *horizontal taxi*), while only having rudimentary first aid skills. However, many early hospital-based ambulance services employed the skills of interns to respond to emergency calls.

Few advances were made during this time to ensure continuity in training qualifications and to require ambulance equipment and vehicle standards, as represented by the many types of ambulances used during this period. (See Fig. 1–2.)

As previously mentioned, the idea of patient care and treatment was based on transporting the patient to the nearest medical facility for definitive care, for it was believed that medically little could be accomplished at the accident scene. Prehospital medical care during this period was based on physician licensure, and the belief that the layman could not respond appropriately to emergency situations. It wasn't until 1966 that the problem of increasing prehospital mortality rate was nationally exposed, in a report of the National Research Council called "Accidental Death and

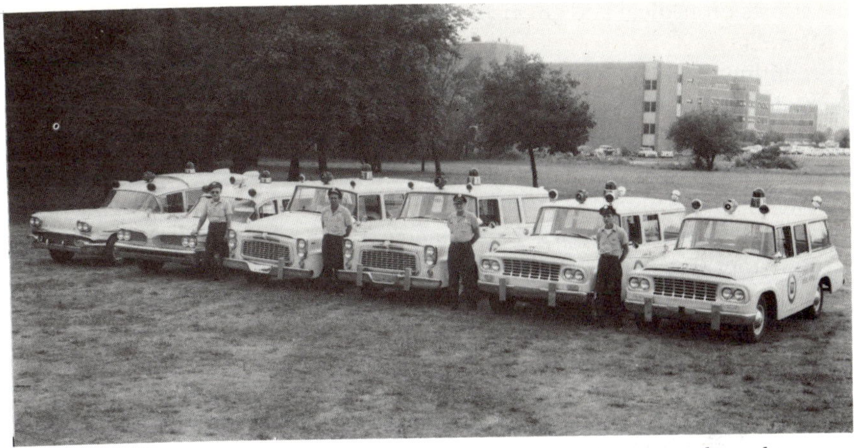

**Figure 1-2.** These International Harvester and hearse style vehicles demonstrate the diversity of ambulances used in the 1950s and 1960s. *(Courtesy of Wishard Memorial Hospital, Indianapolis, Indiana)*

Disability: The Neglected Disease of Modern Society." This was essentially the first such report recognizing that the significant numbers of people killed or disabled by accidents was costing the American people billions of dollars each year. At about the same time, other studies had shown that about one in every four or five patients who died of injury died of survivable injuries. One physician researcher at that time stated that in his experience the majority of unnecessary deaths have been the result of two problems—prolonged hypoxia (little oxygen) and inadequate blood volume (hemorrhage), problems that could be corrected with properly trained medical personnel.

Until 1966, emergency medical services were provided throughout the country in a piecemeal nonsystematic fashion. A strong impetus for emergency medical services to emerge as a system came from the National Highway Safety Act of 1966, passed by the 89th Congress. This Act provided funding for the development of highway safety programs, with the goal of reducing the outrageous number of highway-accident-related deaths. From this Act, many ambulance services of today incorporate defensive driving courses in their training curriculum. A system of emergency medical services emerged throughout the country, as governmental funding programs allowed for additional medical training and basic care equipment for ambulance vehicles.

Also in 1966, a report emerged from the National Academy of Sciences/National Research Council on Trauma. This report recognized the lack of continuity standards in first aid training, vehicle transport, medical direction and local government support of emergency medical services. Reports continued and special committees convened over the next several years that were concerned with the lack of a true EMS system. Spawned by the efforts of medical and governmental indices, EMS began to develop as a system.

In June of 1970, The National Registry of Emergency Technicians was formed in response to the recommendation of the President's Committee on Highway Safety. The report from the Committee stated that "there be a national accreditation agency to establish standards." These standards were to deal with the minimum training of persons needed to work on an ambulance and attested to the competency of these people by establishing written and practical testing criteria. Although these standards were conceived for a better system of care, standards across the country were unequal because no ambulance service was required to have its medical personnel tested for competency.

Congress conducted public hearings in many locations in 1972 and 1973, to try and devise a workable EMS solution. From these hearings, the support of establishing a comprehensive EMS system was realized. During this same period, a National Conference on Cardiopulmonary Resuscitation and Emergency Cardiac Care convened. The conference addressed the topics of emergency medical care and heart attack. National statistics showed that of approximately 600,000 deaths each year attributable to heart disease, approximately 350,000 people died before reaching the hospital. It was realized at the conference that it was probable that a large number of these prehospital victims could be saved by early intermediate treatment.

In response to the national highway and heart disease mortality statistics and of public and professional demand concerning the issue of Emergency Medical Services, Congress enacted the Emergency Medical Services Act in November of 1973, placing responsibility for implementing the Act in the Department of Health and Human Resources. This Act comprehensively defined for the first time an emergency medical services system as "a system which provides for the arrangement of personnel, facilities, and equipment for the effective and coordinated delivery in an appropriate geographical area of health care services under emergency conditions (occurring either as a result of the patient's condition or of natural disasters or similar situations), and which is administered by a public or nonprofit private entity which has the authority and the resources to provide effective administration of the system." To initiate this system, grant money regulations were issued for EMS systems in the Federal Register on July 1, 1974.

Public Law 93-154 called for a three-year program, including the authority to provide grants, contracts to plan, implement, improve and expand comprehensive EMS systems on a regional basis. (Congress has authorized extension of this three-year grant and contracts since that time.)

In 1974, The National Health Planning and Resources Development Act was passed (Public Law 93-641), and programs were developed from a network of entities known as Health System Agencies (HSAs.) Generally, the HSAs are to engage in implementation of programs, but are limited to planning activities. The major intent of such agencies is to urge and encourage a more coordinated use of health care facilities and to regulate the construction or expansion of hospital facilities. Many HSAs throughout the country today play a role in regional EMS systems.

Since the advent of the Emergency Medical Services Act and appropriation of grant monies to emergency medical services systems, a continuity of training, equipment, and transport vehicles has taken a firm footing. Not only are federal requirements necessary to initiate a comprehensive system, but state regulations as well. What used to be federally controlled in the overall EMS System, is now being controlled by state rules and regulations governing such services. (i.e., EMT certification, vehicle inspection, and essential equipment to be carried on ambulance vehicles.)

Today, the "system" of emergency medical services is a continuum of patient care from the onset of injury or illness through maximum patient rehabilitation. Functionally, an effective EMS system can be broken down into three phases:

1. Prehospital
2. Hospital
3. Rehabilitation

and fifteen components inherent to the system as mandated by the EMS Act of 1973.

## EMERGENCY MEDICAL SERVICES SYSTEM COMPONENTS*

### Manpower

Emergency Medical Services System (EMSS) must have an adequate number of health professionals, allied health professionals, and other health personnel, including ambulance personnel, all with appropriate training and experience. There must be sufficient numbers of all types of personnel to provide emergency medical care on a twenty-four hour a day basis, seven days a week, within the service area of the system. These personnel are required:

1. First Responders—fire, police and other public safety elements
2. Communications—EMS/Resources Dispatcher
3. Emergency Medical Technician—Ambulance (EMT-A)—that individual who has successfully completed a prescribed EMT-A course. generally 110–120 of Basic Life Support (BLS)

* This section is taken from International Association of Fire Chiefs, International Association of Fire Fighters AFL-CIO. Emergency Medical Technicians and Paramedics in the Fire Service, Washington, D. C., 1977.

4. Emergency Medical Technician—Paramedic (EMT-P)—that individual who has successfully completed a prescribed Paramedic Course, generally 800 hours or more of Advanced Life Support (ALS)

5. Registered Nurses—Emergency Department

6. Registered Nurses—Critical Care Unit

7. Physician—Emergency

8. Physician—Specialty (medical, surgical, pediatric, psychiatry, cardiology)

9. EMS System Medical Director

10. EMS System Administrator

11. EMS System Coordinators

## Training

Training includes the provision of appropriate training (including clinical training) and continuing education programs for each of the manpower requirements. EMSS-related training must be coordinated with other programs in the system's service area that provide similar training and education.

## Communicatons

Provisions must be made for linking the personnel, facilities, and equipment of the system by a central communications system. In a central communications service requests for emergency health care services are handled by verbal screening. It may have the universal emergency telephone number 911. It has direct communication connections and interconnections with the personnel, facilities and equipment of the system, as well as with other appropriate emergency medical services systems.

The EMS communications system should include a command and control center, which is responsible for establishing communications channels and allocating public resources essential to the most effective and efficient management of the immediate EMS problem. The center should have the necessary equipment and facilities to permit immediate interchange of information essential for the system's resource management and control.

### *Communications and Medical Control*

In most states a physician must assume legal responsibility for all care rendered in an emergency at the scene of an incident and en route to the hospital. Such supervision may take one of several forms depending upon resources available and the configuration of the system in a particular area. In most states, Basic Life Support (BLS) measures are considered to represent emergency first aid and do not require strict medical supervision, although a physician remains responsible for the training and actions of nurses and emergency medical technicians rendering such care. When Advanced Life Support (ALS) is required, physician supervision becomes mandatory. In most systems, physician supervision is provided through voice communications or a combination of radio and telephone linkages between the EMT-P in the field and the physician. Although it is generally agreed that medical supervision may best be given by a physician located in a hospital, it is often not practical to do so, especially in rural areas where frequency of use of the emergency rescue service is low, and hospital-based physicians are not available on a twenty-four hour a day basis. In such areas, the EMT must be patched to a physician, via phone lines, at the major hospital within the region.

In most urban areas, medical supervision is provided through a central base hospital resource. It is emphasized here that it is quite impractical in terms of available frequencies and of expense to have every hospital in an urban area providing medical supervision to ambulances bringing patients to each of these hospitals. Most importantly, personnel at each of the receiving hospitals cannot be expected to be familiar with the radio equipment and communications procedures. Furthermore, where multiple users are sharing a frequency, information may become interchanged, which may lead to errors in diagnosis and treatment. Therefore, for urban areas it is imperative that medical supervision be regionalized and confined to one base hospital communications center as appropriate to the needs of the area. (See Fig. 1–3.)

Transmission of biological signals, through telemetry, primarily of the electrocardiogram (EKG), has been found to be a useful adjunct to voice communications especially in the treatment of the acute cardiac emergency. The absolute need for telemetry of the EKG will vary from system to system, again, depending upon the level of training of available rescue personnel and the frequency of exposure of such personnel to the need to monitor the EKG. In programs which use volunteer rescue personnel, telemetry becomes a more important adjunct than in programs using highly trained full-time EMT-Ps with a high frequency of exposure.

Treatment protocols for each major emergency are an important aspect of medical supervision and control. They provide a basis for the training of all EMT-As and EMT-Ps, affording the opportunity for standardization of training programs on a regional basis. They establish a medical-legal standard of care for the patient with an emergent problem and, through a standardized approach to the patient illness or injury, facilitate cooperation between rescue personnel in approaching a given problem and allowing for meaningful evaluation of training efforts and patient outcome. Such protocols can be simple or complex as required by the patient type and will be influenced by such factors as the level of training of available rescue personnel, the length of transport time to the nearest appropriate medical facility, and the degree to which these treatment protocols must be approved by a consensus of area physicians, based on available national standards and implemented on a regional basis.

**EMS SYSTEM MEDICAL CONTROL**

| *System Phase* | *Activity* | *Medical-Control Technique* |
|---|---|---|
| Access | Service request to communications operator | Communications operator protocol for telephone assistance |
| Communications | Dispatch during disaster situation | Physician monitoring for medical response coordination |
| Pre-hospital care and transportation | • EMT-A/EMT-P on-scene care<br>• Patient distribution and transportation | • Treatment protocol and voice communication with physician or nurse at receiving hospital<br>• Triage protocol and voice communication with physician or nurse at receiving hospital |
| Initial hospital care | • In-hospital care | • Standing orders for ER personnel and direct medical supervision |
| | • Patient transfer decision | • Transfer protocol |
| Transfer care and transportation | EMT-A/EMT-P/ER-RN/specialized transfer team transfer care and transportation | Transfer protocol, direct medical supervision, and voice communication with physician or nurse at receiving hospital |
| Subsequent hospital care | In-hospital intensive/ critical care | Standing orders for ICU/CCU personnel and direct medical supervision |

**Figure 1-3.** EMS system medical control ensures quality in all phases of the system. (*Courtesy of the Central Indiana EMS Council, Indianapolis, Indiana*)

The Communications component should include the following:

Access by the public to emergency resource system

1. 911-Regional emergency access number
2. Alternate single access number (usually seven digits)

Resource Management function

1. Central dispatch-A regional communication system
2. Coordination of EMS and other public services

Medical Control

1. Medical communications to hospital for triage, diagnosis, and treatment

Hospital to Mobile Unit

1. Basic voice
2. Basic voice/advanced biomedical telemetry

Hospital-to-Hospital

1. Basic voice
2. Relayed biomedical telemetry

## Transportation

This component should include an adequate number of necessary ground, air, and water vehicles and other transportation equipment, equipped to meet the transportation and EMS characteristics of the system area. Such vehicles and facilities must meet appropriate standards relating to location, design, performance, and equipment. The operators and other personnel using such vehicles and facilities must meet appropriate training and experience requirements.

The elements of transportation should include the following:

Ground-Basic Life Support Elements

1. Ambulance vehicles meeting DOT/GSA specifications (KKK-A-1822A amended) and including equipment recommended by the American College of Surgeons and HHR/DOT
2. At least two EMTs on each ambulance
3. Locations permitting (for ninety-five percent of all calls) a maximum response time of thirty minutes in rural areas

Ground-Advanced Life Support Elements

1. All elements of a Ground-Basic Life Support component, plus personnel trained to the EMT-Paramedic level must address specific clinical items in medical service plan
2. Extra communications to provide advanced biomedical telemetry
3. Extra equipment for critical care procedures.

Air

1. Helicopters
   —Primary response-unique use depending on geographic constraints
   —Secondary response, 30–150-mile transport radius
2. Fixed Wing
   Greater response for 150-mile transport radius
3. Water
   —Special geographical considerations
4. Snow Mobile
   —Special geographical considerations

## Facilities

This component should include an adequate number of easily accessible emergency medical facilities that are capable collectively of providing service on a continuous (twenty-four-hour a day, seven days a week) basis; that have appropriate standards relating to capacity, location, personnel, and equipment; and that are coordinated with other health care facilities of the system.

The concept of categorization of all emergency care facilities originates from the realization that emergency patients have varying magnitudes of injury and illness and that hospitals have varying capabilities to provide appropriate initial and/or definitive care. It is also realized that a categorization program must address the needs of all emergency medical patients.

Categorization has relevance in urban, suburban, rural and wilderness areas. The categorization concept will have significant effects on the use of EMS manpower and other EMS resources. The basic purpose of categorization is to identify the readiness and capability of each hospital within a region to receive, diagnose, and treat all emergency patients, especially those with serious or critical injuries or illnesses, in an appropriate and expeditious manner. Ambulance personnel, law enforcement, and public safety officers, as well as the public, must be knowledgeable of the designations of the hospital within the region in order for the system to operate effectively.

Categorization elements for hospital consideration include the following:

1. Regional categorization with accepted state or national criteria with at least one hospital providing twenty-four hour physician coverage in the emergency department in each EMS region.

2. Regional EMS advisory groups to plan and carry out the categorization plan. These groups should include hospital administrators, physicians, nurses, other pre-hospital care providers, and health system planners.

3. Regional plans for mutual agreement regarding categorical designation use of critical care units, system linkages (transfer agreements), and resource sharing.

## Critical Care Units

This component requires providing access (including appropriate transportation) to specialized critical medical care units. These units should be in the number and variety necessary to meet the demands of the service area. If such capabilities are not available within the EMS region, then the system must provide access to such capabilities in neighboring regions.

Specialized critical care units should include trauma intensive care centers/units, burn centers/units, spinal cord centers, poison control and alcohol detoxification centers, coronary care units, high-risk infant units, drug overdose, psychiatric centers, and others as appropriate.

The issue here is the availability of critical care units both within the EMS region and in neighboring regions. Specialty care services should provide an adequate number of beds in the region or access to critical care units in neighboring areas. A plan for use of critical care units should be developed, including trained personnel, equipment and transportation, triage and interhospital treatment protocols. The EMS system should include the development of professional advisory groups (trauma, burn, cardiac, etc.) to work with EMS programs to insure that these critical services are being used appropriately within and across political boundaries.

## Public Safety Agencies

Provisions must be made for effective use of appropriate personnel, facilities, and equipment of each public safety agency in the area.

"Effective use" means the integration of public safety agencies into the standard EMS and disaster operating procedures of the regional system. It also includes the shared use of personnel and equipment, such as helicopters and rescue boats, appropriate for medical emergencies.

Public safety agency personnel are most frequently the first responders to the scene of an emergency. The EMS system therefore must involve these agencies to ensure the use of special equipment, proper training of staff, linked communications, and the development of cooperative operating procedures.

## Consumer Participation

The EMS system must make provisions in its system management so that persons residing in the area and having no professional training or experience may participate in the policy-making process for the system. While there is no federally required percentage of consumer participation in EMS planning or advisory organizations, reasonable consumer representation should be provided. One approach would be to involve the advisory council of the local planning agency that has consumer representation.

## Accessibility to Care

The EMS system must not require evidence of the ability to pay prior to care for the services of ambulance, hospital, or critical care units. The system should provide the means to monitor for restrictive measures that may eliminate any person or group of people from equal quality of services within the region.

## Transfer of Patients

The EMS system should provide for transfer of patients to facilities that offer definitive follow-up care and rehabilitation as is necessary to effect the maximum recovery of the patient.

The transfer agreement is necessary to facilitate communication and cooperation of key professional providers (physicians) within the system. Actual letters or mutual agreements that describe the transfer requirements for the critical target patients are essential contracts of regional EMS development. They not only open the lines of communications between physicians in the outlying areas with a patient problem beyond their capability and the center physician with the necessary resources, but they also will establish the manner and mechanism by which critical patients will be initially treated and then transported through the system. Only through this transfer agreement method will physicians and other providers at varying care capability levels come together and decide mutually on treatment, triage, educational, and evaluation protocols.

In urban settings, areawide prehospital treatment and triage protocols will have to be established by councils of key professional providers for the various specialty patient groups. These programs will necessarily bypass the nearest hospital as special critical cases are identified.

## Standardized Patient Recordkeeping

Each EMS regional system should provide for a standardized patient recordkeeping system that covers the treatment of patients from initial entry into the system through their discharge, and should be consistent with patient records used in follow-up care and rehabilitation of the patient.

The minimal patient records necessary for the EMS system are the communication records, the ambulance field records or reports, the emergency department patient records, and critical care records. In order to fulfill requirements of evaluation and reports to Congress, certain information must be available to be derived from these records:

1. *Patient identification information:* the records must be designed so that the communication record, ambulance record, and emergency department record on each patient can be compared for evaluation and management purposes

2. *Patient access information:* how the patient accessed the system (from initial call for service through arrival at emergency department)

3. *Timing of ambulance services:* response time, time at scene, and travel time to hospital

4. *Patient condition:* at scene, upon arrival in emergency department and critical care unit

5. *Patient diagnostic and treatment services:* at emergency department, in hospital, and critical care unit

6. *Disposition of patient:* discharged, referred for out-patient care, referred to another hospital, admitted, died

7. *Condition of patient:* at discharge from emergency department, in hospital, and critical care unit

## Public Information and Education

The EMS system should provide programs of public education and information for all people in the area so they know about the system, how to access it, how to use it properly, and how to pay for it. Successful systems operation depends upon not only the organizers, but also the participants. Continued support, particularly in the arena of competition for dollars, requires community commitment. To secure that commitment, the EMS

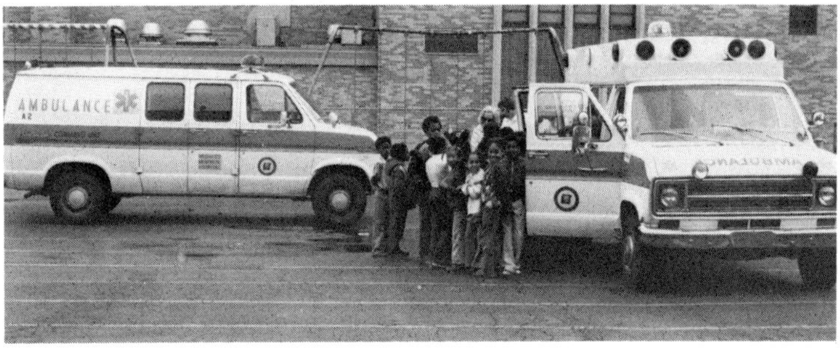


**Figure 1–4.** EMS public education should start at an early age. These grade school youngsters are taking a tour of the ambulance. *(Courtesy of Wishard Memorial Hospital, Indianapolis, Indiana)*

system must keep its public informed. Programs should stress the general dissemination of information regarding appropriate methods of medical self-help and first aid and the availability of CPR training programs and other prevention-oriented resources. (See Fig. 1–4.)

## Review and Evaluation

Each EMS system must provide for a periodic, comprehensive, and independent review and evaluation of the extent and quality of the emergency health care services provided in the system's service area.

It is intended that such review and evaluation be periodic and comprehensive so that changes in emergency health care can be determined. As a minimum the evaluation should include:

1. A description of the EMS resources, capability, and performance measures at the start of the period being evaluated

2. A description of the interventions brought about during the period to include both clinical and EMS components

3. A description of the EMS resources, capability, and performance measures of the period being evaluated

4. Clinical output or impact evaluations of death and disability should include the clinical patient triage groups

## Disaster Linkage

The EMS system must have a plan to assure that the system will be capable of providing emergency medical services in the system's service area during mass casualties, natural disasters, or national emergencies.

The EMS system is not the regional health disaster organization. It is the emergency medical organization that will work with other agencies during a disaster to provide emergency medical care. The EMS system must be linked to the local, regional, and state disaster plans and participate in exercises to test disaster plans.

## Mutual Aid Agreements

Each EMS system must provide for the establishment of appropriate arrangements with EMS systems or similar entities servicing neighboring areas for the provision of emergency medical services on a reciprocal basis where access to such services would be more appropriate and effective in terms of the services available, time, and distance.

Arrangements among EMS regional systems and similar entities serving neighboring areas must be written agreements, signed by individuals authorized to act for the respective parties with respect to such agreements and reviewed and reevaluated at least once a year. Such agreements should cover the exchange of service coverage, communications linkages, licensure and certification, and reimbursement. (See Fig. 1–5 and 1–6.)

The true "systems approach," then, in EMS planning, operations and management is based and evaluated upon:

1. Ready citizen access to the system
2. Effectiveness of prehospital emergency care
3. Communication system and control of equipment
4. Safe transportation services to a medical facility
5. Definitive hospital care capabilities within the EMS region and surrounding areas
6. Availability of definitive care services as well as rehabilitative services to ensure maximum patient care and rehabilitation

The Emergency Medical Services System has evolved slowly, but dramatically since the Napoleonic Wars. The EMT and his responsibilities have grown increasingly more complex with the system as local, regional, state and federal rules and regulations change for continued improvement of the EMS System. It is a system whose cardinal reason for existing is to reduce prehospital mortality by being a crucial link in an effective health care system.

*References*

"Accidental Death and Disability: The Neglected Disease of Modern Society," National Academy of Sciences/Patronal Research Council, Sept. 1966.

Duval, M. K. "*The Hidden Crisis in Health Care*," *Emergency Medical Services: Behavioral and Planning Perspectives.* New York: Behavioral Publications, 1973.

"The EMS System Response Sequence," *Central Indiana EMS Council, Planning Committee Report.* Indianapolis, IN, 1976.

"Emergency Medical Systems Act," Public Law #93–154, 93rd Congress, SB2410, November 16, 1973.

THE EMS SYSTEM CONCEPT

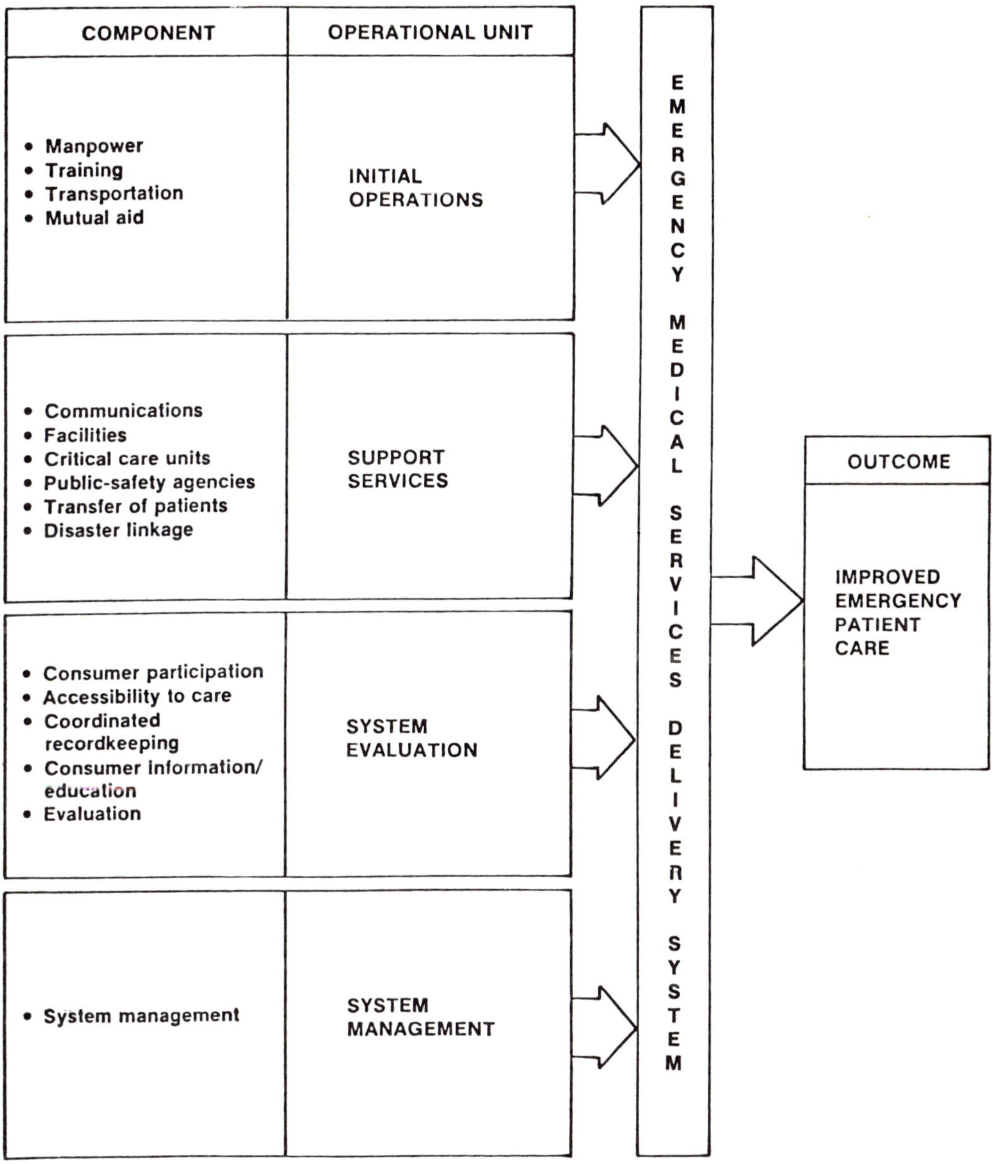


Figure 1-5. The operational linkage of the EMS components and the outcome to be expected if the components are identified, linked, and managed successfully. (*Courtesy of the Central Indiana EMS Council, Indianapolis, Indiana*)

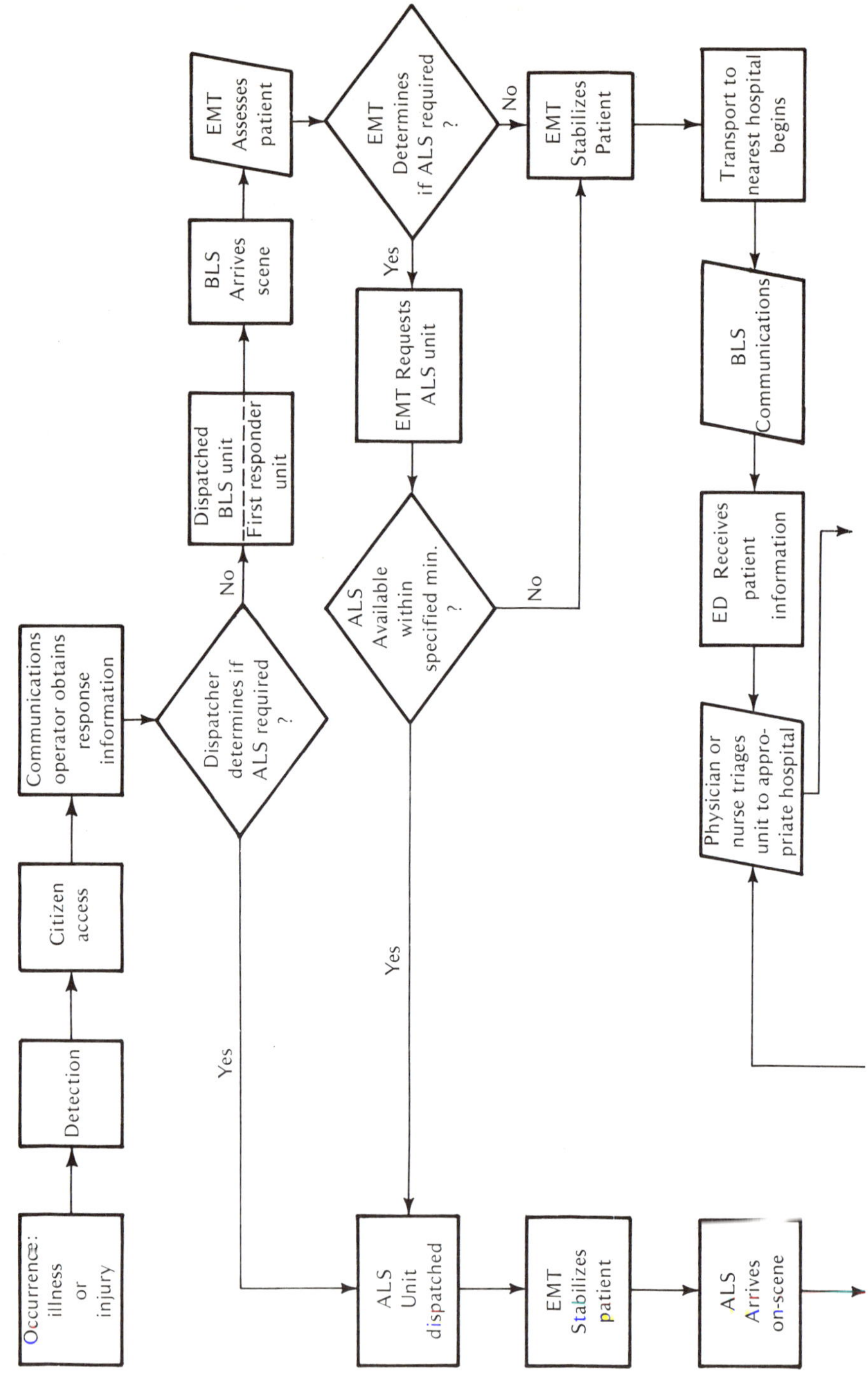

Occurrence: illness or injury
Detection
Citizen access
Communications operator obtains response information
Dispatcher determines if ALS required ?
No
Yes
Dispatched BLS unit
First responder unit
BLS Arrives scene
EMT Assesses patient
EMT Determines if ALS required ?
Yes
No
EMT Requests ALS unit
ALS Available within specified min. ?
No
Yes
EMT Stabilizes Patient
Transport to nearest hospital begins
BLS Communications
ED Receives patient information
Physician or nurse triages unit to appropriate hospital
ALS Unit dispatched
EMT Stabilizes patient
ALS Arrives on-scene

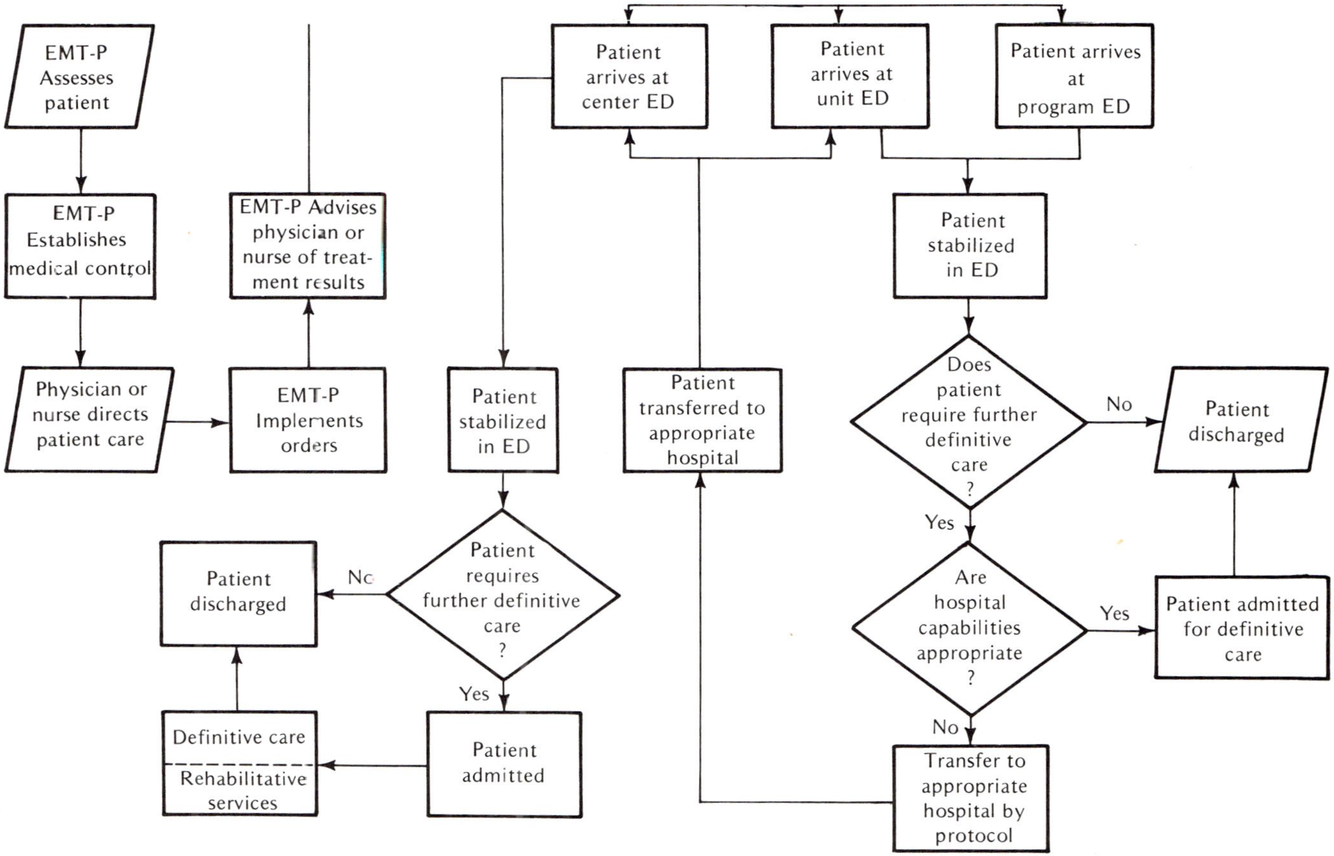


**Figure 1–6.** The EMS system response sequence. (*Courtesy of the Central Indiana EMS Council, Indianapolis, Indiana*)

International Association of Fire Chiefs, International Association of Fire Fighters, AFL-CIO. "Emergency Medical Technicians and Paramedics in the Fire Service." Washington, D. C., 1977.

Jelenko, C. III, and Frey, C. F. *Emergency Medical Services, An Overview.* Bowie, MD: Robert J. Brady Co., 1973.

"Medical Control in the EMS System." *Central Indiana EMS Council, Planning Committee Report.* Indianapolis, IN, 1976.

"Operational Linkage of the EMS Components." *Central Indiana EMS Council, Planning Committee Report.* Indianapolis, IN, 1976.

Page, J. O. *Emergency Medical Services,* 2nd ed. Boston, MA: National Fire Protection Assn., 1978.

Stevenson, K. A. *Emergency Ambulance Services in U.S. Cities—An Overview.* Operations Research Center, Massachusetts Institute of Technology, Aug. 1968.

Waller, J. A. "Urban Oriented Methods, Failure to Solve Rural Emergency Care Problems," *JAMA* 266: 1441–1446, 1973.

# Chapter 2

# Role and Responsibilities of the EMT-A

## ROLE

The days of body snatching and making a mad dash to the hospital with red lights flashing and siren wailing are all but gone. The professional EMT-A today must be able to work as part of the total health care team in an environment that is less than desirable. Today's EMT-A must be knowledgeable in basic life support, so that appropriate medical care and treatment is administered to the patient for stabilization before transport is attempted. The EMT-A must be able to appropriately make independent decisions concerning the physical and emotional well-being of the patient to reduce human suffering and integrate pertinent information so that communication with the rest of the health care team does not lapse.

## RESPONSIBILITIES

The responsibilities of an EMT-A are numerous. Although each EMS system throughout the country has certain aspects that are unique, the EMT-A working and functioning within the system has the following major responsibilities:

1. Patient responsibility
2. Appropriate appearance
3. Professional Code of Ethics and Oath
4. Emotional stability
5. Self-realization of limitations
6. Education and training
7. Understanding of medical and operational equipment

8. Emergency scene control
9. Proper vehicle awareness
10. Recordkeeping (medical and mechanical documentation)
11. Communications
12. Understanding of emergency departments procedure and policy
13. Understanding the local EMS system
14. Patient guidance
15. Community involvement

## Patient Responsibility

The primary responsibility of the EMT-A is to provide proper comprehensive basic life-support treatment and care for each patient. This responsibility is always assumed by the EMT when no other qualified medical authority is treating or caring for the patient at the emergency scene. In so doing, the EMT must be able to rapidly evaluate the patient's condition and intervene by providing proper treatment. The evaluation and examination should be accomplished in an orderly and systematic fashion.

The patient's injuries should be stabilized before vehicle transport. During stabilization procedures, the EMT should provide necessary safety and protection for the patient, even if it means removing the patient from the source of potential injury before complete stabilization procedures are accomplished, (removing the patient from a burning building, the path of gun fire or a volatile crowd). Once the patient is removed to a safer environment, stabilization procedures should be instituted or completed.

The EMT-A should always ride in the patient compartment of the emergency unit during patient transport to the medical facility. During transport, the EMT should continually monitor the patient for changes in medical conditions. If the condition of the patient deteriorates, communications should be established to the appropriate medical facility.

The EMT-A has the responsibility to care for the deceased with dignity. The victim should be shielded from onlookers by covering the victim with a sheet or blanket. If the victim has expired at home and relatives wish to view the body, the EMT-A should respect the request. The victim's body should be prepared by making the body look as normal as possible, and closing the eyelids of the victim. Relatives of the deceased (the EMT-A's secondary patients) should be comforted as much as possible. If only a single relative is present, the EMT-A should inquire as to relatives, close friends or clergyman that could be called. The EMT-A will witness many different reactions from surviving relatives and friends in these situations, and must have an understanding of the reactions of the death and dying process.

The EMT-A should not fall victim to mechanical procedures (obtaining blood pressures, applying splints, shock trousers, etc.) to such an extent that communication is lost with the patient. The EMT-A must listen attentively to what the patient has to say concerning medical complaints. The EMT-A will learn more by listening than by talking. The EMT-A should never assume that a patient cannot hear, even if the patient is in a stuporous or unconscious state. Many health care professionals have been severely embarrassed by chance remarks made in the presence of such patients when they have later learned that the patient heard what was stated. Remember that the sense of hearing is the last sense to dissociate before unconsciousness.

Be honest with the patient. Sometimes an indirect answer to a question is appropriate, for example, when the patient asks "Am I going to die?" One's response should be, for example, "You have serious injuries, but we are doing everything we can for you." Every situation will be a little different, but the EMT-A should not lead the patient into thinking one thing when he is sure the outcome will be another. In the long run, this generates distrust and a false sense of hospitals and physicians.

The medical advisor of the employing emergency service should discuss with the EMT-A how area hospitals are categorized and what policies exist concerning transport of the critically ill or injured patient.

The EMT-A should respect the religious beliefs of patients. Some patients may not wish to be treated because of their beliefs. In these situations, the EMT-A should properly advise these patients of the potential medical risk in not seeking medical attention. If the patient still does not wish to be treated, the EMT-A should document the refusal, either by hav-

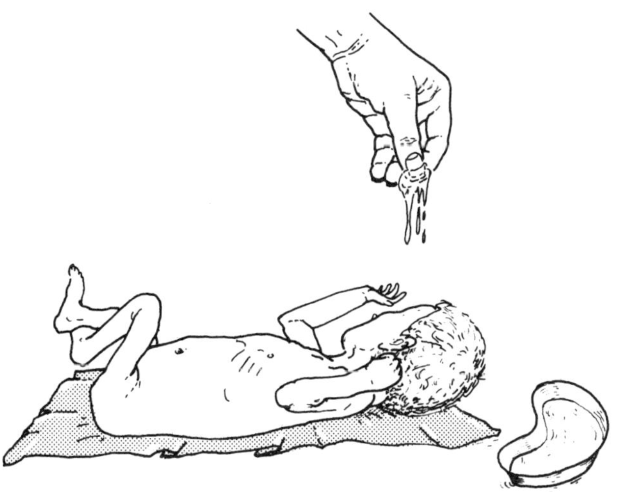

**Figure 2–1.** The rite of baptism. Sprinkle water on the head and say, "I baptize thee in the name of the Father, and of the Son, and of the Holy Spirit."

ing the patient write his refusal or having a witness to the situation, (policeman, fireman, EMT, etc.) countersign the documentation of the refusal.

The EMT-A may have occasion to perform the rite of baptism. The imminent death of a child or stillborn infant is the usual case. The EMT-A of any religious denomination may perform the rite. The ceremony is simply performed by sprinkling several drops of water (although not necessary) on the head and saying "I baptize thee in the name of the Father, and of the Son, and of the Holy Spirit." If resuscitation procedures are underway, they should not be stopped during the ceremony. Although not all Christian parents of the child or infant may think it necessary to perform the baptismal rite, it gives religious comfort to many of them. (See Fig. 2–1.)

## Appropriate Appearance

The professional EMT-A takes pride in his work and his appearance by being neat and clean, and conforming to required uniform policy, as directed by the emergency service. A well-groomed appearance forms trust, enhances cooperation and brings a sense of order to the emergency scene. The EMT-A should never smoke, or chew gum or tobacco, while treating or caring for patients. One must remember that the patient is putting trust in the EMT-A for care and if the EMT-A looks untidy and is uncouth, his patient care is probably on the same order. His image to the general public is important as well.

Personal hygiene is extremely important. Fingernails should be neatly trimmed and clean and long hair should always be restrained so as not to fall into open wounds.

The EMT-A should have at least two uniforms. One day's work may render the uniform nonwearable for the next day! The EMT-A should always wear a name tag over the left breast pocket area so that patients and other health care professionals know the EMT-A by name. The well-prepared EMT-A should always have the following items on his person to assist him with the care and treatment of the patient:

1. Watch with a second timer (for timing pulses, labor pains, etc.)
2. Black pen for documentation (black because it photocopies well when patient reports have to be reproduced)
3. Penlight (for checking pupils, etc.)

Most EMTs purchase the following items for their own personal use, instead of relying on the service to supply them:

1. Stethoscope
2. Ruler (with both centimeters and inches)
3. Bandage scissors

By having a neat and clean appearance and being prepared, the EMT-A produces a professional air that invites the trust of the patient and that the general public can be proud of.

## Professional Code of Ethics and Oath

The EMT must earn the respect and recognition of others as a responsible professional member of the health care team in the EMS system. It is paramount that the moral and ethical standards of the EMT be high, guided by an accepted Code of Ethics (see Fig. 2–2) and Professional Oath. (See Fig. 2–3.)

*THE EMERGENCY MEDICAL TECHNICIAN CODE OF ETHICS*

Professional status as an Emergency Medical Technician and emergency medical technician-paramedic is maintained and enriched by the willingness of the individual practitioner to accept and fulfill obligations to society, other medical professionals, and the profession of emergency medical technician. As an emergency medical technician, I solemnly pledge myself to the following code of professional ethics:

1. The fundamental responsibility of the Emergency Medical Technician is to conserve life, to alleviate suffering, to promote health, to do no harm and to encourage the quality and equal availability of emergency medical care.

2. The Emergency Medical Technician provides services based on human need, with respect for human dignity, unrestricted by consideration of nationality, race, creed, color, or status.

3. The Emergency Medical Technician does not use professional knowledge and skills in any enterprise detrimental to the public well-being.

4. The Emergency Medical Technician respects and holds in confidence all information of a confidential nature obtained in the course of professional work unless required by law to divulge such information.

5. The Emergency Medical Technician as a citizen understands and upholds the law and performs the duties of citizenship; as a professional, the emergency medical technician has the never-ending responsibility to work with concerned citizens and other health care professionals in promoting a high standard of emergency medical care to all people.

6. The Emergency Medical Technician shall maintain professional competence and demonstrate concern for the competence of other members of the health care team.

7. The Emergency Medical Technician assumes responsibility in defining and upholding standards of professional practice and education.

8. The Emergency Medical Technician assumes responsibility for individual professional actions and judgment, both in dependent and independent emergency functions, and knows and upholds the laws which affect the practice of the emergency medical technician.

9. The Emergency Medical Technician has the responsibility to be aware of and participate in matters of legislation affecting the Emergency Medical Technician and the emergency medical services system.

10. The Emergency Medical Technician adheres to standards of personal ethics which reflect credit upon the profession.

11. The Emergency Medical Technicians, or groups of Emergency Medical Technicians, who advertise professional services, do so in conformity with the dignity of the profession.

12. The Emergency Medical Technician has an obligation to protect the public by not delegating to a person less qualified any service which requires the professional competence of an Emergency Medical Technician.

13. The Emergency Medical Technician will work harmoniously with, and sustain confidence in Emergency Medical Technician associates, the nurse, the physician, and other members of the emergency medical services health care team.

14. The Emergency Medical Technician refuses to participate in unethical procedures and assumes the responsibility to expose incompetence or unethical conduct of others to the appropriate authority in a proper and professional manner.

Adopted by the National
Association of Emergency
Medical Technicians
January 21, 1978

**Figure 2–2.** The Emergency Medical Technician Code of Ethics. (From the *EMT Journal*, March 1978, Vol. 2 No. 1, p. 23. St. Louis, MO: The C. V. Mosby Co.)

## Emotional Stability

The EMT-A must be able to work and make independent decisions under stressful situations. One will see and witness scenes involving the corporate business executive to the indigent "wino." The EMT-A will witness accidents and testimony, and see everything from atrocities like body dismemberment to the miracle of birth. Murder, rape, incest, and suicide will not be uncommon situations in which the EMT-A must work.

The multitude of emotional attitudes displayed by patients, relatives, and curious onlookers must be professionally handled with care and respect and yet with a distant neutrality.

The EMT-A must discipline himself to control his emotions, whatever the situation, never losing sight of caring for the patient's physical and emotional injuries. It is extremely difficult, even for the most experienced EMT-A, to zero in on the patient as a person and to block out the cries of pain and injury to properly treat and care for the patient.

*THE EMERGENCY MEDICAL TECHNICIAN*
*OATH*

Be it pledged as an Emergency Medical Technician, I will honor the physical and judicial laws of God and man. I will follow that regimen which, according to my ability and judgment, I consider for the benefit of patients and abstain from whatever is deleterious and mischievous, nor shall I suggest any such counsel. Into whatever homes I enter, I will go into them for the benefit of only the sick and injured, never revealing what I see or hear in the lives of men unless required by law.

I shall also share my medical knowledge with those who may benefit from what I have learned. I will serve unselfishly and continuously in order to help make a better world for all mankind.

While I continue to keep this oath unviolated, may it be granted to me to enjoy life, and the practice of the art, respected by all men, in all times. Should I trespass or violate this oath, may the reverse be my lot. So help me God.

Adopted by the
National Association of
Emergency Medical Technicians
January 21, 1978

**Figure 2–3.** The Emergency Medical Technician Oath. (From the *EMT Journal,* March 1978, Vol. 2 No. 1, p. 39. St. Louis, MO: The C. V. Mosby Co.)

## Realization of One's Limitations

The responsibility of the EMT-A in the prehospital setting is to conserve life and alleviate suffering by stabilizing the patient. It is not the responsibility or role of the EMT-A to act as an extension of the physician, policeman, or lawyer. It is the professional duty of the EMT-A to act as an extension of oneself, realizing the medical and legal limitations that one possesses. The EMT-A must be able to recognize situations where additional help is needed (medical, mechanical, or legal) and call for assistance. When orders by a physician are given, and one does not possess the knowledge or skill to complete the task, the EMT-A should properly decline the order stating the reason why the request cannot be carried out. Medical vocabulary is a language that should be used correctly. Never use terminology that you are not sure of, even though it may seem to fit the context of the situation. One of the quickest ways to tell if a person really knows what he is talking about is to listen to him verbally deliver a patient report. Again, use your medical vocabulary correctly and appropriately. The professional EMT will recognize his limitations and request help or guidance when necessary.

## Education and Training

After the initial state and/or national EMT-A Certification, it is the responsibility of the EMT-A to maintain necessary continuing education to remain certified. The providing hospital, ambulance service, or other educational agency must make available appropriate continuing education for EMT recertification requirements.

The EMT-A should continue to enhance his knowledge beyond the initial education and training, and be atuned to changes and advancements in an emergency medical services system. Every EMT-A should document his continuing educational experiences for his own record and for the record of certifying agencies.

## Understanding of Medical and Operational Equipment

The EMT should know the function and proper use of and how to troubleshoot each medical and operational piece of equipment on board the emergency unit.

All equipment should be checked and inspected when coming on duty, and after each emergency run. Necessary documentation concerning equipment failure or equipment used on the patient that is still with the patient at the hospital should be communicated to the oncoming shift crew, so that replacement or retrieval of equipment can be accomplished.

Certain medical and operational equipment should be tested to ensure that it is working properly at the beginning of each shift. This may include:

1. Sphygmomanometers (sfig "mo-mah-nom' ĕ-ter)
2. Pen light
3. Radio equipment
4. Patient-monitoring equipment (defibrillator [de-fib"ri-la'tor], pulse monitor)
5. Flashlights
6. Oxygen/suction
7. Traction splints
8. Antishock trousers
9. Airway equipment
10. Bandaging and dressing supplies.

All medical equipment in the vehicle and technician's kit should have its own place, so that some element of order exists. It also makes the responsibility of checking the equipment an easier task.

## Emergency Scene Control

Perhaps one of the most difficult and dangerous responsibilities of an EMT-A is to gain control of the emergency scene pertaining to the patient. The EMT-A must be able to put order into the presenting situation without compromising patient care. Interpersonal relationship skills are mandatory. The EMT-A should have a sense of anticipation of possible hazards and remove the patient from situations that might threaten the life of the patient as well as the rescuer.

Coordinated efforts with other agencies (police, fire, Civil Defense, etc.) to ensure proper patient care should be maximized for a good working relationship.

The EMT-A should avoid assuming the functions of the police or other authorities, when present, but should not permit his actions to compromise patient care. Yelling and screaming with one another (whoever it may be) is not only unprofessional, but harmful to patient care.

An interesting challenge that the EMT-A may encounter on the scene is the appearance of a physician. The EMT-A should be able to distinguish his level of emergency medical ability, and depending upon the condition of the patient and the physician's actions, intervene swiftly but politely to stabilize the patient. Most physicians will let the EMT-A do his job and lend a hand if asked. If the EMT-A is not sure of the person attending briskly to the patient, he should ask politely who he is and if necessary ask (again politely) for identification. Most physicians carry some type of medical identification. The EMT-A should realize that even though the physician is the higher medical authority on the scene, it does not mean that the physician is properly stabilizing the patient. Few physicians actually know and realize the inner workings of prehospital care and adjuncts used in patient stabilization. If the physician has actively participated in patient care by giving medication or other invasive treatment before your arrival, you must make sure that you document his treatment and request his signature that he treated the patient. It would be best for the patient and the EMT-A that he accompany you with the patient to the designated hospital. The physician has assumed the medical responsibility of the patient, and needs to communicate to the attending physician at the medical facility what treatment the patient has received. This type of situation demands a common-sense approach on the part of the EMT-A and the ability to recognize above all else whether patient care is suffering.

The EMT-A should not try to be a hero or risk life or limb unduly in any situation, for if he injures himself he cannot be responsible to the patient. He must realize when a situation has or will become out of control and seek additional assistance.

## Proper Vehicle Awareness

Ideally, every EMT who will have the responsibility of operating an emergency vehicle should be certified as having passed a defensive driving course. It is essential that the EMT responsible for operating the vehicle ensure its mechanical safeness before and after each emergency run. He must document those mechanical aspects of the vehicle that are not functioning and follow proper channels to have the mechanical problem corrected.

The EMT driver must abide by local laws and traffic regulations pertaining to emergency vehicles, exercising emergency privileges properly and using flashing lights and siren properly (very few patient conditions require the use of lights and siren.) It is important that the EMT driver drives in such a manner as to minimize further damage to the already existing problem the patient may have (especially fractures). The driver should drive with sense, avoiding sudden stops and starts, letting his partner know when he is about to come to a rough area on the road (pot holes, railroad crossings, etc.) so that the EMT attending to the patient can prepare himself and the patient for such an occurrence.

The driver should know the geographical service area well enough so that the response time to the accident scene is not inappropriate. At the emergency scene, the driver should park the emergency vehicle in an appropriate location so as not to obstruct the flow of traffic, making the area safer for passers-by and helping the local police in traffic and crowd control.

## Recordkeeping

Since the EMT is many times the first to arrive on the scene, medical, legal, and health documentation and reporting is crucial.

*Medical:* The EMT is always responsible for ensuring that every verbal or written patient report is medically pertinent, concise, accurate, and orderly.

*Legal:* The EMT should note circumstances in suicide, homicide, rape, or child abuse. Preservation of the crime scene is important for the local authorities, and the EMT should not move or touch anything unnecessarily while at the scene.

*Health:* The EMT-A should note and report, if necessary, cases of animal bites, radiation hazards, chemical or gas exposures, and health hazards to small children in the home.

Many EMT-As keep their own personal log of emergency calls. However, one should never write anything in the log that one wouldn't want someone else to read. The log not only helps clarify certain situational events at a future date, but it can be subpoenaed in a court of law for evidence. Every word used in the verbal or written patient report should be used and spelled correctly. Remember that the patient report form is part of the patient's medical record. The EMT-A's choice of words, either verbally or written, is a reflection on not only himself but his profession. Unfortunately, some EMT-As use medical terms incorrectly and cannot spell, creating a poor impression on the other EMT-As in their service. Verbal and written communication takes practice and experience. The EMT-A should utilize an accepted standardized reporting system to ensure order and accuracy of information. (See Fig. 2–1.)

## Communications

The EMT-A should have a general knowledge of how the communication system operates on the local, regional, and state level. It is advised that the EMT spend some time observing the functions and respon-

WM. N. WISHARD MEMORIAL HOSPITAL INDIANAPOLIS, IND. EMERGENCY AMBULANCE SERVICE

EMERGENCY PATIENT REPORT FORM

DATE - - | UNIT | UNIT | UNIT | ☐ S.O.R. | ☐ S-9. AUTH.______ | INCIDENT #

EMERGENCY LOCATION | CODE

DISP. TIME | 10-23 TIME | 10-24 TIME | 10-7 TIME | BEGIN ODO. | 10-23 ODO. | 10-7 ODO.

SERVICES ON SCENE | AID PRIOR TO ARRIVAL

PATIENT NAME: FIRST | M.I. | LAST | D.O.B. - - | AGE | RACE | SEX | PHONE

GUARANTOR'S NAME: FIRST | M.I. | LAST | GUARANTOR'S S.S. # | INSURANCE INFORMATION CO.______ #

BILLING ADDRESS: STREET | CITY | STATE | ZIP

DISPOSITION | # OF PAT. | E/R CONTACT ☐ NONE ☐ OTHER______ ☐ PHONE ☐ RADIO, CHNL.______ ☐ NOTIFY ☐ CONSULT | ☐ PHYSICIAN ☐ NURSE: NAME

CHIEF COMPLAINT: ☐ ON THE JOB INJURY ☐ SEE COMMENTS (1)

APPARENT CONDITION WHEN FOUND: ☐ SEE COMMENTS (2)

PATIENT HISTORY: ☐ MEDICATIONS ☐ HEART DISEASE ☐ HIGH BLD. PRESS. ☐ STROKE ☐ LUNG DISEASE ☐ ASTHMA ☐ OTHER ALLERGY ☐ DIABETES ☐ KIDNEY DISEASE ☐ LIVER DISEASE ☐ EPILEPSY ☐ MENTAL ILLNESS ☐ INFECTION ☐ PREGNANCY

☐ TERMINAL ILLNESS ☐ SEE COMMENTS (3) | RECENTLY HOSPITALIZED ☐ Y ☐ N: | WHEN/WHERE/WHY/HOW LONG | ☐ SEE COMMENTS (4)

VITAL SIGNS

| TIME | B/P | PULSE | RESP. |
|---|---|---|---|
| | / | | |
| | / | | |
| | / | | |

MEDICATIONS/IV'S ADMINISTERED ☐ SPECIALS ☐ SEE COMMENTS (15)

| TIME | TYPE | DOSE | ROUTE |
|---|---|---|---|
| | | | |
| | | | |
| | | | |

PATIENT ASSESSMENT | PAIN ☐ Y ☐ N SEE DIAGRAM AND COMMENTS (5)

SKIN: ☐ NORMAL ☐ WARM ☐ HOT ☐ COLD ☐ DIAPHORESIS: ☐ EXTREME ☐ MODERATE ☐ DRY ☐ CYANOSIS (SEE DIAGRAM AND COMMENTS) ☐ COLOR______ ☐ SEE COMMENTS (6)

NEURO: ☐ CONSCIOUS, ALERT ☐ ORIENTED, CONVERSANT ☐ UNCONSCIOUS ☐ DISORIENTED TO ☐ PERSON ☐ PLACE ☐ TIME ☐ NON-CONVERSANT ☐ LETHARGIC ☐ STUPOROUS ☐ REACTIVE TO STIMULI: ☐ NOXIOUS ☐ VERBAL ☐ NON-REACTIVE TO STIMULI: ☐ NOXIOUS ☐ VERBAL ☐ 10-96 ☐ POST ICTAL ☐ SEE COMMENTS (7)

PUPILS (R)(L): ☐ P.E.R.L ☐ NOT EQUAL ☐ CONSTRICTED ☐☐ ☐ DILATED ☐☐ ☐ SLOW TO REACT ☐☐ OTHER:______ ☐ SEE COMMENTS (8)

PATIENT ASSESSMENT CONTINUED

PARALYSIS: ☐ NONE ☐ BELOW WAIST ☐ ONE SIDED ☐ L ☐ R ☐ BELOW NECK ☐ SEE COMMENTS (9)

APPEARANCE: ☐ FLUSHED ☐ NORMAL ☐ SHOCKY ☐ ABNORMAL ☐ SEE COMMENTS (10)

BLEEDING ☐ NONE: ☐ INTERNAL ☐ EXTERNAL ☐ MINIMAL ☐ MODERATE ☐ SEVERE ☐ ARTERIAL ☐ VENOUS ☐ SEE COMMENTS (11)

ABDM./GI ☐ NONE: ☐ RIGID ☐ FLACCID ☐ GUARDED ☐ BLUNT TRAUMA ☐ PENETRATING ☐ NAUSEA ☐ VOMITING ☐ SEE COMMENTS (12)

BREATHING: ☐ NORMAL ☐ LABORED ☐ RALES ☐ BREATH SOUNDS ☐ EQUAL ☐ UNEQUAL ☐ ABSENT ☐ SEE COMMENTS (13)

FX SITE: 1. ☐ SEE DIAGRAM ☐ EDEMA ☐ DEFORMITY ☐ OPEN ☐ CLOSED ☐ POINT TENDERNESS 2. ☐ SEE DIAGRAM ☐ EDEMA ☐ DEFORMITY ☐ OPEN ☐ CLOSED ☐ POINT TENDERNESS ☐ SEE COMMENTS (14)

COMMENTS SECTION

SIGNATURE OF PERSON(S) COMPLETING FORM | M.T.I.D. | M.T.I.D. | M.T.I.D. | SIGNATURE OF PHYSICIAN GIVING ORDERS

PATIENT HOSPITAL NO.

X X

MEDICAL RELEASE

I DO NOT WISH TO BE TRANSPORTED BY A WISHARD MEMORIAL HOSPITAL AMBULANCE TO A HOSPITAL FOR EXAMINATION AND/OR TREATMENT EVEN THOUGH WISHARD MEMORIAL HOSPITAL EMERGENCY MEDICAL TECHNICIANS HAVE RECOMMENDED THAT I BE TRANSPORTED TO A HOSPITAL FOR EXAMINATION AND/OR TREATMENT.

☐ EKG STRIPS ATTACHED ☐ AUDIT PAGE ATTACHED

78810 REV. 1-79

23993—L8 MM

**Figure 2-4.** A patient report form should fit the needs of its system medically, administratively, and operationally. (*Courtesy of Wishard Memorial Hospital, Indianapolis, Indiana*)

sibilities of the emergency medical services communication operator so that the "street" EMT-A can gain an appreciation of that important aspect in the total EMS system.

It is the responsibility of every EMT-A to use the communication system in a proper manner and to establish communications when necessary with the medical facility to provide patient information.

## Understanding of Emergency Department(s)

One of the most serious problems in an EMS system is poor communication. An important part of the EMS network is the hospital emergency department. Every effort should be made to establish a good communicative relationship with all emergency department personnel. A mutual understanding of roles and responsibilities should be fostered. The EMT-A has the responsibility to understand and abide by the general accepted protocols and procedures of each emergency department in each hospital in the system. Each emergency department has different methods of operation in receiving the patient, from paperwork distribution to triage procedures. How the EMT-A is greeted and accepted at the particular emergency department as a member of the health care team, rests a great deal on how the emergency ambulance service and its personnel have communicated, cared for, and treated the patient. It also becomes relatively apparent to the emergency department personnel (especially the nursing triage staff) how well the EMT-A possesses the skills of writing and verbalizing patient information.

Emergency departments play a critical role in the education and training of the EMT-A. It is important that the EMT-A have an opportunity to observe and perhaps become involved in the care and treatment of emergency department patients. In coordination with the emergency service and emergency departments, the EMT-A should make arrangements and observe in as many local emergency departments as possible to gain insight as to the next step of care given to the patient in the EMS system.

Most emergency department personnel are extremely helpful in answering questions and providing necessary feedback for the EMT-A. The EMT-A should attend and participate in continuing education programs offerred by the emergency departments. One may find out if this is possible by contacting the educational offices of the emergency service.

A working relationship and good communication must exist between hospital emergency departments and pre-hospital providers. Through this effort a mutual knowledge and respect for one's role and responsibility is realized.

## Understanding of Local EMS System

All EMT-As should be given an overview of the local, regional and state emergency medical services system. The state level of operations may be presented by a regional or state emergency medical services representative. The local EMS system should be explained in detail by the appropriate person(s) employed in the emergency service system. The EMT-A should be aware and if possible take a part in various local, regional and state commissions, councils and committees concerned with EMS. The EMT-A should attend public hearings concerning proposed rules, regulations and legislation pertaining to the EMS profession and when appropriate, voice concerns regarding such proposals. Leadership by the EMT-A is always needed in the EMS System. If the EMT-A takes an active part and is cognizant of how the system operates, his ability to explain its function to the general public is improved.

## Patient Guidance

In cooperation with the medical advisor of the emergency service, the EMT has a responsibility to appropriately guide the patient, and/or relatives to available social service agencies operating in the local community. The EMT-A should be aware of the various social services available to the general public. These include:

1. Emergency access number (911 or local number)
2. Alcohol abuse clinic
3. Crisis and suicide prevention center
4. Drug abuse clinic
5. Child abuse/neglect center
6. Venereal disease clinic
7. Poison control center
8. American Heart Association
9. Diabetes association
10. Cancer association
11. Lung association
12. Kidney foundation
13. Sickle cell anemia association
14. Sudden Infant death organization
15. American National Red Cross

Although many other agencies may exist in the community, the EMT-A should learn the agencies' functions. If there are hot-line numbers (poison control, suicide prevention, etc.) the EMT should know them and pass them along if requested or needed. Most of these services will provide free literature upon request.

One should remember that it is not the place of the EMT-A to be judge and jury in making social service decisions for the patient or relatives, but only to advise them that the social service or health agency exists should they require information or professional guidance.

### Community Involvement

One of the best ways to carry the message of EMS is for the responsible EMT-A to become involved in community affairs. The EMT should take an active part in health fairs, blood pressure screening clinics, and so on, both to be a service to the community and to explain to the general public the components involved in local emergency service. Public communication concerning the emergency service is one of the best ways to decrease ambulance abuse (when a person calls an ambulance simply because there is no other means of transportation. Terms used to describe this type of run are *clinic run, taxi cab run, crock run.)* Having an opportunity to explain to the public how to utilize the emergency service, (i.e., when, where and how to call the emergency service) gives the consumer a better feel for the emergency service operating in his community, and when to activate it.

It may also be advantageous to communicate to the consumer that certain questions may be asked of them by the communications operator when and if they do call. These questions (phone number, address of emergency, how many people are injured, etc.) are important so that the correct emergency unit(s) can be dispatched to the correct location. Some communication center operators hold the caller on the line after the emergency units have been sent to give correct medical first aid, and tell the caller what to do for the victim(s). (This is one reason why communication operators should be at least an EMT-A.) Giving medical advice by telephone about what to do before the EMTs arrive has saved lives.

## NATIONAL REGISTRY OF EMERGENCY MEDICAL TECHNICIANS

The National Registry of Emergency Medical Technicians is a certifying agency attesting to the education and training of ambulance personnel. It was formed in 1970 out of a need to establish standards and improve ambulance services in the care for patients. Just as other health professionals have a national accreditation organization, so it is with the EMT, one of the newest allied health professions.

The Registry attests to the competency of the EMT through uniform training and qualifying examinations. Although each state may require the EMT-A to pass their state certification examinations, the EMT should be nationally registered as well.

The purposes of the Registry are:

1. To promote the improved delivery of Emergency Medical Services by
    a. Assisting in the development and evaluation of educational programs to train EMTs

b. Establishing qualifications for eligibility to apply for registration

c. Preparing and conducting examinations designed to assure the competency of EMTs

d. Establishing a system for biennial re-registration (every two years)

e. Establishing procedures for revocation of certificates of registration for cause

f. Maintaining a directory of Registered EMTs

2. To develop guidelines and programs to assist individuals who have completed EMT programs to raise their level of competence to assure the provision of improved emergency medical services

3. To do any and all things necessary or desirable for the attainment of the purposes stated above

## EMT–A Identification

The nationally registered and/or state certified EMT-A may be recognized by a shoulder patch. It is to the discretion of the individual and/or emergency service which identifying patch should be worn.

Although the EMT-A may be certified in other courses (first aid, CPR, etc.) one should not decorate the uniform with pins, buttons and patches. This is inappropriate for the professional uniform. Successful completion of courses that award pins and patches should be stated in one's resume and not adorned on the uniform. The National Registered EMT-A shoulder patch, pin, and certificate is shown in Fig. 2–5.

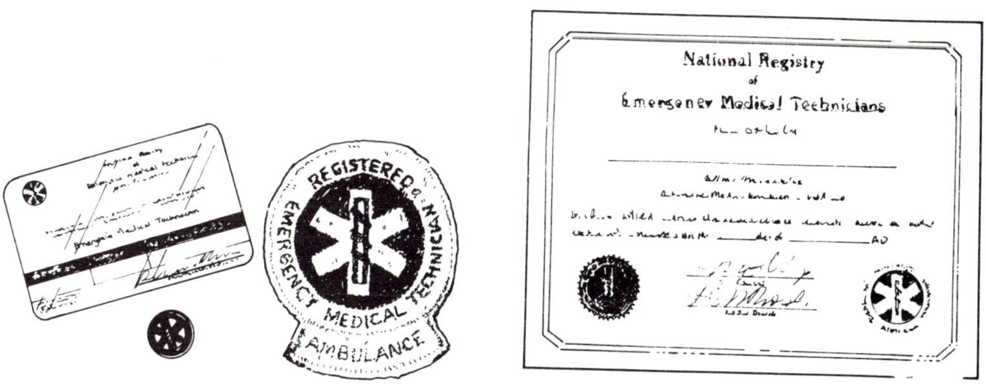


**Figure 2–5.** The identification card, pen, shoulder patch, and certificate of the National Registered EMT-A.

## Emblem—The Star of Life

### *History*

The star portion of the symbol dates back to prehistoric times. The story goes that this asterisklike star represents the four original rivers of earth with the Tree of Life rising from their waters. The Staff of Aesculapeus (Greek God of Medicine) has a serpent wrapped around it with its head at the top. This staff represents the art of healing and was the medical symbol of the ancient Greeks. In 1961, the American Medical Association (AMA) established a committee to develop a universal emergency medical identification symbol (EMI). The AMA holds a Class A copyright registration on the EMI. The AMA granted permission for the National Registry of Emergency Medical Technicians to incorporate the Star of Life into its official emblem and to utilize it as the focal point for the registered EMT emblem. The Registry emblem, its design and lettering, is protected by way of a Registration of Mark with the U.S. Patent Office, reserved for use only by the National Registry and is to be worn only by the Nationally Registered EMT. Permission was also secured to use the EMI symbol as the universal emblem to identify the properly configured, equipped, and manned emergency ambulance vehicle, meeting the Department of Transportation (DOT) specifications. The Division of Emergency Medical Services of the Department of Health and Human Resources (DHHR) requested, and was granted, permission to use the Star of Life emblem on all DHHR publications concerning emergency medical care. The Star of Life Emblem is shown in Fig. 2-6.

### *Logo*

In an effort to standardize the use of the term *emergency medical services,* and the abbreviation *EMS,* the Department of Health and Human Services' Division of Emergency Medical Services devised a logo, shown in Fig. 2-7. The logo will aid the general public to quickly identify with emergency medical services and reinforce the public impact of current ongoing EMS efforts to help the public.

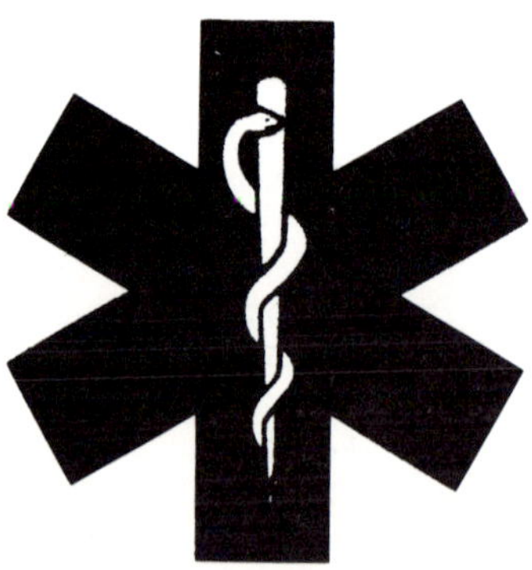

**Figure 2-6.** The Star of Life.

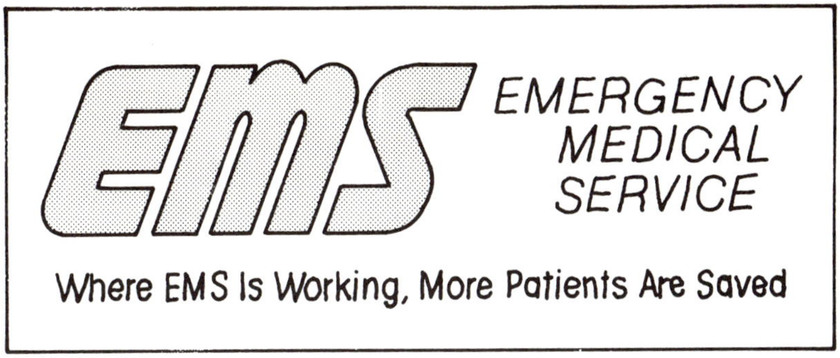


**Figure 2-7.** The EMS logo.

## Professional Society and Professional Journal

The purpose of the National Association of Emergency Medical Technicians (NAEMT) is as follows:

1. To promote and encourage the national acceptance of a uniform standard of recognition for the skills and abilities of the EMT

2. To promote the professional status of the EMT

3. To foster, encourage, and promote the constant upgrading of the skills, abilities, qualifications, and educational requirements of the EMT.

4. To encourage, promote, and support the establishment of EMS systems at the municipal, county, regional, state, and national levels.

5. To offer information and guidance on current concepts of emergency medical care and governmental policies related to the control, certification, and licensure of the EMT.

6. To promote, encourage, and carry out scientific research related to the care and transportation of the sick and injured.

7. To promote the public welfare and education of the general public in emergency medical services.

The *EMT Journal* is the official publication of the National Association of Emergency Medical Technicians. The purpose of the Journal is to provide a means of expression, a source of knowledge, and a catalogue of resources directed especially to the EMT-A. It is important that the EMT-A remain current on new skills, equipment, and ideas related to the field of EMS. The *EMT Journal* and others will satisfy that need.

# THE EMERGENCY MEDICAL TECHNICIAN-AMBULANCE (EMT-A) JOB DESCRIPTION

## Job Summary

The EMT-A responds in an emergency medical unit to the scene of reported medical emergencies; provides efficient and immediate basic life support at the scene and en route to and in the hospital; exercises judgment as to the need for advanced life support and other specialized agencies (if available); prepares accurate reports and participates in continuing education and quality of care assessment activities.

## Typical Duties

1. Provides emergency medical care at the basic life-support level according to the emergency service practices, policies, and established protocols, verbal and written orders, and state regulations; exercises independent judgment as to the need for advanced life support (if available) and in critical emergency situations coordinates activities of involved public safety personnel; and provides medical reports to hospital staff.

2. Medically monitors the patient while in transport and continues treatment begun on the scene; provides information via communication systems as required.

3. Drives an emergency vehicle under emergency conditions; maintains safety, cleanliness and security of the vehicle and equipment; checks and maintains the vehicle's equipment and supplies; performs basic, routine maintenance activities.

4. Prepares accurate, legible records and reports; participates actively in continuing education and medical audit programs.

5. Provides medical care with physician, nursing, and allied health personnel in the hospital and pre-hospital setting in accordance with established practices and protocols.

## Education, Training and Experience

A high school education or equivalency qualification is considered minimal. The person must be eighteen years of age or older.

Minimum training shall be that prescribed in the basic training program for emergency medical technicians-ambulance (EMT-A) of the Department of Transportation and the Public Health Service, or local state equivalency or both.

He must have practical experience in the care and use of emergency equipment commonly accepted and employed, such as suction machines, oxygen delivery systems (installed and portable), spineboards, fracture equipment, emergency medical care kits, obstetrical kits, intravenous kits, shock trousers, stretchers of various types, light rescue tools, and basic automobile mechanics. He has the basic understanding of sanitizing and disinfecting procedures and knowledge of safety and security measures.

The EMT-A acquires a thorough knowledge of the territory within his service area, and the traffic ordinances and laws concerning emergency vehicle transport of patients. He has the necessary driver's and professional license as required by law and the emergency service.

## Special Characteristics



### *Aptitude*

The EMT-A must have motor coordination in administering emergency care of the critically ill and injured, in lifting and carrying patients, and in driving an emergency vehicle. One must have manual dexterity and physical coordination in carrying, lifting, extricating, climbing, hoisting and other similar maneuvers, in a manner not detrimental to the patient, fellow workers, or self. The EMT-A must have the facility to give and receive verbal and written direction and instruction.

### *Physical Demands*

The EMT-A must have normal good health and the ability to lift and carry up to one-hundred pounds. He needs to have visual color discrimination in examining patients and determining by appearance, diagnostic signs that require immediate detection and proper action, as well as to distinguish traffic signs and lights. Both far and near visual acuity is necessary for driving and for examining the patient (correction by lenses is permitted).

## *References*

American Academy of Orthopedic Surgeons, Committee on Allied Health. *Emergency Care of the Sick and Injured*, 2nd ed. Chicago, IL, 1977.

Caroline, N. L. *Emergency Care in the Streets.* Boston, MA: Little, Brown & Co., 1979.

"The Emergency Medical Technician Oath," *The EMT Journal,* March 1978 Vol. 2 No. 1. St. Louis, MO: The C. V. Mosby Co.

Farrington, J. D. "Ambulance Services," *The EMT Journal,* March 1977, pp. 37–39.

Farrington, J. D. "A New and Unique Professional Journal for the EMT," *The EMT Journal,* March 1977, p. 27.

Grant, H. D., and Murray, R. H., Jr. *Emergency Care,* 2nd ed. Bowie, MD: Robert Brady Co., 1978.

Job Description—Emergency Medical Technician-Ambulance. U.S. Department of Transportation, National Highway Traffic Safety Administration, May 1972.

National Association of Emergency Medical Technicians. "The EMT Newsletter," No. 7, October 1979, pp. 1–6.

Smith, P. J. "Job Description—Emergency Medical Technician-Ambulance." Wishard Memorial Hospital Ambulance Service, September 1980.

"A Standarized EMS Logo," *The EMT Newsletter.* National Association of Emergency Medical Technicians. No. 1, January 1979. St. Louis, MO: The C. V. Mosby Co.

"Star of Life History," *National Registry of Emergency Medical Technicians Newsletter,* Vol. 11, No. 1, April 1980.

# Chapter 3

# The Ambulance

The means of transportation for the sick and injured has come a long way since the horsedrawn carriages of the nineteenth century. Time has surpassed the use of the hearse, limousine-style vehicle, and converted station wagons. Today's ambulance is supplied with more sophisticated medical and communication equipment and has more room in the patient compartment for better care. Because of stricter federal and state vehicle requirements, an ambulance today must provide two compartments, one for the emergency driver and one for the patient. The patient compartment must accommodate two EMT-As and two stretcher patients positioned so that at least one patient can be given intensive life support during transport. The vehicle must be able to carry sufficient equipment and supplies for optimum emergency care at the scene, as well as during transport. The ambulance must be equipped with two-way radio communication for reporting the patient's medical condition and for safeguarding ambulance personnel. The emergency unit must carry equipment necessary for light rescue procedures and be designed and constructed to afford maximum safety and comfort to avoid aggravation of the patient's condition, exposure to complications and threat to survival.

## TYPES OF AMBULANCES

The emergency medical care vehicle must meet federal and/or state requirements to be classified as an ambulance. There are three basic types (see Fig. 3–1).

### Type I

This ambulance has a conventional cab and chassis, on which is mounted a modular ambulance body. This type of vehicle is available in both two- and four-wheel drive. The advantage of the unit is that the

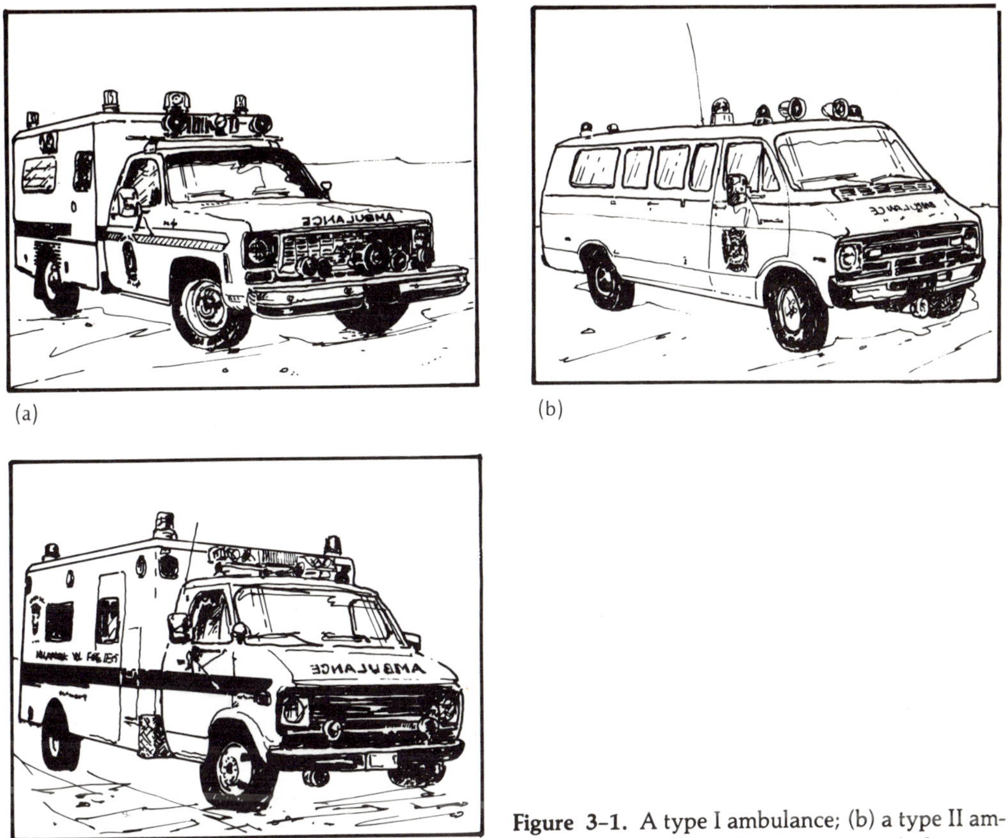

(a) (b) (c)

**Figure 3-1.** A type I ambulance; (b) a type II ambulance; (c) a type III ambulance.

modular body can be replaced with newer models. A disadvantage is there is no passageway between the driver and patient compartment.

## Type II

This ambulance is a van-type constructed emergency vehicle. The cab and body of the unit are integrated. There is a passageway between the driver compartment and patient compartment. This vehicle is available in two- and four-wheel drive and is the most widely used type of ambulance in the United States.

## Type III

This vehicle has a forward control cab and an integral body that is generally larger than that found on a Type II Ambulance. This vehicle is referred to as a specialty van ambulance and has gained popularity as a paramedic unit because of the room offered in the patient compartment.

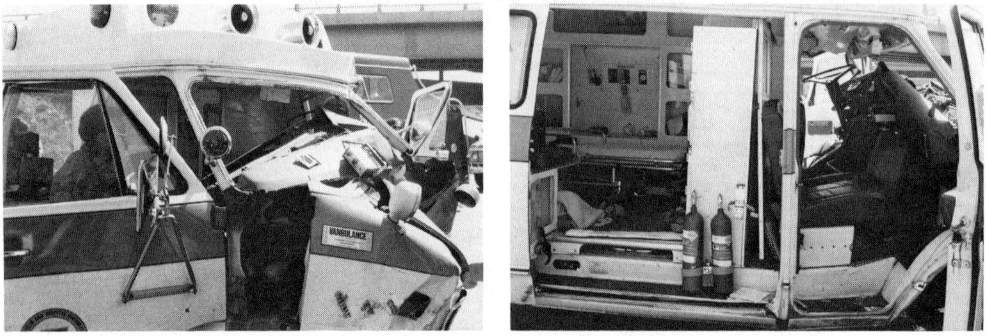

(a) (b)

**Figure 3–2.** (a) This type II ambulance struck a utility pole head-on. (b) A view of the front and rear ambulance compartments. Note the steering column position and the driver's seat. The EMT-A driver of this vehicle sustained multiple fractures of the lower extremities.

Type I and II vehicles, although roomy, usually have a rougher ride and because of the van-type front end, the driver and front passengers are exposed in front-end accidents. (See Fig. 3–2.) Although there are three basic types of emergency units, they may be modified in many different ways. This is often the case given the particular terrain and geographical location of the emergency service. Some of the many ways which the vehicle may be altered would include four-wheel drive, heavy-duty suspension and specialized interior.

## AMBULANCE IDENTIFICATION

### Color

Federal regulations specify that the exterior color of an ambulance be basically white in combination with a horizontal orange stripe parallel to the road. The white and orange colors were chosen over others because they are a more visible color pattern, making the emergency vehicle safer moving through traffic. The band or stripe of orange should not be less than six inches wide nor more than fourteen inches wide and should encircle the entire ambulance body configuration at the belt line (below the lowest edge of the cab windows).

### Emblems and Markings

Federal regulation requires that all emblems and markings on the vehicle be of a reflective color. The word AMBULANCE in blue letters will be mirror-image and centered above the grill, so that motorists will see in their rear-view mirror the word AMBULANCE. The Star of Life emblem is

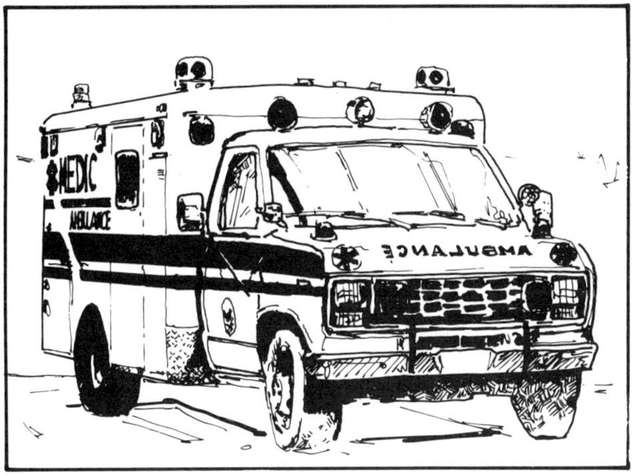

**Figure 3–3.** This type III ambulance shows the parallel color striping, emblems, and markings required by federal specifications.

also used to identify the ambulance. Warning lights must be rotating beacons mounted on the roof, corners, and in the grill of the vehicle. (See Fig. 3–3.) Although the specifications call for blue lights, this often differs from one region to the next. Blue lights are often reserved for the police department; other areas have red lights for all emergency services.

## EQUIPMENT AND SUPPLIES

All emergency transport ambulances should carry the necessary equipment to provide optimum treatment and care for the patient. Obviously, the EMT-A must be able to properly use and troubleshoot all equipment and supplies carried on the vehicle for efficient care and treatment for the patient.

All equipment and supplies utilized during the care and treatment of the patient should be situated in a logical place for easy retrieval. (e.g., airway equipment and supplies should be situated near the head of the patient, traction splints, shock trousers, etc., should be stored at the foot end of the patient.)

Basic equipment that should be carried on all ambulances is listed in Table 3–1.

### Safety Equipment

Safety equipment for ambulances that is necessary to secure an area and provide safety for rescuers and patients until specialized help arrives should include:

1. Reflectorized or intermittent flashing warning devices
2. Flashlights and 6-volt battery powered lantern
3. Floodlights—portable .300W/120V with 100-foot cord
4. Air masks—self-contained (not oxygen generating)
5. Fire extinguisher—B:C dry powder type
6. Insulated gauntlets—foam insulated, vinyl-coated flourescent orange
7. Protective flak vests (armored)—use varies from region to region, often used in inner-city areas where violence is high
8. Warning cones or flags for daylight safety

TABLE 3-1. BASIC AMBULANCE EQUIPMENT

| |
|---|
| Stretchers (also called cot or gurney)—wheeled and adjustable |
| Stretchers—hand carried (also called break-a-way) |
| —scoop (for removing patients who are critically injured with minimum movement) |
| Folding stair chair |
| Pillows |
| Pillowcases |
| Towels |
| Washcloths |
| Blankets |
| Emesis basins or bags |
| Tissue |
| Bedpans |
| Urinals |
| Paper or styrofoam cups |
| Plastic bags (assorted sizes for avulsed and amputated body parts) |
| Body bag |
| Wall-mounted and portable suction units (should provide a vacuum of at least 300 mmHg within 4 sec. The units should be equipped with nonkinking base and a rigid pharyngeal tip) |
| Wall-mounted oxygen delivery system (minimum of 3000 *l* reservoir with an evaporative $0_2$ humidifier) |
| Portable oxygen delivery system (minimum of 300 *l* reservoir and capable of delivering 10 *l*/m) |
| Sandbags |
| Cardiac press board |
| Sphygmomanometer |
| Stethoscope |
| Thermometers—oral, rectal, hypothermia |

## Access And Extrication Equipment

The access (light extrication) equipment listed below is recommended by the American College of Surgeons for the ambulance, unless the ambulance is routinely accompanied by a true rescue vehicle with extrication equipment aboard. The various access tools utilized to lift, pry, cut, pull and batter should be located in compartments accessible from outside the ambulance.

1. One wrench, 12-inch, adjustable, open end
2. One screwdriver, 12-inch, regular
3. One screwdriver, 12-inch, phillips
4. One hacksaw with 12 wire (carbide blades)
5. One pliers, 10-inch, vise grip
6. One hammer, No. 5, 15-inch handle; one fire axe butt, 24-inch handle, one wrecking bar, 24-inch; separate or as one combination tool
7. One crowbar, 51-inch, pinch point
8. One bolt cutter, 39-inch, jaw opening, 1-1/4 inches.
9. One portable power jack and spreader tool (Minimum 4-ton capacity)
10. One shovel, 49-inch, pointed blade
11. One double action tin snips, minimum 8 inches.
12. Two ropes, manilla 50-foot by 3/4 inch in diameter
13. Power wrench (optional). Front-mounted winch minimum 2-ton capacity, recommended particularly in areas where one is not readily available. Chain 15-foot, with one grab hook and one running hook.

### *Additional Suggested Items*

1. One asbestos blanket
2. Two pair goggles
3. Two pair gloves (gauntlets, leather)

## Airway and Resuscitation Equipment

The establishment of an airway in an unconscious patient is important. Airway- and oxygen-related equipment should be versatile to accommodate both the adult and pediatric patient.

### *Airway Equipment*

1. Oropharyngeal (o″ro-fah-rin′je-al) airways (size 0–6)
2. Pocket mask
3. Bag valve mask unit (with oxygen reservoir capable of delivering 100 percent oxygen)
4. Tongue blades or mouth gags
5. Nasopharyngeal (na″zo-fah-rin′je-al) airways
6. Suction unit (wall mounted and portable)

*Oxygen Therapy Equipment*

1. Nasal cannula
2. Simple face mask
3. Venturi masks
4. Nonrebreathing mask and bag
5. Intermittent positive pressure breathing unit (IPPB)—optional

## Dressing and Bandaging Supplies

Supplies for treating small wounds and burns, and for controlling hemorrhage should include:

1. Bandaids® assorted sizes
2. Roller gauze, 2 inches wide (sterile)
3. Universal dressing (Trauma dressing) 10x36 in (sterile)
4. Occlusive dressings:
   —Vaseline-impregnated gauze pads (sterile)
   —aluminum foil 18 x 25 in (wrapped and sterilized)
   —plastic wrap
5. Adhesive tape, 1/2-inch, 1-inch, 2-inch and 3-inch widths
6. Eye pads
7. Gauze pads—4x4 in and 5x9 in (sterile)
8. Bandage shears
9. Triangular bandages
10. Safety pins
11. Sanitary napkins
12. Gloves—sterile (assorted sizes)
13. Gloves—examination (assorted sizes)
14. Burn sheets (sterile)

## Equipment for Fracture Immobilization

1. Long spineboard
2. Short spineboard
3. Cervical collars (assorted sizes)
4. Four sandbags
5. Two traction splints or hinged half ring splint for lower extremity fracture
6. Four long board splints—padded 3 x 36 in
7. Four short board splints—padded 3 x 15 in

Also available are uncomplicated air splints, wire ladder splints, cardboard splints and vacuum splints. Availability, locality and local medical direction will dictate which is to be used.

## Supplies for Pregnancy and Childbirth

These supplies can be wrapped and sterilized as a package for easy access:

1. One pair surgical scissors
2. Three hemostats or cord clamps
3. Umbilical tape or sterile cord
4. Ear syringe or rubber bulb syringe for aspiration of mucus contents from the baby's nose and mouth
5. Towels
6. 12 gauze pads—4 x 4 in
7. Four pairs of sterile gloves (assorted sizes)
8. Baby blanket
9. Sanitary napkins
10. Two large plastic bags or plastic basins

## Supplies for Poisoning

1. Syrup of ipecac (ip′ĕ-kak)
2. Activated charcoal
3. Drinking water for ipecac and activated charcoal

### *Supplies for Venomous Arthropod (ar′thro-pŏd) Bites and Stings*

1. Snake-bite kit—commercially available or include two suction cups (rubber type or ECG suction bulbs), 1 knife handle, 1 #11 surgical blade, 1 lymphatic/venous tourniquet
2. Venomous marine-life kit—supplies carried in the kit will vary from region to region; medical direction will dictate which supplies should be used

## Equipment for the Hypovolemic Shock Patient

1. Antishock trousers—adult and pediatric
2. Intravenous administration kit
3. Intravenous volume expanders—Ringer's lactate or other volume-expanding fluid in 2–1000cc bags
4. Survival blanket (aluminum)

## Miscellaneous Supplies

1. Lubricating jelly
2. Sterile water
3. Normal saline (sterile, 0.9 percent)
4. Razor blades (straight edge)
5. Rubber bands
6. Paper bags (small)
7. Hydrogen peroxide
8. Glucose preparation—commercially available for the diabetic patient
9. Tongue blades
10. Isopropyl alcohol
11. Alcohol swabs (disposable)
12. Iodine swabs (disposable)
13. Chemical cold pack
14. Benzoin—bottle or spray

Most ambulances have supplies and equipment stocked in the unit, and heavily used first aid items are in jump kits or in boxes taken to the patient. Kits vary from small doctor's bags to large multisectioned plastic boxes. Custom-made light aluminum cases usually outlast all other kits where use is heavy.

Certain treatment kits, such as poison and childbirth kits, should be located where they are readily accessible, rather than scattered throughout the vehicle.

All equipment and supplies necessary for airway management should be stored or located near the head of the patient for quick access. The radio communication equipment in the patient compartment should also be located near the head of the patient, so that medical communication can be quickly established.

Depending on location and medical direction, some EMT ambulance units stock advanced life support supplies and equipment for the physician or paramedic, should they be at the scene of the medical emergency and the patient warrants advanced life support intervention.

An advanced life support medical kit and stocked ambulance may include:

1. Intubation equipment
2. Intravenous therapy set
3. Venesection (ven″e-sek′shun) kit
4. Pleural decompression set

5. Tracheostomy (tra″ke-os′to-me) or cricothyrotomy (kri″ko-thi″rot′o-me) set

6. Urinary catheters

7. Portable electrocardiogram monitor/defibrillator

8. Drugs for the cardiac, diabetic, overdose and shock patient

Communication equipment is necessary for a functioning ambulance. This equipment varies from one geographical location to the next, and may range from hand-held portable two-way radio units to a vehicle-based radio network, (i.e., mobile transceivers, mobile telephones and telemetry systems).

## *References*

American Academy of Orthopedic Surgeons, Committee on Allied Health. *Emergency Care of the Sick and Injured,* 2nd ed. Chicago, IL, 1977.

Gazzaniga, A. B.; Iseri, L. T.; and Baren, M. *Emergency Care: Principles and Practices for the EMT-Paramedic.* Reston, VA: Reston Publishing Co., Inc., 1979.

Grant, H. D., and Murray, R. H., Jr. *Emergency Care,* 2nd ed. Bowie, MD: Robert J. Brady Company, 1978.

# Chapter 4

# Emergency Driving

An important aspect of working as an EMT in the emergency medical services field is operating a motor vehicle under emergency conditions. While no one is a born emergency vehicle operator, many individuals feel because they possess a valid operator's license, have flawless driving records and are certified as EMTs that they have the training and experience necessary to safely operate an emergency vehicle. Although this assumption is widespread, it is incorrect, and the false sense of security that is fostered injures and kills a significant number of people each year. In order to adequately prepare for the emergency driving task, the professional EMT must, in addition to having a basic understanding of the highway transportation system, acquire an in-depth working knowledge of emergency vehicles and advanced driving techniques.

## HIGHWAY TRANSPORTATION SYSTEM

There are three major elements which make up the highway transportation system—highways, vehicles, and people. In 1956, the Federal Highway Act was enacted, establishing funds for construction of interstate highways. Over 40,000 miles of highway would be built, linking most cities that have populations greater than 50,000. The goal of this entire project was to upgrade roadways in the United States and hopefully reduce traffic accidents. However, highway improvement alone was not destined to lower the motor vehicle accident rate.

As highways began to improve and speed limits were raised, traffic accidents soared. In 1966, the National Highway Safety Act was passed. This act grew out of the realization that in order to curb the rising death toll, all levels of government—federal, state and local—would have to work together to control traffic accidents. As part of this realization the federal government signed into law the National Traffic and Motor Vehicle

Safety Act. Motor vehicle manufacturers were given safety standards that each motor vehicle must conform to. These standards became effective on all American vehicles manufactured after January 1, 1968. Despite this effort, there remains one element of the highway system which was virtually uncontrollable and was responsible for the greatest cause of vehicle accidents: people.

Each year 50,000 people lose their lives and another 2,000,000 suffer disabling injuries as a result of motor-vehicle-related accidents. Of these traffic accidents, it is estimated that 85 percent result from operator error. The related economic loss in the U.S. is over twenty billion dollars. As an Emergency Medical Technician and highway user, you have the responsibility to be a careful driver both on and off the job.

## DRIVER SELECTION AND TRAINING

Because emergency driving is a specialty, careful consideration must be given to driver selection and education. Little is known about why people differ in their ability to act and drive safely. Of all occupations, few involve a greater need for safety than that of the emergency vehicle operator.

If properly selected, educated, motivated, and supervised, the emergency vehicle driver can usually avoid accidents that result in property damage, injuries, and death.

Before discussing specific screening, there are a few general requirements for emergency vehicle drivers that must be considered before selection.

### Driving Experience

Past driving experience is the most critical indicator of future safe driving ability. It has been fairly well documented that accident repeaters of the past will continue to have frequent accidents in the future.

### Physical Examination

Before a person is allowed to drive an emergency vehicle, he should be examined by a qualified physician. This is usually done as part of hiring procedures; however, it should also be done on an annual or semi-annual basis. The American Medical Association's Committee on Medical Aspects of Automobile Injuries and Deaths has published a medical guide for physicians for determining fitness to drive a motor vehicle. This brochure covers most aspects of the physician's role in ascertaining physical, mental, emotional, and physiological impairments as they relate to safe driving, and can be of great assistance to the examining physician.

Some of the minimum applicant standards for driving an emergency vehicle should be:

1. Mental and physical condition
   a. No loss of foot, leg, hand, or arm
   b. No mental, nervous, organic, or functional diseases likely to interfere with safe emergency driving
   c. No loss of fingers, impairment of use of foot, leg, fingers, hands, or arms or other structural defects or limitations likely to interfere with safe emergency driving
2. Eyesight
   Visual acuity of at least 20/40 (Snellen) in each eye, either with or without lenses and a field of vision in the horizontal meridian not less than a total of 140°; ability to distinguish traffic colors (red, green, amber) (See Fig. 4–1.)
3. Hearing
   Hearing should be adequate in the better ear for conversational tones without the use of hearing aids

## Psychophysical Testing

An often overlooked area of screening for emergency vehicle driver selection is psychophysical testing. Through proper administration of the psychophysical test, the EMT can learn his limitations as related to visual perception, reaction time, and glare recovery. This information is important to the driver as it relates to the driving task and helps a driver arrive at traffic decisions in a more effective manner. Each driver must know and be able to interpret his psychophysical limitations before entering complex traffic situations. Information such as visual acuity, color vision, depth perception, field of vision, complex reaction times, and night vision must be tested. Following these tests, a driver will have a chance to recognize shortcomings in any of these areas and can correct or compensate for these deficiencies, thus putting him at a more advantageous position in the traffic environment.

Depth perception and peripheral vision are critical to a driver's judgment of space relation between vehicles, pedestrians, and other objects in the traffic environment. Additionally, they are needed in order to make successful passing maneuvers. Devices that test depth perception can provide clues to any visual weakness in this area. Since it is not possible for a driver to perceive the entire traffic scene at a glance, peripheral vision in conjunction with depth perception is needed. Peripheral vision is particularly helpful in scanning an intersection, in lane changing, in merging, and when driving near parked vehicles or objects. It is imperative that the

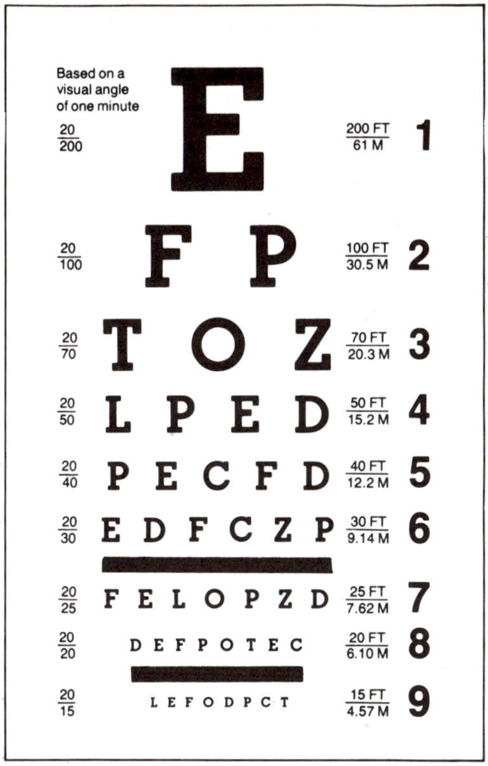


**Figure 4–1.** The Snellen eye chart. Used to determine if a person has normal 20/20 vision. If one can stand 20 feet away and read line 8, he has 20/20 vision.

emergency vehicle operator be tested for and have normal ranges of peripheral vision. There are several devices on the market that can be used for perimeter and depth testing. Most are relatively inexpensive to purchase and are simple to use. (See Fig. 4–2.)

Color blindness should be checked with isochromatic plates rather than color switch tests, as some color blind people can determine primary colors by their lightness or darkness, rather than by their hue. The pseudo-isochromatic testing system is simple to administer and is good for initial screening. This test usually consists of arabic numerals made up of dots on a field of other colored dots. The first card has colors with sharp contrast to be used as a demonstration card. Each of the following cards have closer hues, requiring an increase in one's ability to distinguish colors.

Reaction time can be checked with a device known as a brake reaction timer. (See Fig. 4–3.) As the driver depresses the accelerator, a green

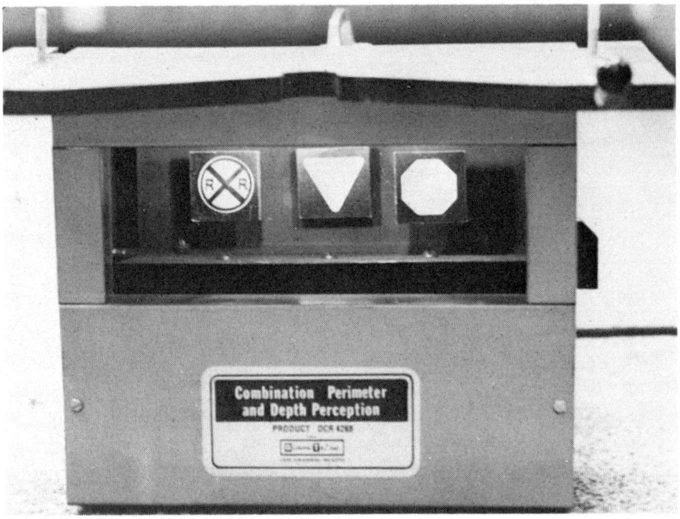


**Figure 4–2.** A perimeter and depth testing device.

light is lit. When the driver sees the red light, he is to move his right foot as quickly as possible to the brake. When the brake is applied, the timer is automatically stopped and the reaction time has been measured to the nearest 1/100 of a second. Average standards are .45 seconds. Persons found to have longer times can be made aware of the increased stopping distance required for various speeds.

Poor night vision and glare recovery are factors for which the driver can compensate, but in order to do so, he must recognize the degree to

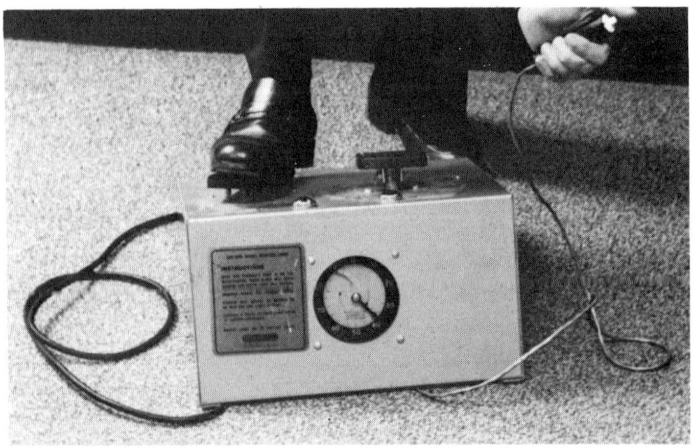

**Figure 4–3.** A brake reaction timer.

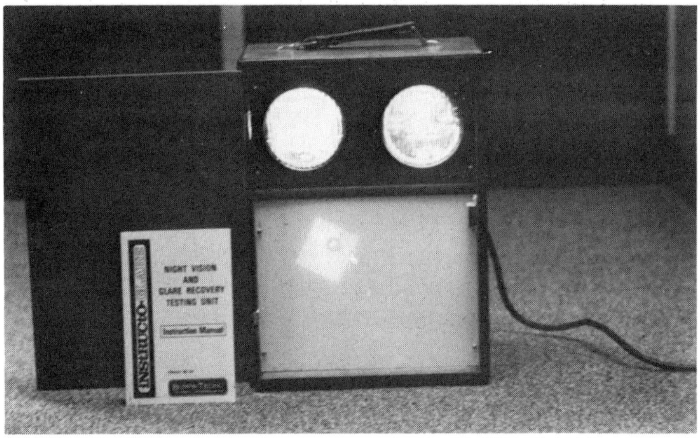

**Figure 4-4.** A night vision and glare recovery testing unit.

which he is impaired. Through the use of potentiometer-controlled (po-ten″she-om′ĕ-ter) lights (see Fig. 4-4) persons can be evaluated on their ability to recognize objects at night and then their ability to recognize the same object after being temporarily blinded by headlight glare. Average glare recovery should range in the area of three to eight seconds. Occasionally a driver may react in an incorrect manner when headlights are shined into his eyes (looks straight into headlights, closes eyes, turns head, etc.) The correct technique is to look downward to the right edge of the roadway until the light passes or is dimmed. It is advisable for all persons who show a below-average glare recovery to have an in-depth eye examination by an ophthalmologist. Translating the period of temporary blindness from seconds into the number of feet his vehicle will travel at highway speeds is a most effective way of viewing compromised night vision. These tests are not a basis by which drivers should be eliminated from driving an emergency vehicle, but rather tools used to develop better drivers.

## DYNAMICS AND DRIVING

As an EMT driving an emergency vehicle you will do more than guide the vehicle over the road's surface. Emergency driving is a full-time job requiring the total attention and skill of the driver. Each moment you will be involved in a complex and constant process of interacting with the surrounding traffic environment. Mastery over this system is, of course, something one cannot learn from reading; however, reading is where you must begin in order to understand those concepts which will have an effect on the vehicle and its occupants. As you gain experience in vehicle han-

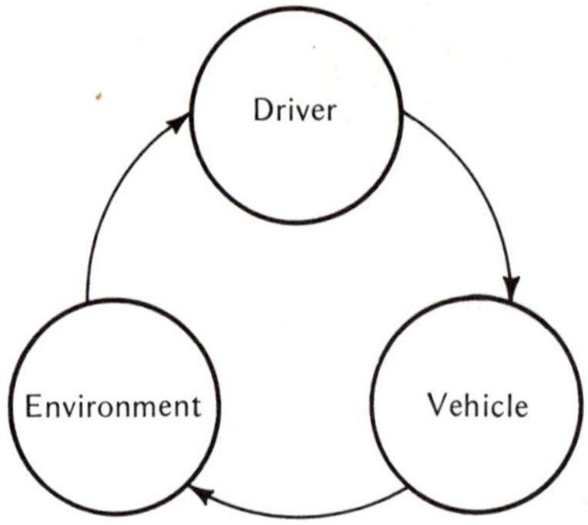


**Figure 4-5.** The EMT-A emergency vehicle driver must react to vehicle conditions as well as environmental conditions.

dling you will begin to realize a special ability critical to long-term safe driving—the ability to anticipate other vehicles by sensing movements and affecting corrective action. (see Fig. 4-5.) This is what professional drivers call being "in rhythm" with the vehicle. Being in rhythm demands smooth and even control so as to avoid loss of control. Understanding the human factors of sensory perception, alertness, judgment, and skill are the essentials of good and safe driving. Of course, there is much more.

A basic law one must understand when driving is that every movement of the vehicle requires a form of force. Generally, the forces one must be concerned with are those that affect starting, stopping, and turning of the vehicle. Vehicle control is almost completely dependent upon the tire and its contact with the ground. (see Fig. 4-6.) In order to control the vehicle properly, the tire must maintain a rolling footprint or adhesion with the road surface. Each tire or set of tires can only provide a specific amount of adhesion (traction). This adhesion or traction to the road's surface is called the *coefficient of friction.* In theory, the highest coefficient of friction that can be developed is 1.0. Practically speaking the highest coefficient of friction that the average driver can experience is 0.9. At any time the amount of friction needed exceeds that which exists, the vehicle begins to slip or skid. (see Fig. 4-7.)

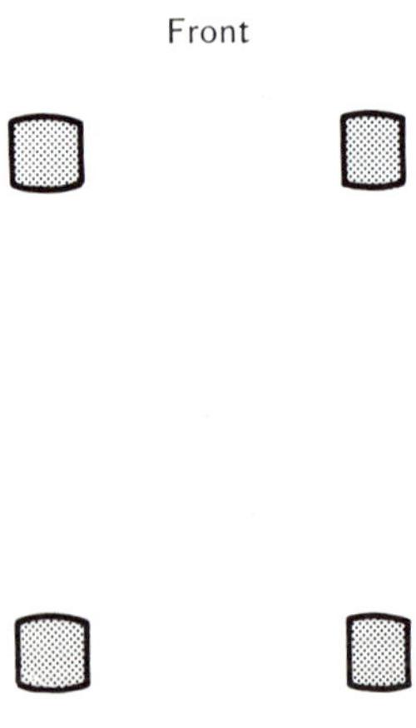


**Figure 4-6.** The EMT-A emergency vehicle driver is almost completely dependent upon these four tire spots.

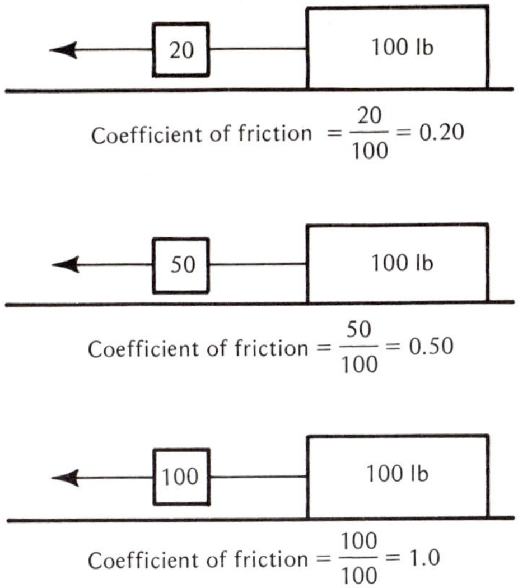


**Figure 4–7.** The calculation of coefficient of friction. A weight scale is attached to a 100-pound block of rubber and an applied force of pull starts the block moving. The reading of the scale when the block starts moving determines the pull required to keep the block in motion. In the first example, 20 pounds is required to keep the block in motion. Therefore, 20/100 = 0.20, the coefficient of friction.

As rotating force is directed from the motor through the drive train to the tires, the vehicle begins to move. With the steering wheel pointed straight, the vehicle tends to move in a straight line. If this force is removed then the vehicle, acted upon by forces of friction, slows and eventually comes to a stop. In order to decrease the amount of distance needed to coast to a stop, braking force is applied to further retard the vehicle's movement. As the road surface or other conditions change, so does the coefficient of friction and one's ability to start or stop. On glare ice for example, the coefficient of friction is less than 0.10. Coefficient of friction on dry-wear polished concrete has been measured as low as 0.10, as slick as ice. (see Fig. 4–8.) This decrease in friction can cause a vehicle traveling at 20 mph to use up almost 150 feet of road surface to stop. Additionally, normal reaction time of 3/4 second can add an additional 20 feet to the total stopping distance.

Of course, not all vehicle movements are confined to a straight line. Where turning is necessary, it is required that a force be applied to the vehicle through the tires at an angle in order to change the vehicle's direction. As the front tires are turned they begin to change their direction of travel. Only when speed is at the 1–2 mph range do the tires actually roll around corners in a guided manner. At higher speeds the tires tend to generate cornering forces by scrubbing sideways on the road surface. This causes the

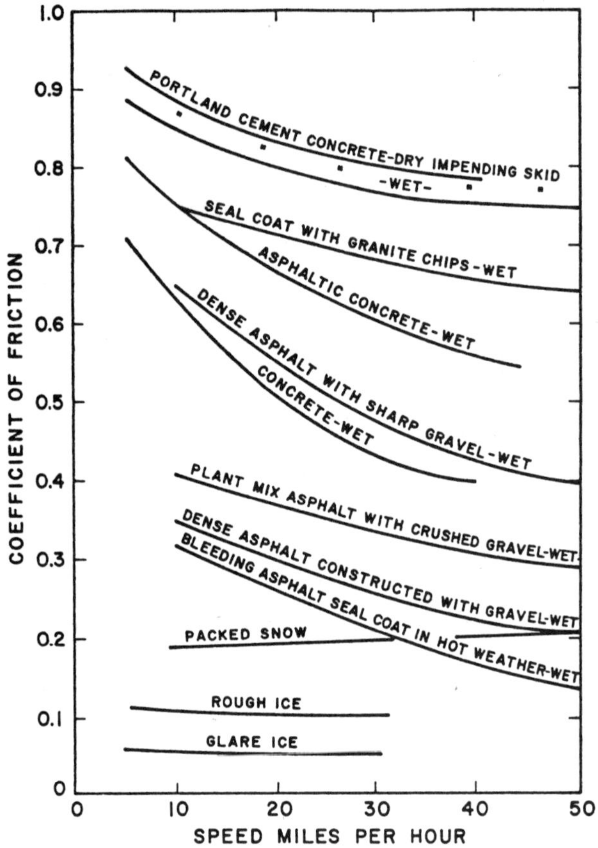


**Figure 4–8.** Friction coefficient variation depends on vehicle speed, road surface, and road condition. (Used with permission of the Society of Automotive Engineers, Inc., Warrendale, PA.)

tire to push at an angle and the vehicle changes directions. Of course, there is always a measurable amount of tire skid as cornering force is generated. We actually establish a drift angle each time we exceed 1–2 mph and turn the steering wheel. Both front and rear wheels are generating cornering forces, supplying part of the total cornering force. We initiate cornering maneuvers by directing the front wheels in the desired direction, but the cornering force from all four wheels is required to turn the vehicle and maintain direction in the curve or turn. The sum of all tire-cornering force must equal and resist another force acting on the vehicle called centrifugal force. (See Fig. 4–9.) Should the wheels stop rotating, the tire will lose most of its cornering force and the vehicle will continue in a straight path off the curve, no matter what direction the steering wheel is turned. On the other hand, if only the rear wheels lose their cornering force, the rear of the vehicle will begin to skid or drift toward the outside of the curve. When operating on wet surfaces, there are additional factors that must be con-

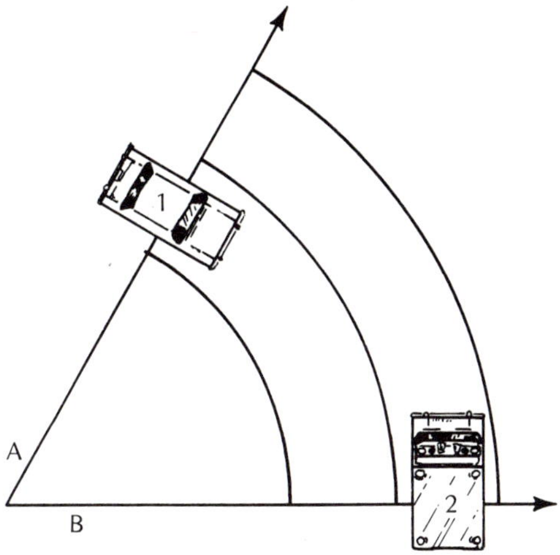


**Figure 4-9.** Centrifugal force can cause vehicles 1 and 2 to move in the direction of the arrows.

sidered. On wet pavement coefficient levels are lowered and therefore, a reduction in the tire's ability to produce cornering force. Compared to dry pavement, the tire's drift angle for the average tire on wet pavement is four to six degrees less. This can become very important especially when the tires are developing maximum cornering force and acceleration or braking forces are added. As acceleration or braking increases, the tires' ability to produce cornering forces decrease. Because of this principle, it is safer for the driver to slow the vehicle before entering a curve than move through the curve without applying acceleration or braking. One of the more difficult habits for any emergency vehicle driver to break is applying brakes or acceleration while cornering at higher speeds. Remember, the vehicle's tires can only produce a given amount of traction; when one demands more traction than the tire can produce, a skid and subsequent loss of vehicle control results.

As you become familiar with the vehicle and its handling characteristics, you will be able to safely control the vehicle in most normal situations. However, it is extremely important that before practicing vehicle handling on an emergency run you drive on a driving range, where the situation is more controlled and the consequences of miscalculation are less devastating.

## VEHICLE INSPECTION

Today's modern ambulances are complicated devices composed of some 15,000 parts, integrated into a number of major mechanical units—braking, suspension, steering, power, fuel, drive-train, exhaust, cooling, and electrical. These units combine to form seven major systems. It is essential that every emergency vehicle operator know the functions, early symptoms of malfunctions, and corrective action for the various systems used on the vehicle. In addition to knowing your vehicle, you must be sure each system is performing properly. To do this, daily inspections must be made. The inspection should be worked into a preshift inspection routine where discrepancies are noted and repairs, or arrangements for repairs, are initiated.

While it is realized that vehicles vary widely from manufacturer to manufacturer, a general guideline for system inspection has been listed below. Additions and deletions in this routine should be made as necessary to cover specific vehicles or needs. The seven systems requiring inspection and examples of units inspected in each system are:

1. Protective system
    a. Items not controlled by driver
        1. Air bags
        2. Exterior glass
        3. Impact-resistant bumpers
        4. Padded surfaces
    b. Items controlled by driver
        1. Seat belts
        2. Head restraints
        3. Ignition interlock system
2. Comfort system
    a. Seat adjustment
    b. Air conditioner
    c. Heater and defroster control
    d. Air vents
    e. Cruise or speed control
3. Control systems
    a. Steering wheel
    b. Accelerator
    c. Foot brake
    d. Parking brake
    e. Selector lever and quadrant
    f. Ignition switch
4. Vehicle check system
    a. Speedometer
    b. Odometer
    c. Charging system gauge or light
    d. Temperature gauge or light
    e. Oil pressure gauge or light

f. Fuel gauge(s)

g. Parking brake indicator light

h. High beam indicator light

i. Emergency warning device indicator lights

j. Door ajar light

5. Visibility system

   a. Headlights

   b. Rear-view inside and outside mirrors

   c. Wipers/washers

   d. Sun visors

   e. Interior lights

6. Comunications system

   a. Parking lights

   b. Horn

   c. Directional signals

   d. Warning flashers

   e. Tail light assembly (includes brake and back-up lights)

   f. License plate light

   g. Side marker lights

   h. Emergency lights

   i. Internal communciations

   j. Back-up warning device

7. Antitheft system

   a. Ignition and buzzer

   b. Steering column lock

   c. Door locks

   d. Compartment locks

## Predriving Check and Procedures

The following is a suggested preshift vehicle inspection routine that may require modifications to be adapted to your particular vehicle or service. The routine suggested below is essentially two separate routines that can be combined into one. The first is designed to give the driver a general overview of the vehicle's exterior condition. This inspection will allow the driver to decide if the vehicle is immediately ready to respond to an emergency. If this inspection proves to be satisfactory and time permits, the driver can make a second or in-depth vehicle inspection to better determine the vehicle's operating condition. During the second inspection the driver may find items that need attention, but may not be serious enough to place the vehicle out of operation. These items should be noted and repairs scheduled. Should the condition of any item inspected show signs of deterioration or damage sufficient to pose an unsafe operating condition, the vehicle must be marked out of service and repairs initiated.

## Initial Inspection

1. Unlock door, insert ignition key
2. Adjust driver seat and inside rear-view mirror
   a. Adjust left and right outside mirror
   b. Set parking brake
   c. Turn accessory switches off
   d. Check gear selector for proper position
   e. Turn battery switch on
   f. Turn ignition switch on
   g. Start vehicle
   h. After engine starts, check oil pressure (if no pressure within fifteen seconds, stop engine)
   i. Check fuel gauge(s)
   j. Turn headlight switch on
   k. Turn hazard warning flashers on
   l. Turn exterior emergency and loading lights on
   m. Turn radio(s) on, check for proper channel
3. Inspect left-front body and fender, note damage if present
   a. Check left-front tire for inflation, scuffs, breaks, etc.
   b. Check wheel rims, valve stem and caps
   c. Check side marker light
   d. Check spotlight
4. Check body, grill, wiper arm and blade
   a. Check left headlight, parking and turn lights
   b. Check emergency lights
   c. Check bumper for security, note damage if present
5. Check that hood is latched and secure
   a. Check windshield for cracks, nicks, etc.
   b. Check under vehicle for major leaks from radiator, engine, etc.

6. Check right headlight, parking and turn lights and check front bumper and grill for damage

7. Inspect left-front body and fender, note damage if present
    a. Check left-front tire for inflation, scuffs, breaks, etc.
    b. Check side marker light
    c. Check outside mirror for security, cracks
    d. Check wheel rim, valve stem, and cap
8. Check side emergency and loading lights and inspect right side of body and compartments, note damage if present
9. Inspect right-rear tire(s), rim(s), and valve(s)
10. Inspect rear emergency and loading lights, tail lights, and license plate lights(s)
    a. Check rear step and/or bumper for security, note damage if present
    b. Inspect rear doors for proper operation
11. Inspect left-rear body; note damage if present
    a. Inspect wheel(s); check rim and valve, side marker light, and emergency and loading lights
12. Inspect left side of body and compartment, note damage if present
13. Check radio(s), siren and horn
    a. Check air conditioner, heater, defroster
    b. Adjust air vents
    c. Check windshield wipers/washers
14. Turn all lighting and accessory switches off
    a. Turn ignition switch off
    b. After engine stops completely, turn battery selector switch to auxiliary battery and restart vehicle
    c. Turn ignition switch off
    d. After engine stops completely, return battery selector switch to normal operating position and/or switch main power or battery switch off
    e. Record odometer reading
    f. Complete forms

## Secondary Inspection

### *Engine Compartment Inspection*

Check fluid levels:

1. Crankcase oil level
2. Transmission fluid level

3. Brake fluid level
4. Cooling system fluid level
5. Windshield reservoir fluid level
6. Battery acid level
7. Power steering fluid level

Visually inspect the radiator for signs of fluid leakage, inspect heater hoses and clamps, check drive belts and pullies, ignition wires, battery cables, wire connectors, etc. Look beneath engine compartment for signs of oil or other fluid leakage. After inspection is completed, close engine compartment hood and check latch for security.

*Body Exterior*

1. Clean windshield and all glass and mirrors

2. Check right-front tire for correct pressure (PSI), tread depth, cuts, and bruises; check valve cap

3. With a flashlight, inspect the back side of the wheel and rim and note any fluid leakage that may appear on the tire

   a. Check flexible brake lines for leakage; check under vehicle for oil, water, fuel and other leaks
   b. Check right-rear tires for correct pressure, cuts, bruises, and rocks between wheels, if equipped with dual wheels
   c. If visible, check wheel nuts, axle studs, and valve caps
   d. Check for leaks around fuel tanks and be sure that gas cap is present and secure
   e. Check right brake lines for damage or leakage
   f. Check for any fresh damage on the underside of the vehicle
   g. Check below rear differential housing for signs of oil leakage

4. Check left-front wheel for correct pressure, cuts, bruises, and valve caps

5. Check spare tire for condition, proper inflation, and valve caps If locked, do you have the key?

   a. Check rear suspension system (spring, U-bolts and shackles)
   b. Check inside left-rear wheel for signs of fluid leakage
   c. Check left brake line for signs of leakage
   d. Check left-rear tire(s) for correct pressure, cuts, bruises, and rocks between wheels, if equipped with dual wheels
   e. Check wheel nuts and valve caps
   f. Check exhaust system for damage, leaks, or looseness

*Vehicle Interior Inspection*

1. Check safety harness and seat belt interior reels for proper operation

2. Check lights, ventilation, heating, and air conditioning in patient compartment to insure proper operation

3. Inspect fire extinguisher and emergency warning devices (flares, reflectors)

*Instruments and Control Inspection*

1. Check intercommunications system (voice or light)

2. Check all radio channels

3. Check steering wheel (more than a two-inch turn before wheels respond may indicate excessive free play)

4. Check accelerator and parking brake for ease of operation

5. Start engine, place foot on brake pedal, move gear selector to "drive" position to see if brakes are holding and transmission is engaging

6. Place gear selector in "reverse" and check to see if transmission engages; additionally, have someone check back-up lights for proper operation and note sounds

7. Complete all reports and secure vehicle

Remember that each vehicle may be different and many items may need inspection in addition to the general ones listed above.

## DRIVING PERCEPTIONS

The senses of sight and hearing are very complex, and the driver of an emergency vehicle sometimes has difficulty understanding why the motorist cannot see or hear the vehicle, despite flashing lights and siren. This section is designed to familiarize the reader with some very real problems relative to visual and hearing perceptions of the driving public and how these can affect reaction to an emergency vehicle.

### Visual Perception

The eye is made up of two visual systems, each specialized for a different function. Each system has its own kind of receptor cells, called rods and cones. The cones function only in daytime, and are responsible for color vision and sharpness of vision. At night, the second system, comprised of the rods, becomes functional. (See Fig. 4–10.) Night vision does not respond to the color of objects. As the eye becomes adapted to the

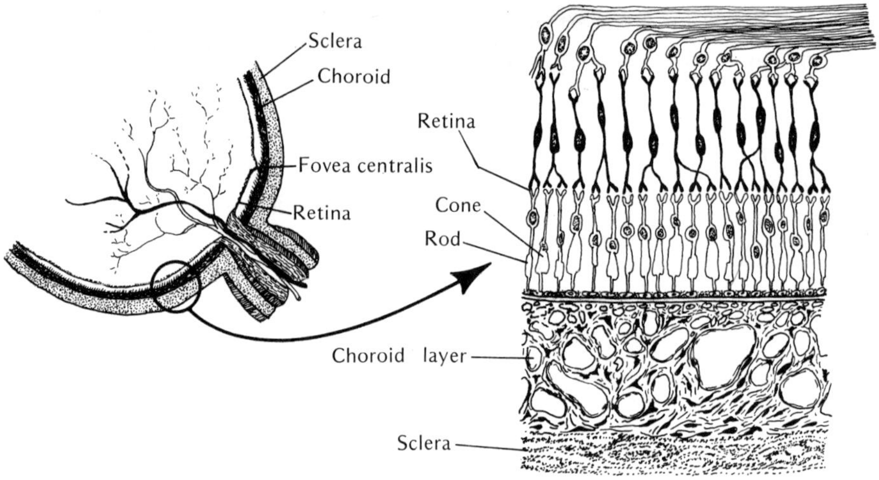


**Figure 4–10.** This enlarged view shows the rods and cones of the eye. These cells are responsible for changing light energy into nerve impulses transmitted to the brain for interpretation.

dark, red is the first color to leave the spectrum and the last to return. This is especially important to those who drive red lighted emergency vehicles. Also important for night driving is glare recovery time. When an approaching vehicle or roadside sign is passed by a vehicle at night, it will take the driver's eye approximately ten seconds to readjust to the dark. This recovery time increases with age. At 50 miles per hour, the distance traveled during a second is approximately 75 feet. Thus, in 10 seconds, the vehicle has traveled about 750 feet before the driver has fully regained night vision. At 80 miles per hour, a vehicle travels approximately 120 feet per second, or 1200 feet in 10 seconds. At 80 miles per hour, therefore, the vehicle travels almost one-fourth of a mile before the driver's eyes readjust.

Another phenomenon of night vision is called the "moth effect," or phototropism (fo″to-trop′ism). This is the tendency for the eye, especially when fatigued, to be attracted to light. This knowledge is beneficial to the emergency vehicle operator in determining flare location. Flares should be placed well down the road from the scene of an accident so that proper protection of the scene is guaranteed.

## Sound Perception

The ear, like the eye, is a very sensitive and complicated organ. The ability to locate sound is due almost entirely to the fact that humans have two ears. A sound coming from an object on the left strikes a person's left ear before it does the right one. Because it is stronger in the left ear, the person is able to determine that the origin of the sound is coming from the left.

A condition characteristic of all humans is the "zone of confusion." Beginning at each ear at approximately a 10° angle, and extending outward in a cone shape, this is an area in which one is unable to distinguish sound origin. The farther away the emergency vehicle is from the motorist, the more difficult it will be for the driver to determine the direction from which the emergency vehicle is coming because of the cone effect. As the emergency vehicle approaches, the cone shape will lessen, and the motorist will be able to determine direction more readily. If the sound changes (e.g., by using an alternate siren), the chances of hearing the emergency vehicle will be greatly increased. This zone of confusion is a physical characteristic which limits driver response, and all emergency vehicle operators should be aware of it.

Another obscure physical characteristic of all human hearing is the "median plain of sound." This condition also limits the human ability to determine sound origin. The condition arises because the sound waves from the source affect both ears the same. The sound reaches each ear simultaneously and with the same strength. It is therefore impossible to determine the origin of the sound without moving the head. By moving the head, the ear position in relation to the sound origin changes, and the individual is then able to determine direction, since the sound wave is stronger in one ear.

If an emergency vehicle is approaching directly from the front or the rear, it is very difficult for the motorist to determine sound origin because of these innate physical limitations, not because of inattention or recklessness. In addition, it must be kept in mind that a person may not respond to a siren because of total deafness, partial loss of hearing in one or both ears, or internal vehicle noises and distractions.

Beyond preoccupation, inattention, or physical limitations, a driver may not respond to emergency warning devices for a number of other reasons. For example, the emergency vehicle operator may be "tailgating" to such an extent that the emergency lights are obscured, and because of the "median plain of sound," direction cannot be determined.

To add further to motorist confusion, various municipalities have different markings, colors, sirens, and even lights on their emergency vehicles. Therefore, in order to reduce motorist confusion and enhance the potential for recognition of the emergency vehicle, it is recommended that when approaching a driver who is not responding to the emergency warning devices, the operator should:

Fluctuate the sound wave.
Sound the horn to assist the driver in determining direction of approach
Flash headlights to add visual input for direction location.
Remain patient and courteous.

In summary, the emergency vehicle operator should at all times realize that the motorist may not be intentionally refraining from moving to the right as the law requires, but, in fact, may simply not be aware that the emergency vehicle is approaching.

*References*

American Automobile Association. *Sportsmanlike Driving,* 6th ed. St. Louis, MO: McGraw-Hill Book Company, 1970.

Clark, John K., Jr. *Emergency and High Speed Driving Techniques.* Houston, TX: Gulf Publishing Company, 1976.

Instructors Manual, *Advanced Driver Education for Emergency Vehicle Operators.* Missouri Safety Center, Missouri State University, 1978.

National Safety Council. *Driver Improvement Program Defensive Driving Course* Chicago, IL, 1975.

National Safety Council. *Motor Fleet Safety Manual,* 2nd ed. Chicago, IL, 1972.

# Chapter 5

# Body Mechanics

Lifting and moving patients or objects is part of the everyday responsibility of a working EMT. One lifts and moves things so often that it becomes an automatic response with little thought given to the constant stresses and strains acting on the body. But if lifting and moving is performed incorrectly, the cumulative effect on the muscles and bones of the body will eventually result in injury, most commonly of the back.

Good posture or body alignment is essential to good body mechanics. In the best mechanical postion, the body parts support each other; one does not have to hold the body upright. However, if the position of the body is not mechanically correct, muscles of the body must work to support parts against the pull of gravity, wasting body energy and producing undue stress and strain.

As an EMT, it is important that you understand and practice good body mechanics to prevent injury during the everyday work that must be performed in the care and treatment of the patient. Remember, the EMT is the most important person to the patient. If the EMT is injured, the patient may suffer from lack of care or treatment.

## POSTURE

When the body is in correct alignment, an imaginary line (representing the pull of gravity) can be drawn from the head through the center of the shoulders, through the center of the hip joint, crossing the center of the knee joint to the center of the ankle joint. The body segments most likely to be out of alignment, when standing or sitting, are the pelvis and the five lumbar vertebrae of the lower back. This malalignment due to poor posture may produce a condition known as lordosis, (lor-do′-sis) creating inappropriate tension of the hip muscles. Lordosis or swayback (see Fig. 5-1) is an increased forward curve of the lumbar vertebrae and is one of the

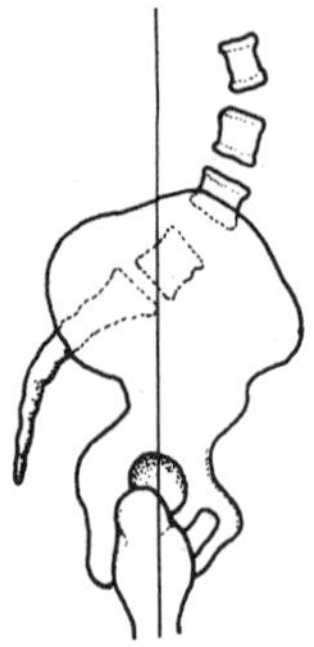

**Figure 5–1.** Positioning top of pelvis forward causes swayback. (Adapted from *Back Care* by Arthur Grant and Murray Swanson. Issaquah, WA: Medic Publishing Co.)

most common causes of injury to the lower back when lifting or moving. Lordosis may occur when the upper part of the pelvis rotates forward and downward, creating the increased curvature of the lumbar spine. In other words, the lumbar spine "falls" forward toward the abdomen, resulting in a swayback position or deformity. Because the abdominal muscles attach to the upper part of the pelvis, weakness of these muscles is the major cause of the swayback condition. Moreover, since the gluteal (buttocks) muscles attach to the back of the lower pelvis, weakness of these muscles also contributes to the forward rotation of the pelvis, helping to create a swayback position. A swayback deformity from poor posture may cause the muscles, ligaments, and other tissue of the back to become shortened, causing pain even though no exertion or injury has taken place. However, with exertion or sudden movement of the lower back, a swayback deformity is an invitation to an even greater pain or injury when compounded by the stress and strain of incorrectly performed lifting or moving.

Another poor posture situation may exist when one sits incorrectly for long periods of time. This tends to lighten hip muscles (flexor muscles), adding to the problem of the increased forward lumbar curvature.

Good posture is achieved by tilting the pelvis upward and backward (see Fig. 5–2), thereby reducing or flattening the curve of the lumbar spine. When walking or standing, it is important to stand erect and flatten the lumbar curve. Shoe heights are critical on and off the job; high heels will increase the lumbar curve no matter how good one's posture may be, and they should be avoided.

When sitting or driving, you should be aware of the height of the seat. An excessively high seat allows the feet to dangle, causing the knees to be lower than the hips. This will result in an increased lumbar curve. The knees should always be higher than the hips when sitting. This can be corrected temporarily by crossing the legs or propping your feet up. When driving, you should not slump forward, as this causes increased stress on the upper back and may create pain.

The position in which you sleep is also important. Sleeping on your abdomen tends to increase the lumbar curve and should be avoided. A

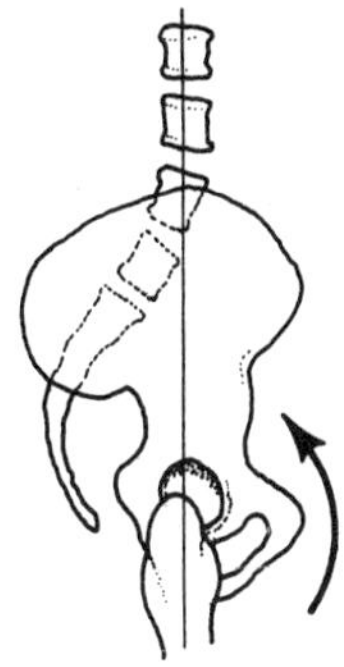

**Figure 5-2.** Tilting top of pelvis backward corrects swayback. (Adapted from *Back Care* by Arthur Grant and Murray Swanson. Issaquah, WA: Medic Publishing Co.)

recommended position while sleeping is sidelying or semifetal position, or lying on the back with a pillow under the bend of the knees.

We have been discussing the curvature of the lumbar spine and postures that are good and bad. Let us now check our lumbar curve. Stand with your back touching a wall. Notice that your hand probably slips into the space between your lower back and the wall (see Fig. 5-3). Now:

1. Move your feet away from the wall about eight inches and rest your back against the wall.

2. Squeeze your buttocks, as if you were gripping a coin between them. Notice that the front of your pelvis (pubic area) moves forward.

3. While still squeezing the buttocks, pull in your abdomen. The space between your back and wall should now be gone. (see Fig. 5-4.)

4. Now gradually shift your feet closer to the wall, while holding your back against the wall.

5. If you can stand straight with no curve of the lumbar spine, try walking around the room with your back in the same position. Then return to the wall and see if your back is still flat.

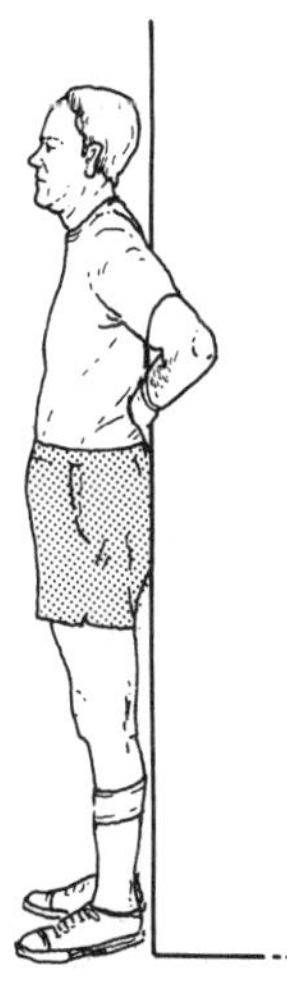

**Figure 5-3.** Check your lordosis.

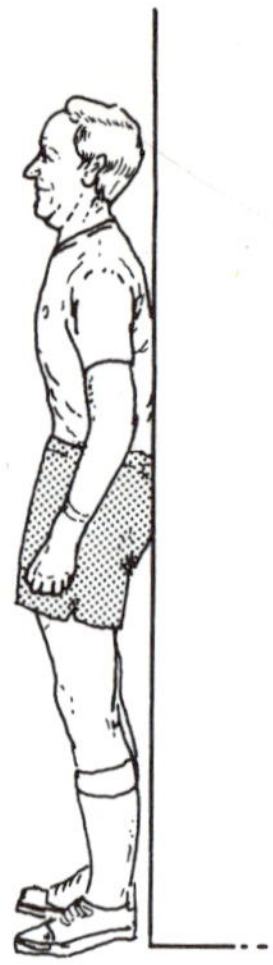

**Figure 5-4.** Flatten your lordosis.

If you are like most people, you cannot easily stand erect with your back flat or assume that posture for a long period of time, but this is the posture that you should have when standing or sitting. You can assume good posture if you follow the exercises listed below for the back. Good posture requires exercise and remembering how to assume a correct stance and sitting position.

All exercises should be performed on a firm surface, preferably the floor. They should be performed daily and accomplished slowly and smoothly. At first, you will have some soreness or mild stiffness, but this usually disappears as you continue to exercise.

## The Pelvic Tilt (Fig. 5-5)

The purpose of this exercise is to strengthen the gluteal (buttocks) and the abdominal muscles and decrease the lumbar curve.

1. Lie on your back with knees bent.
2. Squeeze the buttocks tightly together.
3. While holding the buttocks together, pull in the abdomen. You should feel the lumbar spine (lower back) become flush against the floor. Hold this position for five seconds.
4. Relax. Repeat three times, gradually increasing to twenty repetitions.

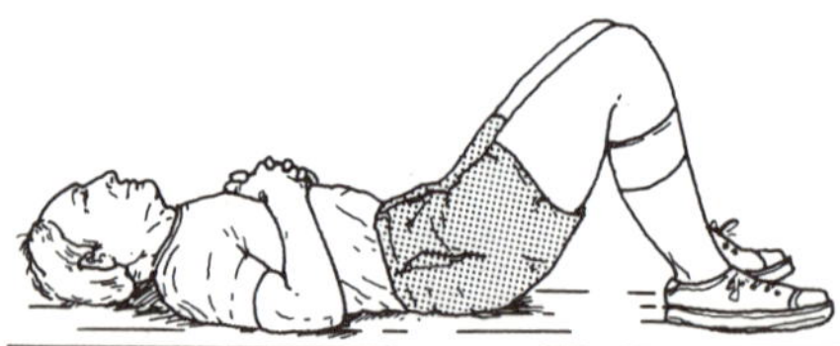

**Figure 5-5.** The pelvic tilt.

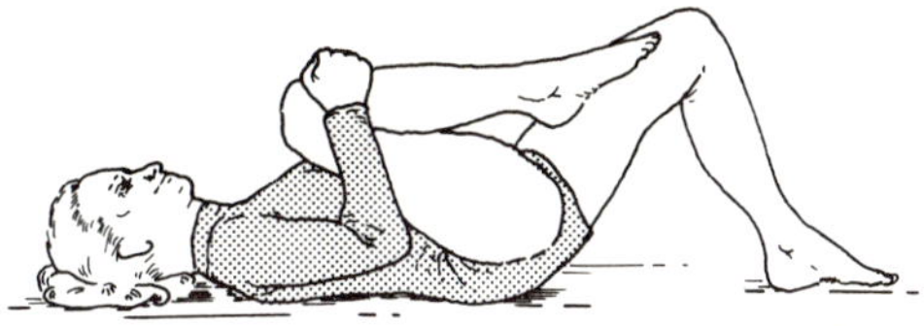

**Figure 5-6.** The single knee raise.

## Single Knee Raise (Fig. 5-6)

The purpose of this exercise is to stretch and strengthen the lower back muscles and hamstring muscles in back of the thigh.

1. Lie on your back with knees bent.

2. Squeeze the buttocks and tighten the abdomen, so that you begin the next step with the lower back flat to the floor or nearly so.

3. Raise one knee over the chest area.

4. With the hands over the knee, pull the knee slowly toward the armpit. Hold this position for five seconds.

5. Return to the beginning position without allowing the lower back to raise off the floor; relax and repeat the exercise, gradually increasing to ten repetitions.

6. Repeat with other leg.

## Double Knee Raise (Fig. 5-7)

The purpose of this exercise is to stretch and strengthen the lower back and hamstring muscles.

1. Lie on your back with knees bent.

2. Squeeze buttocks and tighten abdominal muscles so that the next step begins with the lower back flat to the floor or nearly so.

3. While holding the back flat to the floor, raise both knees over the chest area.

4. With hands over the knees, pull the knees slowly toward the armpits. Hold this position for ten seconds.

5. Return to the starting position without allowing the lower back to rise off the floor; repeat the exercise three more times, gradually increasing to ten repetitions.

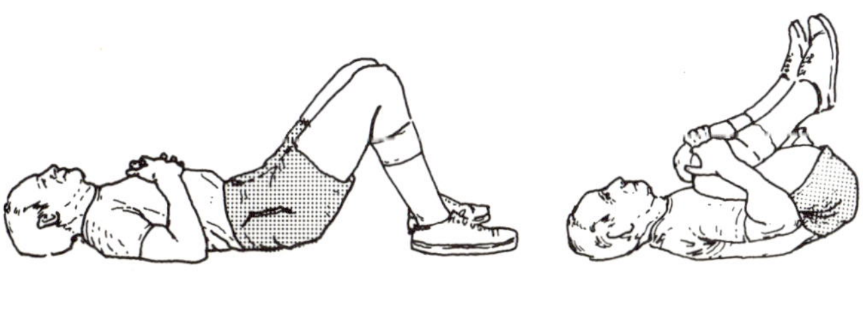

**Figure 5-7.** The double knee raise.

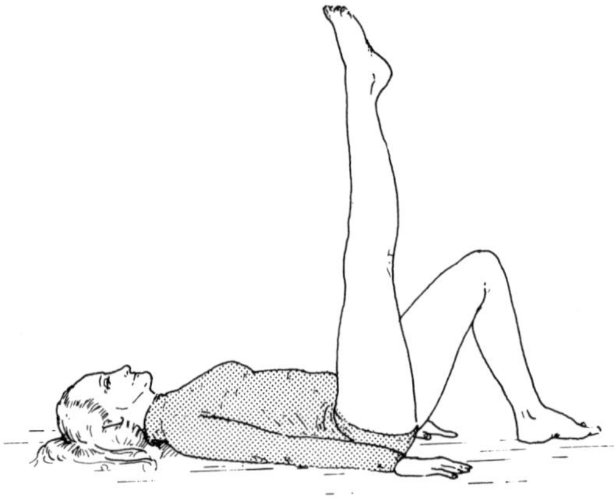

**Figure 5–8.** The single leg raise.

## Single Leg Raise (Fig. 5–8)

The purpose of this exercise is to stretch the lower back and hamstring muscles and strengthen the abdominal and hip flexing muscles. *Caution:* If one suffers from "down the leg" pain (sciatica [si-at'ĭ-kah]), omit this exercise.

1. Lie on your back with one knee bent.

2. Squeeze buttocks and tighten abdomen so that the lower back is flush against the floor.

3. Slowly raise the straight leg, keeping it straight and the lower back flat. Raise the leg as far as possible without causing discomfort.

4. Slowly lower the leg, flattening the lower back as the leg approaches the floor. Repeat this exercise, gradually increasing to ten repetitions.

5. Repeat exercise with the other leg.

## Sit Up—Partial to Full (Fig. 5–9)

The purpose of this exercise is to strengthen the lower back and abdominal muscles.

1. Lie on your back with the knees bent.

2. Squeeze buttocks and tighten the abdomen so that the lower back is flush to the floor.

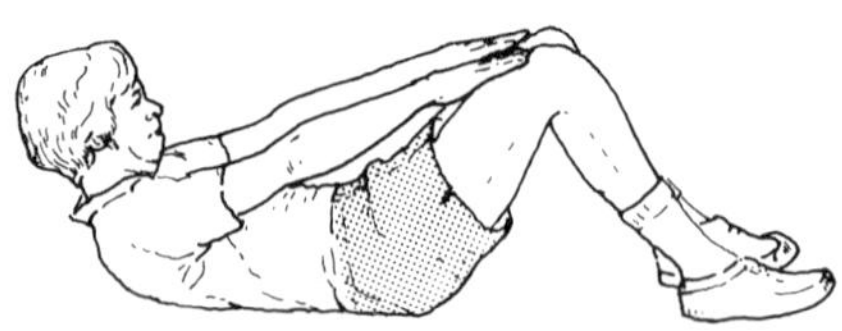

**Figure 5–9.** The sit-up: partial to full.

3. Slowly raise the head and neck and then the shoulders, toward the knees, keeping the lower and middle back to the floor. Hold this position for five seconds.

4. Return to the starting position and repeat the exercise three more times, gradually increasing exercise to ten repetitions.
*Caution:* One should never do sit-ups with the legs straight. This position tends to increase the lumbar curve.

## Sitting Bend (Fig. 5–10)

The purpose of this exercise is to stretch the lower back and hamstring muscles.

1. Sit in an armless chair with the feet flat on the floor, knees should be no more than twelve inches apart and hands at the side.

2. Squeeze buttocks and pull in abdomen so the lower back flattens against the back of the chair.

3. Bend over no further than is comfortable, hands reaching toward the floor. Hold this position for three seconds.

4. Return to starting position, ending with back flat against the chair. Repeat three times, gradually increasing to ten repetitions.

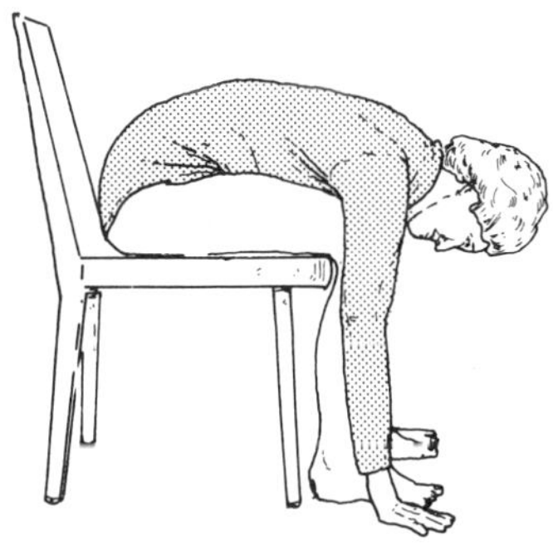

**Figure 5–10.** The sitting bend.

## Knee Bend: (Fig. 5–11)

The purpose of this exercise is to strengthen the hamstring and quadriceps muscles of the thigh. This exercise will prepare the EMT for lifting and moving by using the leg muscles, not the back muscles.

1. Stand erect behind a sofa or heavy chair, and hold on for balance.

2. Squeeze the buttocks and tighten abdomen.

3. Squat down only as far as comfortable.

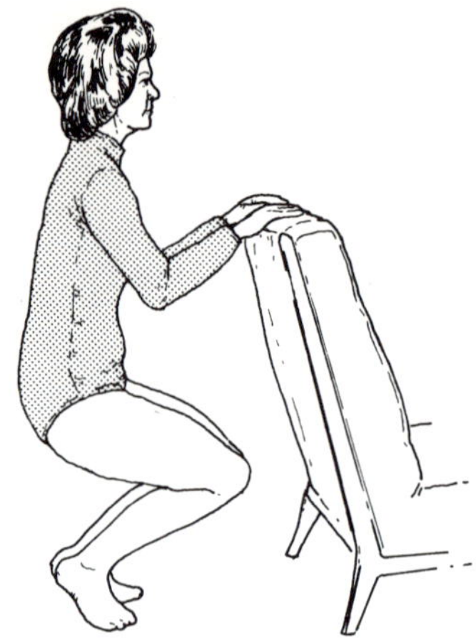

**Figure 5-11.** The knee bend.

4. Stand up using leg power, not hands. Repeat this exercise three times, gradually increasing to ten repetitions. It helps to have someone confirm that the back is held flat during the exercise.

Once the proper muscles have been strengthened by exercise, general principles of lifting or moving should be followed.

## PRINCIPLES OF GOOD BODY MECHANICS

When lifting or moving a patient or object, consider the location of center of gravity—the point of an object at which all its mass is centered. In the human body, the center of gravity is found in the pelvic cavity.

1. The lower the center of gravity, the greater the stability.

2. An object's center of gravity shifts constantly with a change in one's position. If the center of gravity did not change, balance would be lost. Imagine the location of the line of gravity. It intersects the center of gravity in a perpendicular direction, passing through the body's base of support, which is the area between the feet.

3. The farther apart the feet are, the more stable one becomes.

Good body mechanics are accomplished when one performs the task efficiently, safely, and with as little energy expenditure as possible. When faced with the task of moving or lifting a patient or object (see Fig. 5-12):

1. Face the object. Do not twist the body.

2. Bend the knees, going down as far as necessary with the legs, not the back.

3. Stand with one foot forward to give a wide base of support.

4. Keep the back straight—squeeze the buttocks and pull in the abdomen (the pelvic tilt).

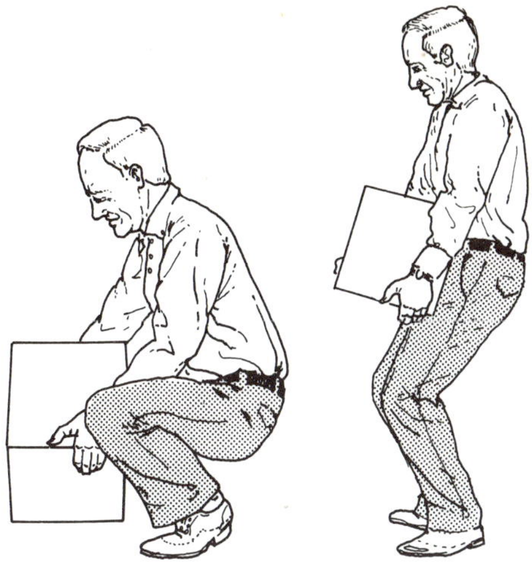

**Figure 5-12.** The correct method of lifting an object.

5. Keep the load close to the body and well balanced. Avoid leaning and stretching.

6. Lift with the legs using the large muscles of the thigh, not the small muscles of the back.

7. Plan the actions to best use the leverage provided by the trunk of the body and legs.

8. Lift a heavy load no higher than the waist, and light loads no higher than the shoulders. Greater height increases lumbar curve.

9. Do not twist the body when carrying an object. Pivot on the feet.

If you are aware of these principles and are willing to practice them, the chance of injury will be greatly reduced. Admittedly, these are ideals to be practiced in ideal situations. As an EMT, some of these principles will have to be modified to deal with awkward situations and positions where patients may be found. It will be a common practice to carry, lift, and move patients up and down different types of stairs. These situations require strength, balance, and the ability to plan a course of action. Before the EMT begins to work in these situations, it is appropriate to practice:

1. Lifting a patient into and out of the ambulance.
2. Carrying a patient downstairs on a stretcher.
3. Trying different lifts to put the patient on or off the stretcher.

Let's discuss each of the above situations.

## Lifting a Patient Into and Out of The Ambulance

In this situation, some physical limitations must be considered. Ambulances in use today make it almost physically impossible for someone under the height of 5′2″ to lift the front end of the stretcher high enough to

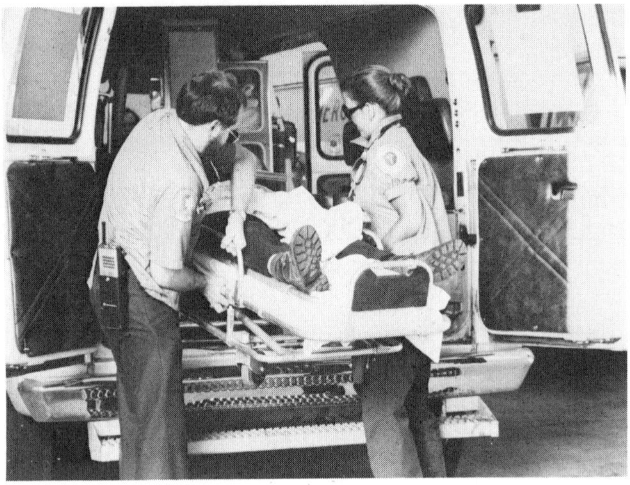

**Figure 5–13.** These EMT-As avoid imbalance by being the same height while unloading the patient from the ambulance. (Courtesy of Wishard Memorial Hospital. Photo by Bob Biehn.)

clear the rear door entry of the vehicle. A person under that height loses leverage and is more prone to back injuries. Ideally, EMTs of this height should avoid imbalance in carrying or lifting the loaded stretcher. (See Fig. 5–13.)

When actually performing the procedure, you should remember to bend down with your knees and lift with your legs, not your back. Then lift the head of the stretcher to clear the back end of the ambulance.

When unloading the stretcher from the rear of the ambulance, you should remember that the stretcher height and the back end of the ambulance are not the same. If you are not careful, back muscles may be excessively stressed at this point. Arm and shoulder muscles are important here to take the stretcher out of the vehicle. Once the stretcher is pulled out and is held for a few seconds for coordinated movement with your partner, it is then placed on the ground gently.

The procedure of lifting and pulling out the loaded stretcher must be accomplished in an equal and coordinated fashion for proper balance. The EMT must remember when placing the stretcher on the ground to use the leg muscles, and not the back. Even though this procedure is done routinely, it is worthwhile to practice with every new partner that may be assigned to the unit.

## Carrying a Patient Downstairs on a Stretcher

This is one situation where partners of different heights are an advantage. The taller person should go down the stairs first and the shorter person should be at the head of the patient. The patient should go down feet

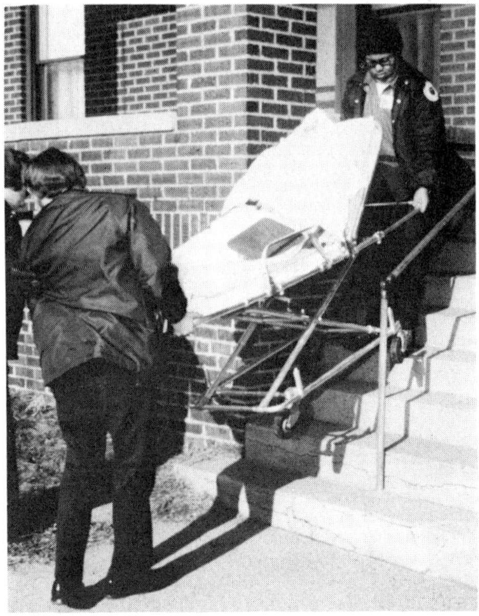

**Figure 5-14.** This EMT-A is being "spotted" so that the safety of the patient and the medical team is assured. (Courtesy of Wishard Memorial Hospital. Photo by Bob Biehn.)

first, whether placed on the stretcher or on a stair chair. The patient should be safely secured to the stretcher or stair chair, so as to not slide off with feet pushing against the EMT. The patient should be secured with strong material that is wide and not binding so as to occlude circulation.

As the patient is being carried down the stairs, and if the manpower is available, it is important that someone stand behind the EMT at the foot of the patient and "spot" him to give the necessary support should it be needed. (See Fig. 5-14.) Because all stairways and stairwells are constructed differently, carrying a patient down them will not be an easy task and must be well planned before starting.

## Moving a Patient On and Off a Stretcher

There are numerous ways this can be accomplished and each situation will be different, depending on where the patient is located and what obstacles are in the path of work. The EMT should always practice the principles of good body mechanics, so that the task can be performed safely without injury to oneself or the patient.

1. When moving or lifting the patient, work together in a coordinated fashion.

2. Keep the patient as close to the body's center of gravity as possible when lifting.

3. Do not twist your body when lifting.

4. Always lift with the legs, and not the back.

5. Keep a wide base of support, with one foot ahead of the other.

6. Think and plan before you move a patient, and get extra help if necessary.

By practicing good body mechanics and planning out each moving situation, the chances of injury to the patient and the EMT will be greatly decreased.

*References*

Finneson, Bernard E., M.D. *Low Back Pain.* Philadelphia, PA: J. B. Lippincott Lippincott Company, 1973.

Grant, Arthur, E. M.D., and Swanson, Murray A. *Back Care.* Issoquah, WA: Medic Pub. Co., 1975.

Rantz, Marilyn, and Courtial, Donald. *Lifting, Moving and Transferring Patients: A Manual.* St. Louis, MO: The C. V. Mosby Co., 1977.

*Recommended Reading*

Drapeau, Janine. "Getting Back Into Good Posture: How to Erase Your Lumbar Aches," *Nursing,* 5:63–65, September 1975.

Ford, Jack, and Duckworth, Bridget. "Moving the Dependent Patient Safely, Comfortably: Part I, Positioning," *Nursing,* 6:27–36, January 1976.

Ford, Jack, and Duckworth, Bridget. "Moving the Dependent Patient Safely, Comfortably: Part II, Transferring," *Nursing,* 6:58–65, January 1976.

Foss, Georgia. "Use Your Head and Save Your Back: Body Mechanics," *Nursing.* 3:25–32, May 1973.

Werks, Roberta F. "Hints on Lifting and Pulling," *American Journal of Nursing,* pp. 260–261. February 1972.

Yates, Judith. "Moving and Lifting Patients: Principles and Techniques," Minneapolis American Rehabilitation Foundation, Inc. 1970.

*Video Tapes*

*Body Mechanics and Transfer Techniques,* Department of Audio Visual Communications, Fairview General Hospital, 18101 Lorain Avenue, Cleveland, OH 44111, Phone: (216) 252–1222, ext. 534.

tional systems. Any growth of the system may have to be compatible with existing components.

*Continuity*

The system should be available for use by all potential users on a twenty-four-hour-a-day, year-round basis. Although all stations may not be staffed continuously (such as the volunteer fire station or rural clinic), the essential components of citizen's access, vehicle dispatch, and medical control should be intact at all times according to the community's needs.

*Expandability*

Disasters and unanticipated heavy demand periods may tax the capability of the system. The ability to handle these demands and those generated by large public gatherings should be built into the system.

*Convenience of Use*

Most of the users of the system will be nontechnical people. Components of the system should be simple and selected on the basis of the more people who have to use it, the simpler it should be and the least training required.

*Coverage*

The entire geographic area should be covered by the telephone and radio systems with the intent of maximum coverage with minimum interference from other systems. The unique geographic and terrain requirements of the area should be taken into account in planning and operating the system.

*Flexibility*

The continuing growth of community needs and services requires that a system be flexible in order to deal with additions and changes in the medical and communications fields. In so far as possible, a system should be developed with the intent of serving as the nucleus for future systems.

*Noninterference Frequency Coordination*

The growth of EMS requires that radio frequencies be selected so as to provide adequate coverage and flexibility, yet reduce interference from and with other systems. Radio waves do not respect geographic, political, or service district boundaries.

*Radio Spectrum Management*

The radio spectrum is a national resource (with international implications as well), that should be utilized properly and efficiently. Indiscriminate use of radio should be avoided and where possible, consistent with operational needs, communications should be effected over other telephone or cable links.

*Regular Use*

All portions of the system, both those used for primary communications and back-up functions, should be exercised frequently—daily in most cases. Not only will this ensure that all systems are in working order, but it serves to keep all involved familiar with the equipment and operation.

## Federal Communications Commission

The Communications Act of 1934 established the Federal Communications Commission (FCC) to develop the effective use of the radio spectrum. It is the regulatory and controlling agency nationwide for allocating frequencies for various uses, licensing individual stations (and operators in certain instances), and assigning call signs, maintaining frequencies and users to ensure compliance with applicable regulations, and setting standards for the operation of equipment. Additionally, it is involved with the regulation of interstate and international telephone operations that may have an impact on EMS communications systems.

A goal of the FCC is to promote the most efficient utilization of radio frequencies and facilities by the maximum number of users. Radio frequencies are shared across the United States and by sufficient distances between users of any one frequency or group of frequencies and the control of transmitting power and direction, interference is minimized.

Within the broad framework of the public safety service category established by the FCC are found the VHF radio frequencies utilized by many EMS services. Since the category is shared with nonmedical activities, and is actually intended for use by agencies operating relatively independently, the VHF frequencies traditionally used by EMS providers have been inadequate to meet the requirements engendered by the need for increasing cooperation between agencies and the increasing use of ambulance to hospital communications.

In 1974, the FCC established a medical services category for the licensing and operation of medical radio communications. The additional frequencies primarily are UHF-paired frequencies permitting duplex operation. The allocation and licensing of these frequencies is designed to encourage a common systems approach where all area users participate in a unified program. Such areawide cooperation permits the individual user to have the most flexibility in the day-to-day operation of the system. Many such systems are in operation today, and the number is increasing.

Because the use of VHF is still so widespread by EMS agencies, and in many cases provides satisfactory service, the FCC does not contemplate that licensees using VHF will be required to abandon their systems.

However, such systems are necessarily limited in their ability to expand or provide more sophisticated service (such as telemetry), and it is believed the advantages of an areawide system will encourage the utilization of the UHF frequencies.

Radio equipment operated by EMS agencies must be licensed by the FCC. Unauthorized transmissions could result in a fine or imprisonment or both.

## SYSTEM CONFIGURATION AND CAPABILITY

Equipment utilized in the EMS communications system merely provides the opportunity for health professionals to improve patient care. But the design of the system and associated hardware can provide increased efficiency in delivering this care, or conversely in the case of a poorly conceived or poorly operated system, create obstacles to the smooth flow of patient care. The EMT should be familiar with the design concepts and equipment functions of the system in which he or she will practice.

Most EMS systems in the United States include radio contact between a dispatch point and ambulances and between ambulances and a medical control point. The sophistication of these systems varies enormously, but it is reasonable to assume that the EMT must increasingly be able to deal with complex electronic hardware as more and more EMS agencies link together in coordinated, regional communications systems.

In localities where the number of ambulance runs is relatively low and only one or two hospitals are routinely served by the ambulance service, the complexity of the equipment utilized by the EMT may be different from that faced by the EMT in an area with a large number of runs and hospitals, but certain equipment elements are common to emergency care providers.

### Portable Radios

Hand-carried portable units are very useful when emergency personnel need to communicate with their communications center, one another, or the hospital from the patient's location or when they are some distance from the vehicle. In some EMS systems, the physician who gives directions to the EMTs is not located within the hospital, but can be located by means of a portable radio as he goes about his daily practice.

Because such portable radios are limited in their power output, the range of communications is likewise limited. Thus, a method must exist for boosting the radio signal or relaying it over longer distances (see below).

Typically the portable unit utilized by the EMT will contain at least the following (see Fig. 6–2):

1. An *on–off* switch usually coupled with a *volume control* that permits the EMT to turn the unit on and adjust the volume of the speaker to the desired level.

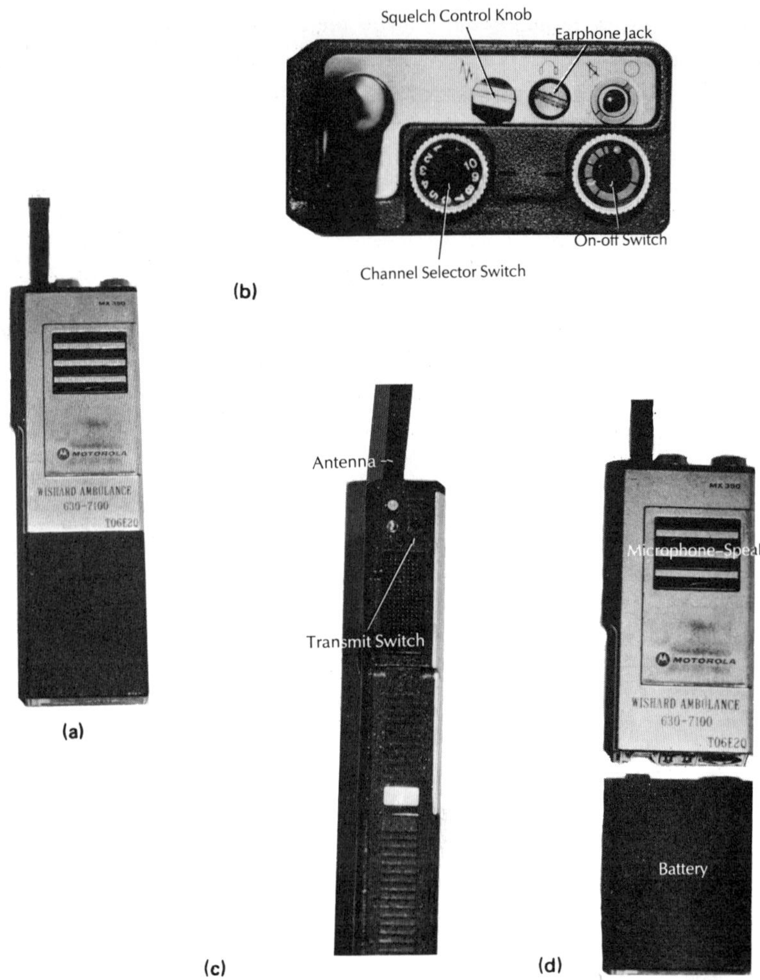


**Figure 6–2.** (a) A 10-channel portable radio unit; (b) the on-off switch, squelch control knob, channel selector switch, and earphone jack; (c) antenna and transmit switch, (d) microphone-speaker; the nickel cadmium battery attaches directly to the radio.

2. A *squelch control knob* to control the circuitry that keeps out unwanted radio noise between transmissions. Additionally, some systems utilize a tone-coded squelch system that permits the EMT to hear only transmissions that are generated within his system and not those that may be carried from a distant system. If a system is so equipped, the portable radio will have a switch to control this function.

3. A channel selector switch to permit the EMT to utilize the various frequencies in his system. In some facilities the EMT may use only one radio frequency in his portable radio. Larger systems may have ten fre-

quencies in the portable radio and be employed by the EMT for dispatch and ambulance to hospital communications.

4. An *antenna,* typically short and flexible, to send and receive the radio signal. The radio may also contain an area for attachment to an external antenna.

5. A combination *microphone/speaker,* typically built into the body of the radio or as a flexible cord, that permits the EMT to speak or hear radio transmissions.

6. A *transmit switch* that, when pressed, allows the EMT to speak into the microphone and transmit his message. A small light may also be mounted in the radio to indicate that it is transmitting.

7. An *earphone jack* that permits the EMT to plug in an earphone for listening to the radio in environments where there is a great deal of background noise.

8. A nickel-cadmium *battery* that powers the radio and may be recharged in a tabletop charger or in a mounted unit in the vehicle. Usually these batteries may be easily charged in the event a fresh battery is quickly needed.

9. A *carrying-case* that allows the radio to be carried on the belt or by a shoulder strap and protects the radio.

Wherever possible, emergency medical personnel should be equipped with portable radio units and such units should be of the highest available quality.

## Radio Spectrum

The radio spectrum is a national and international resource in the public domain. In the United States the Federal Communications Commission (FCC) controls frequency allocations and licensing of nongovernment radio services and individuals.

Radio frequencies are designated by cycles per second, or hertz. Abbreviations are generally used as in the following:

1. hertz (Hz) = cycles per second
2. kilohertz (KHz) = 1000 cycles per second
3. megahertz (MHz) = 1,000,000 cycles per second
4. gigahertz (GHz) = 1,000,000,000 cycles per second

Radio waves are confined to the portion of the electromagnetic spectrum from 3 KHz (three thousand cycles per second) to approximately 3000 GHz (three trillion cycles per second). A normal voice channel takes about 3 KHz (three thousand cycles per second), but many frequency bands are not assigned to land mobile use or are impractical for use. Generally speaking, the lower bands require antennas of rather large dimensions and the much higher bands currently are limited by the expense and difficulty of generating sufficient power for mobile use. Certain portions achieve great range because of the presence of ionization layers in the upper atmosphere.

The most commonly used bands for EMS are the Very High Frequency (VHF) band and the Ultra High Frequency Band (UHF). Both bands are line-of-sight with range essentially a function of transmitter power output, antenna type, and antenna height.

The VHF band extends from approximately 30 MHz to 175 MHz and contains many of the frequencies in use by some EMS and public safety organizations. Arbitrarily, this band has subdivisions designated as low-band (30-50 MHz) and high-band (150-175 MHz).

Characteristic of the low-band frequencies is a somewhat greater

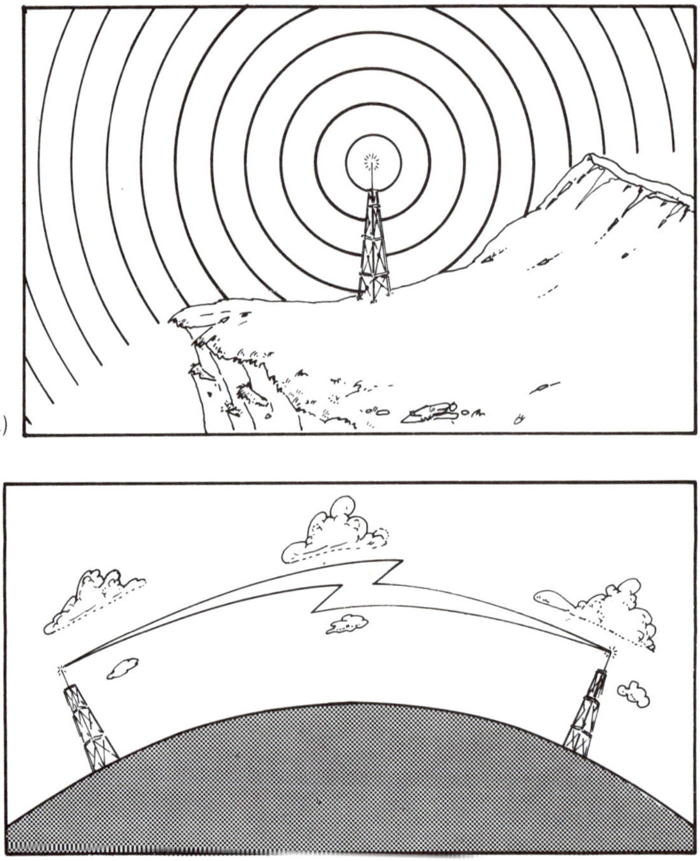

(a)

(b)

**Figure 6-3.** (a) The VHF low band (30–50 MHz) generally provides a greater range than the VHF high band because the waves follow the curvature of the earth. (b) The VHF high band (150–175 MHz) signal can be obstructed by the surrounding terrain due to its straight line nature. This is why the VHF high band signal is often referred to as "line-of-sight."

range than that of the high-band frequencies. Changes in ionospheric conditions may result in unpredictable ranges of 2000 miles or more over the time of day or year. Users of these frequencies may sometimes be plagued by "skip" interference from other systems and patchy communications. (See Fig. 6–3a.)

Most VHF communications by EMS agencies occur within the high band within the 150 MHz to 160 MHz range. These frequencies are considerably less susceptible to "skip" interference than low band, but have shorter ranges, under standard conditions. (See Fig. 6–3b.) Antennas are shorter and the background noise levels are less than those in the low band. However, the spectrum is considerably crowded by users in this region, and the EMS provider will often find less expansion availability. Dispatch, ambulance-to-medical control communications (except telemetry) and paging are possible in this band.

The UHF band spans from 300 MHz - 3000 MHz, with medical communication occurring for the most part between 450 MHz to 470 MHz. At these frequencies there is essentially no "skip" interference and minimal signal distortion. Under the same circumstances, UHF frequencies have less range than VHF frequencies, but a better penetrating power in dense

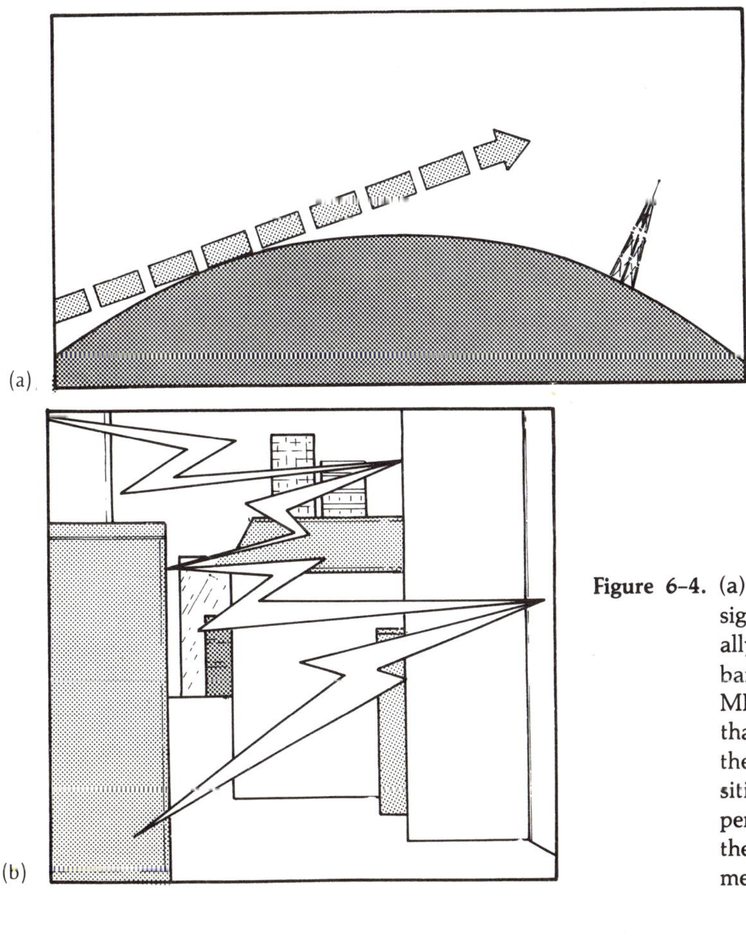

**Figure 6–4.** (a) Because of the straight-line signal, the UHF high band generally has a shorter range. (b) UHF band frequencies (450 MHz–470 MHz) have more limited range than VHF frequencies because they are more "line-of-sight" sensitive. However, they have better penetrating power and are usually the frequency of choice in dense metropolitan environments.

metropolitan environments, although their energy is more readily absorbed by trees and foliage. (See Fig. 6–4.)

Area and regional EMS communications networks are built around a block of UHF frequencies that the FCC has set aside to be shared by all the licensees in a coordinated system. Dispatch and ambulance-to-medical control (including telemetry [tĕ-lem′e-tre]) may take place on these frequencies. However, the number of frequencies and their allocation in pairs provides great flexibility and the medium for areawide coordination. EMS paging is not permitted on UHF frequencies.

The FCC has assigned the following UHF frequencies for EMS, with the lower frequency used for base and mobile service and the higher frequency for mobile only:

1. 463.000/468.000 MHz (Med One)
2. 463.025/468.025 MHz (Med Two)
3. 463.050/468.050 MHz (Med Three)
4. 463.075/468.075 MHz (Med Four)
5. 463.100/468.100 MHz (Med Five)
6. 463.125/468.125 MHz (Med Six)
7. 463.150/468.150 MHz (Med Seven)
8. 463.175/468.175 MHz (Med Eight)

The first three pairs of frequencies are authorized primarily for telemetry, but on a non-interference secondary basis, other types of communication are permitted. The last five pairs are used primarily for communications among EMS vehicles, medical facilities, and personnel related to medical supervision in the rendering of medical care.

## Mobile Transmitter/Receivers

By means of radios mounted within the vehicle, the EMT can contact the communications center, medical facilities, and other units. A variety of power ranges exists, but typically the vehicle-mounted unit will have greater output power and thus greater range than a portable unit in comparable environments.

Because of their greater range, a number of EMS systems utilize the vehicle radio as a repeater to pick up the comparatively weak signal from a portable unit located elsewhere (such as inside a patient's house), and rebroadcast it on another frequency and at greater power. When the EMT is in the vehicle, the vehicle radio itself may be used by pushing a button to take the radio out of the "repeat" mode. (See Fig. 6–5.)

Some systems utilize the portable radio as the vehicle's radio, by sliding the radio into a mount that effectively increases the range of the radio by connecting it to a "gain" antenna affixed to a high point on the vehicle roof, as well as charging the radio battery. (See Fig. 6–6.)

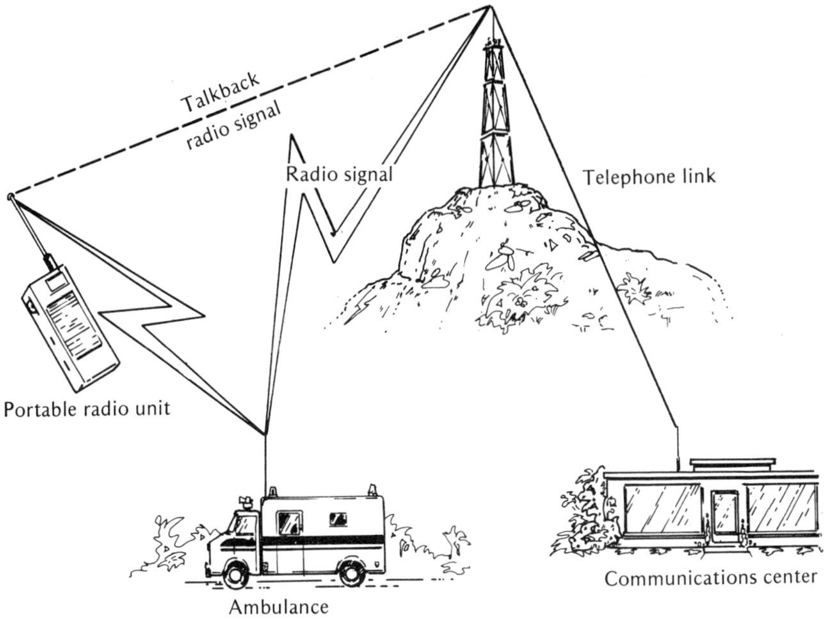


**Figure 6–5.** The vehicular repeater system.

The typical emergency vehicle will contain transmitter/receiver portion permanently mounted into the vehicle (except those systems above that use a portable radio as the transmitter/receiver element in the system), on-off switch and volume control, a squelch control, and an antenna located on a high point on the vehicle so as to effect maximum range. Oftentimes critical controls are duplicated in the driver's compartment and

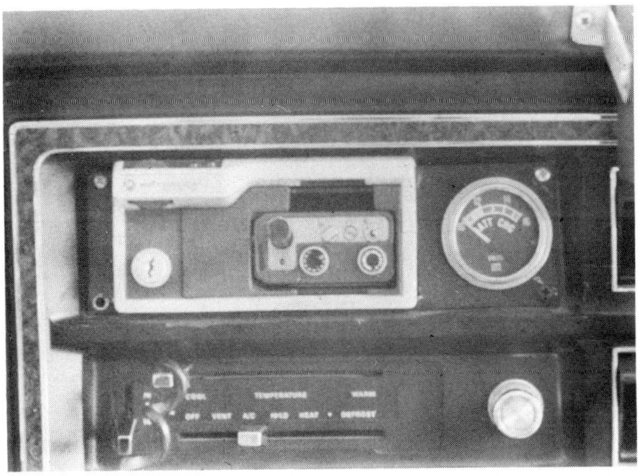

**Figure 6–6.** After the portable radio unit is placed in the slide mount, it can act as the vehicular radio.

patient's compartment so both the EMT driving and the EMT with the patient may utilize the radio. A microphone on a flexible cord with a transmit switch built into the body of the microphone, a transmit indicator light, and a mounted speaker are all usually found in both compartments. In some cases a headset worn by the EMT with the patient permits hands-free operation of the radio system.

A number of variations exist on how the EMT utilizes this equipment to contact a medical facility or individual responsible for medical advice to units in the field. The EMT may contact a central communications center on a predetermined channel (a term often used to denote a pair of frequencies used for two-way radio conversations), and request a channel to the desired medical facility. Then by means of a patching matrix located in the communications center, the assigned channel is linked to a receiver in the medical facility. The EMT need only turn his channel selector switch to the assigned channel and contact the medical facility. (See Fig. 6-7.) In other cases, the EMT may have an encoder in his ambulance that resembles a telephone dial or he may have a series of pushbuttons in the ambulance or on his portable radio. By means of this encoder, a series of pulsed tones is sent over the air to all receivers. A decoder located at the desired medical facility, the hospital, or a remote site capable of being linked to the medical facility (for example, by dedicated or automatically dialed phone lines) receives these pulses and activates the audio portion of the receiver so that medical personnel can hear the message. However the system functions in his area, the EMT will be expected to be competent in its operation.

Systems delivering advanced life suport (ALS) may also utilize telemetry, which when referred to in the EMS context means transmitting certain critical physiological data to the distant station. Most often this means sending to the hospital by radio or telephone, a visual display of the patient's electrocardiogram (ECG). The radio equipment carried by the

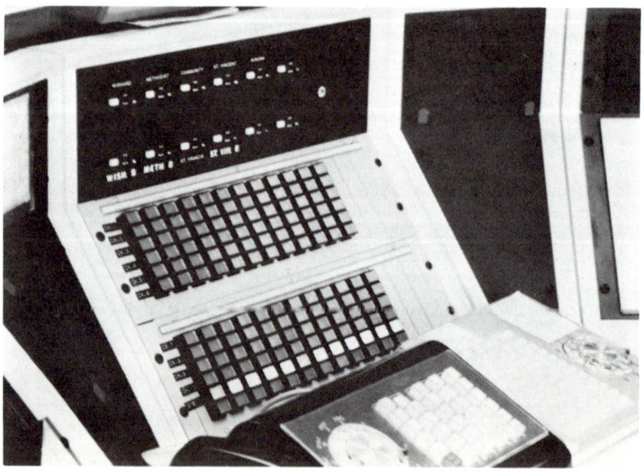

**Figure 6-7.** The patching matrix.

EMT or in the emergency vehicle may be equipped for this function, but special training in interpretation and application are required. (See Fig. 6–8.)

## Receiver/Transmitter Site

The signal sent by the portable or mobile radio will be received by an antenna, generally located at a high point in the geographic area designed to maximize coverage and reception. A number of possible configurations exist for this site. (See Fig 6–5) The antenna may feed the signal into a powerful base station radio transmitter located at the site, which in turn rebroadcasts the signal at a much stronger strength so the desired medical facility or communications center located some distance away can hear the message. This type of system is known as a mobile relay.

In another type of system employing satellite receivers, a base station transmitter at the site does not actually rebroadcast the radio traffic, but feeds it to the desired destination automatically by means of dedicated telephone lines (or by means of a remote telephone switching station—RTSS—that automatically dials a predetermined phone number), or a microwave link that sends the information straight to the receiving facility through a wide band, point-to-point radio signal.

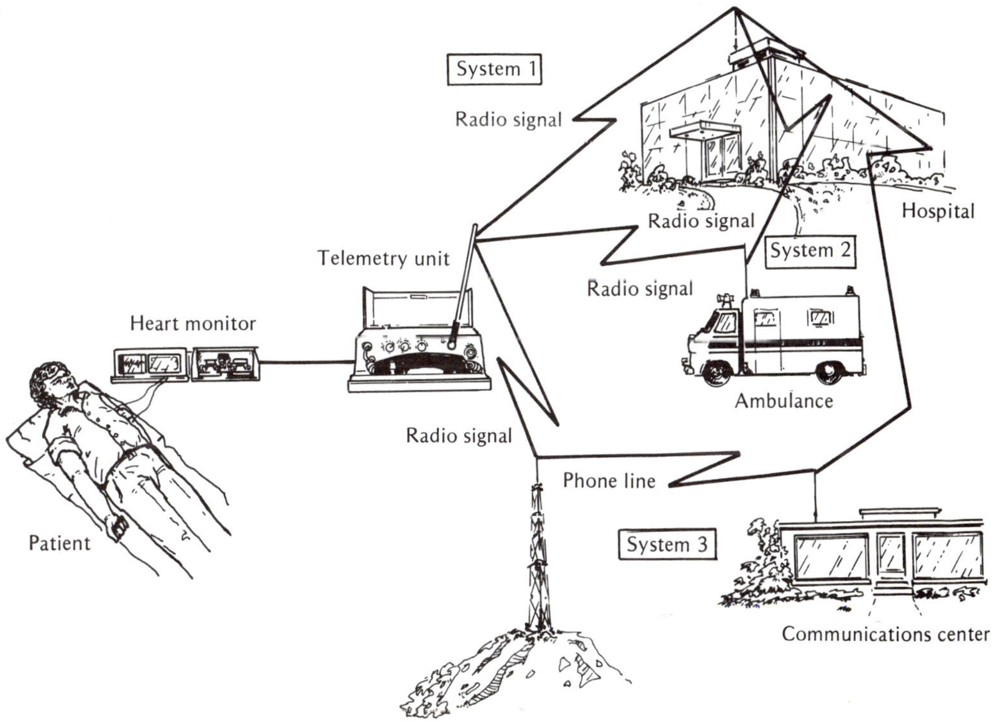


**Figure 6–8.** The various ways by which the telemetry signal may reach the hospital communication base station.

## Extended/Remote Control Center

The extended remote control center controls the powerful base station transmitters in the system, and is usually the desired reception point of the EMT's radio message, generally the medical facility or communications center. In simplest form, the receiver/transmitter site is located on the same premises as the extended/remote control center. For example, the EMT's radio signal is received by an antenna on the hospital's roof and is fed by a cable to a receiver and then (by cable, again) to a speaker in the emergency department, where the physician hears the EMT's comments. When the physician replies, he presses a transmit switch that activates (by cable) a base station transmitter (usually in the same cabinet as the receiver that picked up the EMT's message), that transmits the physician's message back out over the antenna that received the EMT's message. In this simplest system, the physician and EMT cannot speak at the same time as when the unit is transmitting, and the person who is transmitting cannot hear any messages (simplex system). He must release the microphone transmit key to hear.

Base station transmitters are located as close as possible to the transmitting antenna so that power loss that occurs in long connecting cables is minimized.

Other systems may be considerably more complex. An EMT's signal from the field may be received by a number of satellite receivers that all feed their signal in turn, by phone line or microwave, to a centralized comparator (or "voter"). The comparator in turn selects and the "voted" receiver site (continuing to scan all sites at a high speed should one of these other sites suddenly display a better signal or hear another transmission), and feeds the signal into the communications center consoles. If the EMT has requested to speak to a hospital, the communications operators "patch" the signal by means of a multibuttoned patching matrix (attached to dedicated phone lines or a microwave link to the desired hospital) and the physician hears the message. When he in turn keys his microphone, the signal goes back to the communications center and out to a transmitter that is instantaneously activated. The transmitter site may or may not correspond to the receiver site hearing the EMT, since in such systems there are many more receiver sites to pick up the comparatively weak portable or vehicle signal than there are needed powerful base transmitter sites. If the equipment is so designed, the EMT and physician may be able to talk and listen simultaneously in much the same manner as in a telephone conversation (duplex). Sophisticated systems may also send ECG telemetry on the same channel without interrupting the conversation (multiplex).

## Reserve Communications Systems

Most EMS communications systems employ back-up systems to deal with failures of equipment or disaster situations. Key elements of the system may be duplicated and located at scattered sites. The sophisticated, extensive radio network may be backed up by a somewhat less flexible, but highly servicable system in the event of widespread disruption. In addition certain portions of the system may back up other elements. For example, if a hospital loses the ability to operate its remote control in the emergency department, a central communications center may be able to patch radio transmissions to a regular phone in the facility. This function may also be used to patch radio conversations from EMTs in the field to a physician using his phone in his office or at home.

## EMS SYSTEMS

As the EMS system grows, advantages may be found in combining elements of all the systems. For example, an area that has grown enough to develop a series of satellite receivers linking all ambulances and hospitals in a unified network through a regional communications center may elect to maintain digital encoded radios and their frequency so that the area's vehicles could be utilized in communities that have not joined the regional system and to serve as a back-up system.

In many regional systems and plans, the last frequency pair (med eight) is utilized as a "common-calling" frequency for vehicles to request a central communications center to assign a hospital channel.

Two other frequency pairs, contiguous to the eight med channels, have been assigned by the FCC and are used for command, dispatch or mutual assistance type purposes:

462.950/467.950 MHz
462.975/467.975 MHz

Systems exist where the EMT in the field can carry in his hand a 10-channel portable radio that permits him to be totally independent of the emergency vehicle, yet able to contact the communications center, hospital, or any other ambulance in his region, and indeed any telephone, by means of a radio phone patch.

In addition to the frequency pairs, four single UHF frequencies have been allocated for very low power telemetry or voice transmissions from a portable unit to an emergency vehicle for automatic retransmission on one of the med channels delineated above. These frequencies are shared by highway call box operations:

| | |
|---|---|
| 458.025 MHz | 458.125 MHz |
| 458.075 MHz | 458.175 MHz |

All of the EMS radio equipment in the VHF and UHF band is frequency modulated (FM), which more easily suppresses noise and interference than amplitude modulated (AM) stations (such as Citizen's Band radios).

The assigned frequencies can be employed in a number of systems. When both communications stations (such as the hospital and the am-

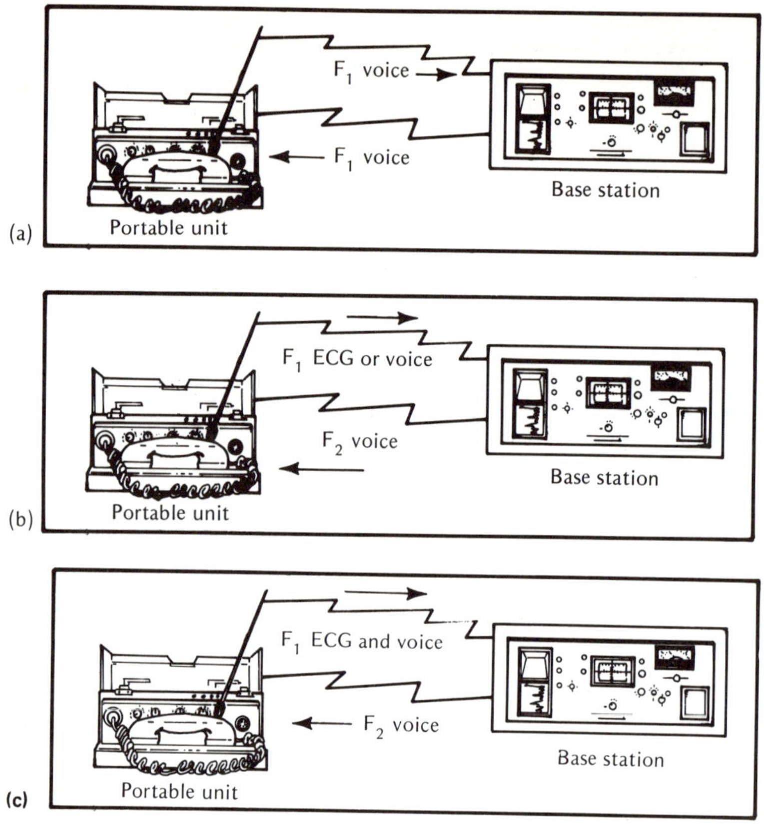


**Figure 6–9.** (a) The simplex mode; (b) the duplex mode; (c) the multiplex mode.

bulance) cannot simultaneously transmit and receive, but can only transmit or receive taking turns, the system is called *simplex.* When two different frequencies are used and simultaneous reception and transmission by both stations is possible, the system is called *duplex.* It is also technically possible to send more than one signal on a channel simultaneously (for example, voice and telemetry); this is known as *multiplex.* (See Fig. 6–9.)

Public safety services have long used simplex systems with no detrimental effects on their operation. Indeed, it encourages radio discipline and, in effect, increases the number of available frequencies (since duplexing requires two frequencies for one conversation). But it is somewhat less flexible than a duplex system, particularly in the delivering of advanced life support (ALS). Within the broad framework outlined by the FCC rules and regulations, the EMT may encounter a wide divergence in the methodology of the frequency utilization, each with its own particular advantages and disadvantages. For example, an EMS system may assign a certain group of frequencies to a portion of the region for use by all ambulances and hospitals in that area, with the rest of the frequencies assigned to the remainder of the region. By means of low power portable radio and repeaters, the EMT may contact a hospital on a prearranged channel with the hospital responding from its own on-premises base station. This system has the advantage of the increased range of the vehicle repeater and the self-sufficiency of the hospital's own base station. As disadvantages, the hospital and ambulance may have only a small number of frequencies that may be overloaded, and the hospital must purchase and maintain its own base station. Further, if the ambulance provider maintains a large fleet of reserve ambulances, each must be equipped with expensive vehicle repeaters even if the frequency of vehicle use is low.

Another type of major system utilizes only a portable radio containing all frequencies and a series of satellite receivers throughout the areas capable of receiving all frequencies, and connected to a central communications center patching matrix that can connect any frequency to any hospital. The advantages to this system is that the EMT need not employ a vehicle repeater (therefore with less cost to the ambulance provider), and can utilize any channel assigned to talk to any hospital, which in turn need not purchase its own base stations, but rather use a common base station dedicated to the community. The disadvantages lie in the cost of maintaining the satellite receiver sites (a significant number of which may be required in a large region), and linking them to the communications center.

The EMT may find in his service area a number of configurations, each of which may be uniquely suited to the terrain and characteristics of the region. It is entirely possible, particularly in a rural area where patients may be transported to a number of large population centers, that the EMT will have a variety of methods of contacting a medical facility depending on his destination. As EMS systems grow and expand, it is likely that communications will become more standardized across the country, but the EMT is expected to be familiar with all configurations and operations he is likely to encounter.

## EMS SEQUENCE

In the operation of an Emergency Medical Service system, there are essentially eight sequential steps. (Actually there are more steps in the total care of the patient after arrival at the hospital. The discussion here is confined to the prehospital and emergency department phases.)

### Prevention

Of course, the ideal way for managing a medical emergency is to prevent its occurrence. While this goal is not fully attainable, EMTs are playing an increasing role in public education. In some areas, between runs, EMTs are working with the local chapter of the American Heart Association to provide hypertensive screening. Cardiopulmonary resuscitation and the risk factors associated with cardiovascular diseases are being taught by EMTs, often under the direction of the American Heart Association or the American National Red Cross, in public classes across the country. EMTs may also be certified by the National Safety Council to teach Defensive Driving Classes (DDC) to interested groups.

## Incident and Detection

The gap between the time the incident occurs and it is detected may range widely, measured in seconds or days. Even when detected, the seriousness may be underestimated as symptoms are misinterpreted or dismissed by the patient as insignificant. Again, EMTs are involved in first aid courses, cardiopulmonary resuscitation courses including early warning signs of coronary problems, and programs that encourage the carrying and wearing of identification that signifies a pertinent medical condition, in an effort to inform the general public of how to detect and cope with medical emergencies. Important also in public education programs is the instruction in how to get help and how to enter the EMS system.

## Notification

All EMS systems must have some means through which the person with a perceived medical emergency can receive help. Most such notifications are made by telephone. Oftentimes, an area may have several separate political jurisdictions, each with its own emergency telephone numbers, a particularly acute problem when an emergency arises away from home and the only available telephone is a pay phone.

To deal with this duplicity of telephone numbers and the attendant possibilities of confusion, an increasing number of communities are implementing the three-digit telephone number 9–1–1 (pronounced nine-one-one, not nine-eleven) as their universal emergency number for EMS, police, and fire. Other communities are using one seven-digit or toll-free telephone number, in the case of very large geographic areas, for all EMS requests.

Those systems that implement 911 often adopt a number of auxiliary services that improve service. One common feature is hold and rering to allow a 911 operator to quickly ring back an excited caller who forgot to give crucial information or to trace bomb threats and false alarms. Another auxiliary service is forcible disconnect to allow the 911 operator to disconnect a nonemergency call that is tying up the emergency lines. Yet another service is dialtone-first that can be extended to coin-operated telephones, thereby allowing the caller to dial 911 without first depositing a coin.

A community that implements 911 may decide to consolidate all emergency dispatching into the same facility, perhaps operated by a specially established communications service that is neither police, fire, or EMS, but serves all three functions. Such a Public Safety Answering Point (PSAP) would not only receive all requests for assistance, but would also dispatch all vehicles. In other cases, the PSAP may only receive requests for assistance and they either pass on the information or directly transfer the call to the persons responsible for the dispatch, located in the same building or miles away. Regardless of how a community manages the notification process, the goal should be to decrease the time from the occurrence of the incident, to the arrival of competent medical help, and to widely publicize the process for attaining help.

In addition to the telephone, the EMS System will receive requests for assistance through a variety of other means. The burgeoning popularity of Citizen's Band (CB) radios has resulted in EMS Communications Centers monitoring CB, or receiving reports through local CB groups. Call boxes along the highway and requests from other government agencies, such as highway crews, police departments, forestry services, and fire departments may be the source of EMS requests.

## Resource Allocation

Once a request for assistance is received by the communications operator, the decision must be made as to which resources in the community will be brought to bear on the situation. A multiple injury traffic accident may require basic and advanced life support ambulances, fire and rescue units to suppress fire and perform extrication, police officers to direct traffic and perform crowd control, utility company personnel to deal with downed power lines, and even a helicopter for transport of some of the patients. All of these units may come from separate agencies, so the EMS communications operator must be extremely well versed in system resource management.

All EMS systems must have some method for dispatching needed units to the scene of a reported medical emergency. The facility from which this is accomplished may take the form of a volunteer's home or a multimillion dollar communications center, staffed around the clock by dozens of operators. While the volume and sophistication may vary, the basic principles remain: *identify* the need and *allocate* the resources.

In most localities the dispatch of emergency personnel is accomplished by radio, either by direct two-way contact or by paging, or by means of a telephone link. Upon the initial dispatch or as soon as the emergency crew acknowledges the run, the communications operator advises the *exact* location of the patient, including cross street, business name, apartment number, etc. Most EMS systems also advise the responding unit of a dispatch time-out and a preliminary assessment of the patient's problem or circumstances by means of special brevity codes or a short verbal description, and relay hazards that may be encountered en route or at the scene, i.e., road closed, hazardous materials present. Local custom may also dictate that other information be given en route.

## On-Site Treatment

On-the-scene treatment, which may include extrication of the patient, is performed with the goal of stabilizing and improving the condition of the patient prior to transport. Further communication with the communications center is required to request additional units and advise of the status of the units on the scene. Additionally, the units on the scene may need to establish communications with a medical facility or person. Basic life support (BLS) does not require the same level of medical supervision as does the advanced life support (ALS) operations, although in most systems a physician retains ultimate responsibility for BLS actions and education. But BLS units may still seek advice or desire to notify the medical facility of status of the patient they are treating.

On-the-scene activities may also involve vehicle-to-vehicle communications for the purposes of coordination or requesting equipment. This is especially important in disaster operations involving vehicles from several jurisdictions, and is facilitated by the presence of an areawide common frequency and the ability of a central communications center to radio-patch units together.

## Transport

Once the patient is secured in the vehicle, if warranted, the EMT may elect to contact the medical facility or continue the communications established back on the scene. In all cases, the EMT should inform his communications facility of his destination and other such information as dictated by local policy (number of patients, whether lights and siren are being used, etc.). As the patient or patients are removed and their EMT duties are accomplished, remaining units on the scene should advise their communications facility that they are in-service available for another run. (See Fig. 6–10.)

## Emergency Department Care

All emergency facilities likely to receive emergency ambulance patients should have a means of communicating with emergency ambulances en route to their facility. (See Fig. 6–11.) A major metropolitan hospital

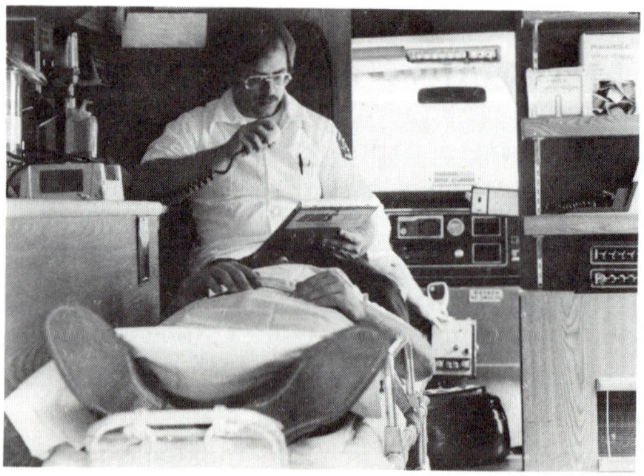

**Figure 6–10.** Communications established in the field to the hospital base station provide an important link for the total care of the patient.

may contain equipment for interfacing with a statewide hospital-to-hospital and hospital-to-ambulance network, and a regional ambulance communications system permitting two or more simultaneous ambulance-to-hospital communications, including the reception and recording of telemetry by radio or telephone. In addition, there is certain to be the presence of an in-house and external paging system for delivering messages to medical personnel.

Unless the hospital has an areawide monitoring responsibility, emergency department radios should be silent unless the radio traffic is specifically directed to that facility. This permits the facility to direct its attention only to its cases, and may be accomplished by means of an encoder-decoder, tone-controlled radio system that activates the speaker only when the ambulance radio sends the appropriate radio tones, or a central patching-matrix facility that disburses radio traffic to the desired facility.

In certain systems, the EMT in the field may not always contact a physician in the emergency department. A physician or other specialist may not be present around the clock, and may be contacted in certain systems by means of a phone patch that connects the EMT's radio with the physician's or specialists's home.

In other systems, specified physicians may carry portable radios permitting the physician to speak with the EMT by means of the radio. Even in these systems where radio medical direction does not come physically from within the emergency department, a radio link to the medical facility is advantageous for advising the hospital of the status of the patient being transported.

Medical facilities also have a need to have a radio link between one another, for purposes of transferring patients and supplies and ascertaining

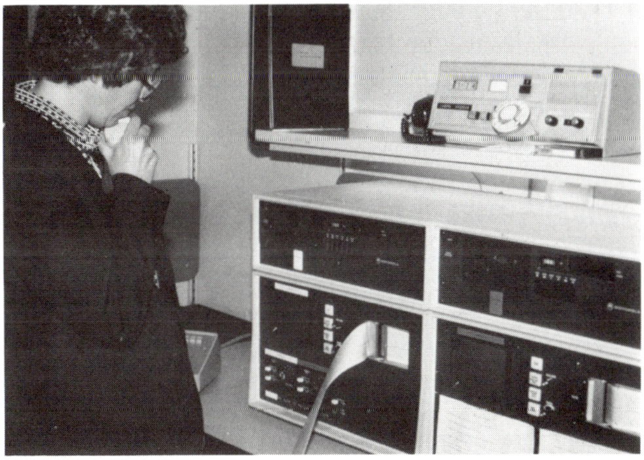

**Figure 6–11.** Medical communications established from the hospital base to the field provide medical control in the EMS system. (Courtesy of Wishard Memorial Hospital. Photo by Bob Biehn.)

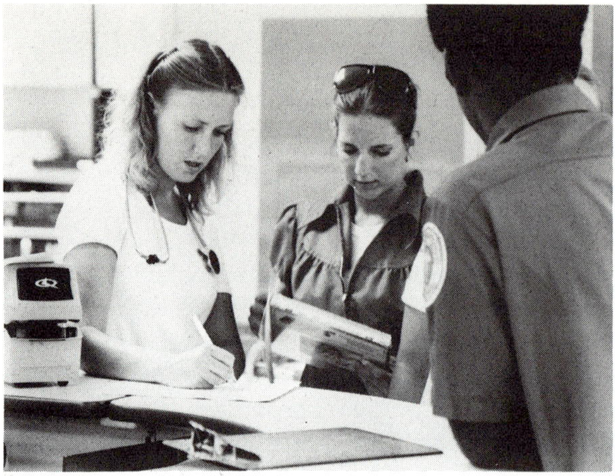

**Figure 6–12.** The patient report given to the triage nurse is the final step in first-line medical communications by the EMT-A.

available beds and personnel. While most such communications may be effected by telephone, particularly in disaster situations, this may not be adequate or functional. Medical facilities should be linked to any central communications center by radio and dedicated telephone circuit. Additionally, the means should exist for medical personnel in the field to communicate with any or all facilities simultaneously in the event of a disaster.

Once the patient is delivered to the medical facility, radio conversations with the institution cease, but communications continue. A briefing or update on the patient's condition and treatment rendered is given to the responsible staff, and a copy of the ambulance run sheet is also left. (See Fig. 6–12.) The EMT may continue to assist with the care of the patient in the emergency department, and advise his communications facility as soon as possible that he is available for another run.

## Evaluation

Following the completion of the run, the EMT and the EMS communications operator will be involved in reviewing how the run was conducted. Immediate feedback may come upon arrival in the emergency facility when the EMT has the opportunity to discuss the management of the patient with the hospital staff. Formal reviews may also be held where the EMT is able to review the run and the patient's hospital progress with his peers and other medical and hospital personnel. Where possible, the EMS communications operator should be included in these reviews, particularly where the operator was able to speak directly with the caller (as opposed, for example, to requests relayed by a CB operator or the police department), and was able to advise the caller of actions to take or not to take while awaiting the arrival of emergency personnel.

The EMS communications operator does far more than dispatch emergency vehicles; thus the term *dispatcher* is not truly descriptive, and may properly be considered archaic. The current concept is that of a manager of system resources, well acquainted with these resources; knowledgeable in emergency medicine and able to apply this knowledge to decide how to manage a call for help, and in some cases advise the caller of actions to take or avoid while awaiting emergency crews; and knowledgeable of the techniques and operations of an electronic communications system.

For most systems, the first contact a caller has with the system comes in the voice of the EMS communications operator. Impressions are formed, and the quality of care may be affected by what the caller is told to do or to avoid doing. A high standard of performance and professionalism must be the rule for all EMS communications operators.

The actual tasks performed by individual EMS communications operators may vary from region to region, but there are responsibilities that are common to most systems:

1. Receive requests for EMS assistance and elicit information about the situation necessary to assess severity of injuries and any hazards associated with the situation.

2. Where appropriate, advise the caller of first aid measures or actions to avoid while awaiting help.

3. Allocate EMS resources to the situation which may include ambulances, public safety units such as police and fire, and utility company units, and provide sufficient information to the responding units to enable them to properly cope with the situation.

4. Establish the communications link between the ambulance and the appropriate medical facility and in the event of a failure of a portion of the system, relay the information between parties.

5. Maintain records of the situation and participate in audit and evaluation programs.

6. Maintain an awareness of all significant public safety and emergency medical activities in the region and surrounding areas.

The EMS communications operator is a critical link in the EMS chain. He or she must be able to think and act promptly in the face of emergencies, analyze a situation accurately and take the appropriate action. Poise, self-reliance, calmness, and alertness are paramount. He must be thoroughly grounded in the concept and operation of his system, and must possess the technical skills required in its operation. A feature often overlooked in the selection or education of the EMS communications operator is that he must possess a clear and distinct speaking voice.

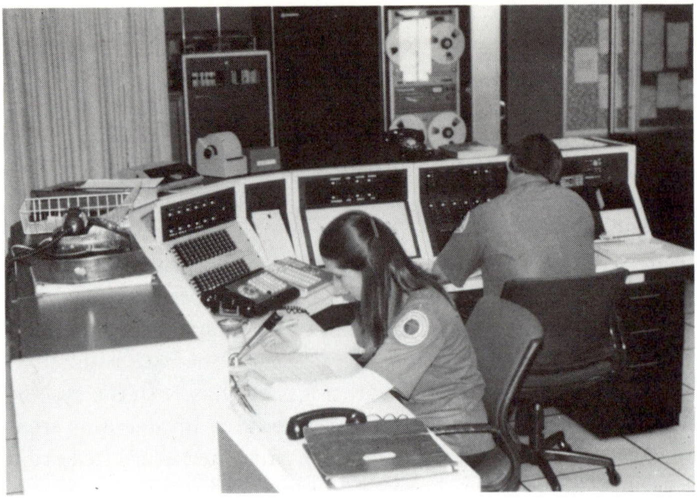

**Figure 6–13.** The EMS communications operator should be an experienced EMT-A. (Courtesy of Wishard Memorial Hospital. Photo by Bob Biehn.)

As important as the communications knowledge is the emergency medical knowledge. The EMS communications operator should be an experienced Emergency Medical Technician and should attend continuing education and audit programs as do other EMTs; thus he will be best equipped to determine the urgency of the call, give the appropriate advice, and decide on the best response. In order to maintain his medical skills he should work periodically on an ambulance or participate in an observer program. It is this medical education that differentiates the EMS communications operator from those of other public safety departments. (See Fig. 6–13.)

In addition to his medical education, the EMS communications operator will have to undergo an education program in the operation of the system coupled with "communications internship," whereby he participates in the actual operation of a communications system under the observation of an experienced EMS communications operator. The format of the education program varies widely and reflects the diversity of EMS communications systems. Regardless of the shape of the program, before assuming his duties, the EMS communications operator should be thoroughly familiar with the concepts of his and adjacent systems, the technical operation of his equipment, the types and operations of EMS resources available, the policies and procedures governing his system, and he must possess the requisite medical skills.

The "street" EMT should likewise be familiar with concepts behind the EMS communications center and, where feasible, be permitted to observe the operation of the communications center. This will aid in decreasing operational problems and increasing the flexibility of the system.

Facilities utilized for the purpose of EMS communications range in size and sophistication from a corner of a volunteer's home to a building housing multiple operators and serving several communities. The growth and complexity of EMS systems is reflected in the operation of their communications centers.

There are multiple ways that various EMS systems configure the resource allocation function of their systems, each configuration found in large and small systems and each with its advantages and limitations. Within one given geographic area, the mechanism for dispatch may vary widely from service to service. Systems exist where all requests for police, fire, and emergency medical assistance are received at one central facility and the dispatch of all units is handled by that same center. In other localities all calls are received at central locations, and the information or call itself is transferred to the appropriate service, located in the same building or miles away. In yet other areas each ambulance service (perhaps as well as each police and fire department) maintains its own telephone number and communications center. Particularly where the population is large and a number of services exist, or where there exists a significant transient population, this latter type of configuration increases the chances of confusion on the part of the caller and a delay in obtaining help. However the system is configured, the design of the communications center is affected.

Most commonly thought of in conjunction with a communications center is the radio equipment. But the center contains a host of other devices for receiving calls, communicating with field units, monitoring other agencies, and maintaining records of EMS activities. In some centers, equipment for establishing the link between the ambulance and the hospital is also found.

Telephone equipment found in the center may be only single, familiar table-top telephone, or it may consist of a hundred push-buttons built into the communications consoles, permitting the center to handle multiple calls and have dedicated telephone line contact to all public safety agencies, medical facilities, airports, etc. The center may also be equipped with a comparatively inexpensive teletype device that enables deaf persons to communicate with the center. (See Fig. 6–14.) Generally all telephone conversations received or emanating from the center are tape recorded for future legal, administrative, and evaluation purposes. (See Fig. 6–15.)

Radio equipment found in the center will permit contact with all field units, and in larger systems, with all medical facilities. More versatile systems may be able to patch one radio frequency to another or patch any radio frequency into standard telephone lines. Specialized radio equipment in the center may permit the EMS communications operator to communicate with aircraft and boats, with other agencies linked in a disaster network, or with persons equipped with Citizen's Band radios. Pagers may

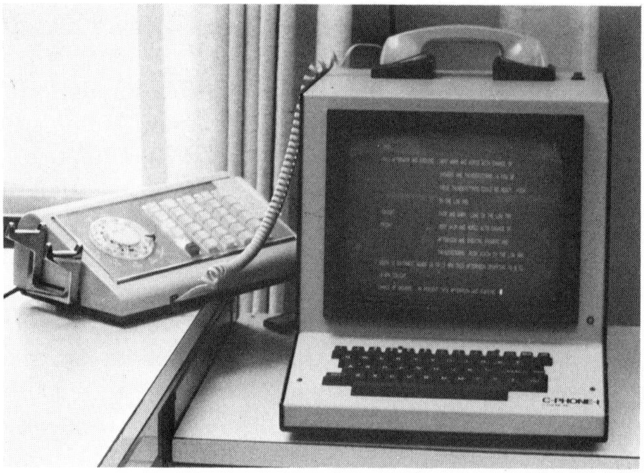

**Figure 6–14.** The deaf teletype device provides emergency communications for the hearing impaired.

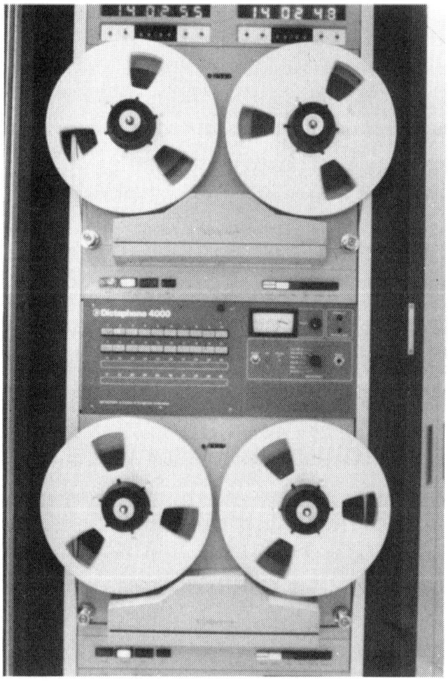

**Figure 6–15.** A tape recording system or device should be utilized in all EMS systems for recall of events should they be needed or lawfully requested.

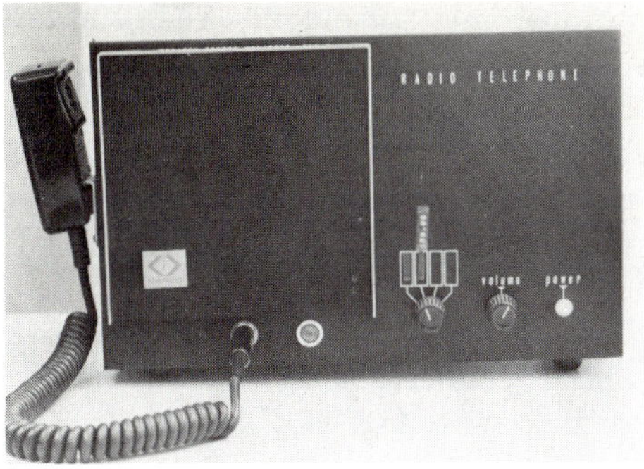


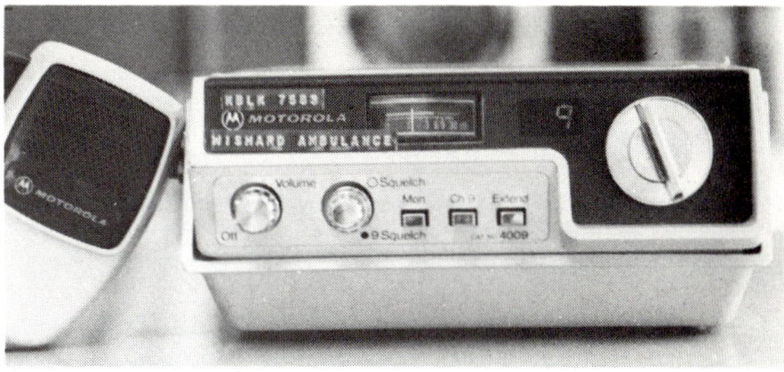


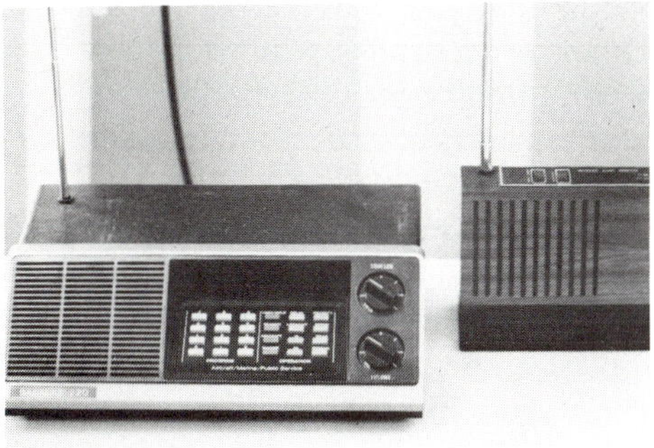

**Figure 6–16.** Different types of monitoring devices allow the communications operator to listen for potential civil, weather, or aircraft emergencies and anticipate proper action to be initiated.

also be controlled by the center, allowing selective contact with operational, administrative, or medical personnel. Crucial radio contacts, especially those with field units and those between field units and medical facilities, are also tape recorded.

Communications personnel are responsible for knowing the status of all units under their control, as well as pertinent information concerning medical facilities, i.e., beds available. Thus the center may be outfitted with status boards or maps that are constantly updated and show at a glance the status of all units. Larger systems may keep track of this information by means of a computer.

The EMS communications center should constantly be apprised of all EMS and public safety activities in their area. Most often this is accomplished by radio monitors and scanners. Especially useful are synthetic, noncrystalled scanners that permit the EMS communications operator to selectively monitor any one of multiple frequencies. Equipment for monitoring National Weather Service broadcasts is also important to the operation of an EMS communications center. (See Fig. 6–16.)

Record-keeping is an important function of the EMS communications center. The EMS communications operators are required in most systems to keep a record of the activities of the center including the location of each run, the units involved, and the judgment of the communications operator concerning the problem and severity of each individual call. For evaluation and administrative purposes, the various times surrounding each run are recorded, such as the time the run was received, dispatched, and acknowledged by the unit; and the time the unit arrived on the scene, left for the hospital, arrived at the hospital, and was in-service available for another run. A variety of information, including how many patients were transported to what facility, other services involved, and any problems encountered, may also be recorded. As well as information surrounding medical runs, the communications center may maintain administrative records such as equipment checks and personnel. All information may be recorded on paper, electronically, or both. (See Fig. 6–17.)

All equipment in the communications center should be checked regularly to make sure that it is operational and that everyone is familiar with its use. This is especially important when dealing with equipment that is not frequently used, but may be vital in disaster operations.

The security of the communications center is of paramount importance. The center should be capable of being secured (locked) so as to prevent unauthorized entrance. Extraneous persons should not be permitted unlimited access to the center and persons should be discouraged from lounging in the center, since this may pose a distraction for the EMS communications operators and interfere with the operation.

As EMS communications centers grow in sophistication, innovative functions are being added to the operation of the center. At least one system has combined into one facility the operation of a statewide poison information center, staffed around the clock by specialized Registered Nurses, with an urban EMS communications center staffed around the clock by experienced EMTs trained as EMS communications operators. Such combined resources facilitate the smooth flow of medical information and coordinate a systems response.

## THE REQUEST FOR HELP

The volume of EMS runs managed by the EMS system significantly affects the method by which the system receives requests for its assistance. Rescue personnel may answer emergency calls in their homes, a nurse at the local hospital may receive such requests, or several full-time operators may man a bank of telephone consoles. No matter the method, the delivery of emergency medical care should properly be considered to begin the moment the phone is answered.

Most requests for assistance will be received by telephone and will be more efficiently managed if the operator utilizes proper telephone technique. Many of those principles are applicable in any telephone conversation:

1. Answer all calls promptly, on the first ring if possible, definitely within three rings.

2. Identify the department. Not only does this reassure the caller

WISHARD MEMORIAL HOSPITAL

AMBULANCE DIVISION COMMUNICATIONS REPORT

DATE____/____/____ SHIFT______

COMM. OP. ____________________

COMM. OP. ____________________

UF–182

| Disp. Probs. | Inj./Ill. Codes | | Screen Codes | Disposition Codes | Hosp. Codes | |
|---|---|---|---|---|---|---|
| 1. EQUIP. | 1. TRAF. INJ. | 10. BURNS | 1. EM-ADVICE | 1. S-9 EXPLAIN | 1. WMH | 11. |
| 2. ACT. OVER. | 2. H. A. | 11. O. D. | 2. EM-NO ADV. | 2. S. O. R. | 2. METH. | 12. |
| 3. NO AVAIL. UNITS | 3. INJ. PUB. | 12. G. S. W. | 3. URG. TRANS. | 3. NO PATIENT | 3. COMM. | 13. |
| 4. CREW RESP. DELAY | 4. INJ. HOME | 13. | 4. NON URG. TRANS. | 4. | 4. ST. FR. | 14. |
| 5. | 5. O. B. | 14. | 5. STAND-BY | 5. | 5. V.A. | 15. OTHER |
| 6. NONE | 6. SICK PERS. | 15. | 6. | 6. OTHER-EXPL. | 6. WIN. | |
| 7. OTHER | 7. SEIZ. | 16. | 7. | 7. | 7. ST. VIN. | |
| | 8. UNCON. | 17. | 8. | 8. RETURN S-8 | 8. I.U. | |
| | 9. ATT. SUI. | 18. | 9. OTHER | 9. | 9. | |
| | | | | 10. RETURN S-10 | 10. | |

| | D.C. | UNIT | DISP. | RESPOND | 10-23 | 10-24 | 10-7 | HOSP. | QTY. | 10-8 |
|---|---|---|---|---|---|---|---|---|---|---|
| Incident No. / Caller I.D. / Reported Problem / Inj./Ill. / Screen | | | | | | | | | | |
| Emergency Location / Tract / Phone / Time call rec. | | | | | | | | | | |
| Comments / Svcs. at Scene / Disp. Prob | | | | | | | | | | |
| Incident No. / Caller I.D. / Reported Problem / Inj./Ill. / Screen | | | | | | | | | | |
| Emergency Location / Tract / Phone / Time call rec. | | | | | | | | | | |
| Comments / Svcs. at Scene / Disp Prob | | | | | | | | | | |
| Incident No. / Caller I.D. / Reported Problem / Inj./Ill. / Screen | | | | | | | | | | |
| Emergency Location / Tract / Phone / Time call rec. | | | | | | | | | | |
| Comments / Svcs. at Scene / Disp Prob | | | | | | | | | | |
| Incident No. / Caller I.D. / Reported Problem / Inj./Ill. / Screen | | | | | | | | | | |
| Emergency Location / Tract / Phone / Time call rec. | | | | | | | | | | |
| Comments / Svcs. at Scene / Disp Prob | | | | | | | | | | |
| Incident No. / Caller I.D. / Reported Problem / Inj./Ill. / Screen | | | | | | | | | | |
| Emergency Location / Tract / Phone / Time call rec. | | | | | | | | | | |
| Comments / Svcs. at Scene / Disp Prob | | | | | | | | | | |
| Incident No. / Caller I.D. / Reported Problem / Inj./Ill. / Screen | | | | | | | | | | |
| Emergency Location / Tract / Phone / Time call rec. | | | | | | | | | | |
| Comments / Svcs. at Scene / Disp Prob | | | | | | | | | | |

**Figure 6–17.** The communications report form should fit the needs of each EMS communication system. (Courtesy of Wishard Memorial Hospital Ambulance Service, Indianapolis, IN)

that he has reached the right place, but a distinct, confident voice answering the phone may have an enormous calming influence.

3. Speak directly into the mouthpiece. Do not speak with anything in your mouth. Speak up.

4. Take charge of the conversation, but observe telephone courtesy. Lead the caller into answering quesitons. Be firm, but extremely polite. Courtesy is always appropriate.

5. Write down all information. Particularly important are such things as the emergency location and the caller's telephone number.

6. Before terminating any conversation, the key information as copied down should be verified, by repeating it back to the caller.

7. Do not make an emergency caller redial. If a caller has reached the wrong agency, the pertinent information should be obtained and relayed to the appropriate department. This should be explained to the caller. The wait should be explained if the caller is put on hold while this is being done.

8. Avoid codes, jargon, and slang. Terms that are frequently used by ambulance personnel, such as 10–4, 10–20, ETA, etc., will not be meaningful to most callers.

9. Treat each call as an emergency. While EMS and public safety personnel tend to become used to medical emergencies, for most callers this will be a new and frightening experience.

10. Terminate each call positively and courteously. Advise the caller of what action is being taken and reassure them help is on the way.

Persons placing a call to an EMS communications center are often distraught and agitated, occasionally hostile. The EMS communications operator must develop the ability to calm callers, but merely telling the caller to calm down rarely is sufficient and may be counterproductive if the caller gets the impression the EMS communications operator does not appreciate the seriousness of the situation. Several measures may prove useful:

1. Answer all calls promptly and in a calm, competent voice identify the department.

2. Listen carefully and patiently, but do not let the caller ramble. Always be courteous and strive to convey a sense of competence to the caller.

3. Let the caller know help is on the way. If the caller must be placed on "hold" while the units are being dispatched, explain what is about to happen and state again what was accomplished while he was on hold. In most instances, if there is more than one EMS communications operator, one can dispatch the units while the other continues to get information or give advice to the caller.

4. Do not allow emotions to interfere with the conversation. If the caller becomes agitated, the EMS communications operator should not speak sharply or reply in a harsh tone of voice, but rather in a calm, competent manner. Even if the caller displays anger or abusiveness, the EMS communications operator should not argue back, but calmly explain what information is needed and what is happening to meet the caller's needs.

5. If appropriate, advise the caller of what first aid measures can be taken or what actions should be avoided until help arrives. The anxiety displayed by many callers is a result of their feeling of helplessness. If the EMS communications operator is able to explain ways in which they can help, he may markedly decrease their anxiety. These explanations should not delay dispatching the emergency units.

Two major purposes of obtaining information from callers is to permit the decision on appropriate units and advise them of what to expect upon arrival (a third purpose is to initiate medical care over the phone).

It is imperative that the EMS communications operator obtain rapid, accurate information from callers. At no time should accuracy be sacrificed for speed, but the information should be obtained as quickly as possible and the units dispatched immediately. The type and sequence of information varies somewhat from community to community, but each system should have an organized, established format for gathering such information. An example of one sequence for eliciting information is outlined below:

1. Obtain the exact location of the patient. This is obtained first so that in the event the communications with the caller is cut off, an emergency unit could proceed to the scene to investigate. In urban areas this usually involves the street name, direction, number and possibly the city, apartment number, name of business, nearest cross street, etc. In rural areas this may entail establishing landmarks or any readily identifiable feature that can point the way for the emergency crew. Enough information should be garnered by the EMS communications operator that he himself could proceed to the scene. If the EMS communications operator would not know how to find the location, it is likely that the emergency crew would not either.

2. Obtain the phone number of the caller. This should be obtained next so that the caller may be redialed in the event the connection is broken. Ultimately this may be necessary if the ambulance cannot find the address and needs better directions.

3. Obtain the caller's perception of the patient's problem and any specifics of the patient's condition, i.e., unconscious, breathing, severe bleeding. This may be important in the EMS communications operator's decision on what units to dispatch and any special equipment or services needed.

4. If the caller is reporting a vehicle or industrial accident other information may be required:

a. Type of vehicles or equipment involved

b. Number of persons involved

c. Hazards at the scene—dangerous chemicals, downed electrical wires, traffic hazards, fire, submerged vehicles, etc.

5. Once all of the above information is obtained and recorded, and the units dispatched or being dispatched, the EMS communications operator may elect to advise the caller of appropriate first aid measures.

## RADIO PROCEDURES

The radio has become a ubiquitous part of the EMT's practice. If a volunteer, the EMT sleeps with a radio monitor not far away. If full time, he does not move without a portable radio on his hip or without being in earshot of a radio speaker. Because the radio is so important, it is imperative that the EMT be thoroughly familiar with radio procedures.

Years of experience with public safety communications has resulted in the widespread adoption of certain conventions that have been adopted or appropriated for EMS use also:

1. Before transmitting, listen for other radio traffic. Only one operator may use a radio channel at any given instant of time, regardless of any other capabilities of the radio system.

2. Keep all transmissions as brief as possible, but consistent with clarity. Brevity is very important with so many users of the airwaves, but accuracy should not be sacrificed. Do not use superfluous words or phrases.

3. Pronounce each word clearly and distinctly. Some authorities feel a rate of fifty to sixty words per minute is best. Normal speech is from 100–200 words per minute and this may greatly increase if the speaker is excited. While too-slow speech can actually sound boring or convey apathy, in most cases the EMT will find he must slow down his rate of speech and enunciate for maximum effectiveness.

4. The radio voice should be emotionless, with a deliberate, decisive pitch. As the amount of emotion increases, the intelligibility decreases. Anger, sarcasm, impatience, humor—all are *totally inappropriate*, regardless of the situation, and are the hallmark of a lack of professionalism. Radio conversations should be impersonal, with unit identities being used in the place of names. Obscene language is illegal.

5. Speak distinctly into the microphone, although some microphones are best utilized by holding them at an angle and speaking across the face of the microphone. Too loud a voice will be distorted; too soft a voice, unheard. In heavy background noise environments, the EMT may

have to speak up slightly; shouting simply makes the transmission unintelligible. The EMT should never speak with anything in his mouth or try to transmit while sitting back in the ambulance seat and shouting while keying the microphone still in its dashboard hanger.

6. Do not be hesitant. The EMT should know what he is going to say *before* keying the microphone. Vocal pauses indicate that the EMT is unsure of what he is trying to say. Depressing the microphone transmit key momentarily before speaking will insure that the first part of the EMT's transmission is not cut off.

7. Courtesy and politeness are understood. Words or phrases such as "sir," "please," "thank you," etc., are clearly superfluous and should not be used on the radio.

8. Reliability and accuracy are very important in EMS communications. Important information should be written down when transmitted or received. This will decrease later misunderstandings and the need to have messages repeated over the radio.

9. Radio transmissions should be confined to emergency-related traffic. Nonemergency traffic, including personal messages and announcements, should be relayed over the telephone whenever possible.

10. With the advent of low cost receivers and scanners, more and more persons are monitoring public safety and EMS transmissions. Radio professionalism is always in order.

The EMT may also benefit from avoiding phrases or words that are poorly understood or less desirable on the radio:

| *Use* | *Avoid* |
|---|---|
| Advise | Let me know. Tell me. |
| Affirmative | Yes. OK |
| Apply | Put on |
| Check | Call and see |
| Clear | Out. End of transmission. |
| Confirm | Did I understand |
| Continue | Keep doing . . . . . |
| Copy | Receive. Understood |
| Desire | Want. wish |
| ETA | Estimated time of arrival |
| Negative | No |
| Obtain | Get |
| Repeat | Didn't get that |
| Request | Please |
| Stand-by | Wait |
| Unable | Can't |
| Understand | Know what you're trying to tell me |
| We | I |

The EMT should also be aware of techniques for utilizing his radio for maximum effectiveness and ensuring his transmissions are received. Instructions furnished by the manufacturer of the radio equipment and policies established by the EMS system should be followed carefully. General techniques that may be useful are the following:

1. In most cases the higher the antenna, the greater the range. In many cases merely moving the radio or vehicle a few feet may dramatically increase the reception.

2. The antenna should be pointed straight up. When using certain comparatively low powered portables, the antenna on the portable should not be kept close to the EMT's body when transmitting as the transmission quality may be affected by the body's absorption.

3. Reception in buildings and transmissions from within certain types of structures are apt to be poorer than outdoors. Even in the best of radio systems there are likely to be "dead spots" in certain buildings. Transmissions near windows or from upper floors tend to be clearer. Sometimes high power electrical lines may also contribute to distortion.

## Code System

Many EMS communications systems use some variation of a signal or "10-code" system. Originally these systems were developed to provide some degree of security for public safety radio information. To some extent this is still valid, and many EMTs find it useful to have some code to signify harsh terms or terms that may upset an already volatile situation, such as codes for "corpse," "prisoners," etc. However, for the most part, codes have lost their usefulness as a security measure and are now used chiefly for making messages brief and clear between persons well trained and experienced in their use.

Some EMS systems question the value of code systems, since in many areas various ten codes mean different things to each department, thus increasing the potential for error. Local policy should be followed and the EMT should be careful not to use codes when transmitting to parties that would not understand them. Precisely because no code system has been universally adopted, the EMT should be wary of using them unless it is certain his listener will understand.

The Associated Public-Safety Communication Officer, Inc. (APCO), the professional society of public safety communications, has developed a standard set of aural brevity ten codes under contract with the Office of Telecommunications Policy. While these codes are recommended for use throughout the United States, they are not in universal use and the EMT should be aware of local differences:

10-Codes

| | | | |
|---|---|---|---|
| 10- 1 | Signal Weak | 10-21 | Call ______ By Phone |
| 10- 2 | Signal Good | 10-22 | Disregard |
| 10- 3 | Stop Transmitting | 10-23 | Arrived at Scene |
| 10- 4 | Affirmative (OK) | 10-24 | Assignment Completed |
| 10- 5 | Relay (To) | 10-25 | Report to (Meet) |
| 10- 6 | Busy | 10-26 | Estimated Time of Arrival |
| 10- 7 | Out of Service | 10-27 | License/Permit Information |
| 10- 8 | In Service | 10-28 | Ownership Information |
| 10- 9 | Say Again (Repeat) | 10-29 | Records Check |
| 10-10 | Negative | 10-30 | Danger/Caution |
| 10-11 | ____ On Duty | 10-31 | Pick Up |
| 10-12 | Stand By (Stop) | 10-32 | ____ Units Needed Specify |
| 10-13 | Existing Conditions | 10-33 | Help Me Quick (Emergency) |
| 10-14 | Message/Information | 10-34 | Time |
| 10-15 | Message Delivered | 10-35 | - Reserved - |
| 10-16 | Reply to Message | 10-36 | - Reserved - |
| 10-17 | Enroute | 10-37 | - Reserved - |
| 10-18 | Urgent (Quickly) | 10-38 | - Reserved - |
| 10-19 | (In) Contact | 10-39 | - Reserved - |
| 10-20 | Location | | |

Users of this particular aural brevity should not alter the 10-codes assigned through 10-39. Signal numbers beginning with 10-40 and upward can be assigned meanings according to local needs.

## Numbers

In Emergency Medical Services numbers are an intergral part of messages. Misunderstandings and confusion can have serious consequences; therefore care is indicated in their pronunciation.

1. "WUN" . . . with a strong W and N
2. "TOO" . . . with a strong and long OO
3. "TH-R-EE . . . with a slightly rolling R and long EE
4. "FO-WER" . . . with a long O and strong W and final R
5. "FIE-YIV" . . . with a long I changing to short and strong Y and V
6. "SIKS" . . . with a strong S and KS
7. "SEV-VEN" . . . with a strong S and V and well sounded VEN
8. "ATE" . . . with a long A and strong T
9. "NI-YEN" . . . with a strong N at the beginning, a long I and a well-sounded YEN

0. "ZERO" . . . with a strong Z and short RO

The use of twenty-four-hour time (military time) is preferred over the usual twelve-hour time. A.M. and P.M. are easily misunderstood and are repetitious when used over the radio. Accordingly most EMS communications systems utilize the 2400 hour time system as in the following examples:

| *2400 Hour Time* | *Pronunciation* | *12-Hour Time* |
|---|---|---|
| 2400 | twenty-four hundred | Midnight |
| 0001 | zero zero zero one | One minute past midnight (12:01 a.m.) |
| 0015 | zero zero one five | Fifteen minutes past midnight (12:15 a.m.) |
| 0045 | zero zero four five | Forty-five minutes past midnight (12:45 a.m.) |
| 0100 | zero one-hundred | One a.m. |
| 0130 | zero one three zero (zero one-thirty) | one thirty a.m. |
| 0200 | zero two hundred | two a.m. |
| 0300 | zero three hundred | three a.m. |
| 0400 | zero four hundred | four a.m. |
| 0500 | zero five hundred | five a.m. |
| 0600 | zero six hundred | six a.m. |
| 0700 | zero seven hundred | seven a.m. |
| 0800 | zero eight hundred | eight a.m. |
| 0900 | zero nine hundred | nine a.m. |
| 1000 | ten hundred | ten a.m. |
| 1030 | one zero three zero | ten thirty a.m. |
| 1100 | eleven hundred | eleven a.m. |
| 1200 | twelve hundred | Noon |
| 1201 | twelve zero one | one minute past noon (12:01 p.m.) |
| 1300 | thirteen hundred | one p.m. |
| 1400 | fourteen hundred | two p.m. |
| 1500 | fifteen hundred | three p.m. |
| 1545 | fifteen forty-five | three forty five p.m. (3:45 p.m.) |
| 1600 | sixteen hundred | four p.m. |
| 1700 | seventeen hundred | five p.m. |
| 1800 | eighteen hundred | six p.m. |
| 1900 | nineteen hundred | seven p.m. |
| 2000 | twenty hundred | eight p.m. |
| 2100 | twenty one hundred | nine p.m. |
| 2200 | twenty two hundred | ten p.m. |
| 2300 | twenty three hundred | eleven p.m. |
| 2345 | twenty three forty five | eleven forty five p.m. |

* following 1200 in this system the time may be quickly visualized by adding 1200 to the 12 hour time equivalent. For example: one p.m. in 2400 hour time is 1300 (100 + 1200).

## Alphabet

Unusual words may have to be spelled out. For this reason, phonetic alphabets have been developed so that letters are understandable over the radio. It should be used as "A"—Adam; "K"—King, etc. Never "A" as in Adam, "K" as in King, etc. Words should be spelled slowly with a slight pause after each letter. A common phonetic alphabet is as follows (there are others):

| | | | |
|---|---|---|---|
| A | Adam | N | Nora |
| B | Boy | O | Ocean |
| C | Charles | P | Paul |
| D | David | Q | Queen |
| E | Edward | R | Robert |
| F | Frank | S | Sam |
| G | George | T | Tom |
| H | Henry | U | Union |
| I | Ida | V | Victor |
| J | John | W | William |
| K | King | X | X-Ray |
| L | Lincoln | Y | Young |
| M | Mary | Z | Zebra |

## Reporting Patient Information

Reporting medical information by radio to an emergency facility has become commonplace for EMTs across the nation. It is important to come to the realization that the ability to make a good presentation over the radio is dependent on the EMT's ability to use patient assessment skills. An EMT who does a poor on-the-scene assessment will deliver a sketchy, confusing report to the medical facility. While it is true that an EMT who performs an excellent on-the-scene assessment and treatment also may give a poor radio presentation, the application of a few basic principles and the utilization of a prior agreed upon standardized reporting format will likely prevent this occurrence.

In most EMS systems, EMTs require less radio contact with medical facilities than do advanced life support personnel, such as paramedics, since EMTs do not require orders to perform their authorized skills, as do paramedics in most states. Nevertheless, particularly in certain communities and when dealing with smaller hospitals, EMTs may use radio transmissions to alert the hospital of the transport of a patient who will clearly require the services of a special unit, such as burns, or a specialist who may not be immediately available in the emergency department, such as an ophthalmologist.

To be most effective, radio conversations in the medical facility should adhere to certain basic principles and a standardized format. For the most part, basic radio procedures outlined previously are applicable to medical conversations, but elaboration and reiteration are in order.

1. Speak slowly and distinctly using standard medical terminology. Generally speaking, abbreviations should be avoided unless the EMT is absolutely sure the receiving facility will understand. A good simple description of the patient conveys far more than attempting the use of specialized terminology.

2. The EMT should identify his unit with each transmission. While this is less important in systems that can assign individual, clear radio channels to each conversation (thus ensuring only one EMT unit is speaking with a given medical facility), it is of paramount importance in those systems that may have several conversations taking place at any given time on one channel. In any system it is a good habit to cultivate and prevents confusion.

3. Codes, signals, and other language commonly used in dispatching should be avoided in ambulance-to-hospital communications. Unless all involved are well versed in their use, the consequences may be serious. Some systems have been able to successfully implement a code system between ambulance and hospital, but in most instances the large number of ambulance personnel and the existence of numerous hospitals and changing medical personnel precludes their successful adoption.

4. Clarity, accuracy, and brevity are important in radio communications. Prior to initiating a call to the hospital, the EMT should take time to organize his thoughts and data so that the emergency department will receive sufficient information without having to ask numerous questions, punctuated by pauses as the EMT gathers the information. Phrases that may create doubt should be avoided. For example, when an EMT reports that he is "unable to obtain a blood pressure, " does he mean the patient has no blood pressure or that the patient is combative and will not permit the taking of a blood pressure?

5. Labeling the patient should be studiously avoided. For example, once the EMT reports that he is on the scene of a "stroke" he may cause the personnel at the medical facility to develop "tunnel vision" when perhaps the patient is not really suffering from a cerebrovascular problem. Instead the patient's problem should be carefully described.

6. The radio should be used when absolutely necessary. If available, the telephone may be more appropriate for conversation with the medical facility, although some systems discourage the practice.

Telemetry is an integral part of many EMS communications systems, although it is more widely used to support advanced life support operations. If the EMT functions in a setting where telemetry is utilized, he should be familiar with its usage.

## Reporting Format

A standardized reporting protocol greatly expedites the communications flow between the prehospital and hospital links in the EMS chain. All essential information is provided and efficiency is greatly enhanced. Again, it bears repeating that a successful radio presentation will depend on the assessment and treatment skills of the EMT and the taking of a few moments by the EMT to organize his thoughts. One suggested outline is as follows:

I. Unit Identification
II. Age, Sex, and level of consciousness (LOC)
III. Description of Incident and Patient Location
IV. Chief Complaint or Problem
V. Patient History and Medications
VI. Examination Findings
VII. Vital Signs
VIII. Treatment
IX. Estimated Time of Arrival (ETA)

*I. Unit Identification*

Prior to delivering any patient information, the EMT should clearly establish the identity of his unit.

*II. Age, Sex, and LOC*

The EMT must attempt to paint a mental picture of his patient to the medical personnel of the receiving facility. If necessary, the patient's age should be estimated. For some medical conditions, the patient's race may be important and can be inserted here. Level of consciousness is one of the first things to be noted on the scene. It should, therefore, be communicated to establish the context for the rest of the information.

*III. Description of Incident and Patient Location*

In general terms where, and perhaps how, the injury or illness occurred should be added to the mental picture being painted by the EMT. It may be important to the care of the patient and may also describe to the medical facility why certain actions are being taken. For example, advising that a patient is trapped on top of a silo, at the bottom of a well, or even lying on the corner of a busy intersection, may describe to the hospital the circumstances in which the EMT will be treating the patient and may be useful in ascertaining the mechanism of injury.

*IV. Chief Complaint (CC) or Problem*

Simply stated, this is the reason why the patient called for help. Insofar as possible, the patient's own words should be reported. It should be limited to one or two symptoms and should also include the duration of the symptoms. Significant findings from the EMT's primary survey may be appropriate as the chief complaint.

*V. Patient History and Medications*

The presentation of the history should be given in two parts: a history of the present problem and any pertinent past medical history.

The history of the present problem will have been gathered from the patient and perhaps bystanders. Symptoms reported by the patient should be characterized by quality, location, and severity. It is also important to report symptoms that are denied by the patient, but may be expected to be present. Any medications taken by the patient should be reported. The past medical history should include any significant illnesses or injuries that could be expected to influence the patient's care. Any known allergies should be reported.

*VI. Examination Findings*

A summary of the observations gleaned during the EMT's secondary survey is appropriate at this point. Particularly not to be overlooked is a report on the position of the patient on arrival (i.e., lying in bed, sitting up). Remember, the personnel at the hospital cannot see the patient.

*VII. Vital Signs*

Vital signs, including pulse, respirations, and blood pressure, should be reported in every case.

*VIII. Treatment*

The care rendered by the EMT and any others who arrived before him should be described.

*IX. Estimated Time of Arrival (ETA)*

All presentations should be concluded with an estimate of time until the patient arrives at the medical facility. If some time will elapse until the patient is able to be transported, this should be explained prior to giving the ETA. This will prevent misunderstandings and will minimize the medical facility's inquiries as to what is transpiring.

*References*

American Academy of Orthopedic Surgeons, Committee on Allied Health. *Emergency Care and Transportation of the Sick and Injured*, 2nd ed. Chicago, IL: American Academy of Orthopedic Surgeons, 1977.

Bell, Samuel V., and Baxter, Verne E. "A Beginning Training Manual for Radio Operation of the Emergency Medical Services of the State of Kentucky." Contract with Kentucky Department of Human Resources, September 1977.

Bush, Stan G. "Sending and Receiving Signals: The Art of Communications," *Emergency*, March 1978.

Drury, Coln G., and Schico, Samuel George. "Evaluation of an EMS Communications System," *JACEP* 6:4, April 1977.

Elliott, Max. "EMS Communication's Role," *APCO Bulletin*, August 1976.

Gazzaniga, Alan B., M.D.; Iseri, Lloyd I., M.D.; Baren, Martin, M.D. *Emergency Care: Principles and Practices for the EMT-Paramedic*. Reston, VA: Reston Publishing Co., Inc., 1979.

Gerald, Kevin B. "Guidelines for Reporting Medical Information to the Resource Hospital (A Basic Life Support Approach)," *EMT Journal*, September 1979.

Grant, H. D., and Murray, R. H., Jr. *Emergency Care*, 2nd ed. Bowie, MD: Robert J. Brady Co., 1978.

"A Guide for Hospital Participation in an Emergency Medical Communications System," American Hospital Association, 1973.

McCorkle, James E.; Nagel, Eugene L.; Penterman, Donald G.; Mason, Robert. *Basic Telecommunications For Emergency Medical Services*. Cambridge, MA: Ballinger Publishing, 1978.

*National Training Course Emergency Medical Technician Paramedic, Instructors Lesson Plans, Module XV*. U.S. Department of Transportation, NHTSA.

*911: A Handbook for Community Planning*, Executive Office of the President, Office of Telecommunications Policy, May 1973.

Stewart, Ronald. *Field Assessment and Reporting: A Systematic Approach for Paramedics*. Handout given at a 1975 California Conference.

"Training Program for Emergency Medical Technician: Dispatcher," Instructors Lesson Plans and Student Study Guide. U.S. Department of Transportation, *NHTSA*, November 1976.

Wilford, C. L. "Communications" (Column), *Emergency Medical Services*, Jan/Feb. 1977.

Wilford, C. L., "Communications" (Column), *Emergency Medical Services*, Jan/Feb. 1978.

# Chapter 7

# Legal Concerns for the EMT

EMTs, like other health team members, should be aware of the legal implications in their day-to-day practice. They should be cognizant of the legislation that governs their practice, and they should possess a sensitivity to the problems that are most likely to result in legal action.

Two or three decades ago, it would have been quite unusual for a physician, nurse, or other health care worker to be sued. Today, however, it is not uncommon for patients and their families to wait and watch for a "vulnerable spot" in care to initiate a legal action. Most legal action is aimed at receiving compensation (money) for injuries or wrongdoings.

Legal action is usually prompted by a dissatisfied consumer. He is seeking retribution for injuries, death, or emotional trauma that was supposedly caused by the person being sued. The most common cause of a lawsuit in the health care field relates to unhappiness of the patient about how he is treated. This anger and malcontent about treatment is far more likely to lead to legal action than any other cause, including the quality of care delivered. Before discussing specific legal problems in prehospital care, some basic terms must be defined:

*Plaintiff:* The person who *complains* or who sues (for the EMT, this would probably be the patient or his family).

*Defendant:* The person being sued or who is defending himself against a complaint (for example, the EMT or his employer).

*Duty:* In legal actions the person who sues must prove that an individual or agency failed in a duty involving him, or that there was a *breach* of duty. Furthermore, the plaintiff must prove that *damage* or harm was done as a result of the breach of duty and that the defendant was the *proximate cause* of the damage or injury. These four elements must be proven by the plaintiff in order for him to win the suit or be awarded compensation:

- duty
- breach of duty
- harm or damage resulting
- proximate cause

*Malpractice:* Professional misconduct, unreasonable lack of skill in professional duties, evil practice, or illegal or immoral conduct. Malpractice means that wrong or poor care resulted in the suffering, further injury, or death to the patient, and that it proceeded from ignorance, carelessness, disregard of rules or principles, neglect, or malicious or criminal intent to do harm.

*Negligence:* Failure to do something which a reasonable and prudent person would do under the same or similar circumstances. (Distinguishing negligence and malpractice is difficult, so many authorities consider them synonymous.)

## UNDERSTANDING THE COMPONENTS OF A LAWSUIT

The best defense of the EMT or any other health care worker is to conduct himself according to the standards of practice expected of a well-trained, skilled and prudent peer under the same or similar circumstances.

### Duty

An EMT has a very specific duty as he functions in the prehospital care environment, not only to the patients being served, but to all others in the environment. For example, the EMT has a *duty* or obligation to provide prompt transport of a critically ill patient, but he also has a *duty* to his fellow man in the streets or on the highway. Driving at excessive speeds, failure to take all precautions at intersections, or careless handling of the vehicle could result in harm to others; thus, the EMT would be considered *negligent* in the performance of duty.

The environment that an EMT finds himself in affects his obligation to provide care. If in street clothes and off-duty, there is no obligation to provide care to a person in distress. If in uniform or recognized as an EMT (by bumper stickers and emblems on clothes or vehicles), there is a duty to treat a stranger according to the standards of care for the given situation. This means that the treatment rendered is prudent, that appropriate judgment has been rendered, and that skillful performance of tasks ensues. On the other hand, if the EMT was under the influence of alcohol or drugs, was careless, or lacked the appropriate training to execute the care, it would represent serious liability.

The EMT should be alert to the fact that there is a *duty* when he is recognized as an EMT. The general public has a right to expect intervention in emergencies by qualified individuals. If the EMT is anonymous and could not be identified as an EMT, there is no legal obligation to provide care. (Most EMTs, however, would probably have a sense of moral obligation to a fellow man in a life-threatening situation, thus choosing to provide care even though there is no legal obligation.)

The *duty* of health care personnel is also influenced by statutory law of a state. For example, if a state law forbids providing certain care without licensure or certification, the EMT would be practicing illegally, unless he possessed the given licensure or certification. The laws that govern ambulance personnel and equipment in the various states are examples of statutory legislation (man-made).

A breach of duty is exemplified by an EMT whose conduct does not represent a reasonable standard of care. For example, if an EMT has not been taught to place an endotracheal tube, it would be considered a breach of duty for him to do so, because it would represent an unnecessary risk to the patient. If the state laws forbid endotracheal intubation by an EMT, any attempt to place an endotracheal tube would be a breach of statutory duty.

### Proximate Cause

Proximate cause means that there is a cause and effect relationship between the care and the results of care. For example, if an EMT fails to stabilize a cervical spine before extrication from a vehicle and the cervical spine is transected in removing the victim, the EMT's actions (and lack of reasonable and prudent care) could be directly linked to the outcome of irreversible spinal cord injury.

If a pulseless and nonbreathing patient is encountered and the EMT performs CPR and fractures a few ribs, there would be no easy way to prove that the patient died from fractured ribs! The care given did not obviously make the situation worse. The provision of CPR is always safe if it is done on a pulseless, nonbreathing patient.

Every practicing EMT has only one duty to the patients he encounters. That duty is to perform as other well-trained and prudent EMTs would under the same or similar circumstances. Furthermore, he should not execute any procedure unless he has had the training and is authorized to do the procedure under the terms of statutory law (e.g., within the scope of licensure or certification).

## GOOD SAMARITAN LEGISLATION

Good Samaritan legislation exists in most states to ensure protection for persons who render emergency care to strangers. Laws are predicated on the fact that the individual providing aid is acting in good faith.

EMTs as health care providers are bound by "duty" as previously described. The so-called Good Samaritan laws were designed to protect individuals with right intentions, but there are no documented cases in which a medical "Good Samaritan" has been protected by such legislation. It seems that laws such as these are useful primarily to reduce the legal anxiety level of emergency care givers who provide nonofficial services to strangers. Good Samaritan legislation is not of a practical concern for the qualified EMT.

## PROTECTION AGAINST BEING SUED

The EMT can avoid being involved in a lawsuit primarily by displaying reasonable action, skill, and sensitivity toward the patient and his loved ones. Most suits are the result of angry, unhappy people who are "getting even" with the individuals whom they perceive as "wrongdoers" —not just in the care provided, but by the attitude and concern as they interact with the ill and injured.

EMTs can protect themselves against suits in several specific ways that reflect their commitment to the public.

First, they should be cognizant that their training and skill maintenance is paramount. Documentation of in-service activities, continuing education, and conformity to care standards are important. If an EMT can demonstrate that his education and work record reflects sound performance, these factors alone will be important if a defense of performance is required.

Recordkeeping cannot be emphasized enough! The EMT must document his activities as he assesses a patient and provides care. If obtaining orders or medical direction is necessary, this must be noted carefully according to a specific format. It is essential to note times, environmental conditions, basic care provided, and observations about the responses to treatment. Care that is not documented is considered not given. For example, if an EMT does not chart "all peripheral pulses intact," it could be assumed that they were not even assessed. If postural vital signs are not recorded, there is reason to believe that they were not elicited. Charting is a critical task of every EMT.

Charting should convey what can be supported by objective evidence. Do not note that the patient was combative and uncooperative. Rather, indicate what behavior occurred that led you to your conclusion. For example, state, "The patient hit me in the face twice as I tried to take his blood pressure. Blood pressure not recorded on the scene." Do not say, "The patient was drunk." State, "Empty whiskey bottle on table. Patient smells of alcohol." Do not record, "Patient is shocky." State, "Unresponsive, BP 70/40, P 146, R 44 and shallow. Skin pale, cool, and clammy. Peripheral pulses easily obliterated." Essentially, avoid subjective statements that you cannot support with objective data. Record the objective data and let others draw their conclusions.

When there are unusual circumstances, such as a patient refuses to be transported after your advising him that it is necessary for proper care, have your partner witness the patient's refusal to obtain definitive treatment by placing his signature with yours noting "witness." Be certain to note instructions that are given in the prehospital care setting for alternate care, referral, or follow-up. For instance, "Refused transportation for child to hospital via ambulance," or, "Advised parents that fever and vomiting can indicate serious illness. Urged them to contact private pediatrician and/or arrange transport to hospital this evening." Avoid global statements such as, "Parents advised," or "Parents given follow-up instructions."

When charting care, use only approved abbreviations. Do not incorporate codes or cryptic messages into documentation of care, since others will be required to decipher your record later, and chances are you will not be available to interpret your notes.

## Consent for Treatment

Individuals who are competent have an inherent right to decide what will happen to their bodies. They may choose to be treated or not be treated. If the patient himself summons the services of an emergency medical crew, it is implied or assumed that he is asking for care or consenting to treatment. *Implied consent* is nonverbal and represents a willingness for an act to occur. However, if another interested person (i.e., spouse, friend, neighbor) calls the EMTs, the patient may choose not to submit to care. If an individual says or indicates that he does not want care, the EMT cannot force his services without risking charges of *battery*, or the unlawful touching of another person without consent. *Informed consent* means that the patient understands what is being done for him and if there are risks, that he is aware of them. For example, an individual who agrees to ambulance transport to a hospital implies that he understands the hazards of transport and the consequences of nontransport. This consent does not require a signature, but the EMT has an expressed obligation to fully explain what is happening, why, and the risks of not doing what is being proposed. Immediate treatment may be given to safeguard health or preserve life—even without a consent. When the age or condition of an individual makes a consent impractical, it is considered implied.

If minors younger than fourteen are involved in an emergency, consent should be obtained from parents when possible for all care beyond immediate lifesaving care. The consent must be an *informed* consent. Children who are fourteen years old or older must give consent along with a parent or guardian, unless a condition exists that would render them unable to provide consent.

*Emancipated minors* (fourteen or older) may be a sole consenting party to treatment if they are married, self-supporting, and maintaining their own home.

EMTs should provide basic life support and emergency care in any situation which poses a serious threat to life or health (regardless of an implied, informed, or written consent) since a failure to do so would ordinarily constitute a breach of duty. However, if a competent adult refuses additional care or transportation, he should not be further cared for but advised of the risks inherent in a failure to continue care at a definitive treatment center. Even most psychiatric patients retain a right under the law to refuse treatment because the majority of states permit them to continue to manage their own affairs. Of course, if they are endangering themselves or others, certain emergency measures are in order under the doctrine of implied consent.

Furthermore, adults under the influence of drugs or alcohol may not be competent to grant consent either, and thus implied consent is used to justify emergency care in the prehospital arena.

## Withdrawal of Consent

If consent is withdrawn, direct care must cease unless the patient's life would be directly threatened, of if the withdrawal of consent is done in an instant of pain or anger, thus not representing a rational mind. An EMT, who is applying pressure to control arterial bleeding, for example, should not release the pressure if a patient says, "Stop squeezing my arm. That hurts, now get away from me!"

## False Imprisonment

False imprisonment is the intentional confining of a person without legal justification or consent. Impeding freedom of movement can result in harm under certain cases, and if it does, an EMT could be sued. For instance, consider an EMT who locks a patient in the ambulance and hauls him to a hospital against his will, and the patient is injured during the course of the treatment en route. Since the patient had no escape from the wrongdoing, the act of the EMT might be considered *false imprisonment*. Threats of confinement, as well as locked doors or restraints, constitute false imprisonment under certain circumstances, as well, so it is imperative to avoid threats in order to obtain a patient's cooperation or compliance.

## Child Abuse Reporting

In every state it is a legal responsibility for health professionals to report suspected child abuse or neglect. There is no requirement for the reporter to be able to prove the occurrence; the only element is a *suspicion* that wrongful acts have occurred, and the report has been made in good faith. States guarantee immunity from legal recourse for the reporter in such reportings. Furthermore, most states make it a crime to fail to file a report of suspected abuse or neglect, e.g., a statutory duty. The failure of duty is therefore *negligence* if further harmful abuse or neglect of the child occurs after the issue of suspicion has been raised. In some states, a child may be retained for protection by health professionals. The EMT should be familiar with the statutory requirements of the state in which he practices. (See page 122.)

## Sexual Assault (Rape)

The victim of rape or sexual assault may be encountered by the EMT. *Informed consent* is essential to treat this individual. The EMT is obligated to notify the police, but the patient does not have to talk with them or to permit a rape examination to be completed at the hospital.

In completing forms, the EMT should take care to note: "Patient states that she was raped." Do not say, "Patient raped," since you cannot determine this in the field. Objective evidence of a struggle, however, should be charted.

Usual emergency measures should be taken as needed for nongenital injuries, but the EMT should *not attempt any genital examination in the field.* Furthermore, no probing questions should be asked about the incident. Specific documentation of the rape account should only be obtained by a police officer or qualified rape crisis counselor at the hospital.

Ensure the patient's privacy and provide support and comfort en route to the hospital. Avoid any judgmental comments about her actions or the alleged rapist's actions. A quiet, caring approach will be appreciated by the individual who has suffered this grave psychological and physical insult.

*Summary*

Many fine legal points are beyond the scope of this book. The EMT will need to be knowledgeable about his own state's laws and how they relate to a role in prehospital care.

The EMT's best defense is to be skilled and operating in good faith in the provision of emergency care. Careful communications, indicating sensitivity to the patient, and precise objective documentation of care will be useful in limiting liability associated with emergency medical technician practice.

*References*

Armington, Catherine L. "Legal Implications in Emergency Services," *Nursing Clinics of North America*, 9:445–451, September 1974.

Moritz, Alan R., and Morris, R. Crawford. *Handbook of Legal Medicine*, 4th ed. St. Louis: The C. V. Mosby Co.,1975.

Murchison, Irene A., and Nichols, Thomas S. *Legal Foundations of Nursing Practice*. New York: The Macmillan Company, 1970.

Page, James O. "Legal Issues Involved With Basic and Advanced Life Support." Lecture given at Paramedic Parameters '77 (National Conference on Pre-Hospital Care). University of Southern California School of Medicine, September 2, 1977.

Willig, Sidney H. *The Nurse's Guide to The Law*. New York: McGraw-Hill Book Company, 1970.

# Chapter 8

# Assessment: General Principles and Skills

Prehospital patient assessment skills are among the most demanding yet important an EMT can possess. It is the basis for good patient care. Patient assessment in actuality is more than a skill; it is an art. It requires the senses of seeing, hearing, touching, and smelling. Patient assessment requires the EMT to be an investigator, interviewer, identifier, adjustor, and at times an intermediary, integrator, and reporter. The EMT must perform all these roles quickly, yet be able to change the line of reasoning or the treatment when cued to do so by medical changes in the patient or situational circumstances.

In the field there is more than just the patient. You will have to cope with the environment in which you find your patient, as well as the situation surrounding his illness or injury. Unlike the controlled atmosphere of an emergency department you will have to deal with weather conditions, poor lighting, bystanders, and obstructions to your maneuverability, as well as the movement of the patient. In spite of these obstacles, you cannot lose sight of your primary responsibility—the patient!

The process of patient assessment begins long before the emergency call is received and continues after the patient is delivered to the emergency department. The starting point of patient assessment is in the fundamental medical knowledge an EMT has to enable him to suspect, recognize, and properly treat the illnesses or injuries. As an EMT, you cannot expect to perform a good patient assessment unless you are cognizant of the signs and symptoms that accompany certain illness or injury. You must be able to integrate presenting information into proper lines of reasoning that will help you determine immediate and future care of your patient. For example, if you do not have the ability to recognize signs and symptoms of a heart attack, you cannot expect to ask pertinent questions concerning the patient's medical problem. From the basis of medical knowledge, the EMT can evaluate, examine and interview the patient, identify and prioritize medical problems, and intervene accordingly.

Life or death situations should be promptly recognized and managed without question. Injuries must be looked at in terms of what is visible to you, what else may be injured, and what complications you might expect because of the particular injury, even though presenting signs and symptoms may not be obvious.

The whole patient assessment is then continued by a follow-up of the patient at the hospital and feedback given you on the final diagnosis of the patient by the attending physician. It is important to your self-safisfaction to know that you treated the patient appropriately. The effectiveness of an EMT is reflected by feedback, and depends upon an ability to perform a complete patient assessment and then utilize that information to reduce suffering and prolong the life of the patient.

The EMT cannot be expected to perform without some experience. The art and skill of patient assessment takes months of practice before the EMT develops a feeling of comfort and possesses a "streetwise" intuition about the patient.

## CONSIDERATIONS IN COMMUNICATION—PREARRIVAL PHASE

Ideally, every call for medical assistance should be answered by an EMT. When the call is received it is necessary to find out more than just the location of the patient. Information about the patient, his particular problem, condition, and extenuating circumstances can be vital to the survival of the patient and possibly, the safety of the responding EMT. When an EMT receives the emergency call, he can give instructions so the caller can initiate proper treatment and the responding unit can be informed as to the number of patients, hazardous conditions, directions to the scene, and other helpful pertinent information. Should hazardous conditions exist, such as fires, toxic fumes or violent crimes, appropriate agencies must be notified as soon as possible for the protection of everyone involved. (See Fig. 8-1.)

While en route to the emergency scene, the EMT should utilize the information received from the EMT communications operator and mentally prepare and adjust for the situation he may encounter. The EMT (non-driver) should review in his mind the various illnesses or injuries that may be present, and the signs and symptoms by which they can be recognized. For instance, if the call is to an auto accident, head, spinal, and internal injuries associated with rapid deceleration may be present and the EMT can mentally remind himself to take all spinal cord damage precautions and anticipate possible hypovolemic shock. On the other hand, if the call is to a patient with chest pain, the signs, symptoms and treatment of heart attack should be reviewed.

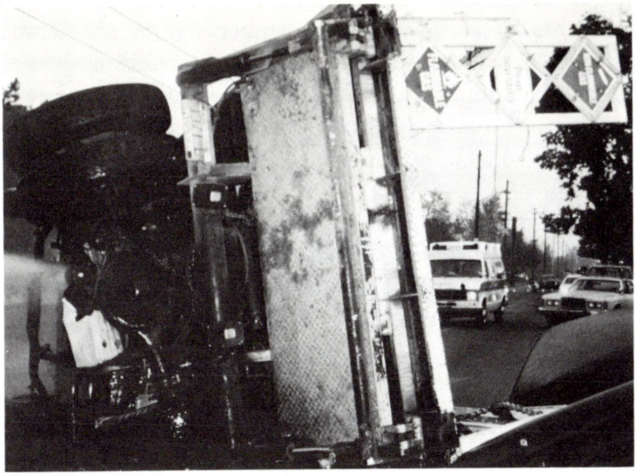

**Figure 8–1.** When specific hazardous conditions exist on the scene, the EMT-A should notify the communications center so that appropriate safety and rescue agencies can be notified of the situation. (Courtesy of Wishard Memorial Hospital. Photo by Bob Biehn.)

The EMT should develop assessments for medical as well as trauma patients, and utilize mental checklists to go over important points concerning each. Very rarely does every emergency run turn out the way you think it will, and oftentimes what you think the problem is, is not at all what you actually encounter. Mental preparedness is essential. The EMT should expect the worst circumstances and be prepared to deal with them. He should *never assume* anything concerning the medical stability of the patient. Only a thorough assessment of each patient will satisfy your responsibility.

## ON-THE-SCENE ASSESSMENT—ARRIVAL PHASE

Upon arrival at the emergency scene, many bits of information must be gathered and numerous tasks performed in an atmosphere that is generally less than ideal. As a result, a sense of teamwork among all emergency medical personnel on the scene is vital for efficient assessment and treatment of the patient. Among the basic elements of teamwork are (1) one EMT should be in charge of patient care; (2) one EMT should talk to the patient; and (3) no more than four EMTs should be directly involved with the treatment of the patient. Cooperation by all persons involved insures a small, organized team working with continuity and efficiency.

Basic observations should be made upon the initial approach to the scene. These observations will not only be helpful in the overall patient evaluation, but will supply helpful information to the physician and nurse back at the hospital. The EMT must remember that the physician and nurse are not with you, so all pieces of information surrounding the patient must be documented. This information starts with environmental conditions: Is it raining? snowing? Extremely hot or cold? Is it day or night? foggy? muddy? icy? Is the inside of the house dirty and disorganized? Might it breed disease and poor hygiene? Are there animals? As you approach the patient, look around. Are there liquor bottles? medicine containers? drug paraphernalia? Is the inside of the house unreasonably hot or cold? Are there insects, lice, bedbugs, cockroaches? Is there evidence of violence, such as weapons, blood spills, and broken furniture? Are there other people in the house? Who do they appear to be—friends, family, outsiders? What kind of neighborhood are you in? It is always wise whenever approaching any door to stand to the side of it and knock. Do not put yourself directly in front of it. Some people may not be expecting an EMT, and may fire a weapon through the door! All types of information that you can elicit will be important to the medical personnel at the emergency department. Certainly a history of alcohol or drug abuse, and domestic violence, for example, is an important factor in caring for the patient in the emergent phase and to plan for appropriate follow-up with other health care agencies and personnel, i.e., the social worker or drug treatment center.

It is important that the EMT preserve crime scenes. If, upon your arrival, the police are not present and you find the patient a victim of a violent crime, take care to not tamper with evidence that may aid the police. Weapons should not be handled and if your patient is dead on arrival, do not attempt to move him or anything around him. If the police are not en route, have the communications operator notify them.

The family of the patient or bystanders in the area may show an air of indifference, anger, fear, or panic. It is important that the EMT recognize that these feelings may or may not be appropriate for the situation, and may have a dramatic effect on the patient. In many cases, the patient's apparent condition will change dramatically when moved from a hectic, crowded home or accident scene to a calm and controlled atmosphere inside the ambulance.

## GENERAL OBSERVATIONS AND INITIAL DATA COLLECTION

The EMT should note the dress, facial expression, mood, and general appearance of the patient. The location of the patient, his position, and initial apparent condition, as well as interviews with the family and bystanders, will help in determining the three vital factors contributing to the patient's condition.

1. *History of the incident (what happened).* In any situation, (especially accidents), a brief explanation of the overall incident that

resulted in the injury or illness is quite helpful. If the patient was in an auto accident, it is helpful to note where the patient was seated, the angle of impact, the kind of vehicles or other structures involved in the accident. Besides satisfying natural curiosity, this information is very helpful in understanding the mechanism of injuries and in predicting specific consequences.

2. *Mechanism of injury (what caused the injuries).* The mechanism of injury refers to exactly what aspect of the situation caused injury. In most cases this can only be inferred by evidence around the patient. For instance, in an automobile accident, the mechanisms of injury might include the head striking the windshield, the chest hitting the steering wheel, or the abdomen or chest compressed sharply by the seat or shoulder belt. The mechanism of injury is necessary to understand the injury potential. (See Fig. 8–2.)

3. *Injury potential (what injuries may have occurred and how severe might they be).* The injury potential means those injuries that may have been caused by the mechanisms of injury, and the potential severity of those injuries. It is at this point that the EMT must know his topographic and internal anatomy, and how they relate with what may have been injured internally. The injury potential is the key that shows the EMT just what injuries to suspect and check for. It is extremely important, however, for the EMT to realize that if the mechanism and the potential for an injury exists, but no signs or symptoms are seen, the injury may exist anyway. Many of the body's protective mechanisms against shock may hide discernible signs and symptoms of significant injuries. As a result, the history of the incident, the mechanism of injury, and the injury potential may be the only clues that the EMT has to a serious injury or illness.

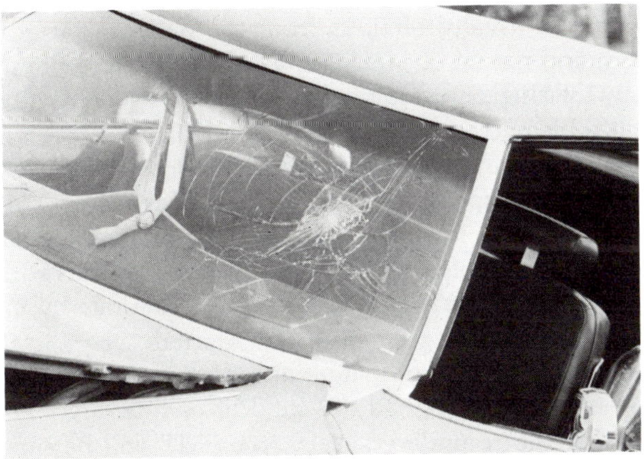

**Figure 8–2.** The EMT-A should try to determine the mechanism of injury in all trauma. In this case, the driver's portion of the windshield has been fractured, possibly indicating head or cervical spine trauma to the patient.

The primary survey of the patient starts the moment your eyes make contact with him. The primary survey consists of a rapid evaluation of the ABCs (*A*irway, *B*reathing, and *C*irculation,) and immediate correction of any compromise that may be found. This is the first and most important process of patient assessment.

Patient care is futile without an open airway, adequate breathing, and circulating blood. Regardless of what other problems exist, any compromise of the airway is the first problem that the EMT must correct. (See Chapter 10 for a complete discussion.)

## Vital Signs

The vital signs should be observed and measured upon starting the patient assessment and retaken every ten minutes for as long as the EMT is with the patient. In those cases where the patient's signs and symptoms are changing rapidly, vital signs should be observed and measured every five minutes. The EMT must realize that one set of vital signs actually provides a very limited amount of information. The true value of vital signs comes when a number of sets are taken and compared. It is the change or lack of change in a patient's vital signs that is truly meaningful. Each patient that the EMT transports to the hosptial should have vital signs measured a minimum of two times. (See Chapter 9 for a complete discussion of vital signs.)

## Pain

While pain is usually obvious from the patient's facial expression, body position, and nature of injury, it should be explored in more detail. Pain is usually the single most important clue as to what is actually causing the patient's problem.

Location of the pain is of primary importance. The patient should be encouraged to try to pinpoint the exact location of the worst pain area. It is helpful to ask the patient to point to the spot of worst pain with one finger. The point of worst pain, often, but not always, corresponds with the site of the primary illness or injury. The EMT should continue by exploring all aspects of the pain including where it first started; where it radiates; the quality, severity, tenderness on palpation; what makes the pain better or worse; and if the patient has had this kind of pain before.

Throughout the secondary survey, the EMT will be simultaneously interviewing the patient and performing a complete head-to-toe physical examination. Starting with the head and neck, palpate for deformities and painful areas, moving downward to the chest, abdomen and back, and then the upper and lower extremities. Major problems should be treated immediately. Make notes of the problem areas, and then return to those points for a more detailed survey.

With practice, the entire process that we have discussed so far, including blood pressure, pulse, and respiration measurements can be completed in two to three minutes. Then the EMT can move on to a more detailed assessment of problem areas.

## THE SECONDARY SURVEY

Since the EMT has established the presence or absence of the basic components of life and intervened where necessary, he now has more time to do a thorough and systematic assessment of the patient. The secondary survey consists of the examination of the patient's level of consciousness; an interview of the patient, exploring the patient's perception of the problem; and a detailed examination of each body system. In actual practice, many of the components of the primary and secondary surveys take place simultaneously. Teamwork is important. With an organized team, each facet of patient assessment can be carried out quickly and with little duplication.

### Level of Consciousness (LOC)

Because it is usually obvious, the level of consciousness is often overlooked as an important vital sign. The brain is the most sensitive organ of the body to a lack of oxygen and of vital nutrients such as sugar, and to injury. The level of consciousness is controlled by the brain and therefore, is one of the first signs to change in the face of chemical imbalance and injuries to the body. Anytime that a patient's level of consciousness is anything but totally conscious, alert, and oriented to time, place and person, the EMT can be certain that something is acting to hinder proper brain function. Again, a change in the level of consciousness is one of the first signs to appear before any other vital sign. A decreasing level of consciousness (that is, a progressive inability of the patient to stay awake and to orient himself to time, place or person), may be indicative of alcohol or drug intoxication, swelling of the brain due to injury, or reduced oxygen available to the brain. In any case, the EMT should keep a close watch on the changes that take place and consider what may be causing the problem. Since the brain is most sensitive to oxygen levels, the proper administration of supplemental oxygen will improve the brain's ability to function as well as give vital organs additional oxygen.

The EMT must realize that the outward behavior of a patient is greatly influenced by his physical condition and oxygen level. For instance, an injured patient may be agitated and possibly violent, simply due to a loss of blood which means that less oxygen is being transported to the brain. Such situations require a strong, professional attitude on the part of the EMT to treat the patient carefully and completely and not take the actions of the patient as a personal attack. (See section on Management of the Unconscious Patient.)

## Patient Interview

One of the most important functions in patient assessment is that of interviewing the patient. The patient interview should be performed by one EMT who stays with the patient from the beginning until the patient is transported to the emergency department.

From the patient's point of view, a medical emergency, especially outside the hosptial, is extremely frightening. As such, the patient needs to have one person with whom he can speak, ask questions, trust, and receive assurance. By using a single interviewer the patient's fears are greatly reduced. Information received in a calm, supportive interchange usually will need to be said only once.

In his approach to the patient, the EMT must be friendly, gentle, and tactful but firm and confident in what he is doing. The first thing the EMT should do is introduce himself and establish a relaxed but concerned rapport with the patient. The conversation should aim to find out from the patient what medical problems he has and other related information. Realize and respect the patient's need for quiet, but also realize that certain medical information is necessary for treatment and care. When questioning the patient as to specific problems, try to avoid questions that the patient can answer by "yes" or "no". Let the patient talk and describe his injury or illness. We sometimes try to answer the question for the patient and end up knowing less than when we started. The EMT should use open-ended questions such as, "Where do you have pain?" and, "What were you doing when the pain began?" instead of, "Do you have pain in your chest?" and, "Did the pain start after you ate dinner?" The EMT must try to determine as much information as possible surrounding the medical problem of each patient. The following points should be explored in each patient's interview:

### *Chief Complaint(CC)*

The chief complaint refers to what the patient feels is his main problem. The EMT can ask the patient, "What seems to be your problem?" or, "Why did you call the ambulance?" The chief complaint should be recorded in the patient's words. For instance, "I can't make water," "I've got high blood," "I fell", or, "My heart is fluttering." Some patients may use language that should not be fully written on your patient's report form, for example, "I can't sh--." In such cases write the first two letters and add blanks as written above. To the side of the patient's quotes, write your description of the patient's problem. So, if the patient states "I can't sh--," write next to it, "unable to move bowels" or "constipation." It is important to write the chief complaint in the patient's own words because we want to know the patient's perceived problem, and how he relates to it. Often the chief complaint is not the most serious problem. What is important is the fact that the patient thought it was bad enough to call for help. The chief complaint is the first part of the overall information given to the physician when transmitting or writing your patient report. When radio transmitting the chief complaint, the EMT should state the patient's problem in medical terminology. This should also be done when giving information to the nurse or physician upon arrival at the emergency department.

*History of The Present Illness*

The history of the present illness is an objective exploration by the EMT into exactly what the real problem is and how it came about. Basic guidelines of what needs to be asked of the patient are listed below. We will use chest pain as an example.

1. *Location.* The exact location of the pain is necessary. This also includes where the pain goes or radiates to.

2. *Quality or quantity.* The EMT should ask the patient to describe what kind of pain he is having. Character of the pain is important in differential diagnosis of the particular problem. Try to avoid suggesting words such as "sharp," "dull," "heavy," or "crushing." Let the patient use his own words. The patient should also be questioned as to how many episodes of pain he has had in the last twenty-four hours.

3. *Intensity.* The severity of pain is quite subjective and will vary from patient to patient. The EMT should remember that pain is a warning system to the body. Because of this, the body's reaction may include the triggering of the autonomic nervous system which results in diaphoresis (di″ah-fo-re′sis) (sweating). When visible perspiration is detected on the skin, the patient is probably really experiencing tremendous pain. Look at the patient's overall expressions and positions. All of these signs may help in determining the intensity of the pain. Ask the patient if the pain has ever been that bad and when.

4. *Time and situation of onset.* What time the problem started and what was the patient doing at the time are valuable pieces of information in determining the source of the problem.

5. *Comparison.* The patient will often describe pain by comparing it to previous pains. If the patient was hospitalized before, ask the patient why he was hospitalized. Many patients may tell you that they had a heart attack and were put in the hospital. If they tell you they stayed a couple of days, the odds are good it was *not* for a heart attack. Patients who have been in a coronary care unit can tell you just about all you want to know about them! In any case, do not draw premature notions about the credibility of the patient's story; keep an open mind. The pain could be from an ensuing heart attack.

6. *Aggravation and alleviation.* The EMT should ask the patient what makes the pain better or worse. He will get answers such as "I feel better when I sit down and rest" or, "The pain gets worse after I eat spicy foods."

7. *Attempts to modify.* It is important to find out what the patient has done or taken to relieve his medical symptoms. All medications taken by the patient should be noted on the patient's report form.

### *Associated Complaints*

Often, there are other complaints in addition to the chief complaint that may prove to be important in determining the problem such as fainting, feeling dizzy, and vomiting. These problems should be explored in relation to the chief complaint.

### *Past Medical History*

The medical problem that the patient has had in the past can have a relationship upon the present illness. Ask the patient if he has been hospitalized recently or in the past, and for what reason.

### *Medication and Allergies*

The EMT must be sure to obtain a complete list of all medications that are being taken by the patient. Often a patient will stop taking medication or take someone else's medication. It is easy to forget common medications, such as aspirin, birth control pills, cough syrups, and allergy or cold pills. All medications of the patient's and others that the patient is taking must be listed and noted on the patient report form. Because of the vast number of drugs available today, many have similar names. Make sure your spelling is correct when noting them. The EMT should also note any allergies that the patient may have, to certain medications, foods, animals, or other substances. If the patient has an allergy, make sure it is noted on the patient's report form as well.

## Physical Examination

The physical examination of the patient, aside from what has been discussed up to now, includes the measurement of vital signs and an assessment of each body system that may be involved in the illness or injury. It is important that you communicate with the patient and let him know what you are doing. You should try to ask questions about a body system before you examine it, rather than vice versa. For example, if you take the patient's blood pressure and then ask him if he has high blood pressure, he will think that you have found that he has high blood pressure, whether or not you have. This may tend to escalate his overall anxiety.

### *Skin Color*

The color of the skin is an indicator of the amount of circulating blood and oxygen being delivered to the tissues. The skin color of every patient should be assessed. Since the vascularity of the face is great, the lips, tongue, mucous membranes, cheeks, chin, ear lobes, and conjunctiva (kon″junk-ti′vah) are the quickest and easiest locations to check color changes. The extremities—the fingers and toenails—should also be assessed. When the peripheral vessels are dilated the skin is warm and red. When they are constricted the skin is cool and white. The various color changes of the skin can be observed under the following conditions:

1. *Pallor* (whitish tint). The skin is termed *pallid* (pal′ĭd) when the blood vessels have severely constricted. This may be seen in shock, decreased blood flow, anemia, and edema. It occurs in edema because the escaped fluid overlies the vessels and decreases normal color.

2. *Red.* A red color can occur from alcohol ingestion, diabetic coma, allergic reaction, infection, external heat, and cold weather. The skin turns red in cold weather because the oxygen is being used less and since hemoglobin gives the red appearance to the skin there is more of it that shows.

3. *Blue (cyanosis).* A patient that is cyanotic is suffering from decreased blood flow to the tissues. This can be seen in congestive heart failure, airway obstruction, embolism, emphysema, pulmonary edema, and cold weather.

4. *Jaundice (yellowish tint).* Jaundice is caused by an accumulation of bile pigments in the skin and mucous membranes due to liver or gallbladder problems.

5. *Bright Pink—cherry red.* This discoloration occurs in heat stroke and early in carbon monoxide poisoning. In late stages of carbon monoxide poisoning, the skin is cyanotic.

6. *Mottled.* The color pattern here is a mixed pattern of white and blue created by pooled venous blood and circulatory collapse. This is typically seen in cardiac arrest patients who have been "down" for a protracted period of time.

### *Pupils*

The pupils of the eye are valuable indicators of injury and illness. The pupils and eye muscles are controlled by cranial nerves located in the brainstem. Because of this, any injury or illness affecting this area will also affect the pupils and eye movements. Pupils are examined by carefully lifting the upper eyelid and comparing one pupil with the other. Initially, the pupils should be compared for equality in size and shape and then reactivity to light. (See Fig. 8.3.) Reactivity means that when bright light is

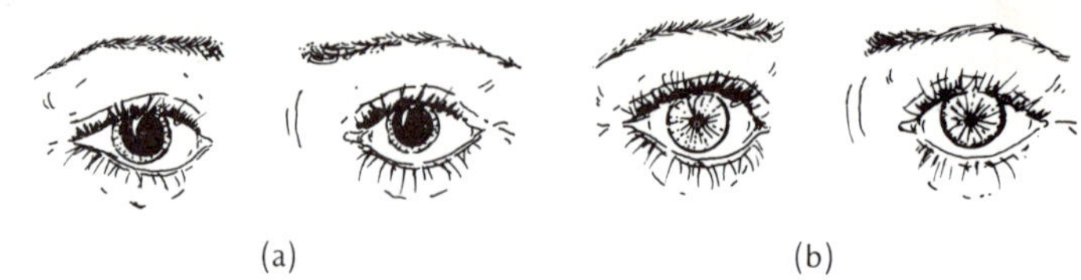


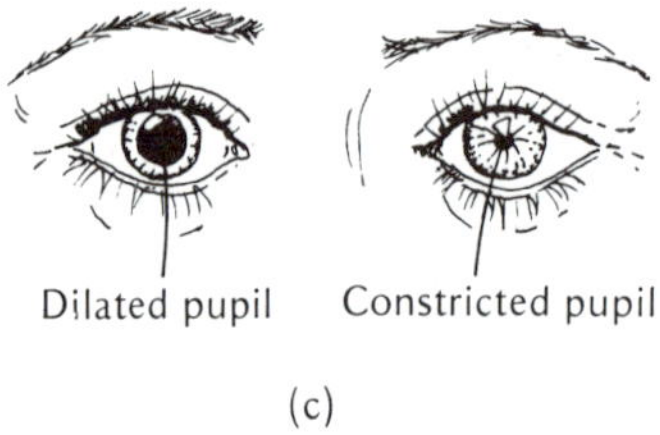


**Figure 8-3.** (a) Dilated pupils; (b) constricted pupils; (c) unequal pupils.

shown in the eye, the pupil gets smaller or constricts. This is a normal reflex mechanism and should be checked in both eyes. When the bright light is removed, the pupils return to their resting state and get bigger or dilate. It should be noted whether the pupils react to light by constricting and whether that constriction is brisk or sluggish, and if it is the same in both eyes. The EMT should be careful not to check pupils for reactivity to light when the patient is in direct sunlight. Instead, the eyes should be shaded and a penlight should be flashed briefly into each pupil separately. Conditions that cause the pupils to remain constricted include some narcotics such as heroin, codeine, morphine; other drugs such as Darvon® ; and central nervous system disease. Conditions that cause the pupils to remain dilated include pain; cardiac arrest; drugs such as atropine (at′ro-pin), LSD, amphetamines (am-fet′a-minz); and fright. Unequal pupils are often seen in patients with head injuries, cerebral edema, and stroke. The EMT must remember that 2 to 4 percent of the population normally have unequal pupils and that cataract surgery may cause one pupil to be smaller than the other. Eye movements should also be assessed. If the patient is conscious, ask him to follow your index finger with both of his eyes focused on the target finger. Move your finger in all planes of vision, moving it up, down, and to both sides while watching if both of the patient's eyes move in unison. Eyes that move together are called *conjugate* (kon′-ju-gāt). The patient with a fracture to the eye orbit (socket) may not be able to move one of his eyes and will have a paralyzed gaze, usually upward.

When the eyes do not move together and turn in different directions, then the movement of the eyes are *dysconjugate* (dis-kon′-ju-gāt). This may be seen in head trauma. Some patients may have a paralyzed gaze to the right or left side of the head. This may also be seen in the stroke or seizure patient. The EMT should be alert for the possibility of a prosthetic (pros-thet′-ik) eyeball (glass eye). If the patient is unconscious, and is wearing contact lenses, they should be removed. The eyes may become dry with contact lenses in place, and serious eye damage may result.

*Other Specific Organ Systems*

The EMT should proceed to evaluate the neurological, cardiovascular, abdominal, and skeletal systems. (See Specific chapters for details.)

## RADIO COMMUNICATION

The communication of information between an EMT in the field and the physician or nurse at the hospital must always be concise and completely understood by both parties. In most cases, the communication is primarily to inform the hospital that you are en route to their facility with a patient(s) and to state his major illness or injury. Sometimes, however, medical instructions are relayed from the hospital to the EMT as to proper treatment. In order to facilitate all types of conversation, the EMT who initiates the communication should do so in a brief, but very informative initial medical report. The initial report can set the stage for the rest of the conversation and often affects the care the patient receives. A clear, concise report that gives the physician or nurse a clear picture of the situation inspires confidence in the EMT from the radio and greatly influences and facilitates patient care. The initial report given by the EMT should be approximately fifty words and should not exceed one minute in transmission duration. In order to include all pertinent patient information in the initial report, it is necessary to assemble all information gained in the assessment survey and sort out what is pertinent for the opening report. Your goal as an EMT is to "paint a picture" for the persons at the hospital of the situation that both you and the patient are in, as well as a description of the patient's condition. The initial report should always follow a set pattern, giving information in an arrangement that will best give an accurate picture of the patient.

### Unit identification

The first part of the report should tell who you are so that the hospital can respond appropriately. For example,

*Ambulance*: "Rescue 14 to Regional Hospital," or if several ambulance services transport patients to area hospitals, "District 11 to Regional Hospital."

*Hospital:* "This is Regional Hospital. Go ahead District 11."

*Ambulance*: "Yes, this is Wishard Ambulance Service District 11, and we are on the scene of a - - - -".

## Age, Sex and Level of Consciousness

These three items are among the first things noticed upon arrival at the patient, and therefore need to be among the first points communicated in order to provide a context for the rest of the information.

## Description of the Incident and Patient Location

The description of the incident and patient location will help "paint the picture" for hospital personnel, and help them realize why you may not be able to answer your radio. If an awkward situation exists, such as patient entrapment, you should contact the personnel as soon as possible.

## Chief Complaint

The chief complaint refers to exactly why the patient (or bystanders) called for medical assistance. Although the chief complaint is often not the most serious problem the patient may have, it is important for the hospital to know what the patient's perception of the problem may be.

## History and Medications

The history of the present problem is the EMT's evaluation of the chief complaint with a brief outline of information gathered during the interview and assessment. The history of the incident and mechanism of injury is included here as well. The patient's pertinent past medical history should be obtained and presented in relation to the present problem.

A list of medications that the patient takes should be included as well as prescription medications that should have been taken but were not.

## Examination Findings

The physical examination report should include signs and symptoms that relate to the chief complaint and other pertinent physical findings. The positioning of the patient, skin color, breath sounds, fractures, wound locations, and so on are included here.

## Vital Signs

The vital signs, including pulse, respiration and blood pressure, need to be reported and then updated when significant changes take place.

## Treatment

The EMT should describe all his treatment rendered to the patient. This may include hemorrhage control, CPR, position of patient during transport, oxygen therapy, application of splints, and shock trousers. The

EMT should also describe treatment given to the patient by bystanders or relatives before his arrival.

### Estimated time of arrival (ETA)

The estimated time of arrival should always be given to the designated hospital physician or nurse so that the hospital can anticipate or prepare for your arrival. In some cases, contact with the hospital is established prior to leaving the scene. In such a situation, the hospital should be informed of the estimated time to transport and then arrival at the hospital. The hospital should also be notified when transportation is initiated.

Throughout the process of patient assessment and treatment, the EMT is often presented with unusual or unexpected circumstances that may hinder treatment, slow the return to the hospital, or interrupt communications. Unless the hospital is informed of these conditions, it will be difficult for them to understand long pauses in radio communication or delays in transportation.

## THE UNCONSCIOUS PATIENT

When EMTs encounter an unconscious or seemingly unresponsive patient, it is imperative that a systematic approach be used in the initial assessment and in field management. There are many conditions that can lead to an unconscious state. It is less important for prehospital personnel to determine the *cause* for the unresponsive state, however, than to plan to protect the victim from further complications in the field and to ensure a safe transfer to a receiving hospital.

### Initial Considerations

#### *Airway Breathing and Circulation*

The ABCs of basic life support are always the first priorities in assessment. Cardiac arrest is a possibility in every event that involves an unresponsive state. (See Chapter 10.) If the airway is patent, breathing is apparent, and the carotid (kah-rot'id) pulse is detectable, the EMT can proceed to subsequent steps in the assessment process.

#### *Response to Verbal Stimuli*

Call the patient's name if known, or offer other verbal stimuli such as asking for a name or determining if the individual knows where he is. This simple contact can tell you if the victim is alert and oriented, confused, or drowsy. It may be necessary to use loud, repeated verbalization to evoke a response. It is wise to combine this with "shaking" or other physical provocation to guard against reaching a wrong conclusion when dealing with the "heavy sleeper" or hard of hearing. (The EMT should always exercise caution when shaking a patient if injuries, especially spinal injuries, are suspected.) If a verbal response is obtained, be alert to speech difficulties or apparent confusion as you listen. If no response is obtained from verbal stimuli, then employ painful stimulation.

*Response to Painful Stimuli*

Do not use cruel or unusual forms of painful stimuli in evoking a response, even if you suspect that the patient is pretending to be unconscious. Slapping the face or pulling pubic hair are not acceptable methods to attempt arousal. The recommended methods of evaluating a response to pain involve exerting pressure on certain nerves that are quite vulnerable to stimuli. Sternal *compression* using your knuckles (not abrasive "rubbing"), thumb pressure over the orbital ridge, and trapezius muscle pinching are acceptable. (See Fig. 8-4.)

Describe the response to the pain rather than just stating that there is a response. For example, note that "the patient responds to sternal compression by moaning and shaking his head."

It is extremely valuable to note whether or not the response to stimuli elicits a bilateral response. Does the patient attempt to withdraw or "strike out" using only one arm? Does only one portion of the body seem affected? It is important to test all extremities and both sides of the body before concluding that indeed the victim is truly unconscious.

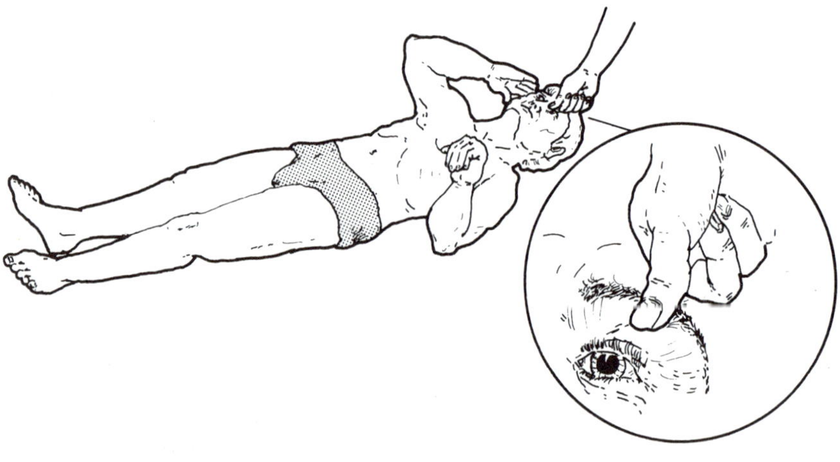

**Figure 8-4.** Orbital ridge pressure. Thumb should press on bone just above the eyeball near or on the midline.

## Use of the Glasgow Coma Scale to Rate Level of Consciousness

The Glasgow coma scale has been designed to quantitatively relate consciousness to motor responses, verbal responses, and eye opening. Coma is defined as no response and no eye opening. Scores of seven or less on the Glasgow scale qualify as "coma"; scores of nine or more do not qualify as "coma." The examiner determines the best response the patient can make to a set of standardized stimuli. Higher points are assigned to responses that indicate higher degrees of arousal.

1. *Best motor response.* (Examiner determines the best response of either arm.)

   a. *Six points.* Obeys simple commands. Raises arm on request or holds up specified number of fingers. Releasing a grip (not grasping, which can be reflexive) is also an appropriate test.

   b. *Five points.* Localizes noxious (nok′shus) stimuli. Fails to obey commands but can move either arm toward a noxious cutaneous (ku-ta′ne-us) stimuli and eventually contacts it with the hand. The stimuli should be maximal and applied in various locations, i.e., sternal compression or trapezius pinch.

   c. *Four points.* Flexion withdrawal. Responds to noxious stimuli with arm flexion but does not localize it with the hand.

   d. *Three points.* Abnormal flexion. Adducts shoulder, flexes and pronates arm, flexes wrist, and makes a fist in response to a noxious stimuli (decorticate [de″kor-ti-kāt] rigidity).

   e. *Two points.* Abnormal extension. Adducts and internally rotates shoulder, extends forearm, flexes wrist, and makes a fist in response to a noxious stimuli (decerebrate [de-ser′ĕ-brāt] rigidity).

   f. *One point.* No motor response. Exclude reasons for no response, e.g., insufficient stimulus or spinal cord injury.

2. *Best verbal response.* (Examiner determines the best response after arousal. Noxious stimuli are employed if necessary.) Omit this test if the patient is dysphasic (cannot speak), has oral injuries, or is intubated. Place a checkmark after other two test category scores after totaling to indicate omission of the verbal response section.

   a. *Five points.* Oriented patient. Can converse and relate who he is, where he is, and the year and month.

   b. *Four points.* Confused patient. Is not fully oriented or demonstrates confusion.

   c. *Three points.* Verbalizes. Does not engage in sustained conversation, but uses intelligible words in an exclamation (curse) or in a disorganized nonsensical, manner.

d. *Two points.* Vocalizes. Makes moaning or groaning sounds that are not recognizable words.

e. *One point.* No vocalization. Does not make any sound even in response to noxious stimulus.

3. *Eye opening.* (Examiner determines the minimum stimulus that evokes opening of one or both eyes.) If the patient cannot realistically open the eyes because of bandages or lid edema, write "E" after the total score to indicate omission of this component.

a. *Four points.* Eyes open spontaneously.

b. *Three points.* Eyes open to speech. Patient opens eyes in response to command or on being called by name.

c. *Two points.* Eyes open to noxious stimuli.

d. *One point.* No eye opening in response to noxious stimuli.

## MANAGEMENT OF THE UNCONSCIOUS PATIENT

### Airway

The airway should be protected by placing the patient in the left, lateral semi-prone position with the head slightly dependent. (See Fig. 8–5.) Remove dentures if they are loose. Use the jaw thrust or chin-lift maneuvers to open the airway and place an oral-pharyngeal airway if it does not produce gagging. Suction the airway as necessary to remove secretions. Oxygen by nasal cannula at 6–8 *l*/min. should be administered. If there is need for assisted ventilations, use a bag-valve mask.

### Vital Signs

Measure the blood pressure, pulse, and respiratory rates and take the patient's temperature if feasible. (See Chapter 9.) If signs of shock are present such as tachycardia, tachypnea, (tak″ip-ne′ah) hypotension, pale, cool skin or cyanosis, place the patient in shock position and transport.

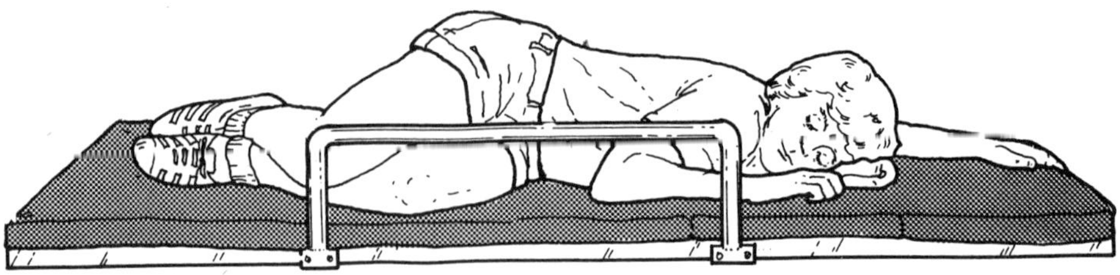

**Figure 8–5.** Semi-prone, or side-lying, position for a comatose patient. The head is elevated slightly and turned so that the secretions may drool from the dependent corner of the mouth.

## History-Taking

As the EMT cares for the unconscious patient, a history should be elicited if there are friends or family members present to provide data.

The timing and nature of the onset of the unconscious state is valuable to learn. Illnesses, complaints, injuries, problems experienced just prior to the episode, or recent drug or alcohol comsumption should be noted. If there are no personal contacts who can provide clues to the present episode, be sure to check for Medic-Alert tags or wallet cards with medical information. Even a bottle of medicine on a bedside stand or a prescription drug in a bathroom cabinet or purse may provide valuable clues to the unconscious state.

# CAUSES OF UNCONSCIOUSNESS

Unconsciousness can result from primary problems in the brain or can be a response to brain disturbances caused by generalized illness. Let us explore some of the typical causes of the unconscious state:

*Circulatory Failure.* The brain is dependent upon a constant supply of blood to supply oxygen and nutrients so vital to its functioning. Any factor which interferes with its circulation can lead to unconsciousness. Hypotension (low blood pressure), a blockage of major blood vessels in the neck or head, brain hemorrhage, or poor cardiac pumping action are common causes. Any history of cardiac or circulatory problems (e.g., heart attacks, dysrhythmias [dis-rith′me-ahz] high blood pressure, blood clots, previous strokes) would be predisposing factors.

*Metabolic Problems.* The brain cells need to be surrounded by a chemical environment which sustains their life processes. When the composition of this environment is adversely altered, electrical activity of cells is modified, and brain dysfunction ensues. Drug overdose, excessive alcohol ingestion, inhalation of toxic chemicals, fluid and electrolyte disturbances, and diabetic states which alter blood sugar levels are examples.

*Mechanical Insult.* Like any vital tissue, the brain needs a certain space where it can be protected from injury. The cranial vault provides a bony shield for the delicate structure and the cerebrospinal fluid serves as a "shock absorber." Despite these protective features, the brain can be injured in trauma states and becomes compressed if there is any swelling, tumor growth, or abnormally high intracranial pressure. A high level of generalized intracranial pressure or structural damage to certain vital areas can lead to unconsciousness.

*Other Causes.* Many seizure patients remain in an unconscious state for several minutes or even hours after the attack. Severe infections, carbon monoxide poisoning, and hypoxia from any cause can lead to unconsciousness. It is valuable, therefore, for medical personnel to consider a comprehensive evaluation of all body systems in determining the cause.

## Protecting the Unconscious Patient

Although an individual is unconscious, he can often receive messages by sight and hearing, even though he is incapable of responding. Talk to the individual and reassure him even though he seems totally unresponsive. He may hear and understand since these senses are often the last ones to be affected.

Be extremely careful to protect the unconscious patient from further injury during transport. Remember, he cannot tell you that he is lying on his dentures or that this hand is caught under your stretcher railing! Be especially gentle in lifting and moving, since the patient is totally dependent on you and cannot help himself. If the blink reflex is absent, the eyes should be closed and covered with gauze squares to protect the cornea.

Throughout transport, the EMT should continue to assess the patient's level of consciousness and monitor vital signs. However, as always, the airway and breathing should receive top priority.

*References*

Barber J., and Budassi, S. *Mosby's Manual of Emergency Care: Practice and Procedures.* St. Louis, Mo: The C. V. Mosby Co., 1979.

Bates, Barbara. *A Guide to Physical Examination.* Philadelphia, PA: J. B. Lippincott Co., 1974.

Caroline, N. *Emergency Care in the Streets.* Boston, MA: Little, Brown and Co., 1979.

De Jong, R. N. *The Neurological Examination,* third ed. New York: Harper and Row Publishers, Hoeber Medical Division, 1967.

Eliastam, Michael, and Souza, Charlene. "Examination of the Patient in the Field: A Physical Examination to be Used by Paramedics," *Paramedics International,* Spring 1977, pp. 24–25.

Gazzaniga A.; Iseri, L.; Baren, M. *Emergency Care: Principles and Practices for EMT-Paramedic.* Reston, VA: Reston Publishing Co., Inc., 1979.

Gillies, Dee A.; and Alyn, Irene B. *Patient Assessment and Management by the Nurse Practitioner.* Philadelphia, PA: W. B. Saunders Company, 1976.

Hinterbuchner, L. P. "Evaluation of the Unconscious Patient," *Medical Clinics of North America,* Vol. 57, No. 6, Nov. 1973, pp. 1363–1372.

Julihn, Miles. "Patient Assessment," *Journal of Emergency Medical Services,* March 1980, pp. 44–46.

Lanros, N. *Assessment and Intervention in Emergency Nursing.* Bowie, MD: Robert J. Brady Co., 1978.

Macleod, John. *Clinical Examination,* 4th ed. Edinburgh, London and New York: Churchill Livingstone, 1976.

Sherman, J. *Guide to Patient Evaluation.* New York: Medical Examiner Publishing Co., 1976.

Stewart, Ronald D. "From Nose to Toes: The Initial Assessment of the Injured Patient," *Paramedics International*, Fall, 1977, pp. 18–21.

Stewart, Ronald D. "The Initial Assessment of Multiple Trauma," *Paramedics International*, Summer 1977, pp. 18–23.

Stewart, Ronald D. "A Paramedic Approach to the Patient with Abdominal Trauma," *Paramedics International*, Fall 1976, pp. 15–17.

Walraven, G., *et al. Manual of Advanced Prehospital Care.* Bowie, MD: Robert J. Brady Co., 1978.

Warner, C. G., Editor. *Emergency Care: Assessment and Intervention*, second ed. St. Louis, MO: The C. V. Mosby Co., 1978.

Chapter 9

# Assessing Vital Signs

The EMT will record the patient's pulse rate, respirations, and blood pressure as part of the initial data gathering on the scene. These three factors reflect the functioning of the heart and lungs and provide information about the overall cardiovascular and circulatory efficiency of the body. The pulse rate, respirations, and blood pressure are termed *vital signs*, or merely *vitals*. Sometimes the temperature is also considered to be a vital sign. The accurate recording of these four values will provide important data for both field and hospital care.

Three tools essential in assessment of vital signs will be discussed in this chapter: the stethoscope (steth′o-skōp), the sphygmomanometer (sfig″mo-mah-nom′ĕ-ter), and the thermometer.

## THE STETHOSCOPE

The stethoscope is an essential tool for the EMT. It is used to listen to breath sounds, to record blood pressure, to count the heart rate of an infant prior to birth, and to count the apical heart rate. (See page 151.) Each EMT should become familiar with the instrument and its use.

The stethoscope consists of a listening surface connected to ear pieces. Depending upon the type of instrument, there may be two sides to the listening surface, the *diaphragm* (di′ah-fram) and the *bell*. The diaphragm screens out low-pitched sound and transmits relatively high-pitched sounds. It is used for listening to breath sounds and for blood pressure recording. The bell is designed to transmit low-pitched sounds and is used primarily for listening to the heart. It is essential that you become familiar with your own stethoscope since many have slightly varying design features. For example, some require rotating the listening device when changing from use of the bell to the diaphragm, and others are designed to use either part without manipulation since both are connected to the ear

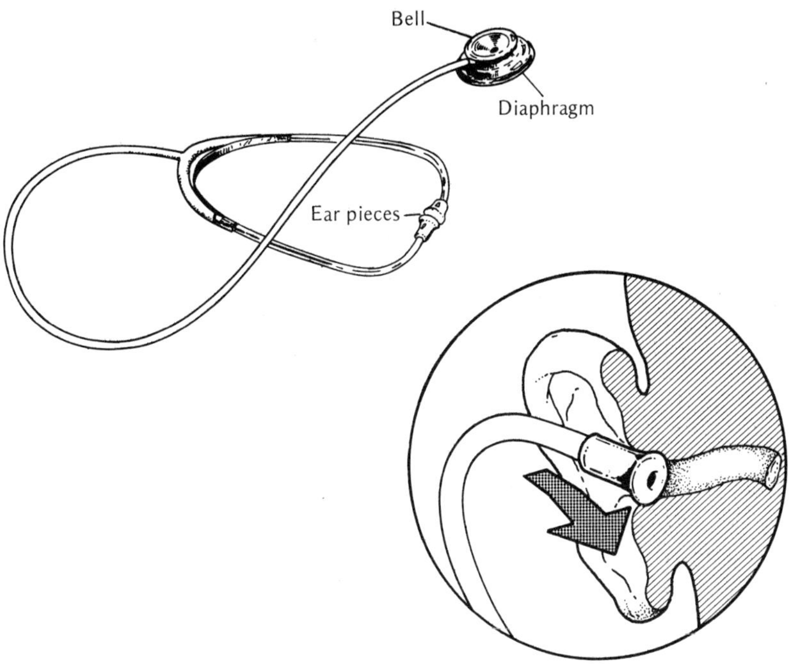


**Figure 9-1.** Stethoscope parts. Inset shows proper position of earpieces with the curve directed downward and slightly forward.

pieces in the same way. Electronically amplified stethoscopes are now available, too, and may be helpful, especially in the ambulance when noise level is high and it interferes with hearing of the pulsations.

The ear pieces are slightly curved. Be sure that you position the ear pieces so that they fit in your ear with the curve directed downward and slightly forward. (See Fig. 9-1.) This subtle maneuver is sometimes all that is required to detect a formerly undetectable blood pressure!

## Pulse Rate

The pulse rate is a reflection of the heart rate and is obtained by feeling the pulsation of an artery as it responds to the heart's pumping action. When the heart contracts and forces blood through vessels, there is an expansion (rise) and relaxation (fall) of the artery for each ventricular (ventrik'u-lar) contraction. This rising and falling is a *pulse* wave which can be easily felt in superficial arteries which overlie bony prominences. The rate (number of beats per minute,) rhythm, and quality of the pulse are important factors for the EMT to assess.

The *rate* of the pulse varies with age, state of health, emotions, the intake of certain food or drugs, and level of activity. Normally it is rapid in an infant (120 beats per minute) and decreases throughout childhood as the heart and lungs become more efficient. Most healthy adults have a rate of 60–90 beats per minute. Unusually rapid heart rates are termed *tachycardia* (tak″e-kar′de-ah); unusually slow rates, *bradycardia* (brad″e-kar′de-ah).

The *rhythm* of the pulse is simply described as *regular* or *irregular.* Ideally, the heart rate is reflected as a steady and evenly paced beat. If the beating is unsteady or unevenly timed, an arrhythmia (ah-rith′me-ah) (without rhythm) or dysrhythmia (dis-rith′me-ah) (abnormal rhythm) exists.

The *quality* of the pulse is also assessed and is described as *strong* (or *full*) or *weak* and *thready.* If it is difficult to feel or disappears when compressed, the phenomenon is sometimes described as "barely palpable (pal′pah-b′l)," or "an easily obliterated (ob-lit′er-a-t′d) pulse."

The pulse rate is assessed by placing one's three middle fingers directly over the artery using light touch. Too much pressure may completely obliterate the pulsation. Count a regular pulse for 15 seconds and multiply it by four in order to get the rate per minute. An irregular pulse should be counted for at least 30 seconds (and multiplied by two) or preferably for a full minute.

The most common sites used for pulse assessment in the field are noted in Fig. 9–2. Note that the pulse is described according to its anatomical (an″ah-tom′e-kal) landmark.

## Respirations

Assessment of respirations involves counting the number of breaths an individual takes per minute. This information is derived from the cycles of breathing in (inspiration) and breathing out (expiration) that occur in a minute. The chest and abdomen are carefully observed to detect the movement which indicates respiration. One inspiration and one expiration constitutes one respiration for the purpose of recording. The EMT will find it easy to note inspiration by the rise of the chest and thus will focus on this feature to facilitate counting. Adults usually breathe fourteen to eighteen times per minute, but stress, exercise, emotions, certain drugs, and fever will accelerate breathing. Certain disorders of the nervous system or of the body's metabolism may affect the rate or character of respirations. Infants and children have more rapid respirations than adults. Normally infants breathe thirty-five to forty times per minute and older children, twenty to thirty-two per minute.

When the EMT assesses respirations it is important that the depth and rhythm also be noted. Since breathing can be voluntarily controlled, it is often desirable to count respirations while still pretending to be counting the pulse. Some patients tend to hold their breath or breathe more rapidly when they are thinking about it.

There are terms which are used to describe patterns of breathing, and the EMT should be familiar with the most common ones. Difficult or labored respirations are referred to as *dyspnea* (disp′ne-ah). If an in-

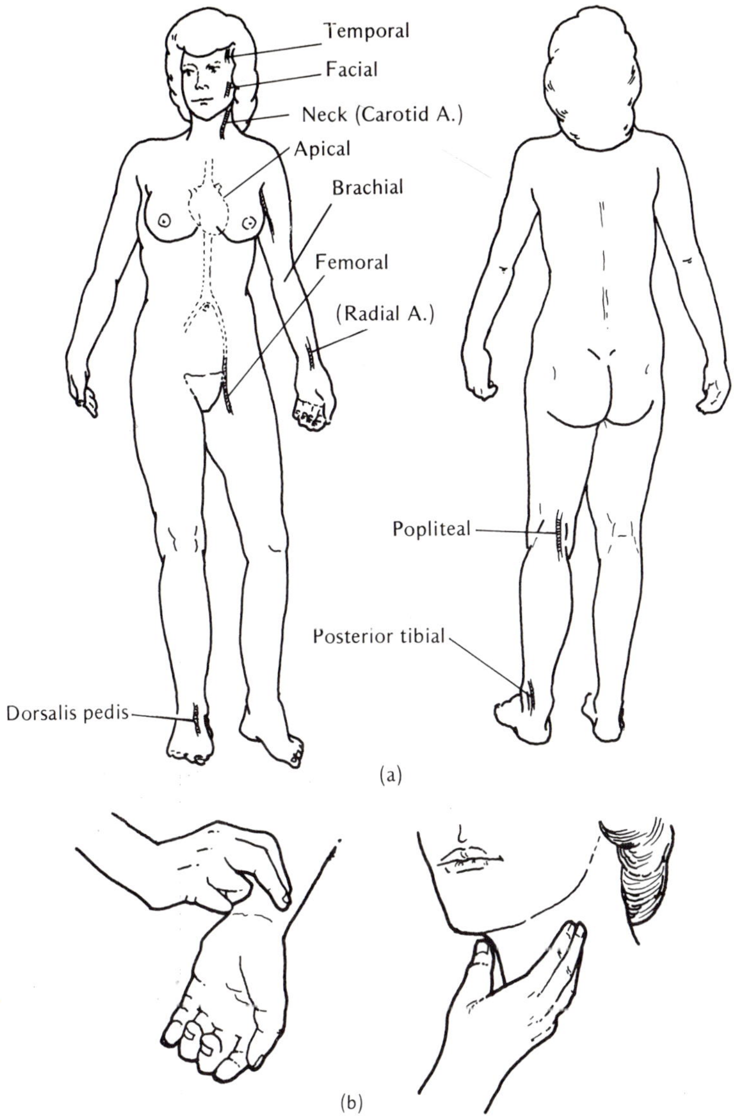


**Figure 9–2.** Sites for assessing pulse. Inset shows technique for palpating radial and carotid pulses.

dividual feels a need to sit up to ease the work of breathing, it is termed *orthopnea* (*or*″thop-ne′ah). Words such as *regular*, *irregular*, *shallow*, *heavy*, *sighing*, or *agonal* (ag′o-nal) are also used to describe characteristic types of breathing.

When an EMT becomes more skilled, he can also assess breathing by listening to breath sounds with the aid of a stethoscope. With this instrument it is possible to evaluate air exchange more specifically. For example, obstructions of air flow or moisture in the lungs can be detected by characteristic sounds.

## BLOOD PRESSURE

The blood pressure is a most important vital sign which the EMT must learn to assess. The blood pressure is an indirect measurement of the force exerted by blood against the wall of an artery during the contraction and relaxation of the ventricles (ven'trĭ-k'lz) of the heart. (See page 160.) Thus, the blood pressure consists of two readings—the one characteristic of pressure during the contraction of the ventricles (termed *systolic* [sis-tol'ik] pressure and one which reflects pressure during relaxation (*diastolic* [di"ah-stol'ik] pressure). A *stethoscope* (see page 148) and a special instrument called *sphygmomanometer* (commonly referred to as a blood pressure cuff) are required to determine these readings.

There are two types of sphygmomanometers that are commonly used to measure blood pressure: the mercury manometer (mah-nom'ĕ-ter) and the aneroid (an'er-oid) manometer. (See Fig. 9–3.) EMTs usually use the aneroid (springtype) since it does not require a fixed vertical position to ensure accuracy as the mercury device does.

A sphygmomanometer consists of (1) a pressure manometer, (2) a compression cuff, and (3) a pressure source equipped with a rubber hand bulb for inflation of the cuff and a pressure control valve for cuff deflation. (See Fig. 9–3.)

The blood pressure reading is usually obtained by applying the compression cuff to the upper arm, inflating the cuff to occlude the brachial (bra'ke-al) artery by compression, and then slowly decompressing the compression cuff while listening for characteristic sounds using the stethoscope over the antecubital (an"te-ku'bĭ-tal) fossa.

The EMT should follow the steps below when recording a blood pressure.

### Steps in Recording Arterial Blood Pressure

1. Apply the compression cuff to the upper arm, being certain that the artery being compressed is essentially at the level of the heart. The cuff should fit evenly and snugly with the lower edge one inch above the antecubital fossa to leave room for stethoscope placement over the artery. (See Fig. 9–4.)

2. While palpating the radial pulse (see page 151) note the rate and rhythm. Leave fingers in palpating position.

3. Inflate the cuff by compressing the hand bulb to approximately 30 mm Hg *above* the point when the pulse disappears, i.e., no longer can be felt.

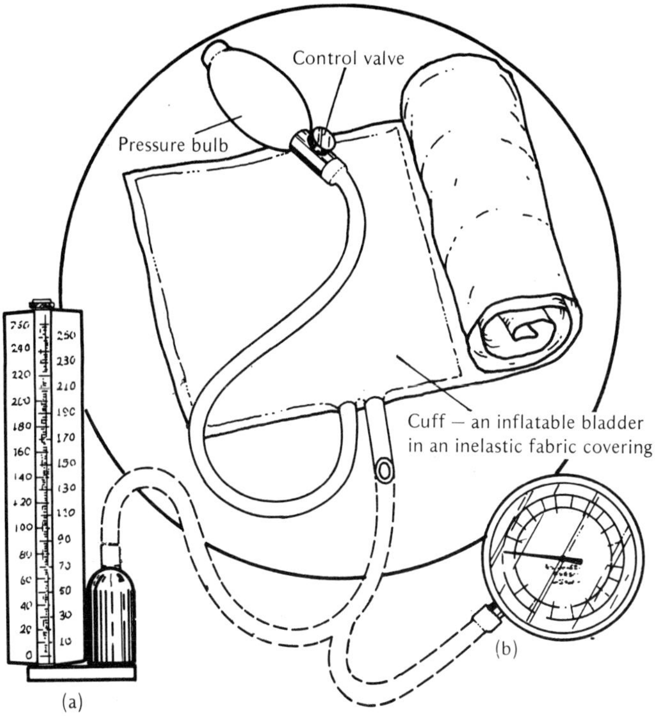


**Figure 9-3.** (a) Mercury pressure gauge sphygmomanometer; (b) aneroid pressure gauge sphygmomanometer. Inset shows details of cuff and control valve.

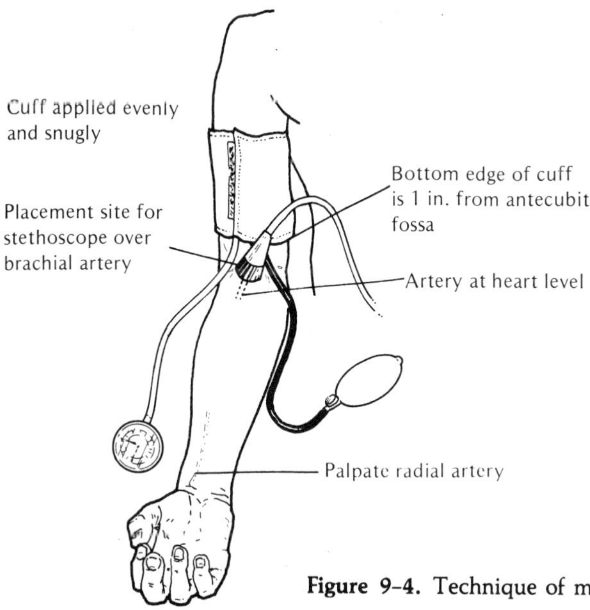


**Figure 9-4.** Technique of measuring blood pressure.

4. Release the pressure valve slowly (2–3 mm per heart beat) and note when the first heartbeat can be felt (palpated) or heard (auscultated [aws-kul′ta-ted]). This reading is the *systolic* blood pressure. Continue to watch the falling manometer. The faint, but clear beats will increase in intensity and then become muffled and the sounds will disappear. The point at which sounds disappear is the *diastolic* pressure. The readings are recorded as a fraction with the systolic reading being the numerator and the diastolic, the denominator, e.g. 120/80. Occasionally a blood pressure will be so low that it does not produce an audible sound which the EMT can hear via the stethoscope. In this instance, a systolic reading is obtained by palpation only. As a pulse is detected over the artery being tested, the manometer reading at that point is recorded as the systolic blood pressure. Diastolic readings cannot be obtained, however, since they depend on changes in *sound* during the cuff decompression.

5. Deflate the cuff and remove, or leave in place (deflated) for continued monitoring of the arterial blood pressure.

Although the technique for measuring blood pressure is relatively easy to learn, there are some common causes for error which deserve discussion.

## Improper Cuff Size

The cuff of most devices is designed for the average adult, so if the patient is very thin or extremely obese, errors in readings can occur. The cuff should encircle the extremity and fit snugly over two-thirds of the upper arm. A cuff that is too narrow will cause an erroneously high reading, and one that is too wide will produce a misleading low reading.

The artery being compressed should be approximately at the level of the heart. If the cuff has been carelessly applied allowing the rubber bladder to bulge or "balloon" within the covering, the reading will be excessively high since much greater force will be required to totally compress the artery.

## Improper Deflation of Cuff

The pressure should be released at a rate of about 2 mm Hg per heartbeat. If the pressure is released very slowly, venous congestion will occur and the diastolic reading will be erroneously high. If deflation is too rapid, the reading may fall up to 10 mm between heart sounds and false low readings might occur.

## Normal Variations in Blood Pressure

Anatomically, the blood pressure is usually slightly different in each arm, perhaps 5–10 mm. A greater deviation, however, is to be noted since it may be indicative of an important vascular problem. If time permits, the EMT should record the blood pressure in both arms.

The blood pressure is often affected by sudden changes in posture, particularly from a lying to a standing position. It is useful to wait a few minutes before taking a reading when a patient experiences a sudden change in posture. A variation of 30 mm or more between lying and sitting or standing pressure is indicative of a hypovolemic (hi″po-vo-le′mik) state. (See page 205.)

Age also affects blood pressure. The normal adult has a range of 90–140 mm systolically and 60–90 mm diastolically. Table 26-2 presents the normal range for pediatric blood pressures. Note that the infant reading is very low compared to an average adult and that throughout childhood it gradually increases to adult levels.

Unusually high blood pressure is called *hypertension* (hi″per-ten′shun) and low blood pressure, *hypotension* (hi″po-ten′shun).

### Other Variations

Blood pressure variations often signal that the body is in trouble or is making adjustments necessitated by disease, the effects of drugs, blood loss, and so forth. Since the blood pressure may be one of the earliest indicators of compromise, it is important to understand how the blood pressure reflects what is going on in the total body.

The blood pressure reflects three factors, all of which are interrelated. These are: (1) the action of the *heart* as a *pump*, (2) the *volume* of blood being circulated and (3) the *peripheral* (pĕ-rif′er-al) *vascular response* to blood flow. Any one of the factors, when altered by disease, injury, or drugs can change blood pressure. Furthermore, when any one factor is affected, the other two will modify their actions to attempt to maintain a blood pressure that will support life. For example, if the heart loses its ability to pump forcefully enough to circulate blood after a heart attack, the vessels in the periphery will tend to relax their resistance to blood flow to make work easier for the failing heart. If hemorrhage (hem′or-ij) causes a serious loss of blood, the heart will beat faster and pump harder to circulate and reoxygenate (re-ok′sĕ-je-nat) the remaining blood. The vessels will constrict and make themselves smaller to ensure that blood flow retains a high velocity through the extremities. Furthermore, the constriction of vessels in the periphery will force more blood back into the chest, head and abdomen to nourish the vital organs such as the heart, lung, brain, and kidneys. The EMT will often be able to judge how well a patient is coping with a disease or injury by assessing vital signs and their adjustments.

## TEMPERATURE

Body temperature provides meaningful information about a patient's condition too, and an EMT may encounter situations in which this vital sign must also be recorded. For example, specific treatment may be instituted for very high or very low body temperature states.

Heat is produced in the body as a result of metabolism (mĕ-tab′o-lizm), or the "burning up of food" to produce energy. This heat production is regulated by the brain in a special control center called the *hypothalamus* (hi″po-thal′ah-mus). The hypothalamus is essentially a thermostat to maintain normal body temperature by balancing heat production and heat loss. When the body produces heat faster than heat loss occurs, fever results. An elevation above 99°F. (37.2°C.) is considered to be a fever state. Unusually high elevations (above 105°F or 40.5°C.) are termed *hyperpyrexia* (hi″per-pi-rek′se-ah) or *hyperthermia* (hi″per-ther′me-ah). Severe infections, heat reactions, (see Chapter 29) drug reactions, and brain injury may cause unusual rises in body temperature.

Low body temperatures may result from environmental cold exposure, shock (see Chapter 30), and medical conditions that affect metabolism or brain functioning. If a patient's extremities are unusually cool, it may be important to check body temperature since heat loss occurs earliest in the periphery of the body. Cold hands, arms, feet, and legs may indicate that the body is conserving blood flow and concentrating on preserving vital organs, for instance, in shock states. It is not uncommon to find a normal temperature when assessing it, however, since the central organs are more richly supplied with blood during both normal and compensatory (kom-pen′sah-to″re) (adjustment to stress) states.

## Recognition of Fever

Fever can be detected in many situations merely by assessing the skin. It will appear dry and feel warm to touch. The skin color is usually paler than usual due to constriction (kon-strik′shun) (or narrowing) of the peripheral blood supply and the onset of sweating. In advanced fever states when the condition is grave the skin may appear cherry-red due to resultant dehydration (de″hi-dra′shun) (loss of water) and vasodilation (vas″o-di-la′shun) (vessel relaxation) in an attempt to lose heat in response to accelerated heat production.

Individuals who have fever are generally listless (without energy) and experience weakness, thirst, headache, aching, and nausea. The pulse is usually elevated and respirations are rapid to aid in heat loss. Delirium (de-lir′ĭ-um) and seizures are more serious consequences and are noted primarily in children from one to six years and thus have an immature hypothalamus or thermostat. (See page 492.)

The EMT will probably assess temperature by using a disposable thermometer since it is safer for field use. An ordinary glass clinical thermometer may also be used. (See Fig. 9–5.) The temperature may be taken orally in alert, cooperative older children and adults. The rectal route is preferred for infants or young children or adults who are unable to safely comply with oral temperature taking, for example, for the recently seizing or unconscious patient. An additional alternative that is sometimes used is

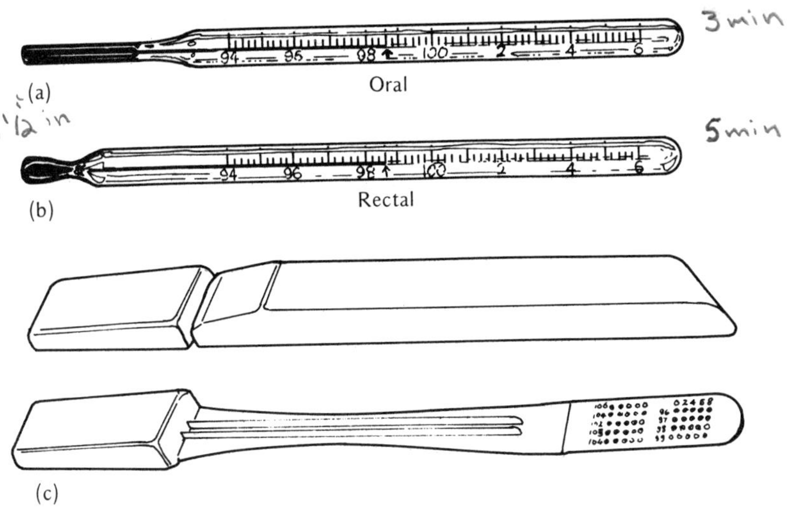


**Figure 9-5.** Clinical thermometers: (a) glass oral; (b) glass rectal; (c) disposable type.

the axillary (ak′sĭ-lar″e) method (under the armpit). Although disposable skin temperature sensors are currently popular, their reliability is questioned by certain authorities.

## Taking Temperature

*Oral Route.* The thermometer should be checked (glass thermometers shaken until the mercury is 94°F or 37°C or below.[1]) Insert the bulb under the tongue, well back under the base so it is in contact with a generous blood supply. Leave it in place for three to four minutes. When it is removed, wipe it off (toward the tip) with a tissue and read it at once.

*Rectal Route.* Check the thermometer and shake down as described. Lubricate the tip with a water-soluble lubricant or petroleum jelly. Insert it just far enough inside the anal sphincter (sfingk′ter) that the bulb is in contact with the mucous lining of the rectum. Leave it in place for three to four minutes taking care to restrain the patient and thermometer as needed to prevent accidental glass breakage. Remove the thermometer, wipe with a tissue and record the reading. Rectal temperatures are usually 1° higher than the oral temperature, so the route should be recorded. Of course, rectal thermometers should be cleaned separately from oral ones, stored in a well-marked container, and *never* used for oral temperatures at a later time!

---

[1] To "shake down" a thermometer, use a quick, wrist action while keeping a firm grasp on the thermometer. It should be held by the top, not by the bulb that is inserted into the patient's mouth.

*Axillary temperatures* are recorded using a rectal thermometer. Place the device well under the armpit and leave it in place for at least five minutes.

The cleaning and restocking of glass (nondisposable) thermometers will vary widely based on institutional or system policy. The EMT should be familiar with the procedure for his unit since each thermometer must be carefully disinfected before use for another patient.

*Summary*

The EMT must be skillful in assessing vital signs and must be able to accurately record and interrelate the data. The pulse, respirations, blood pressure, and temperature reflect important information on general body response to disease or injury, but are especially useful in measuring cardiovascular activity.

*References*

Barber, Janet; Stokes, Lillian; and Billings, Diane. *Adult and Child Care; A Client Approach to Nursing*, second ed. St. Louis: The C. V. Mosby Co., 1977, pp. 766–767.

Chaney, Patricia S. (series editor). *Assessing Vital Functions Accurately*, Nursing Skillbook Series. Horsham, Pa.: Intermed Communications, Inc., 1977, pp. 15–32.

White, Dorothy T.; Rubino, Edith; and DeLorey, Philip E. *Fundamentals: The Foundation of Nursing*. Englewood Cliffs, NJ: Prentice-Hall, Inc., 1972, pp. 80–92.

Chapter 10

# Basic Life Support

## ESTABLISHING AN AIRWAY AND CARDIOPULMONARY RESUSCITATION

There is no role of the EMT that is more critical than being skilled in basic life support. Thousands of lives could be saved each year with a system of public education, professional education, and community programs which deal with cardiac health (e.g., diet, exercise, hazards of smoking) and actions for survival in the event of airway obstruction or cardiac arrest. The American Heart Association has been instrumental in developing a dynamic plan for teaching lay persons and health care team members the fundamentals of basic cardiac life support (BCLS). Other organizations, such as the American National Red Cross, have cooperated in teaching and community awareness campaigns, too, and have stimulated widespread interest within schools, organizations, business and industry, the military services, and hospitals to train their people in the techniques of basic life support.

This chapter will present a brief overview of the anatomy and physiology of the heart, lungs, and airway structures and will provide the knowledge and skills pertinent to the EMT regarding airway establishment and maintenance and cardiopulmonary (kar″de-o-pul′mo-ner-e) resuscitation (re-sus″ĭ-ta′shun).

## ANATOMY AND PHYSIOLOGY OF THE CARDIOVASCULAR SYSTEM

The blood supply is contained within the cardiovascular (kar″de-o-vas′ku-lar) system comprised of the heart, arteries (ar′ter-ez), capillaries (kap′ĭ-lar″ez), and veins.

The heart is a hollow, muscular organ, approximately the size of a fist. It lies within the center of the chest behind the sternum (ster′num) (breastbone) and anterior to the thoracic (tho-ras′ik) spine. It is surrounded by the lungs and is positioned just above the diaphragm (di′ah-fram).

The heart is responsible for pumping blood throughout the body. It is actually divided into a "right heart" and a "left heart" by a septum

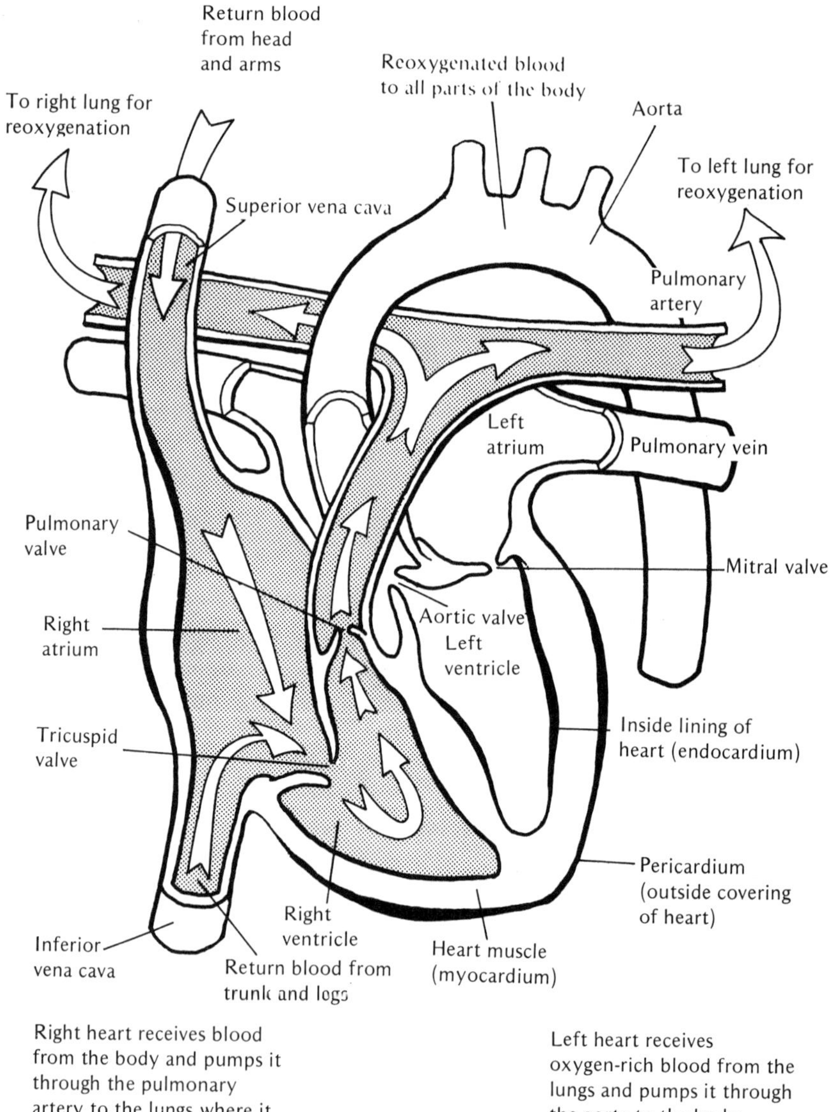


**Figure 10–1.** Anatomy of the heart.

(sep′tum) or wall. Each side of the heart has an upper chamber called an *atrium* (a′tre-um) and a lower chamber called a *ventricle* (ven′trı-k′l). Valves regulate the blood flow between chambers, as well as into the pulmonary (pul′mo-ner″e) artery and the aorta (a-or′tah). The largest artery, the *aorta* delivers blood to other arteries all over the body under high hydrostatic (hi″dro-stat′ik) pressure, created by *volume* and *peripheral resistance*, as well as the *pumping action of the heart.* (See Fig. 10–1.) The coronary arteries arise directly from the aorta and are the vessels that supply the heart with its blood supply.

## Microcirculation (mi″kro-sir″ku-la′shun)

The heart pumps blood throughout the body via arteries to capillary beds where it gives up oxygen and nutrients to support the life of cells and their processes. Capillaries are in a circuit-like pattern and eventually form the venous network which carries blood back to the heart, after reclaiming waste products, especially carbon dioxide from the cell. The essence of all life processes is dependent upon the perfusion (blood flow) and constant exchange at the cellular level. (See Fig. 10–1.)

The left side of the heart pumps blood throughout the body. The right side of the heart receives venous blood from the vena cavae (ve′nah ka′ve) and pumps it to the lungs where carbon dioxide is eliminated and a new supply of oxygen is picked up. Study Fig. 10–2 and trace the blood flow from the left side of the heart and back again.

The adult heart beats about seventy times per minute and delivers about seventy milliliters to the aorta at each ejection (e-jek′shun) from the left ventricle (that is, cardiac output). This output at seventy beats/minute

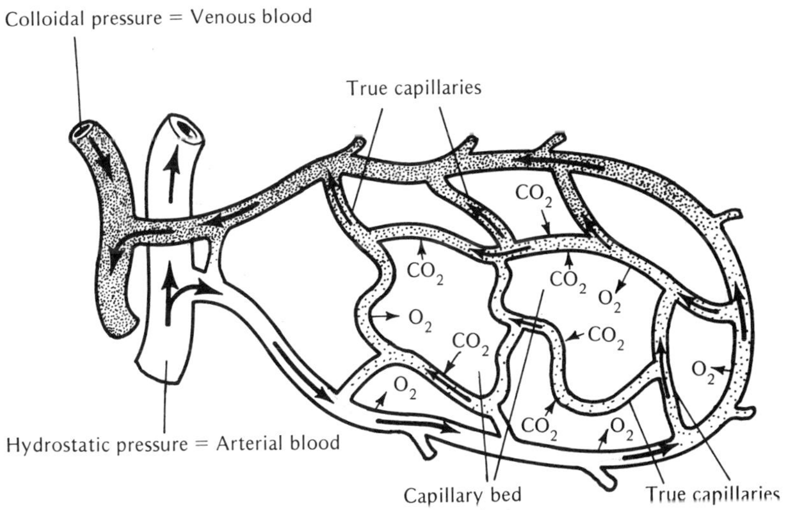


**Figure 10–2.** Microcirculation.

means that about five liters of blood is pumped every minute. This represents all but one liter of the average adult's total blood volume!

There is a complete electrical energy system (nervous tissue) that supplies the heart with impulses to beat in an organized manner, adjusting rate and rhythm to meet the body's changing demands. The exciting nerve fibers that create a contraction (or pumping) make up what is called the *pacemaker*. The pacemaker is dependent upon a nutritive environment with a balanced chemical composition and oxygen supply conducive to its normal activity.

### Respiratory System

The process of breathing (external respiration) is discussed thoroughly in Chapter 17. *Internal respiration*, i.e., the gas exchange process is a function of the alveoli.

The alveoli (al-ve′o-li) (air sacs) are surrounded by both arteries and veins. Arteries carry blood to the capillaries that envelop the alveoli; the veins carry it back to the heart. This exchange mechanism permits continuous intake of oxygen and elimination of carbon dioxide.

Breathing is stimulated by an increasing level of carbon dioxide in the blood. When the carbon dioxide concentration declines, the rate and depth of respirations will decline. The air we breathe ("room air") normally contains a concentration of 21 percent oxygen and negligible carbon dioxide. Expired air contains about 16 percent oxygen, 5 percent carbon dioxide and water vapor. Exhaled air contains sufficient oxygen to support life processes. This fact is an important principle as one studies the techniques of basic life support.

## AIRWAY OBSTRUCTION

The airway can be blocked by the tongue or any type of foreign body. The tongue falling back towards the pharynx (far′inks), particularly in unconsciousness, is the most common airway obstruction that the EMT will encounter. Trauma, inhaled foreign bodies, swelling of airway tissues from any cause, strangulation, and drowning are other causes which may be encountered.

### Foreign Bodies

Foreign objects can lead to partial or complete obstruction of the airway. A partial airway obstruction will be accompanied by forceful coughing and perhaps wheezing, but there will be air exchange. If the victim is able to cough and breathe, the EMT should not attempt to interfere. However if the individual becomes weak, unable to cough, appears cyanotic (si-ah-not′ik) or has high-pitched, "crowing" sounds while inhal-

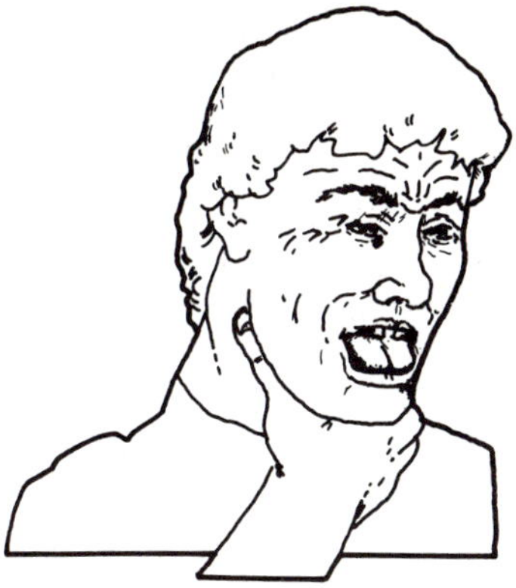

**Figure 10–3.** Universal distress signal for choking.

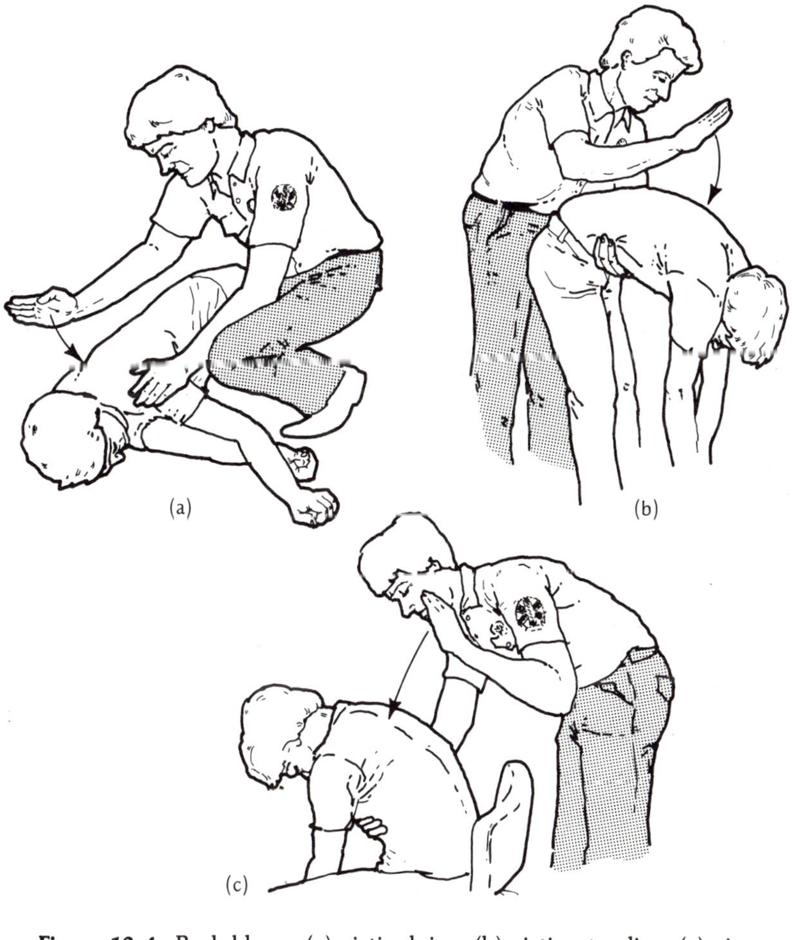

**Figure 10–4.** Back blows: (a) victim lying; (b) victim standing; (c) victim sitting.

ing, there is a need for immediate intervention, identical to that for a complete obstruction.

In a complete airway obstruction, the victim is unable to speak or cough. Cyanosis and respiratory struggle may be evident, but there is no air exchange. The EMT must recognize this need for immediate intervention or the individual will become oxygen starved (*anoxic*, without oxygen), rapidly unconscious, and death will ensue.

The common factors causing foreign bodies in the airway are eating without chewing well, dentures, and alcohol consumption. The signs may mimic heart attack, and thus the term *cafe coronary* has been given to this type of airway crisis. Fainting, strokes, seizures, drug overdose, or other problems may be confused with airway obstruction. The key points in recognition of total obstruction are: (1) inability to speak, (2) inability to cough, and (3) inability to breathe. The victim may clutch his neck, the universal distress signal to denote choking. (See Fig. 10-3.)

The following manual maneuvers are recommended by the American Heart Association and the American National Red Cross to relieve airway obstruction: *back blows* (Fig. 10-4 and 10-5), *manual thrusts* (Fig. 10-6 and 10-7), and *finger sweeps* (Fig. 10-8).

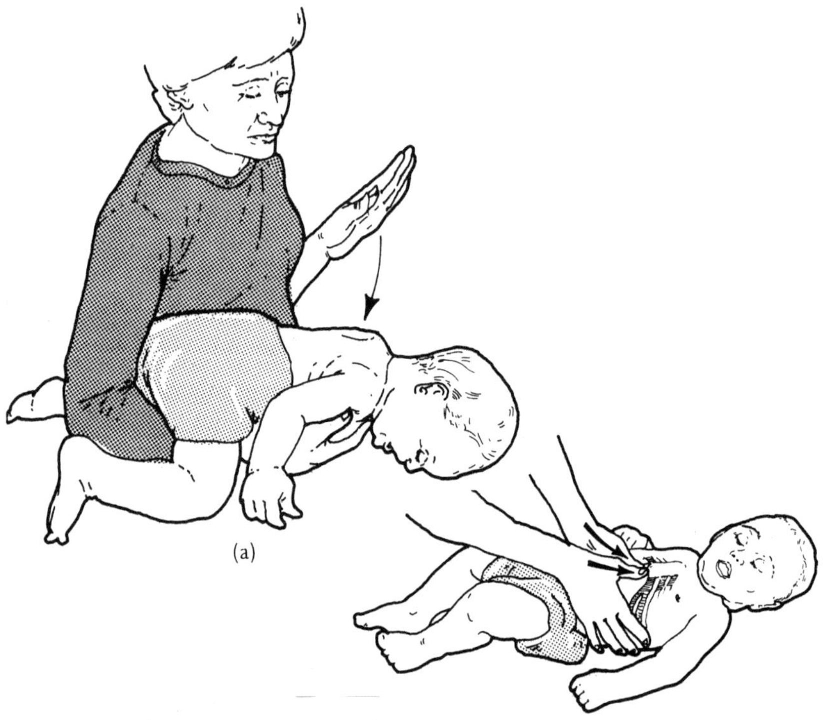

(a)

(b)

**Figure 10-5.** Back blows for the infant. (a) Note that the infant is prone and the head is tilted down. (b) Chest thrusts for infant.

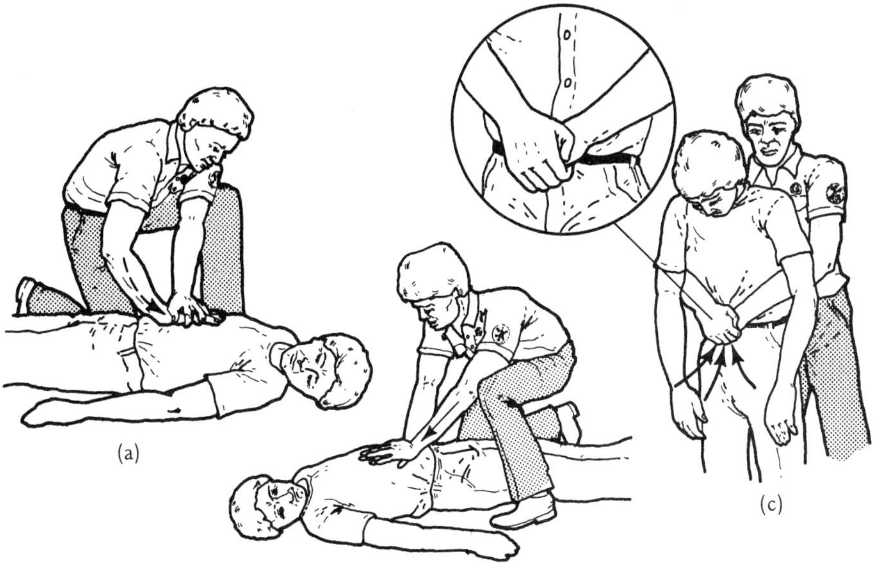

(a) (b) (c)

**Figure 10–6.** Abdominal thrusts (Heimlich Maneuver): (a) victim lying; (b) alternate position for lying victim; (c) victim standing (inset shows details of hand position).

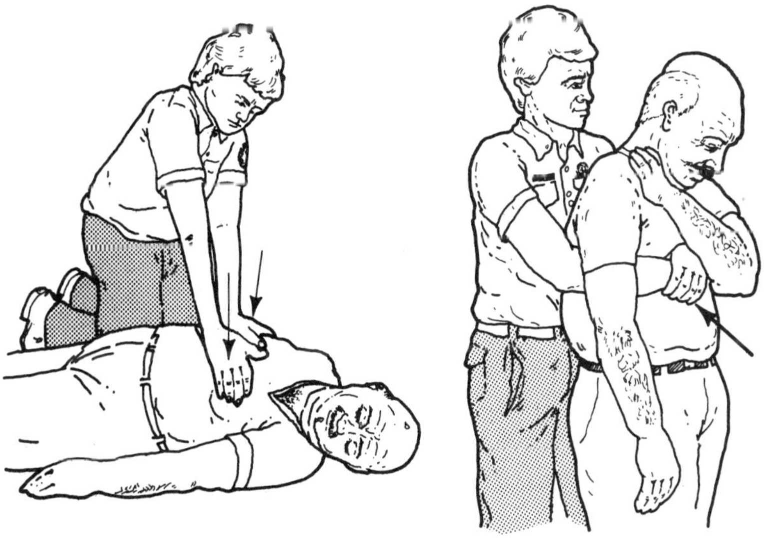

(a) (b)

**Figure 10–7.** Chest thrusts: (a) victim lying (unconscious); (b) victim standing (conscious).

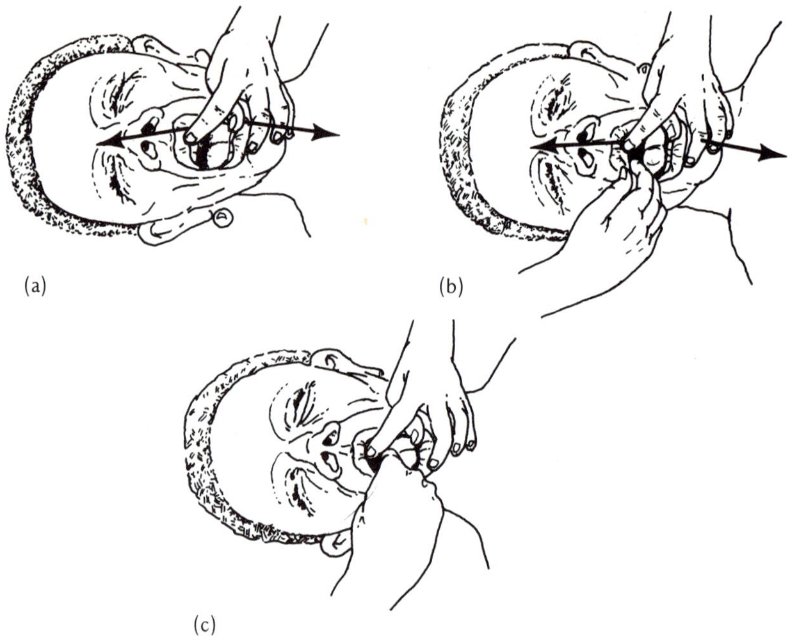

Figure 10-8. Crossed-finger technique for opening mouth. (a) Wedge created by index finger crossed over thumb. (b) Separation of fingers to open airway. (c) Finger sweeps. The index finger should sweep along the oral cavity walls deep into the airway. Any foreign material should be hooked from underneath and brought upward (forward). This approach prevents pushing objects deeper into the airway. The finger should rake along the surface of the mouth as it is being withdrawn to check for any other foreign material.

A combination of back blows and manual thrusts are more effective than either maneuver used alone. Back blows produce a rise in pressure within the respiratory passages that can dislodge a foreign body. Manual thrusts create a prolonged increase in pressure and airflow within the respiratory passages and assist in dislodging a foreign body.

*Back-Blows (Victim Lying)*

1. Roll the victim onto his side facing you with his chest against your thigh.

2. Administer four sharp blows in rapid succession between the shoulder blades with the heel of one hand.

3. Turn the victim to the prone position and explore the mouth and posterior pharynx to locate any dislodged foreign body.

4. Repeat attempts to breathe mouth-to-mouth.

*Note:* If the victim is conscious and standing or sitting, [Fig. 10–4 (b) and (c)] position yourself at the side and slightly behind the victim. Place one hand on the chest to support him while delivering blows as described above. If possible, the victim's head should be lower than the chest to take advantage of gravity.

### *Back Blows for Infant and Young Child*

1. Turn the infant prone (face down) over your forearm with the head tilted down. Support the head with a hand around the jaw and chest.

2. Rapidly deliver four back blows with the heel of the hand between the shoulder blades. (Of course, use less force than for an adult victim.)

3. After the back blows, place your free hand on the infant's back, "sandwiching" the victim between your hands. (One hand supports the neck, jaw, and chest; the other supports the back.)

4. Place the infant on your thigh with the head lower than the trunk. Continue supporting the head and neck. Rapidly deliver four chest thrusts.

5. The airway may be explored and any *visible* foreign body removed. However, *"blind" finger sweeping must be avoided* to minimize the risk of pushing back any obstructing body.

### *Adaptations for the Larger Infant or Young Child*

The rescuer may kneel and place the child across the thighs with the head down for back blows. Rolling the victim to the floor will facilitate chest thrusts.

### *Abdominal Thrust (Heimlich Maneuver)*

#### *Victim Lying*

1. Position the victim on his back with your knees close to his hips. Open the airway and turn the head to the side.

2. Place the heel of one hand against the victim's abdomen, between the xiphoid (zif'oid) and the navel. Place the other hand over the first one.

3. Move forward so that your shoulders are directly over the victim's abdomen.

4. Press into the victim's abdomen, *in the midline,* with a *quick inward and upward thrust.*

*Alternate position:* Rescuer straddling the hips or one thigh of a victim. Both body weight and arm pressure are applied to the upward thrust.

*Victim Standing or Sitting, Conscious* (Fig. 10–6c.)

1. Stand behind the victim and wrap your arms around the waist.

2. Grasp one fist with your other hand, and place the thumb side of your fist against the victim's abdomen between the waist and the rib cage.

3. Press your fist three or four times into the victim's abdomen with a *quick inward and upward thrust.* Having the victim lean over will make the most effective use of gravity.

*Modification: Victim Alone*

1. Press your fist into the upper abdomen as described above using a *quick upward thrust*

or

2. Lean forward and press the abdomen quickly over any firm object such as the table, chair back or railing.

*Important Note: Do not attempt abdominal thrust on infants or small children since the liver and other adjacent organs could be injured. (See page 183.)*

*Chest Thrusts*

(Modification of technique for obesity, advanced pregnancy, or other situations in which the abdominal girth is so large that the rescuer cannot fully wrap his arms around the victim's abdomen.)

*Victim Lying*

1. Position the victim on his back and kneel close at his side. Open the airway and turn the head to the side.

2. Place the heel of the hand on the lower half of the sternum.

3. Exert four quick downward thrusts that will compress the chest cavity.

*Victim Standing or Sitting, Conscious*

1. Stand behind the victim, placing your arms directly under the armpits and encircle the chest.

2. Place the thumb side of your fist on the sternum above xiphoid. Avoid compression on the margins of the rib cage.

3. Grasp your fist with the other hand and exert four quick backward thrusts.

*Finger Sweep*

1. Open the mouth using a tongue-jaw lift. (See Fig. 10–15.)

2. Insert the index finger along the side of the cheek and into the throat at the base of the tongue.

3. A "hook action" should be used to pull out a foreign body. However, be careful to avoid pushing an obstruction deeper into respiratory passages.

### Respiratory Arrest

Any condition that results in inadequate blood flow to the brain will depress and destroy the brain's respiratory center. Shock and cardiac arrest are among the more common causes, but a stroke, drug overdose, head trauma, and diseases or injuries (e.g., cervical spinal cord trauma) which interfere with the function of the muscles of respiration may also lead to a respiratory arrest.

### Cardiac Arrest

A cardiac arrest is a sudden unexpected cessation of breathing or circulation. It may occur as a result of a "heart attack" or may be due to other illnesses and injuries, including adverse drug reactions, electrocution, chest and brain injury, or metabolic disturbances.

The EMT must be skilled in CPR (cardiopulmonary resuscitation). Usually an intensive training course is provided for the mastery of this technique, and opportunities for periodic practice are provided to ensure an efficient and effective management of arrest states. The following steps in CPR techniques are extracted from the American Heart Association and American National Red Cross guidelines and represent their current recommendations. Every EMT should be aware of the need to refresh knowledge and skills regularly, since the science of resuscitation is ever changing.

## CARDIOPULMONARY RESUSCITATION

When breathing ceases and the heart stops pumping blood, the patient is essentially dead, from a clinical standpoint, unless CPR is instituted within four to six minutes.

Properly executed CPR during these first critical minutes may prevent irreversible brain damage or *biological death.* This brief "safety zone" between "clinical death" and "biological death" suggests that lay persons, as well as EMTs, and other medical personnel ought to be skilled in the techniques of cardiopulmonary resuscitation.

### Establishing Unresponsiveness

The first step in CPR (see Fig. 10-9) is to identify a victim who is pulseless and nonbreathing. Since many individuals are "found down" the

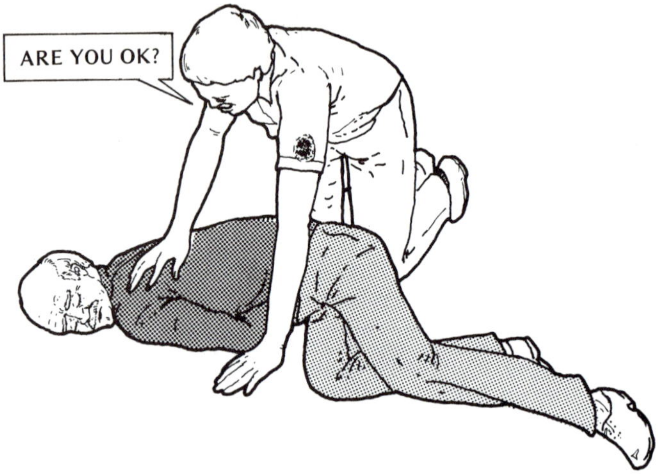


**Figure 10–9.** Establishing unresponsiveness. Gently stimulate the victim and ask "Are you OK?" Do not shake the victim vigorously, since this action could compound injuries.

EMT must determine if there is unconsciousness or if the person is just sleeping soundly. Start by touching the victim and saying, "Are you OK?" Touching is crucial, since some individuals may be deaf and thus not aroused by verbal stimuli alone. Avoid violent "shaking" and "shouting" though. A coexistent neck injury could be compounded by any vigorous motion of the head, neck and shoulder regions. If there is no response with touching and verbal stimulation, summon help. (See Fig. 10–10.) Position

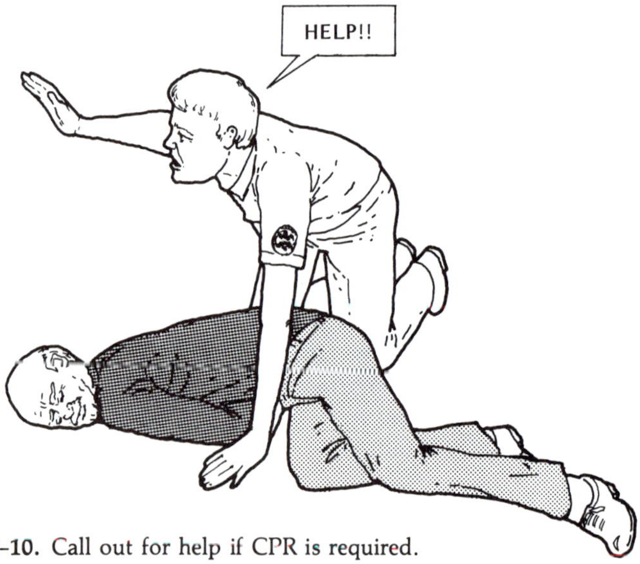


**Figure 10–10.** Call out for help if CPR is required.

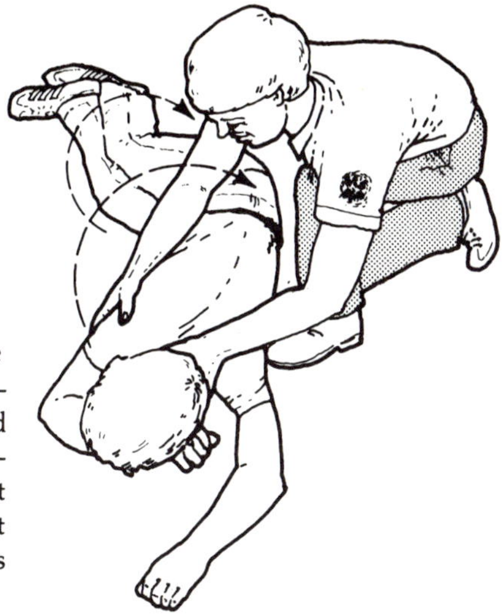

**Figure 10–11.** Positioning the victim. Use log-rolling technique to position the victim who is found on his side or face down. Ensure head and neck support while turning to prevent compounding other injuries which might be present.

the patient so that you could begin CPR. (See Fig. 10–11.) Consider the presence of other injuries and "log-roll" the victim. Note the instructions in conjunction with Figure 10–11.

## Opening the Airway

The tongue is a frequent cause of airway obstruction in an unconscious individual. The airway can be opened by moving the lower jaw forward. (See Fig. 10–12.) If there is tone in the jaw muscles, merely tilting the head back may effect the airway opening. (See Fig. 10–13 for technique.) This approach to establishing an airway is contraindicated for patients who are suspected of having cervical (ser′vĭ-kal) spine injury. (See

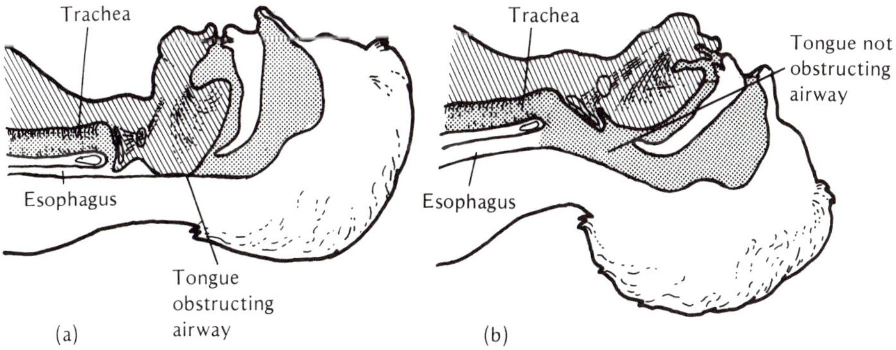


**Figure 10–12.** Lateral view of airway showing (a) tongue obstructing the airway; (b) airway that has been opened by repositioning the head.

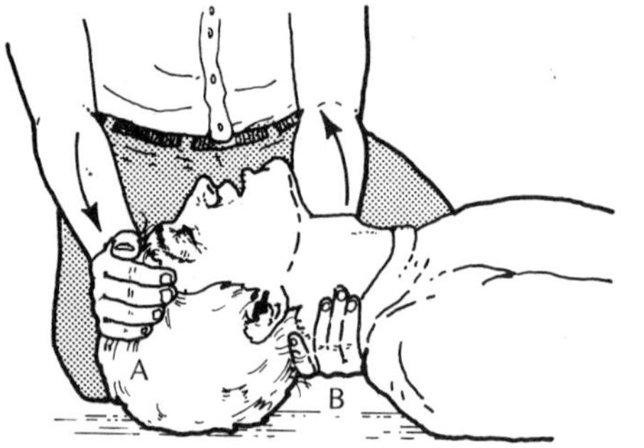


**Figure 10–13.**
Head tilt neck lift maneuver. (a) Place one hand on the victim's neck (close to the back of the head) and the other hand on the forehead. (b) Lift the neck with one hand and tilt the head by backward pressure on the forehead. BE GENTLE: Excess pressure can cause trauma to the cervical portion of the spinal cord.

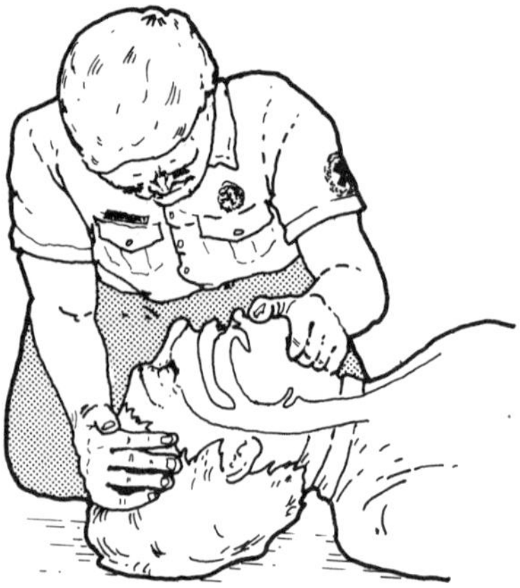

**Figure 10–14.**
Head tilt chin lift maneuver. (a) Place the fingers of one hand under the lower jaw on the bony region near the chin, and the other hand on the forehead. (Take care to avoid compressing the soft tissue under the chin, since this could obstruct the airway.) (b) Lift the chin forward while tilting the forehead backward. (The thumb may be used to lightly depress the lower lip only—*never* to lift the chin.) Avoid completely closing the mouth with this maneuver. Hold loose dentures in place for rescue breathing.

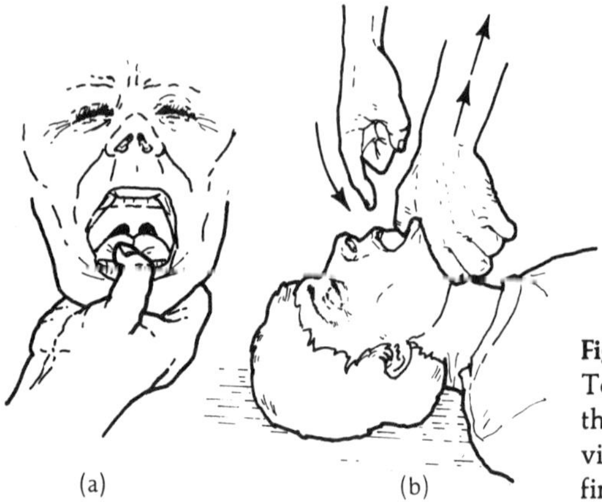

(a) (b)

**Figure 10–15.**
Tongue-jaw lift. Grasp tongue and lower jaw between thumb and fingers and lift. (a) Anterior view; (b) lateral view. This maneuver is valuable in conjunction with finger sweeps for a foreign body.

page 284.) The cervical vertebrae are *not to be hyperextended;* rather, the head and neck are *extended* while the neck is gently being lifted. Denture wearers may require the head tilt, chin lift maneuver (Fig. 10–14). Lifting the chin opens the airway by lifting the tongue away from the back of the throat. The maneuver also supports the lower jaw and assists in tilting the head back. Figures 10–15 through 10–18 exhibit alternate modes of opening the airway.

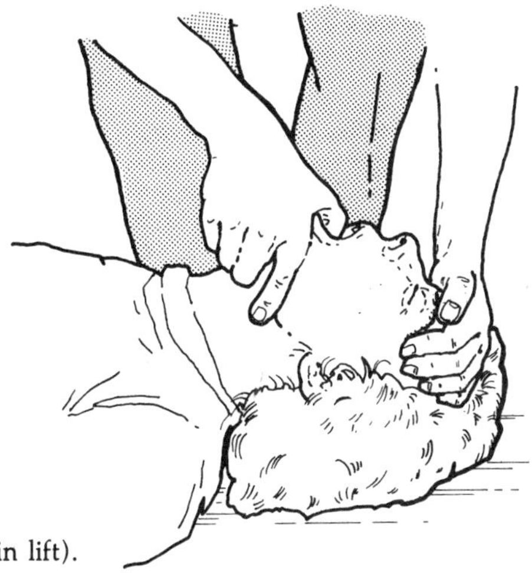

**Figure 10–16.** Jaw lift (variation of chin lift).

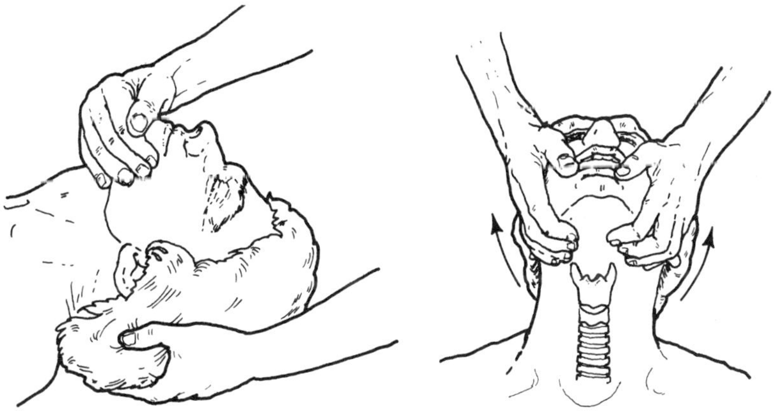

(a) (b)

**Figure 10–17.** (a) Neck extension. Place the hand behind the head and extend the neck by pulling the chin upward. (b) Modification of airway opening for victims with neck injury. Do not flex or hyperextend the neck. Note that the jaw is lifted as the thumbs open the mouth.

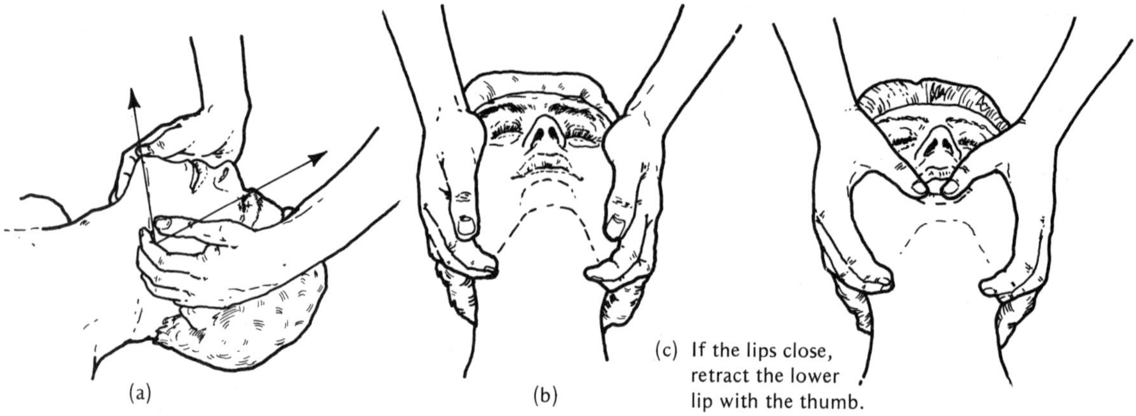


**Figure 10–18.** Jaw thrust (for suspected neck injury). (a) Leave the head in a neutral position. (b) Rest elbows on the surface on which your victim is lying. Grasp the victim's lower jaw (using both hands) and lift. The mandible will be displaced forward. Support the head carefully without tilting it backwards or turning it to the side. (c) If the lips close, retract the lower lip with the thumb.

## Establishing Breathlessness

While maintaining the "open airway," the EMT should place his ear over the unconscious person's nose and mouth and look toward the chest and stomach to note rising and falling of the chest (Fig. 10–19). Listen for air escaping during exhalation and feel for any air flow on the patient's cheek. Respiratory efforts do not necessarily mean that ventilation is occurring. Ensure that air is "moving" into and out of the chest. If not, rescue breathing must be initiated.

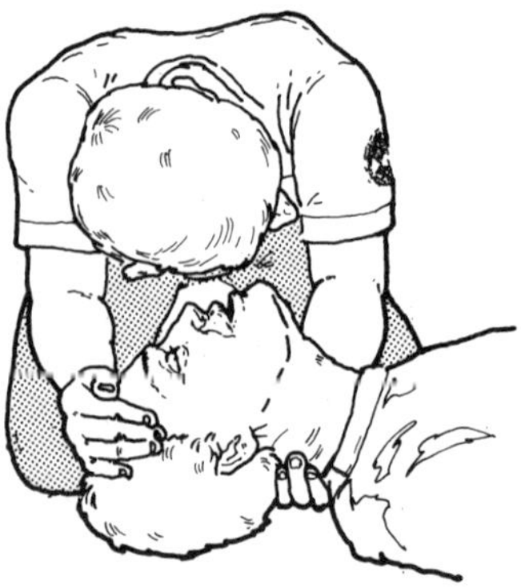

**Figure 10–19.** Establishing breathlessness. Note that the rescuer is listening for air and watching for respiratory movements of the chest and abdomen.

## Rescue Breathing

If spontaneous breathing is not present, the EMT must breathe for the victim. The fundamental method is mouth-to-mouth breathing. This technique requires no special equipment and employs the EMT's expired air to ventilate the non-breathing victim's lungs. The victim's nose is pinched shut and the EMT places his mouth over the victim's and forces air into the lungs.

Initially, four full breaths are delivered without allowing for the victim's lungs to deflate between breaths. (These four full breaths help to open the smaller airways, which tend to collapse as soon as spontaneous breathing ceases.) (See Fig. 10–20.) The EMT should watch for the rise of the victim's chest on inflation as a sign of an open airway. If the chest fails to rise, the head should be repositioned before further attempting ventilations.

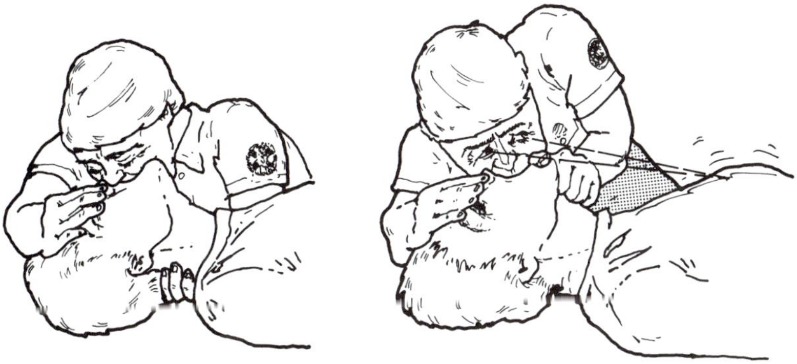

**Figure 10–20.** *Rescue breathing.* The nostrils are pinched off. The rescuer takes a deep breath before sealing his mouth over the victim's, and watches for a chest rise during breath delivery to ensure that the lungs are being ventilated. Four full breaths are delivered quickly without allowing lung deflation to assist in opening smaller air passages, which tend to collapse readily after spontaneous breathing ceases.

The EMT will remove his mouth after each delivered breath to allow for the taking in of fresh air and to permit a passive exhalation for the victim.

*Note:* The EMT who has a pocket-mask or bag-valve mask may, of course, use them in preference to the mouth-to-mouth technique. (See pages 197–200.)

If there is severe trauma to the mouth or lower jaw, and the mouth-to-mouth technique is not feasible, employ the head tilt maneuver, with *care not to hyperextend* the neck. Keep one hand on the forehead while using the other to lift the chin and keep the lips closed. Cover the victim's nose with your mouth and deliver the ventilations. Passive exhalation between breaths must be through the mouth, so the EMT should open the mouth after each breath to permit this process. Be certain to watch for the rise of the chest to indicate successful ventilation.

Ventilations are normally delivered at five-second intervals until there is a resumption of spontaneous breathing.

See pages 514–517 for mouth-to-stoma technique for patients with a laryngectomy or tracheostomy.

## Rescue Breathing for Infants

The EMT should cover the infant's nose and mouth with his mouth while leaving the head in a relatively neutral position. *Do not hyperextend* the neck, since this tends to block the posterior airway passage. (See Fig. 10–21.)

## Airway Obstruction

The attempts to ventilate the patient may be thwarted by a blocked airway. If this occurs, try repositioning the airway and ventilating again.

If ventilations meet with resistance once again, it is likely that a foreign body is obstructing the airway. Try employing the cross-finger technique to manually clear the airway. (See Fig. 10–8.)

Turn the victim to the side and use the cross-fingered maneuver to open the mouth. Explore the mouth and posterior pharynx with the index and middle fingers in an effort to locate an obstructing foreign body.

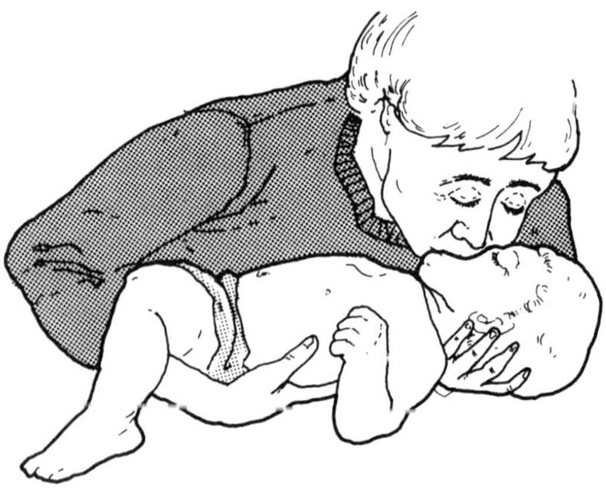

**Figure 10–21.** *Rescue breathing for infants.* The head is maintained in a relatively neutral position. *Do not hyperextend the neck.* The rescuer should cover both the infant's nose and mouth with his mouth when delivering the breaths.

Again, if there is not success in establishing an airway, the back blow procedure should be used. (See Fig. 10–4 and 10–5.)

If the back-blow procedure is equally unsuccessful, the abdominal thrust (or Heimlich) maneuver should be tried up to three or four times before starting over with a sequential repeat of all the procedures for the obstructed airway. (See Fig. 10–6.)

The combination of back blows and manual thrusts seem to be the most effective method of clearing upper airway obstruction. Back blows produce an instantaneous increase in pressure in the respiratory passages which may assist in dislodging a foreign body. The manual thrusts produce a more sustained increase in the pressures within the respiratory passages and may further assist in dislodgment of a foreign body.

## Establishing Presence or Absence of Pulse

The EMT rescuer should feel for a carotid pulse after completing ventilatory efforts. At least five to ten seconds should be spent to confirm pulselessness, since a pulse could be very slow or weak and hard to detect. If the pulse is present, rescue breathing should be continued, reassessing the pulse after every twelve ventilations. The absence of a carotid pulse signals a cardiac arrest, and CPR must be instituted promptly. (See Fig. 10–22.)

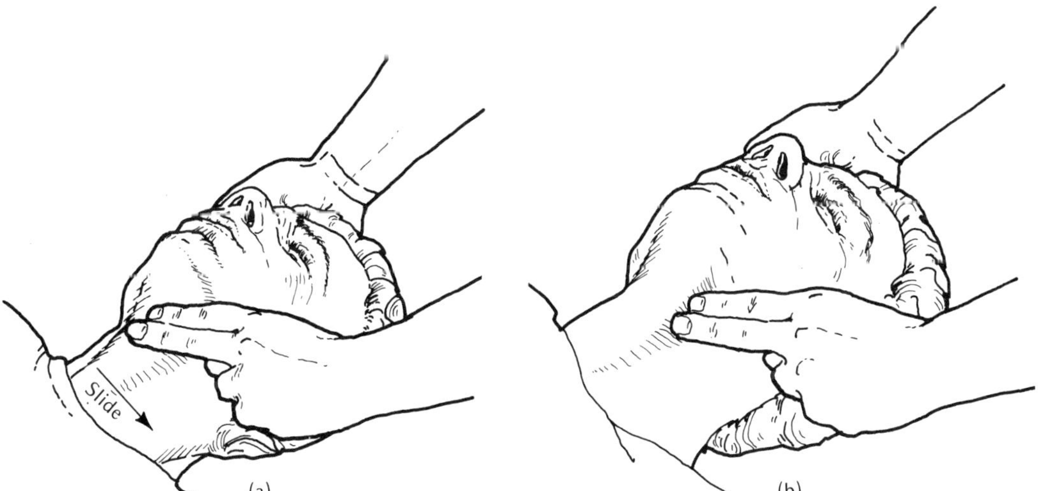


**Figure 10–22.** *Establishing the presence or absence of a pulse.* (a) Palpate the trachea with the index and middle finger, and (b) slide fingers laterally toward the soft portion of the neck. When the pulse is located, palpate for at least 5–10 seconds.

## Cardiac Compressions

Cardiac compressions should be initiated only after the EMT has a functioning airway. The circulation of unoxygenated blood is futile!

Cardiac compressions circulate blood by "squeezing" the heart between the sternum and the bones of the vertebral column. The EMT must be skillful in this technique for successful execution of CPR. (See Fig. 10–23.)

The proper method for compression requires the rescuer to be kneeling at the victim's side next to the chest. A firm surface for the victim is imperative. If a CPR board or similar device is unavailable, the best site for the resuscitation may be the floor! Some authorities recommend a 30 to 40 degree elevation of the legs to increase venous return and perhaps stimulate the heart, improving cardiac output. The victim's chest should be exposed both for landmark identification and for observation of the rise and fall of the chest, as a result of rescue breathing. Two other factors are critical before beginning compressions: (1) locating the proper site for compressions on the sternum, and (2) hand and body positioning for compressions. (See Fig. 10–24 and 10–25, respectively.)

When landmarks have been identified and hand placement assured for proper compressions, the rescuer can initiate the compressions. (Rescue breathing should, of course, still be underway.)

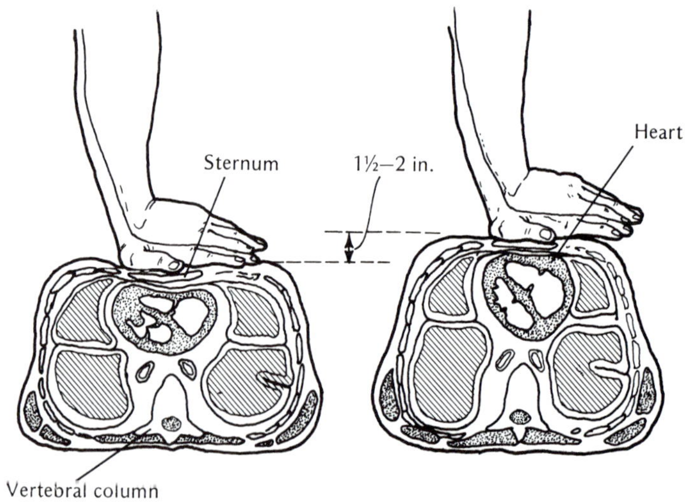


**Figure 10–23.** Cutaway of thorax showing results of cardiac compression. The adult heart empties blood with a downstroke of 1½–2 inches as the heart is squeezed between the sternum and the bones of the vertebral column. The heart refills with blood when sternal pressure is released. Note that hands are *not* lifted off the chest after compressions.

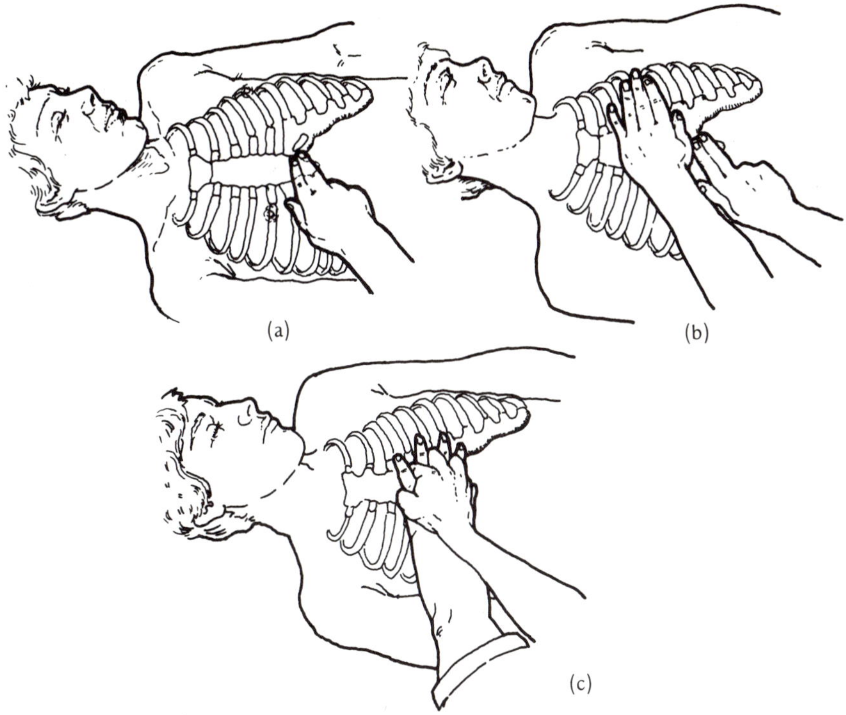


**Figure 10–24.** Location of the proper site for sternal compressions. (a) Locating Xiphoid landmark for compressions, two finger-widths above the Xiphoid. (b) Placement of hand for compressions. (c) Hand position using interlocked fingers.

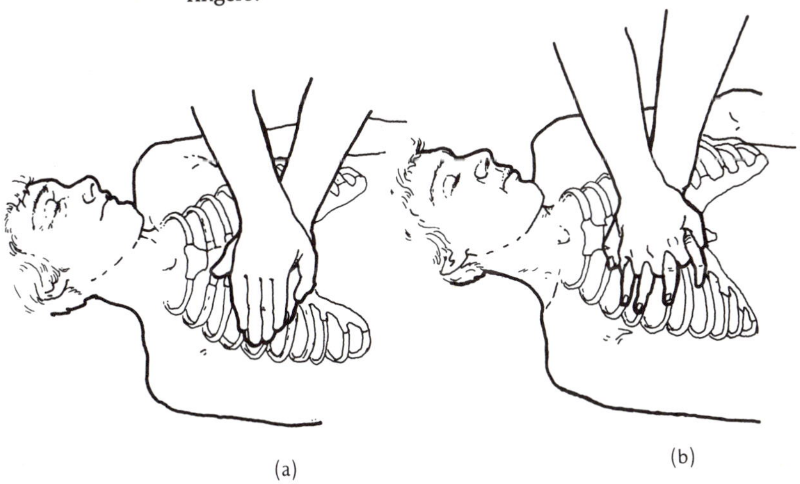


**Figure 10–25.** Hand positioning for CPR. (a) Fingers extended; (b) fingers interlocked. Note that in both (a) and (b) the fingers *do not* exert any pressure on the ribs adjacent to the sternum.

Compressions are made over the lower third of the sternum, two finger-breadths above the xiphoid, at a rate of 60–80 per minute. The sternum should be depressed one and one-half to two inches with each compression.

Chest compressions for an adult require a downward force sufficient to depress the sternum one and one-half inches. The EMT should ensure that his elbows remain locked and that all bending motion is coming from the waist. (See Fig. 10–26.) The interlocked fingers should not touch the chest wall with compressions. When a compression is completed, the rescuer should relax sternal pressure, but the heel of the hand should not lose contact with the victim's chest. The relaxation permits the heart to fill with blood and ready the chambers for the next compression.

While performing CPR, it is likely that air may enter the esophagus and the stomach, creating pressure on the diaphragm, interfering with full lung inflation, and compromising the effectiveness of ventilatory efforts. Furthermore, gastric distention may cause food to be regurgitated. Regurgitation (re-gur″jı-ta′shun), of course, threatens the airway, and so the EMT must be alert for stomach distention, which interferes with breathing, and relieve it by applying gentle pressure to the upper abdomen while the victim is turned to the side. It is imperative to have suctioning at hand, however. (See Fig. 10–27.)

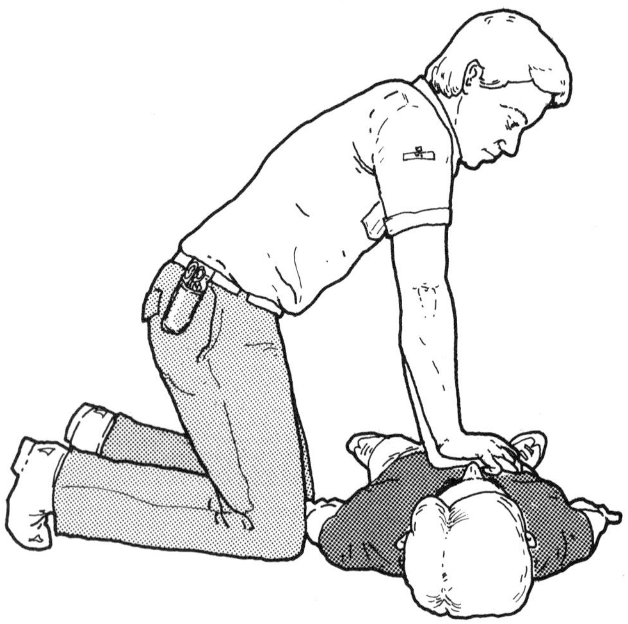

**Figure 10–26.** Rescuer–victim positioning for CPR. Note that the rescuer's elbows are locked in a straight position. Kneeling with the knees separated provides stability and good body mechanics for the rescuer.

Proper execution of chest compressions provides up to one-third of the normal cardiac output and generates a blood pressure compatible to life.

The rate and alternation cycles of breaths to compressions varies with single and two-person rescue. (See Fig. 10–28.) The American Heart Association and American National Red Cross standards for one and two-person rescue are outlined in Appendix 2.

## CPR Modifications for Infants and Children

CPR techniques for infants and children vary somewhat due to the size of their body and some anatomical variations. For example, the heart of a child lies higher in the chest than in an adult, and the sternum and neck muscles tend to be much more pliable (pli′ah-b′l). These differences form the basis for the following modifications in resuscitation.

### *Infants*

The infant who arrests usually has a respiratory arrest as a primary event. Attention to the airway is paramount. The airway should be opened by a slight extension of the head, not hyperextension. Exaggeration of a head tilt kinks off the airway and actually serves to obstruct ventilation.

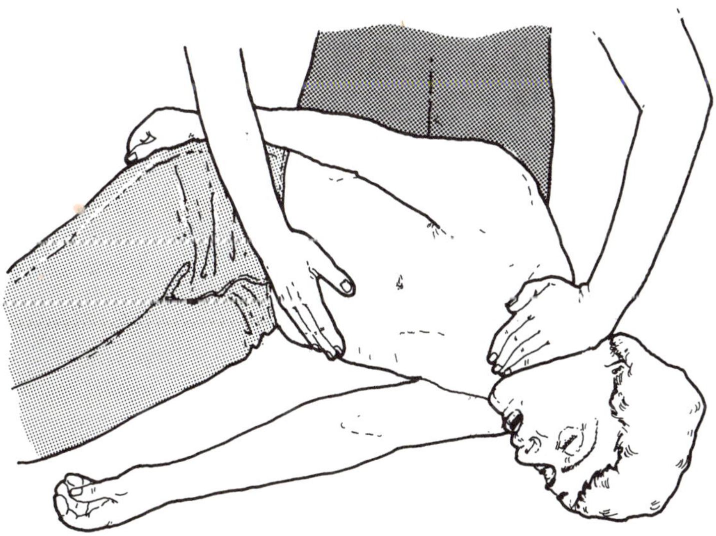

**Figure 10–27.** Relieving gastric distention by applying gentle pressure to the upper abdomen using the flat surface of the hand. Note the victim's side-lying position and dependent mouth to protect the airway in the event of regurgitation of gastric contents. Suction must be on hand for immediate use, however.

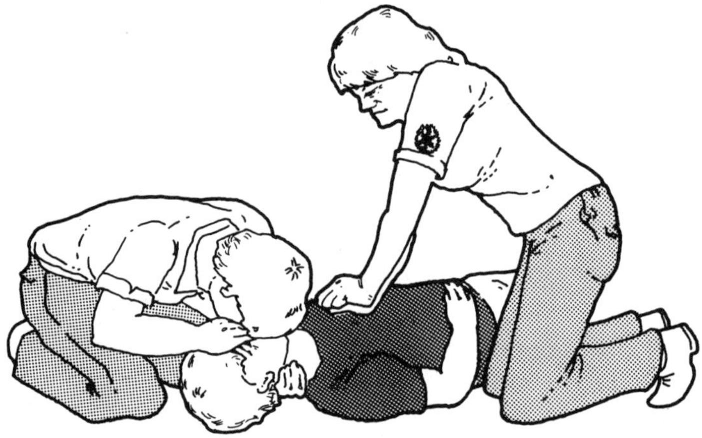

**Figure 10–28.** Rescuer positions for two-person CPR.

Air should be delivered initially by using a mouth-to-mouth technique. Small puffs of air are all that are required to create a satisfactory rise of the chest wall with each ventilation. The rate should be ten to thirty breaths per minute.

If cardiac arrest occurs, external compressions are to be delivered at eighty to one-hundred per minute over the mid-sternum. The middle and index fingers should be used to achieve a one-half- to three-fourths-inch depression of the sternum. (See Fig. 10–29.) An alternate technique is to encircle the thorax with the hands and use the thumbs. (See Fig. 10–30.) Care

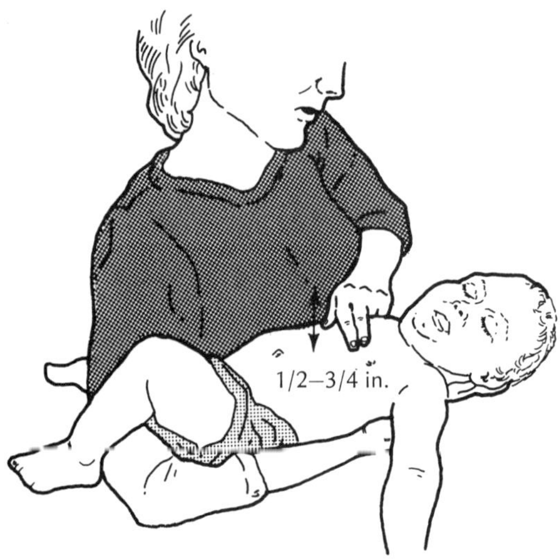


**Figure 10–29.** Positioning for infant CPR. Note that two fingers are used to compress the sternum in the midline. A depression of ½–¾ inch is sufficient for cardiac compressions.

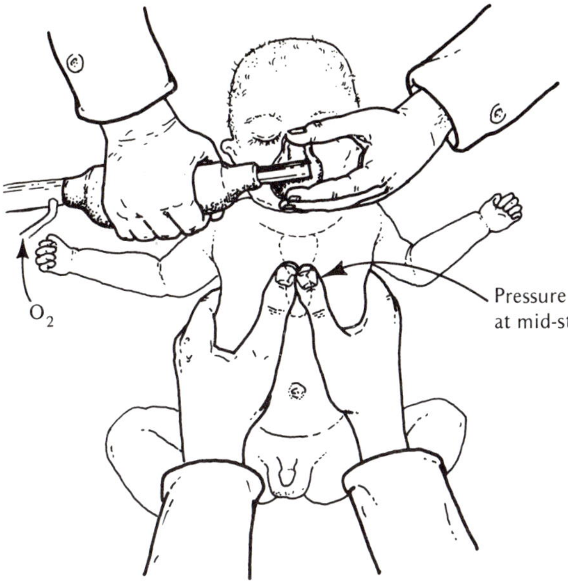


**Figure 10–30.** Infant CPR using thumbs. Care must be exercised to avoid compression of the lower ribs, which could injure the liver or spleen. Technique requires two rescuers.

should be taken to ensure that the *sternum only* is being depressed, since compression on the lower ribs in this latter technique could cause injury to the liver or spleen which lie high in the abdominal cavity. The brachial artery is the recommended site for monitoring the pulse.

*Older Children*

The lower one-third of the sternum is the landmark for compressions in children over five years of age. (See Fig. 10–31.) (Younger children require mid-sternal compressions to protect the high-lying liver and spleen.) Compressions should be delivered using the heel of one hand. Children under five should have eighty to one-hundred compressions per minute, depressing the sternum one-half to three-fourths inch. Children over five require a rate of sixty to eighty compressions per minute, depressing the sternum three-fourths to one inch.

*Continuing CPR*

Once EMTs have initiated CPR, they are obligated to continue until they reach a hospital or are relieved by advanced life support personnel.

Supplemental oxygen at high flow should be given en route. The airway can best be secured by placing an oral-pharyngeal airway in addition to proper head-neck position and the use of a bag-valve mask.

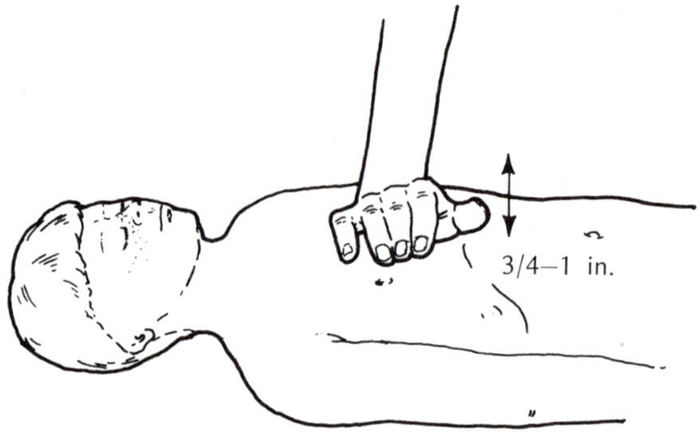


**Figure 10-31.** Children under age 5 require only the heel of one hand for compressions. Compressions are done along the midline of the sternum. A downward stroke of ¾ to 1 inch is recommended.

There should be constant monitoring of the airway and care to prevent airway obstruction from regurgitated stomach contents. Suction should be at hand for immediate use to clear the airway if necessary.

Careful coordination between the EMT driver and the individual(s) doing CPR should be ensured. For example, railroad tracks, bumps, and abrupt stops should be announced so that the EMT doing compressions is not subject to injury. A braced position (feet wide apart) should be used to ensure firm footing for the person doing chest compressions. Even with the best of body mechanics, however, CPR in an ambulance is a strenuous process if it needs to be continued for a long distance transport. "Keeping in shape" with periodic practice sessions is one way for EMTs to prepare themselves for this eventuality, and will serve too, of course, to improve skills required for effective resuscitation efforts.

## AIRWAY ADJUNCTS

### Artificial Airways

Artificial airway devices are used to secure and maintain an open airway, and as an adjunct to facilitate mechanical ventilation. The ones most commonly encountered by the EMT are the oropharyngeal, nasopharyngeal, and esophageal obturator airways.

The *oropharyngeal (OP) airway* is useful for unconscious patients who have a good respiratory effort. It is placed in the oral cavity to prevent the tongue from falling back and blocking the airway. Its placement also aids in suctioning the upper airway and enhances airflow during bag-mask ventilation. An oropharyngeal airway is occasionally used as a "bite stick" for a seizure patient, since it is soft and pliable, thus protecting the teeth.

The oropharyngeal airway should not be used for patients who have

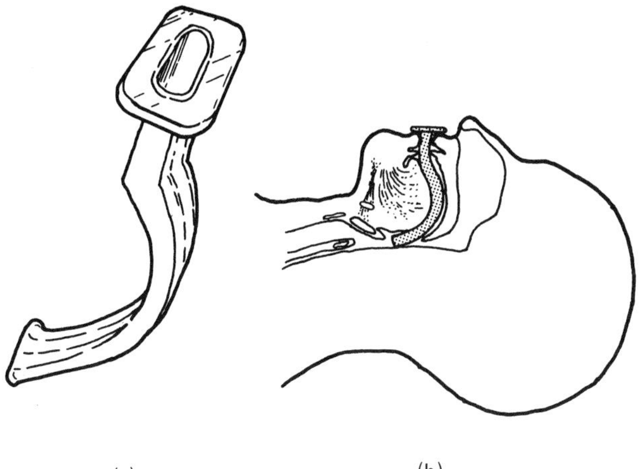

(a) (b)

**Figure 10–32.** (a) Oropharyngeal airway; (b) oropharyngeal airway in place.

an intact gag reflex, since it could induce vomiting and aspiration of gastric contents.

Oropharyngeal airways are available in many types and sizes. The proper size for a patient is determined by measuring the airway from the tip of the earlobe to the corner of the mouth. If the airway extends beyond the corner of the mouth, it is too long. If it does not reach the corner of the mouth, it is too short.

The airway is placed directly by following the curvature of the tongue or by inserting it sideways and rotating it 90° into position. (*Do not* place it in the mouth upside down and rotate it 180° for placement, since such a maneuver can injure the soft tissue in the back of the throat.) A tongue blade is a helpful aid, since it serves to retract the tongue and prevents it from being pushed backward as the airway is placed.

When the airway is in place, the head tilt or jaw thrust position must be maintained to secure a patent airway. (See Fig. 10–32.)

*Nasopharyngeal airways* may be useful for patients who have upper airway problems, but who are responsive and could not tolerate an oral pharyngeal device. The nasopharyngeal airway is a soft rubber tube that is lubricated and inserted gently close to the midline along the floor of the nostril into the posterior pharynx. It creates a passage for air into the lower pharynx and larynx. Careful advancement is advised, since it can easily induce nose bleeding if forced abruptly into place. Correct head tilt or jaw thrust must be maintained with this airway as well to insure unobstructed ventilation. (See Fig. 10–33 a and b.)

*Esophogeal obturator airways (EOAs)* are useful in apneic, unconscious adult patients who require assisted ventilation. The tube is about 15 inches in length, and is designed for insertion into the esophagus and

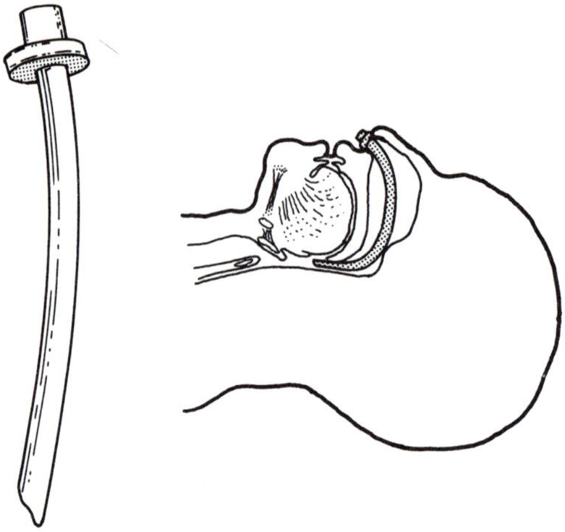

(a) (b)

**Figure 10–33.** (a) Nasopharyngeal airway; (b) nasopharyngeal airway in place.

maintained in position with an inflatable cuff at the blind esophageal end. The upper end has several holes for air to escape into the pharynx and enter the trachea. The unit is completed by a face mask, which accommodates the tube and fixes the unit in proper position. (See Fig. 10–34.) The patient can be ventilated by the rescuer's mouth, or a bag-valve unit.

The airway placement is tested by checking for the rise of the chest upon delivery of positive pressure. If the tube is properly placed, the cuff is then inflated to maintain the EOA in position using a maximum of 35 ml. of air. If by remote chance the tube has entered the trachea, the chest will not rise and the tube must be removed and re-inserted. (See Fig. 10–35.)

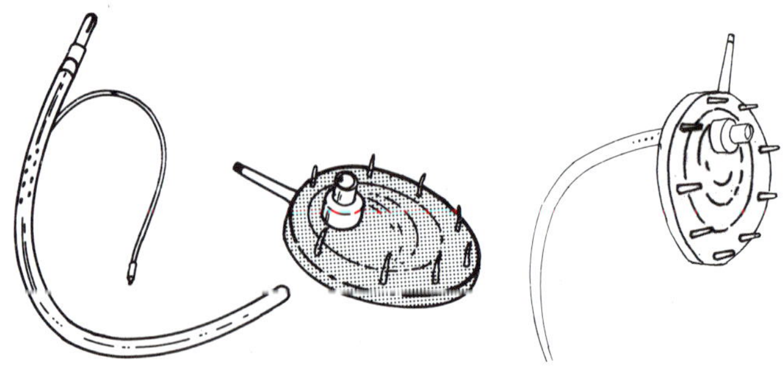

(a) (b)

**Figure 10–34.** (a) Esophageal obturator airway and mask components; (b) device assembled for use.

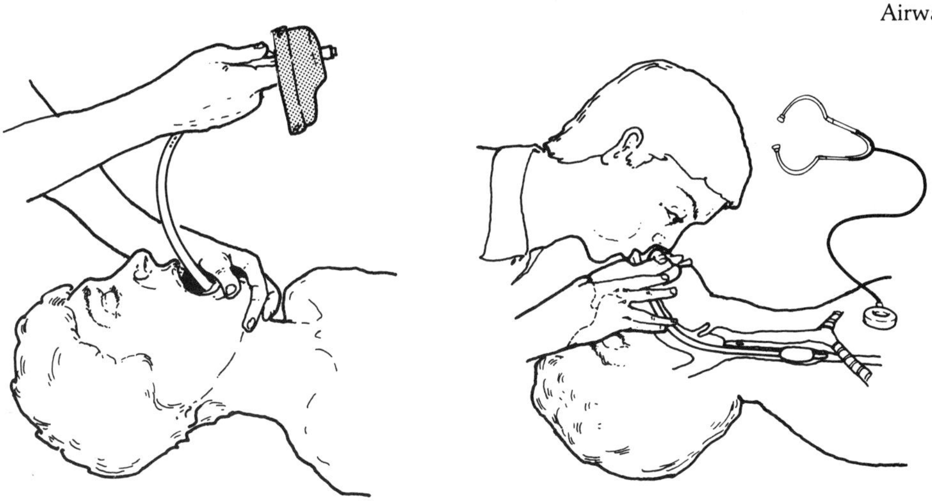

(a) (b)

**Figure 10-35.** (a) Inserting the EOA; (b) ventilating the patient with the EOA.

The EOA is advantageous in preventing stomach contents from being regurgitated and aspirated into the respiratory tract. It also blocks off the esophagus so that air cannot enter the stomach during rescue breathing. (Certain new adaptations of the EOA have a gastric tube within the device to permit decompression of the stomach when indicated.)

The EOA must be removed if the patient initiates spontaneous breathing. Otherwise, the EOA is never removed until the patient's trachea is intubated at the hospital. The removal procedure requires that the patient be turned on his side and the balloon deflated. Suction should be at hand, since vomiting is likely during removal.

The EMT must remember that the EOA is contraindicated if there has been an ingestion of a caustic substance or a history of esophageal disease. In these cases, serious bleeding and even rupture of the esophagus could be induced by attempts to place the EOA device. The EOA is contraindicated in infants and children.

## Other Airway Techniques

There are other modes of establishing an airway in the field, such as endotracheal intubation or cricothyrotomy. (See Fig. 10-31.) These are considered advanced approaches to airway management and are not usually considered within the scope of the basic EMT's practice. However, at times an EMT may encounter massive facial trauma or an airway obstruction that is not relieved by any procedures discussed thus far, and

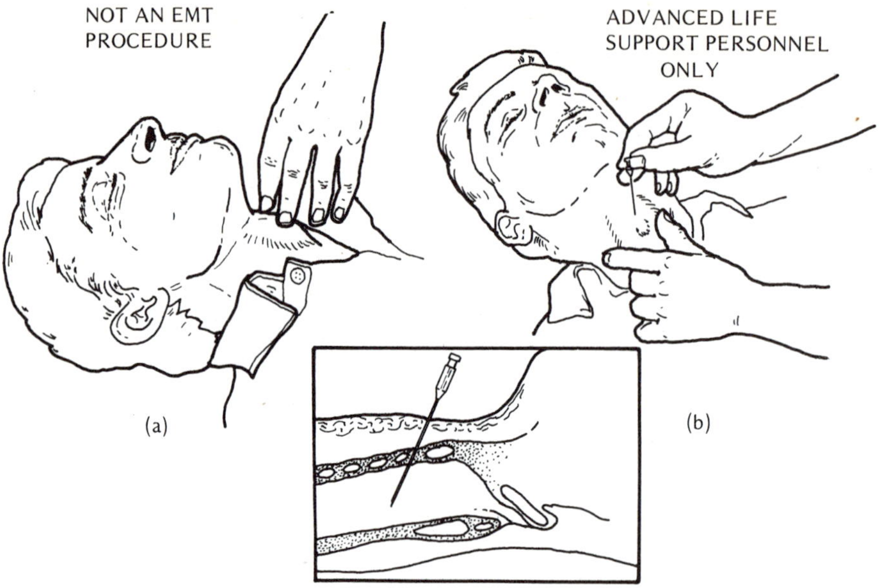


**Figure 10-36.** (a) Locating the cricothyroid membrane for cricothyrotomy; (b) technique for cricothyrotomy.

may observe EMT-Paramedics or physicians performing endotracheal intubation or cricothyrotomy. Of course, EMTs should not attempt any procedure in which they have not been carefully instructed and have had the opportunity to practice with supervision.

### *Suctioning*

When the airway is threatened by blood, vomitus, or accumulating secretions, suctioning must be employed to clear the respiratory passages.

Portable suctioning devices used by the EMT may be foot-operated, hand-operated, or battery-powered. Ambulance units are powered by an electric motor or the vehicle's manifold. (See Fig. 10-37.) A few older vehicles have oxygen-powered units, but these are considered less desirable, since they can rapidly exhaust the oxygen supply on board if the suction is used frequently throughout transport. In all units, regardless of the power source, the basic principle is the production of a vacuum (negative force) for aspirating. (See Fig. 10-38.)

Suction units consist of a power source, a length of tubing, catheter or suction tip, and a trap bottle to collect the aspirate. Suction is created in most set-ups by placing a thumb over a Y-connector in the tubing, and is discontinued by releasing the thumb pressure. (See Fig. 10-38.)

In order to suction the mouth, the head should be turned to the side before introducing the catheter. Do not apply any suction until the catheter is in the desired location for aspirating, since it is nearly impossible to ad-

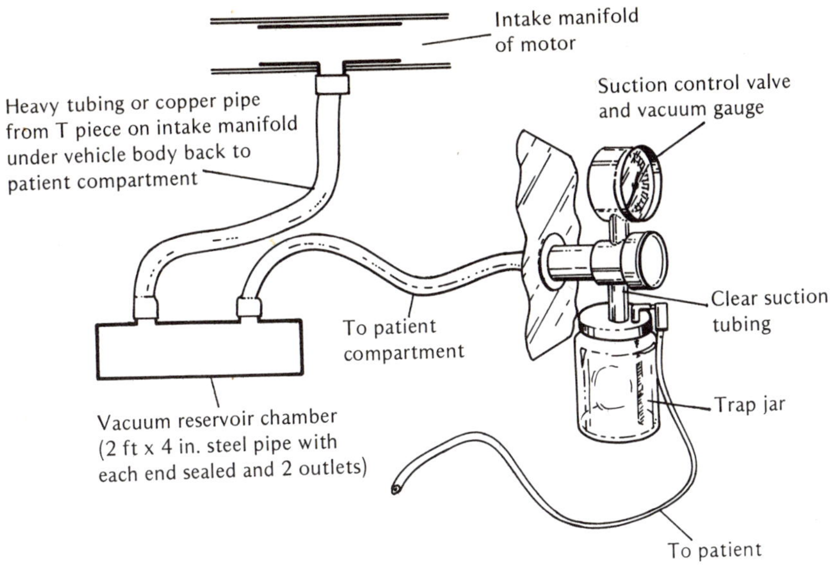


**Figure 10–37.** Diagram of ambulance suction unit.

vance the catheter when suction is in force. The catheter should be rotated gently when it is being withdrawn.

When the nasopharynx or trachea is aspirated, suction should not be applied for longer than 5 to 10 seconds at a time in order to prevent hypoxia. If possible, the patient should be "bagged" with a high concentration of oxygen immediately before and after aspirating to reduce the effects of suctioning out oxygen that is desperately needed in the event of a compromised airway.

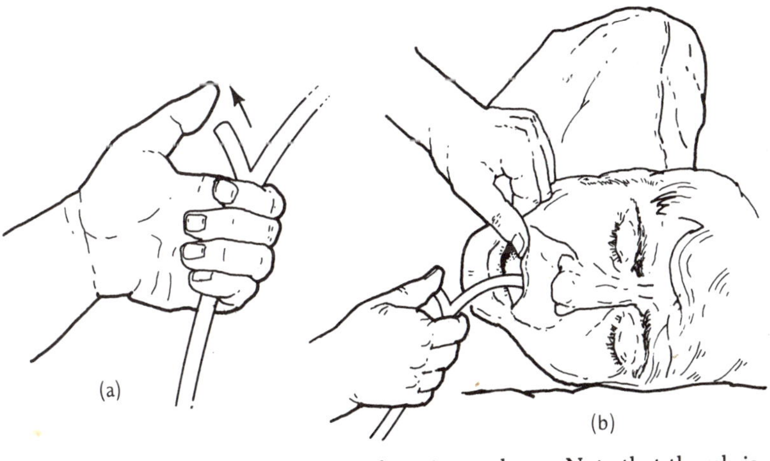


**Figure 10–38.** (a) Introduction of suction catheter. Note that thumb is off the port of the Y-connector. (b) Suctioning in progress. Thumb creates vacuum as port of Y-connector is sealed off.

Suctioning often produces gagging and vomiting and irritates the delicate linings of the upper airway. It also contributes to a rise in intracranial pressure and must be used cautiously for patients with head injury. (See page 287.) If nasal bleeding is induced, it can usually be controlled by slight pressure.

Although the EMT may have little time to attend to details in a true airway emergency, it is ideal to change catheters if both the mouth and trachea must be suctioned to prevent cross-contamination. Clearing the catheter with water or saline between suctionings also is useful in maximizing the efficiency of the catheter and for ensuring good respiratory hygiene.

### Oxygen Therapy

Patients who are short of breath or who have other signs of *hypoxia,* (i.e., tachycardia, cyanosis) should be given oxygen. There are several important factors that the EMT should know about its properties and its administration.

Oxygen is considered as a therapeutic agent, i.e., a drug. It is imperative that an EMT understand some basic properties of this "drug" which have an important relationship to its safe, effective utilization.

#### *Properties*

Oxygen is an odorless, tasteless, colorless substance and is heavier than air. It may escape from supply or delivery apparatus without being noticed. Since it supports combustion, "no smoking" rules must be enforced in the environment while it is in use. Oil, grease, wool, and alcohol, which have low combustion points may ignite spontaneously in the presence of oxygen. Therefore, the use of these products should be avoided while oxygen is being administered. Wool blankets should not be used, for example. Oxygen also has a very drying effect on mucous membranes in the nose and mouth and on the lining of the respiratory tract. Therefore, oxygen should be humidified by bubbling it through distilled water just prior to its administration.

## OXYGEN EQUIPMENT AND SUPPLIES

In the field, the EMT will utilize various equipment and supplies for oxygen therapy. As already stated, oxygen is a drug that must be given properly, depending on the patient's medical condition and past medical history. The equipment and supplies used to allow for the flow of oxygen are just as important as the oxygen given, because the EMT must be able to mechanically prepare the equipment for therapeutic delivery of oxygen.

The components that make up an oxygen delivery system are: source, pressure regulator, flow regulators, humidifiers (hu-mid'i-fi"yerz), and the device for delivery. (See Fig. 10-39.)

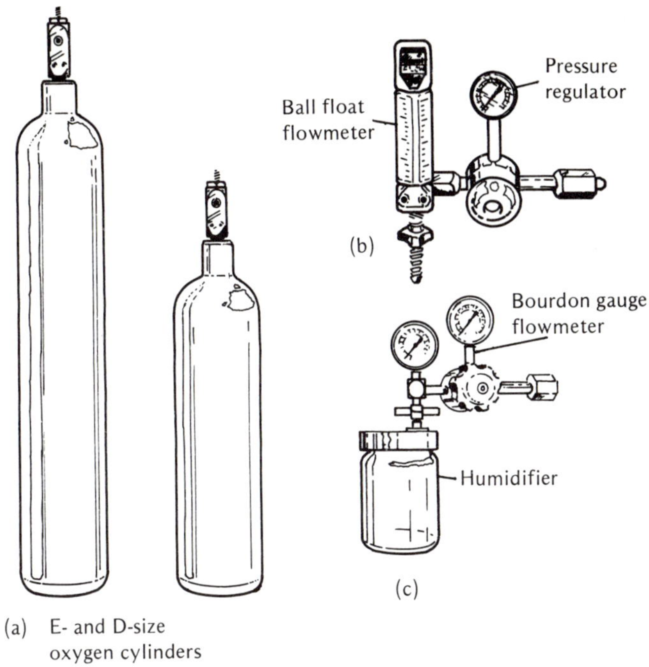


**Figure 10–39.** Components of oxygen administration system: (a) oxygen cylinders; (b) ball float flowmeter and pressure regulator; (c) Bourdon gauge flowmeter and pressure regulator. Note humidification unit.

## Oxygen Source and Regulators

Oxygen comes as a dry compressed gas, stored in varying sized seamless steel containers. Cylinder sizes that the prehospital EMT will most commonly work with are the D, E, and M size oxygen cylinders.

The D size cylinder contains about 350 liters of oxygen when filled to specific limits and has a pressure of 2000 to 2200 pounds per square inch (psi). This size cylinder is usually favored in portable resuscitator units.

The E size cylinder is also generally found in portable oxygen units, because of its size. It contains about 650 liters of oxygen when filled to specific limits and it has a pressure of 2000 to 2200 pounds per square inch (psi).

The D and E size cylinders are considered portable units because their size allows the EMT to carry them to the victim, should oxygen be required. The EMT should never be caught without oxygen to give to the patient. Portable oxygen units should be available to carry to the emergency scene.

The M size cylinder is usually a fixed cylinder, usually located near the head of the patient in the ambulance. Most ambulances today have an oxygen compartment whose access is outside the vehicle. The oxygen regulator and tubing is operable through an access window within the patient compartment. The M cylinder is large and heavy and not designed to be carried by the average person. It contains 3000 liters of oxygen when filled to specific limits, and also has a pressure of 2000 to 2200 pounds per square inches (psi).

Pressure regulators are attached to gas cylinders in two ways. Yoke pressure gauges are attached to E size and smaller cylinders by outlet valves designed to reduce oxygen pressure. The yoke assembly contains a pin-index safety attachment so that the gauge cannot be attached to other gas cylinders that are not filled with oxygen. Pins of various configurations (designated by a combination of any two numbers between one and six) are affixed to all gas cylinders. Each different gas has a different pin-index and only that particular yoke pressure gauge assembly will fit on them. (See Fig. 10–40.)

Threaded connections are used for cylinders larger than E size. High pressure regulators which must be attached to administer such gases must conform to the American and Canadian Standards for compressed gas cylinders. Every conceivable type of gas and gas mixture has been assigned a threaded inlet and outlet combination, to insure against interchanging administration apparatus or regulators calibrated for other gases. This system involves the mating of a hexagonal nut with a corresponding threaded connector. (See Fig. 10–41.)

## High Pressure Regulators

Pressure regulators must be used on oxygen cylinders to regulate the extremely high pressure contained within them. Pressures of 2000 to 2200 could not be therapeutically (ther″ah-pu′tik-le) used for oxygen delivery under any circumstance. Pressure regulators reduce the very high cylinder pressure to a working pressure between 30 to 70 psi. For routine administration of oxygen to patients 30–70 psi is further reduced to achieve a

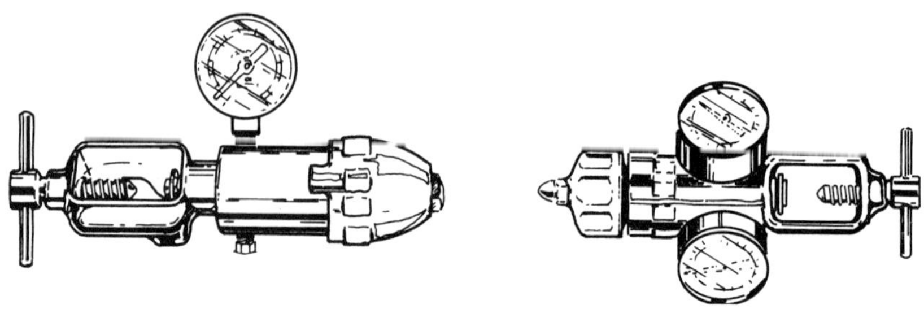

**Figure 10–40.** Two types of yoke assemblies for oxygen administration.

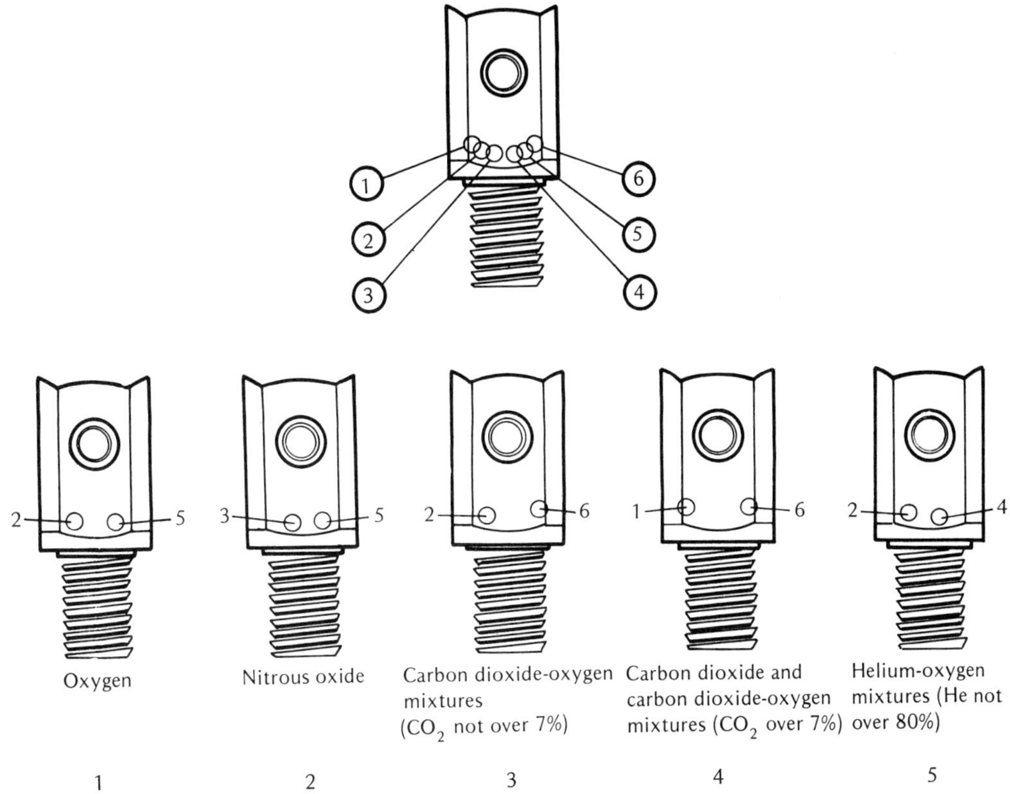


**Figure 10-41.** Examples of the pin index safety system.

more precise rate of flow, measured in liters per minute (l/min). The pressure in the oxygen cylinder is measured by the high pressure regulator. The gauge will indicate the pressure in the cylinder in pounds per square inch. Regulators may be single or double stage. A single-stage regulator will reduce the cylinder pressure in one stage by passing it through a single chamber with one diaphragm and seat. A double-stage regulator is set so that the pressure is dropped in two stages or more gradually, first to about 175 psi and then to about 50 psi. Once the pressure is dropped to a more workable pressure, a flow meter is added to the cylinder so that the release of oxygen can be regulated in liters per minute for definitive therapeutic use.

## Flowmeters

There are two common types of flowmeters that the EMT will use.

*Pressure—Compensated Flowmeter*

The pressure-compensated flowmeters are glass or plastic tubes with the flow setting etched on the surface of the tube. In the glass or plastic tube is a tapered hollow tube containing a light weight ball or "float." The position of the float with respect to the calibration on the tube indicates the flow rate being delivered. The flow of gas is regulated by a needle valve placed downstream from the float ball. The ball or float will record only actual delivered oxygen flow. Therefore, if back pressure develops from an obstruction such as kinked tubing, the ball or float will drop to zero. This is because pressure-compensated flowmeters are gravity dependent and must always be maintained in an upright position. (See Fig. 10–39.)

*Bourdon Gauge Flowmeters*

Unlike the gravity dependent pressure-compensated flowmeter, the Bourdon (Boor′den) gauge flowmeter may be used in any position since it is not affected by gravity. Obviously, this type of gauge hooked to a small oxygen cylinder is extremely useful when transporting the patient from the accident scene to the ambulance. The oxygen unit system should be small enough to fit on the stretcher next to the patient or comfortably between the patient's legs. (See Fig. 10–39.)

In this manner, oxygen therapy is not interrupted during patient transport. Once inside the ambulance, oxygen connecting tubing can be changed from the portable unit to the large stationary cylinder if desired. Then once at the medical facility, the tubing can be changed back to the smaller, portable unit to continue oxygen therapy during transport.

Because the Bourdon gauge is actually a pressure gauge, it is calibrated to record flow rate. In the presence of back pressure from an obstruction downstream, the gauge will actually read a higher flow rate than what the flow actually is. This is the major disadvantage of this type of flowmeter.

## Duration of Oxygen Flow

The EMT should always exchange oxygen cylinders once they reach a certain pressure level. This level is called "residual (re-zid′u-al) safe pressure," and is 200 psi. A method to calculate the remaining life of any oxygen cylinder is shown in the following table.

Formula For Calculating Duration of Oxygen Flow For Any Size Cylinder

$$\frac{\text{(Actual gauge pressure in psi - safe residual pressure)}}{\text{Desired flowrate (liters per minute)}} \times \text{Constant} = \text{Duration of flow in minutes}$$

Constants Used For Various Size Cylinders

| Cylinder Size | D | E | G | H | K | M |
|---|---|---|---|---|---|---|
| Constant | 0.16 | 0.28 | 2.41 | 3.14 | 3.14 | 1.56 |

Safe Residual Pressure is Always 200 psi

Example of how to use the above formula: You have an E cylinder with a gauge pressure showing 900 psi. The patient must have an oxygen flow rate of 6 liters per minute. How long will the flow rate last?

$$\frac{(900 - 200) \times 0.28}{6} = \frac{196}{6} = 32.6 \text{ minutes (or approximately } \tfrac{1}{2} \text{ hour)}$$

COLOR CODES FOR GAS CYLINDERS

| *Gas* | *Cylinder Color* |
|---|---|
| Oxygen ($O_2$) | Green |
| Air ($O_2 + N_2$) | Green or Silver |
| Carbon dioxide ($CO_2$) | Gray |
| ($CO_2 + O_2$) Mixture | Gray/Green |
| Nitrogen ($N_2$) | Silver or Yellow |
| Helium (He) | Brown |
| (He + $O_2$) Mixture | Brown/Green |
| Nitrous oxide ($N_2O$) | Blue |
| Cyclo-propane ($(CH_2)_3$) | Orange or Orange/Chrome |

The EMT should abide by the following safety precautions when using oxygen:

1. To ensure that the proper gas is being utilized the EMT should check the:
   a. label on the cylinder that states the type of gas contained
   b. color of the cylinder (oxygen should always be in a green cylinder)
   c. pin-index system
2. Oil, grease, or any other combustible supporting substance should never be used on oxygen cylinders. The cylinder may explode when oxygen comes in contact with the substance.
3. Smoking should never be permitted around oxygen cylinders or when oxygen is in use. Warning signs should be placed in the appropriate areas that read "Oxygen—No Smoking."

4. Regulators should be inspected routinely for cracks, faults, and corrosion. One should never use a regulator in need of repair under any circumstances.

5. One should gradually turn the cylinder valve wheel slowly to allow the gas to enter the regulator. Avoid a sudden rush of high pressure into the regulator.

6. Regulator inlets and connectors should be kept free from dust and debris.

7. When the gas is entering into the regulator, turn the glass or plastic tube away from the body and never point the regulator in the path of others when opening the cylinder valve wheel.

8. Oxygen cylinders should be stored in an upright position and secured safely. Valve assemblies have broken off cylinders after falling, sending the assembly through the sides of the ambulance walls!

9. The cylinder should be hydrostatically (hi″dro-stat′ik-le) tested every five years. This information appears on the label on the front of the cylinder.

10. All cylinders should have an O-ring or washer attached to them by the plastic dust cover. If the washer is not on the cylinder, do not use it, since the washer seats the pressure regulator.

## OXYGEN DELIVERY DEVICES

Oxygen may be administered by several types of devices, the selection dependent upon the age, general condition, and ventilatory needs of the patient. Oxygen delivery apparatus used in the field may vary slightly from that found in hospitals, but types described below are the basic kinds used in pre-hospital care situations.

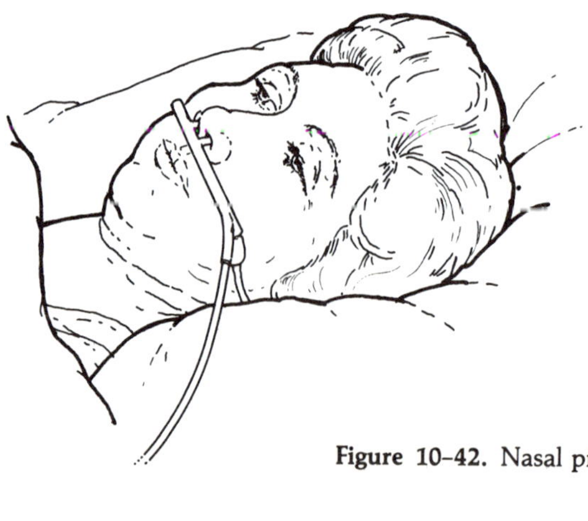

**Figure 10–42.** Nasal prongs for oxygen delivery.

## Nasal Cannula or Prongs

The nasal cannula (kan′u-lah) (see Fig. 10–42) is the most frequently used device for patients who have spontaneous breathing. The flow rate (*l*/min) will determine, to a degree, the ultimate concentration being delivered. Two to six *l*/min will result in oxygen concentrations of 25 percent to 40 percent. Nasal cannulas are well tolerated by most patients and prevent rebreathing of expired air, which occurs when mask-type devices are employed. Nasal devices permit the patient to talk and do not exaggerate the "smothering" feeling experienced by some dyspneic (disp-ne′ik) patients. Even mouth breathing with the nasal cannula in place does little to reduce the concentration of oxygen being delivered.

## Face Masks

Several types of face masks are currently used by EMTS; these include the simple mask (Fig. 10–43), the oxygen reservoir mask, the Venturi (ven″tu′re) mask or variable concentration mask, the pocket mask, (Fig. 10–44), and the bag-valve mask.

Face masks are poorly tolerated by some patients who are short of breath, because they tend to create a feeling of suffocation. They may be used when concentrations of 35 percent to 60 percent are desired (8–12 *l*/min). Face masks should not be used with a flow of less than 5 *l*/min because the mask will not be well flushed and there will be excessive breathing of expired air. Furthermore, with a flow less than 5 *l*/min, *less* oxygen will be delivered than is available in room air. (Room air contains 21 percent oxygen.)

The oxygen reservoir mask provides for the rebreathing of oxygen-enriched air. As the patient exhales, approximately the first third of the air is trapped in the bag for rebreathing. Since this air has been in the "dead space" of the upper airways and has not been involved in gas exchange at the lung level, it is oxygen rich. This air, added to the flow from the supply source, will provide very high concentrations for the patient. The mask, of course, contains numerous exhalation ports to permit the escape of carbon dioxide. The mask seal must be tight for the system to function effectively.

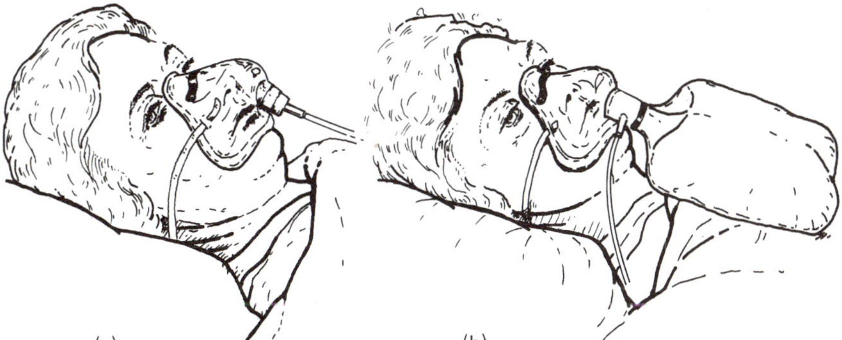


**Figure 10–43.** Face masks for oxygen delivery: (a) simple mask; (b) oxygen reservoir mask.

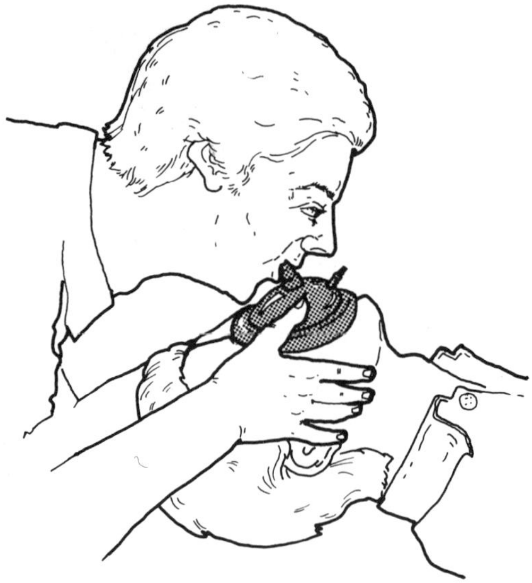

**Figure 10-44.** Pocket mask in use. Note inlet for supplemental oxygen administration.

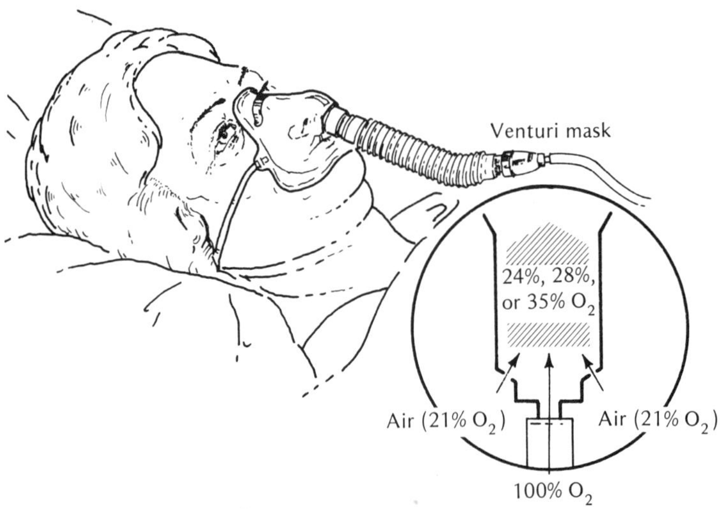


**Figure 10-45.** A Venturi or variable concentration oxygen mask. The inset demonstrates the principle of the Venturi mask. As oxygen is delivered via the inlet tube, a negative pressure is created to the side of the delivery tube. Room air is drawn in through the ports and entrapped. The oxygen delivered to the patient is thus decreased in concentration and accurately calibrated.

Concentrations of 60–90 percent can be achieved with a flow of 6–12 *l*/min.

The Venturi mask is designed to create a carefully controlled and fixed oxygen concentration. The device permits delivery of set percentages by adjusting a flow rate dial on the mask unit. The Venturi mask is especially useful for patients with a history of chronic obstructive lung disease, whose condition may be worsened by highly concentrated oxygen, which further depresses respirations. (See Fig. 10–45.) Low settings, such as 24 percent, are used initially and the concentration is increased based on the patient's tolerance. One important advantage of this mask is that the oxygen concentration delivered is not affected by changes in the rate or depth of respirations.

## Bag-Valve Masks

A bag-valve mask device (Fig. 10–46) is useful to assist the patient in breathing or to ventilate an apneic patient. Oxygen concentration can be increased greatly when used in conjunction with supplemental oxygen or oxygen accumulator (reservoir) tubing. A concentration of 21 percent (room air) can be achieved without any supplemental oxygen. By adding a liter flow of 12 *l*/minute, a 40 percent oxygen source can be obtained. By the addition of oxygen accumulator (reservoir) tubing, it is capable of providing a 90 percent oxygen concentration.

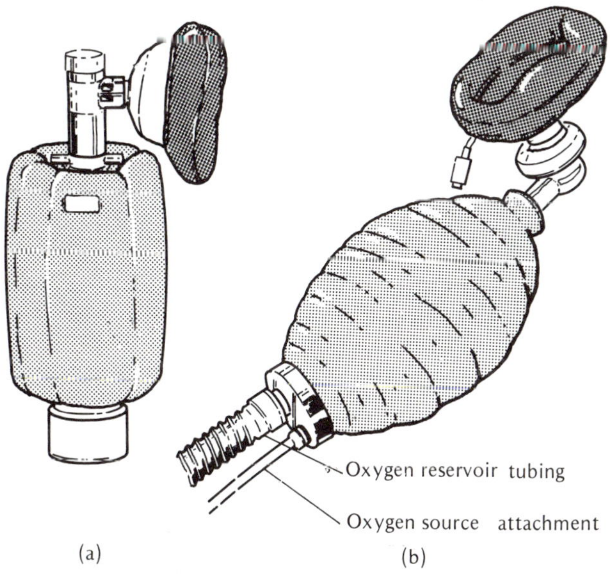


**Figure 10–46.** Two types of bag-valve-masks. Both units are non-rebreathing and self-inflating. Both can be adapted for use of supplemental oxygen and oxygen reservoir (accumulator) tubing.

A tight seal of the face mask is imperative, and it is recommended that an oropharyngeal airway be used in conjunction to ensure an open airway.

As the mask is applied, the EMT should place his last two or three fingers on the patient's mandible. The thumb and index finger are positioned on either side of the valve connection to achieve a good mask fit. Such a seal of the mask rim is imperative and takes considerable practice to perfect. Of course, the head should be tilted as previously described for maximum ventilatory efficiency. The opposite hand is used to compress the bag. The chest should rise with pressure (inhalation) and fall with exhalation.

Since the bag-valve mask technique often causes air to be introduced into the stomach, gastric distention may occur and the EMT should be alert to this hazard.

As EMTs become skilled in the use of the bag-valve mask, they will be able to judge lung compliance and the effectiveness of the ventilatory assistance.

Special units have been designed for neonates and infants which limit pressure with release valves or which control the operator's delivery of air volume, thus protecting the tiny lungs. (See Fig. 10–47.)

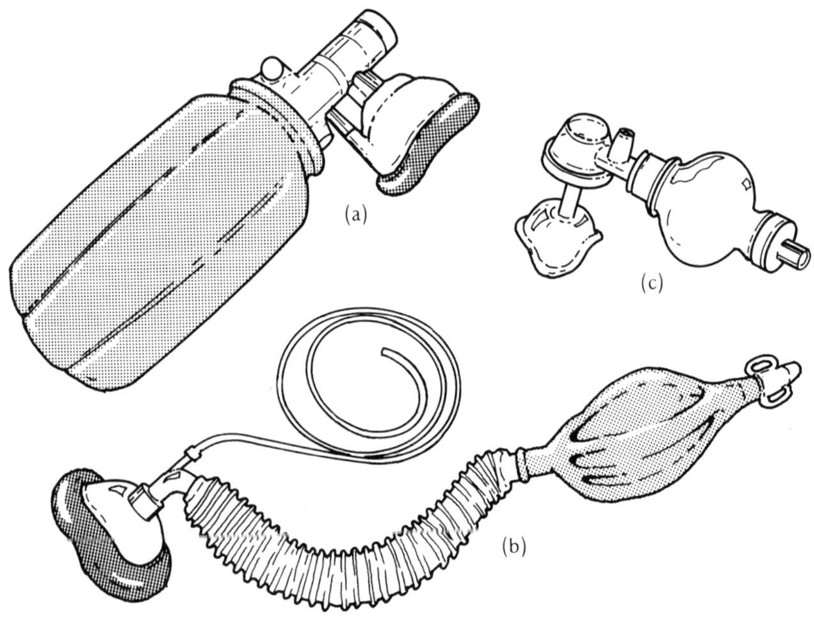


**Figure 10–47.** Special bag-valve-masks for neonates and infants. (a) Infant Ambu-bag (limits pressure with release valve); (b) Mapleson bag (bag limits operator pressure); (c) infant bag-mask (limits pressure with release valve).

## Oxygen-Powered Breathing Device

A few EMTs may find themselves in a locale that uses an oxygen-powered breathing device. (See Fig. 10–48.) One-hundred percent oxygen can be delivered since the flow rate is approximately 100 *l*/min. under positive pressure. The device must be very carefully used since overinflation of lungs can be disastrous! Delivery is regulated by manual triggering of a demand valve using carefully controlled timed intervals. The oxygen-powered device is seldom used in children under ten; however, a special low-flow adapter is available for use in these cases.

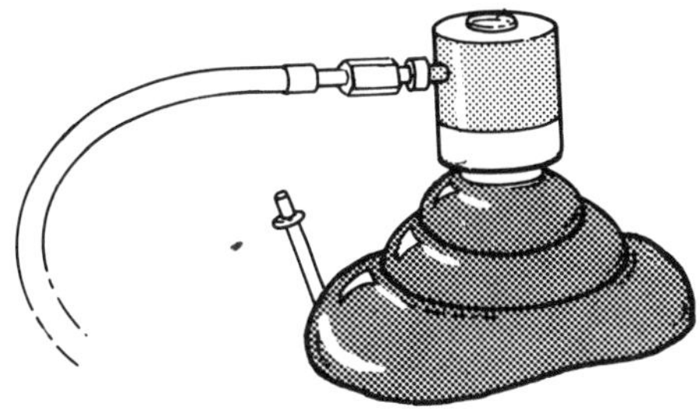

**Figure 10–48.** Oxygen-powered pressure beathing unit. The button is manually operated to deliver at least 100 *l*/min. to a face mask or other airway device.

## Other Considerations in Delivery of Oxygen

### *Humidity*

Oxygen should be humidified during administration to prevent excessive drying of mucous membranes. Moist mucous linings do become dry, and they tend to crack, inviting infection. Furthermore, secretions in the respiratory tract will become dry and thickened which tend to deter their being "coughed up" and consequently, they serve to obstruct vital air passages. Moist oxygen also, of course, contributes to the patient's comfort since dry oxygen irritates delicate upper respiratory structures.

### *Positioning*

Patients who are short of breath ordinarily do not tolerate flat positions well and should be permitted to sit up. Some who are alert may choose to sit on the side of the stretcher and lean over slightly to assist their breathing effort. The EMT should permit the patient to assume the most comfortable position.

## *References*

Bander, Joseph J.; Kimmerle, Linda; and Eie, Knut F.; eds. "Cardiac Arrest," *Topics in Emergency Medicine,* Vol. 1, No. 2, July 1979.

Barber, Janet M. "Pediatric Medical Emergencies," *The EMT Journal,* 4:70–71, June 1980.

Barber, Janet M., and Budassi, Susan A. *Mosby's Manual of Emergency Care,* St. Louis, MO: The C. V. Mosby Co., 1979.

Budassi, Susan A., "Cardiopulmonary Resuscitation," *Critical Care Quarterly*, Vol. 1, No. 1, May 1978.

Dube, Shiv K., and Pierog, Sophie H. *Immediate Care of the Sick and Injured Child*. St. Louis, MO: The C. V. Mosby Co., 1978.

Ellis, Patricia D., and Billings, Diane M. *Cardiopulmonary Resuscitation: Procedures for Basic and Advanced Life Support*. St. Louis, MO: The C. V. Mosby Co., 1980.

Levin, Daniel L.; Morris, Frances C.; and Moore, Gerald C., eds. *A Practical Guide to Pediatric Intensive Care*. St. Louis, MO: The C. V. Mosby Co., 1979.

Pascoe, Delmar J. and Grossman, Moses. *Quick Reference to Pediatric Emergencies*. Philadelphia, PA: J. B. Lippincott Co., 1978.

"Standards and Guidelines for Cardiopulmonary Resuscitation (CPR) and Emergency Cardiac Care (ECC)," *JAMA*, Vol. 244, No. 5, Aug. 1, 1980, pp. 453–78.

Stephenson H., Jr. *Cardiac Arrest and Resuscitation*, 4th ed. St. Louis, MO: The C. V. Mosby Co., 1974.

Todres, I. D., and Rogers, M. C. "Methods of External Cardiac Massage In The Newborn Infant," *Journal of Pediatrics*, 86:781–782, 1975.

# Chapter 11

# Shock

*Shock* is a condition in which blood flow to tissues (perfusion [per-fu′-zhun]) is inadequate to meet the oxygen or nutritional needs of the cell. Shock is not a disease entity. It is a response to injury or illness and is classified according to the event that evokes it. Before discussion of the various kinds of shock, it is in order to review the mechanisms which normally regulate blood flow to tissue.

## CIRCULATION

There are three primary components essential to ensuring circulation: *blood volume, the pumping force of the heart,* and *peripheral resistance.*

### *Volume*

In order for all body cells to be properly nourished, an adequate amount of blood must be available for circulation. The quantity of blood must be sufficient to "prime the cardiac pump" and to reach even the most distant vascular beds. The quality of blood is also important. It must contain an abundant supply of hemoglobin (he″mo-glo′bin) (oxygen-carrying red blood cells), protein, and other vital nutrients within its fluid mass.

### *Pump*

Blood would be incapable of supporting cellular life if it were not being constantly propelled throughout the body to pick up oxygen and nutrients and dispose of waste products at various points along the way. The pumping action of the heart ensures this constant flow. Within the heart's four chambers, there must be a dynamic balance of blood for its pumping efficiency. Essentially, the intake and output of blood at each cardiac cycle must remain fairly constant. Since the heart can only deliver the blood it receives, the circulation must ensure a steady return of venous blood to the right side of the heart. The strength, regularity, and rhythm of the heart's pumping action are all crucial factors in its ability to maintain vital blood flow.

### *Peripheral Resistance*

Blood vessels throughout the body have the ability to constrict (become smaller) or dilate (expand) in circumference. There are nervous system and hormonal interplays that maintain a vascular tone that is appropriate for handling the blood volume in the body and to adapt to changing pumping patterns of the heart. For example, if there is hemorrhage and low volume, the blood vessels constrict to reduce their capacity and increase their resistance to the heart's pumping in order to keep blood flowing at high speed and into even remote, peripheral vascular beds. If they did not have this capacity to constrict, there would be a deceleration of flow and essentially a stagnant circulation, especially in remote areas of the body. Of course, blood that is not flowing is like nonflowing water in a stream; it becomes polluted with waste products and is unable to get rid of them or to replenish itself with fresh supplies. Furthermore, blood that is not moving tends to coagulate or clot, creating an obstruction to further flow.

All three of these factors, *volume, pumping,* and *peripheral resistance* must function together to ensure the maintenance of normal blood pressure and thus cellular perfusion.

## CELLULAR PERFUSION

The EMT must understand what shock's devastating consequences are to the individual cells. These cells are actually responsible for life processes, and demand a dependable supply of energy-giving resources such as oxygen, fluid, electrolytes, protein, and other nutrients. Certain cells have more important activities than others. It is easy to appreciate that brain cells are more vital to life than cells of the feet or hands. Therefore, the intrinsic wisdom of nature has built-in defenses to protect vital organs during circulatory failure. We will talk about these later. First, though, let us study what happens in the smallest components of the circulatory network.

Blood enters the capillary bed as a result of the hydrostatic pressure (fluid pumping pressure) of the blood. As it makes its way around the microcirculatory unit, it pushes off water, oxygen, and other elements vital to the life processes of the cell. Since the blood is giving up water, it becomes concentrated with cellular elements which are rich in protein. Protein exerts an attracting or colloidal (kŏ-loi′dal) pressure within the blood vessel which pulls carbon dioxide and other waste products from the cells to return to the central part of the body for "recycling" or disposal. As long as this process works in a dependable manner, life processes are well supported. If, however, the blood volume is reduced the pump does not work, or if there is too little protein in the blood, compensations must be made, at once, to preserve the cell. In order to appreciate the sequence and types of adjustments, let us look at what happens in hypovolemic states.

## HYPOVOLEMIA

Hypovolemia is a low-volume state resulting from any condition in which body fluid is lost in sufficient amounts to reduce the circulating blood to a point at which some organs or cells are deprived of oxygen and essential nutrients. Burns and crushing injuries, as well as hemorrhage, can result in hypovolemic shock.

During the early phases of body fluid loss, the body makes adjustments to compensate for the state of lowered fluid volume. The urine output is reduced, and vasoconstrictor (vas″o-kon-strik′tor) substances (epinephrine [ep″ĭ-nef′rin] and norepinephrine [nor″ep-ĭ-nef′rin]) are released into the bloodstream to create an increase in peripheral resistance. Blood is shunted (diverted) from the periphery of the body to vital organs in order to sustain circulating volume. There is no significant drop in blood pressure due to adjustments in circulatory dynamics. This initial phase is termed *compensated* shock. When the body can no longer compensate for the lowered volume state, the blood pressure will drop and the skin will be cool and clammy. These latter signs and symptoms mean that the body's defenses have been overwhelmed and that cardiovascular collapse has occurred. In healthy individuals, up to 25 percent of the circulating volume (1–2 liters) must be lost in order for blood pressure to fall!

In acute blood loss states, there is often a twenty minute or longer time period of *compensated* shock before cardiovascular collapse is evident. It is during this interval that the EMT must be alert to early signs and symptoms of hypovolemia.

### Understanding Fluid Loss Adjustments

Sixty percent of the body weight of an average adult is fluid. Sources of this fluid are: water between and within cells and tissues, spinal fluid, blood, lymph, and a variety of essential secretions from glands. Ordinarily the type and amount of body fluid in all spaces is regulated by a varying blood pressure, changes in renal activity, and a series of hormonal-nervous system influences. Normally, there is a constant adjustment of body functions to maintain a delicate fluid balance, that is, a state in which the intake equals the output. For example, when one is deprived of fluids on a hot day, the thirst mechanism encourages us to drink. In the meantime, the kidneys are curbing urine output in an effort to conserve water. If the individual does not correct his fluid level by drinking, the hormones epinephrine and norepinephrine would be released. The purpose of these substances is to constrict peripheral circulation and to enhance the cardiovascular function in a way that it can maintain circulation, even with the reduced volume of available fluid. These hormones tend to excite or stimulate the individual and he may experience a state of anxiety or a feeling of "jumpiness." The heart rate would accelerate in an attempt to circulate the reduced blood volume in the most efficient manner possible. As blood is shunted from the skin to vital organs, the warm, dry skin soon looks pale and feels cool. At this point, the EMT will promptly recognize that there is something wrong. In addition to the rapid pulse rate and skin changes, there may be evidence of poor circulation to the brain. For instance, the patient may be confused, mentally dull, or exhibit other clues of a depressed state of consciousness. All of these changes may precede an actual drop in the blood pressure.

The time period in which the body adjusts to a lowered volume state varies considerably, depending upon how much fluid is lost, what kind, and over what period of time the loss occurs. For example, in dehydration, or a slow loss of blood from a vein, the process may take several hours or days. However, if the blood loss is rapid as in arterial bleeding or associated with large wounds, profound shock may be evident in a matter of minutes.

The EMT should appreciate that shock can occur from any fluid loss, not just blood. Prolonged vomiting, diarrhea, draining wounds, burns, profuse perspiration, and low fluid intake can also result in shock. This is particularly true in the small child or the elderly. If an EMT suspects shock, all clues to hypovolemia should be investigated, not merely bleeding.

## CARDIOGENIC SHOCK

Cardiogenic (kar″de-o-jen′ik) shock is due to a failure of the "pump." It may be due to a failure of the myocardium after an infarction or due to a disturbance in rhythm which creates a failure of tissue perfusion. Cardiac tamponade (tam″pon-ād′) (see page 318) or a pulmonary embolus (em′bo-lus) (see page 328) can also impair cardiac performance, resulting in cardiogenic shock.

The EMT can recognize cardiogenic shock by the following signs and symptoms:

1. Hypotension
2. Diminished peripheral pulses
3. Pale, cool, and possibly cyanotic extremities
4. Changes in level of consciousness
5. Tachycardia

The prehospital treatment is the same as for hypovolemic shock. (See pages 212–215.)

## OTHER TYPES OF SHOCK

There are other shock states which result from a failure of peripheral resistance and a maldistribution (mal″dis″trĭ-bu′shun) of circulating volume. There is no fluid loss or pump failure; however, the circulating volume is in the wrong place to support vital life processes. Allergies, infections, spinal cord injuries, drug overdoses, fainting, and the "third space syndrome" are among causes of collapse in the peripheral vascular system where blood vessels dilate and permit the leakage of fluid into surrounding tissue spaces. Even though the circulating blood volume has not been lost outside the body, it is not supporting circulation. As it pools in the arms, legs and abdomen, for instance, it is essentially useless and the volume remaining in circulation is insufficient to support the blood flow to vital parts of the body. This is when perfusion of cells is compromised and when signs and symptoms of shock become evident. Some common examples of this type of shock should be familiar to the EMT.

### Anaphylactic Shock

Anaphylaxis [an″ah-fĭ-lak′sis] is an acute systemic allergic reaction that commonly results from insect or snake venom or from an adverse drug reaction, e.g., penicillin. It produces dramatic signs and symptoms within three to fifteen minutes after the allergen (al′er-jen) has been introduced into the body. The patient will have a sudden sensation of anxiety and restlessness and may experience itching, particularly at the injection site of the allergen and in the hands and feet. A pounding headache, difficulty in breathing, tightness in the throat, hoarseness, nausea, vomiting, incontinency (in-kon′tĭ-nen-se) of stool and urine, flushing of the skin, and seizures may also be noted. A profound drop in blood pressure occurs promptly. The EMT must act promptly if the victim is to survive until he reaches the hospital. The airway should be assured and basic life support needs attended. Some authorities feel there may be some value in isolating the injection site from circulation by application of a venous lymphatic tourniquet (toor′nĭ-ket). Such action may slow down absorption somewhat, but chances are enough allergen is already in circulation to produce death at the time the EMT arrives.

This is an emergency that must be promptly detected by detailed assessments or signs and symptoms and history if the patient is to survive. The EMT should be familiar with the presentation of anaphylaxis, because there is little or no time for detailed assessments or radio communications. Airway management must be the highest priority. Transport must be prompt. No treatment other than basic life support should be undertaken prior to "packaging" the patient for rapid delivery to a hospital.

## Septic Shock

Septic (sep′tik) shock is due to an endotoxin released by disease-producing microorganisms in the blood stream. This particular endotoxin (en″do-tok′sin) creates a dramatic decrease in peripheral vascular resistance and loss of blood pressure.

Septic shock should be suspected in patients with infections of any type. Urinary tract infections, the presence of a urinary catheter, tooth abscesses, or a history of chronic illness of any type should alert the EMT to the potential for septic shock. Signs and symptoms are similar to other shock states, except that chills and fever may be evident as a by-product of overwhelming infection.

Prehospital treatment is the same as for other forms of shock.

## Neurogenic Shock

Neurogenic (nu″ro-jen′ik) or spinal shock is a transient form of shock, due to transection (tran-sek′shun) of the spinal cord.

The spinal cord carries nerve fibers that are responsible for maintaining peripheral vascular resistance. When these nerves are compressed or cut, vessels relax and there is a sudden loss of blood pressure. In multiple trauma situations, neurogenic shock can be differentiated from hypovolemic shock by its characteristic slow pulse rather than the rapid pulse associated with hemorrhage. (See Chapter 15 for a complete discussion of the management of spinal cord injuries.)

## Fainting

Fainting (syncope—sin′ko-pe) is a sudden loss of consciousness due to inadequate perfusion of the brain. It may be invoked by factors as serious as cardiac arrest or as simple as emotions such as fear, excitement, or the receipt of bad news. These problems create a sudden reduction in cardiac output and/or venous return to the heart, causing a rapid fall in blood pressure. The EMT should be careful in ruling out serious causes of unconsciousness before assuming that the fainting was due to an attendant emotional response. (Review Chapter 8.) Fainting victims will recover promptly in a flat position without definitive care. Merely permit the patient to rest for a few minutes and gradually support the return to an upright position.

## Third Space Syndrome

The so-called third space syndrome is due to a pooling of fluid in a body space which makes it unobtainable to circulation. Ascites (ah-si′tez) (massive fluid accumulation in the abdomen), which often accompanies cancer, can trap several liters of protein-rich vascular fluid in the abdomen and result in dehydration and shock. Tissue infections (cellulitis [sel″u-li′tis]), crushing injuries, vascular occlusions (ŏ-kloo′zhunz), and intestinal obstructions are also typical causes.

The EMT should transport the patient to the hospital for definitive treatment after employing the usual approaches appropriate to the field management of shock.

## SIGNS AND SYMPTOMS OF SHOCK

The EMT should be knowledgeable about the signs and symptoms of shock and be able to detect a developing shock state during the period of compensation.

Early shock states (in which the compromise in fluid volume, pumping acting of the heart or peripheral resistance is being managed by the body's adaptive processes) will produce a different clinical presentation from profound shock, indicating decompensation. Recalling the processes by which the body adjusts to perfusion difficulties, the earliest signs and symptoms may be quite subtle and this could be missed in initial assessments without a systematic data-gathering approach.

*Do not rely on vital signs or evidence of hemorrhage to suspect shock!* The obvious visible bleeding with a dramatic drop in blood pressure and rapid heartbeat and respirations can be readily detected by even the layman! The EMT should be skilled, however, in recognition of early shock states, so that definitive management can begin before the onset of massive vascular collapse.

The early signs and symptoms of shock suggest that specific adaptive processes have already been set in motion. The body's nervous system has triggered the emergency "fight and flight" response, which maximizes the potential for the patient to defend himself in danger. This phenomenon is thought to be a primitive protective system. Let's take a look at the classic reactions of various body parts when the hormones epinephrine or norepinephrine are released as one portion of the compensation process and imagine for a moment their value in emergency "fight or flight" situations that the human organism might face when he is threatened by danger. We can look at these and find the signals which are vitally important in recognition of early shock states.

When the body releases these emergency hormones, the following phenomenon occurs on a rather predictable basis. Imagine yourself being pursued by a hungry bear in the north woods for a moment. How would you feel? How would your body react? When the hormones are released quickly and in large amounts, it produces a dramatic, intense response.

The response is not unlike the sensation when these agents (epinephrine and norepinephrine) are given IV in emergencies to combat shock.

As blood is shunted promptly to vital organs and to large muscle masses, the cardiovascular system is automatically dealing with an additional volume of circulating fluid at once. You detect your heart pounding to circulate this increased volume and you feel that your throat has a lump in it, as neck vessels engorge, sending an increased blood supply to the problem-solving centers in the brain to mobilize its ability to help you cope with the impending doom. You feel a quick chill as the blood in your arms, legs, and other areas goes deep to the muscle masses that do the work of helping you fight or move away from the danger. You surge with energy and strength you never knew you had, even though your palms are sweating and your mouth is dry. You are breathing rapidly to oxygenate this increased volume of circulating blood. Perhaps there are "butterflies in the stomach" as blood is redirected away from these nonvital regions for the duration of the emergency. Some individuals vomit or have diarrhea during extreme stress (or right after they experience a crisis), to empty the stomach and intestines of a burden that cannot be handled during the stress of the circulatory adjustments, calling for a reduced gastrointestinal blood

TABLE 11-1. SIGNS AND SYMPTOMS OF SHOCK

| *Sign or Symptom* | *Early (Compensated)* | *Late (Decompensated)* |
|---|---|---|
| Patient's Behavioral Reaction | Oriented; slow to respond when thinking is required; focus is limited. Seems anxious. | Confused; speech slurring; incoherent; unable to problem solve. May be unconscious. |
| Skin and Mucous Membranes | Skin is pale, but probably dry and reasonably warm. Mouth is dry; patient expresses thirst. Skin blanches under thumb pressure, but color returns. | Cool, pale skin which feels clammy to touch. No color return after skin blanching. |
| Eyes | Pupils may be normal or slightly larger than usual; reaction to light is rapid. | Widely dilated pupils; may be sluggish or non-reactive to light. |
| Pulse | 100–150; Full and even bounding in some patients. | Above 150; thready, peripheral pulses disappear with pressure. |
| Respirations | Normal to deep. Rate is accelerated slightly. | Rapid, shallow |
| Blood Pressure | Normal with postural hypotension. | Marked hypotension; and may be palpable only. |

flow. If you looked in the mirror, you would note that the pupils of your eyes were as "big as dollars!" (Perhaps nature built in a mechanism to help us by improving our capabilities for vision.) Finally, most individuals under duress have a "one-track mind" and cannot focus on anything other than their own "impending doom." This oversimplified example of our responses to stress points out several clues worthy of the EMT's attention in recognizing early shock states.

Study Table 11–1 which outlines the visible or detectable signs and symptoms of early (compensated) and late (decompensated) shock states.

## Postural Vital Signs

The EMT should assess postural (pos'tu-ral) vital signs on patients suspected of hypovolemia from any cause, unless their general condition would suggest that the procedure could not be safely carried out.

Postural vital signs include an assessment of blood pressure and pulse rate with the patient lying, sitting, and standing. The purpose of comparing these readings is to detect whether or not the patient has already maximized his vasoconstrictor capabilities, which are stimulated in response to the loss of fluid volume.

Ordinarily when a patient assumes a vertical position, gravity fills certain vessels of lower extremities and the trunk. If the patient has not used all of his reserve ability to vasoconstrict these vessels, they will promptly constrict to enhance peripheral resistance and thus, there is no appreciable change in blood pressure. A volume-depleted patient no longer possesses this ability, and there is a marked drop in blood pressure as body fluid volume is shifted by postural changes.

Postural changes which create a decrease of 20 mm Hg or more in the systolic or disastolic readings *or* which increase the heart rate by twenty more beats per minute are considered *positive* for hypovolemia.

The EMT should be aware that the patient may become weak, dizzy, or faint during these postural changes, so be certain to protect the patient from injury during the test.

The test should be done as follows:

1. Record the blood pressure and pulse with the patient lying down

2. Have the patient sit up and record the blood pressure and pulse after waiting a minute or two

3. *If feasible, have the patient stand and record the blood pressure and pulse after waiting a minute or two.

---

* Step 3 should be omitted if the test is positive or if the patient's symptoms become acute during Step 2.

## Airway and Breathing

The airway and breathing of the patient in shock is of paramount importance. The natural airway should be ensured by proper positioning and suctioning employed as necessary. (see Chapter 10) Supplementary oxygen should be administered at high flow rates (i.e., 10 *l*/ by nasal cannula). A face mask and ventilatory assistance using a bag-valve device may be required if the airway or ventilatory status is compromised.

When the EMT identifies or suspects shock, the patient should be positioned in the shock position. (See Fig. 11-1.) The body should be flat with the legs elevated to maximize venous return to the heart. Although a Trendelenburg (tren-del′en-berg) position (see Fig. 11-2) was once favored,

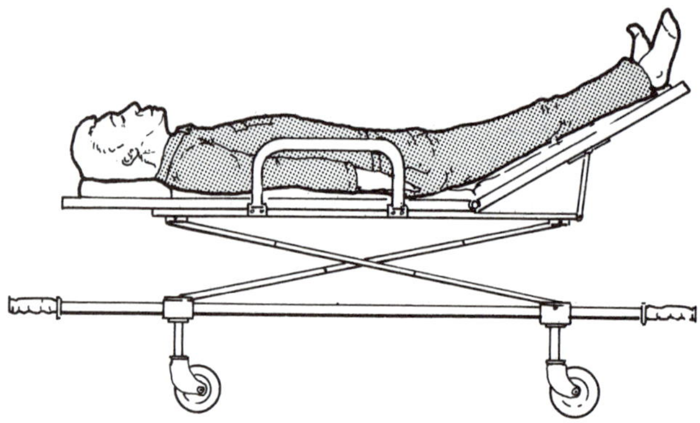

**Figure 11-1.** Shock position; legs only are elevated to encourage venous return.

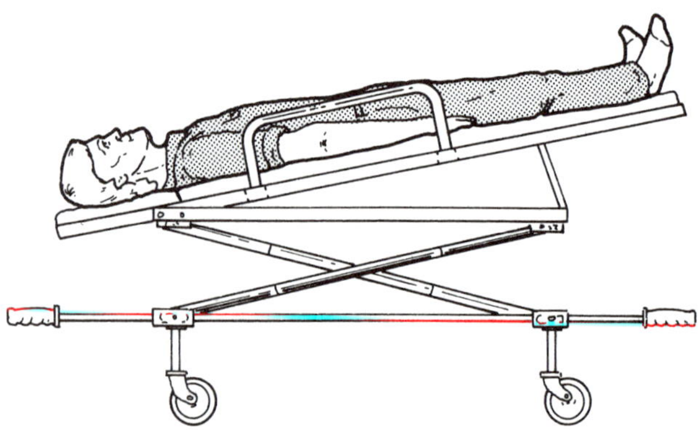

**Figure 11-2.** Trendelenburg position. This position is seldom used, since it may compromise ventilation when abdominal contents push against the diaphragm.

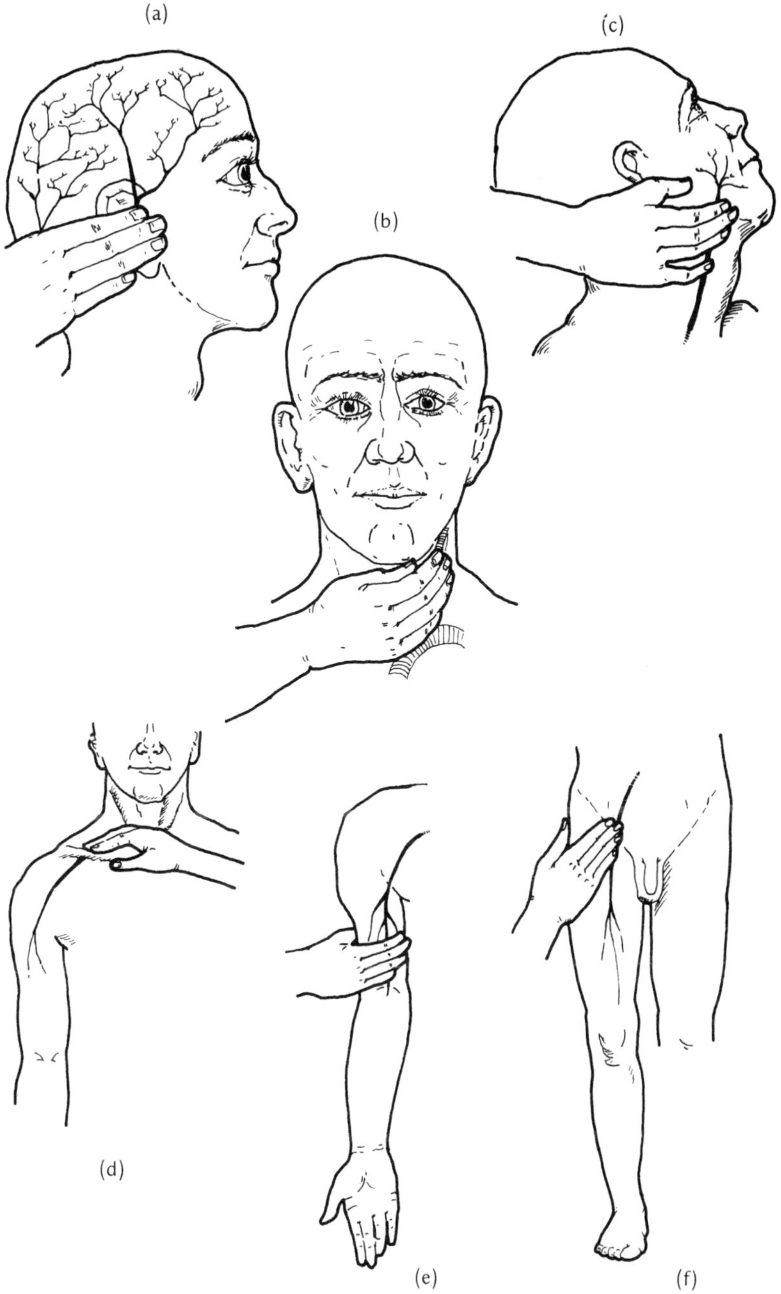


**Figure 11-3.** Pressure points to control bleeding: (a) temporal artery (scalp bleeding); (b) carotid artery (neck wounds); (c) external maxillary artery (facial bleeding); (d) subclavian artery (shoulder and upper arm bleeding); (e) brachial artery (lower arm bleeding); (f) femoral artery (leg bleeding).

it has been largely abandoned since it may cause the diaphragm to move upward and thus compromise room for breathing.

If there is obvious evidence of bleeding, direct pressure should be used to control it. (See Fig. 11–3.) If there is an impaled (im-pāl'd) foreign object, do not remove it. Stabilize it with a bulky dressing and transport the patient promptly. Removing a foreign object can increase bleeding and possibly create additional trauma to body tissue.

The patient should be kept warm to prevent the unnecessary loss of body heat that causes an avoidable expenditure of oxygen and glucose. But do not "overheat" the individual, since this causes the body additional stress and may actually worsen vascular relaxation and fluid loss.

EMTs who possess advanced skills may initiate IV fluid therapy or apply antishock trousers.

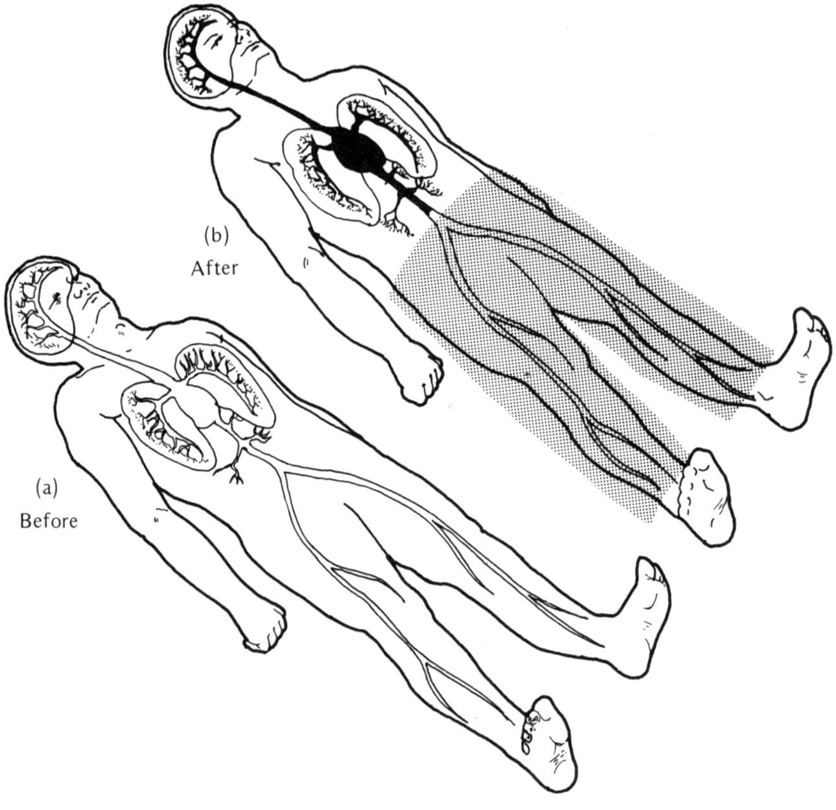


**Figure 11–4.** Vascular response to anti-shock trousers application: (a) before application; (b) after application. Note improved flow to upper portion of body.

## Antishock Trousers

Antishock trousers are designed to apply counterpressure to the lower extremities and the abdomen for the purpose of redirecting venous blood flow in those body parts to the vital organs of the chest and head.

The purposes of antishock trousers are to:

1. Decrease blood flow to the lower extremities
2. Reduce blood loss by the application of direct pressure
3. Autotransfuse (aw"to-trans-fuz) the upper portion of the body with at least 1,000 cc of blood within one or two minutes by redirecting blood from the lower body.

*Application of Antishock Trousers*

1. Assess the environment for objects that could puncture the suit (i.e., needles, glass, rocks) and remove them. Fold open the suit, open the stopcock valves, and attach the foot pump. (See Fig. 11-5.)
2. Place the suit so that the abdominal section will be applied just below the lowest rib.
3. Logroll the patient onto the antishock trousers.
4. Wrap the legs of the trousers around the lower limbs and fasten them.
5. Inflate the suit initially until the gauge reads 25–30 mm Hg *or* until the patient's blood pressure is within acceptable limits. It may be necessary to increase the gauge pressure still more to increase blood pressure. The EMT should monitor the patient's blood pressure, and not the gauge pressure, to ensure its effective use. (The use of the abdominal section is optional.)
6. Close the stopcocks, but do *not* detach the foot pump.
7. Monitor the vital signs; anticipate vomiting.
8. The suit should not be deflated until the patient is well stabilized in the hospital setting.
9. Deflation (NOT A FIELD PROCEDURE)
   a. Deflate the chambers gradually. When the BP drops 5 mm HG, stop deflation, accelerate IV fluid flow, and wait until the BP reaches the predeflation level.
   b. Continue deflation by 5 mm Hg increments, accelerating IV fluids, and stabilizing the blood pressure until the trousers are loose enough to remove easily.

*References*

Barber, Janet M. "Early Detection of Hypovolemic States," *EMT Journal*, 2:72–75.

Bookman, Lawrence B., and Simoneau, Joan Kelley. "Early Assessment of Hypovolemia Postural Vital Signs," *JEN*, 3:43, 1977.

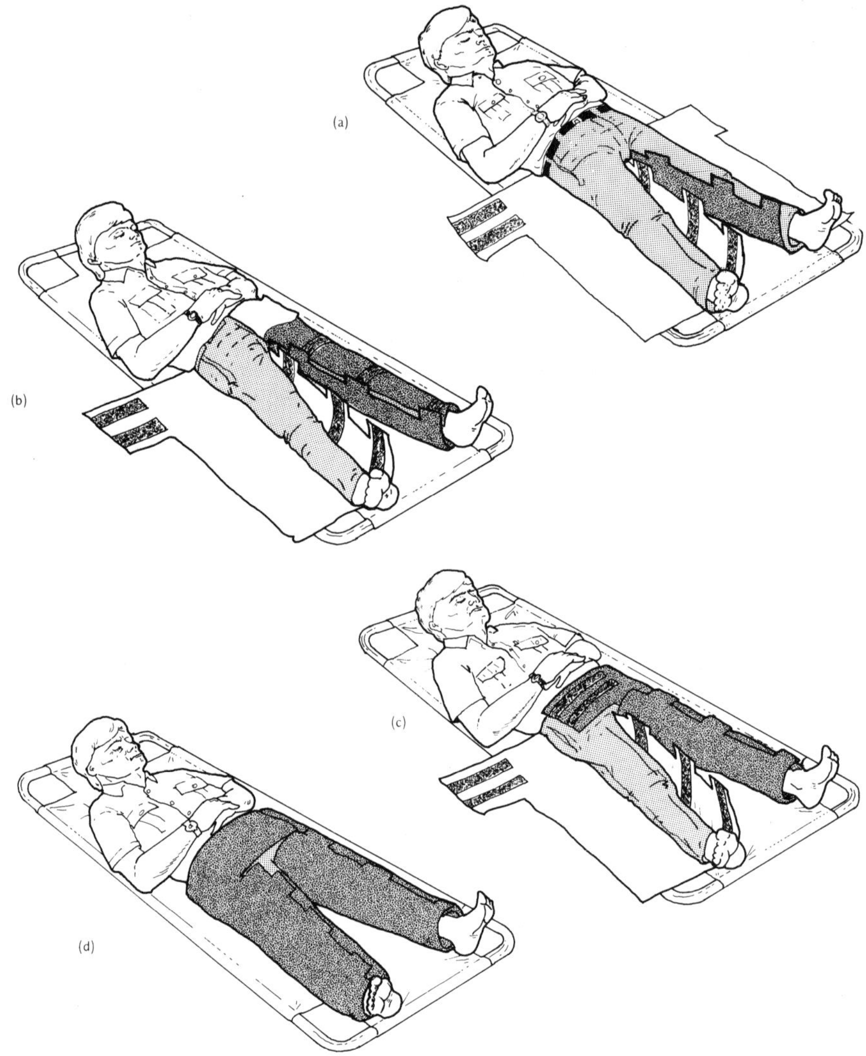


**Figure 11–5.** Steps in applying anti-shock trousers.

Denny M. "Septic Shock," *Jen* 3:19–23, January/February, 1977.

Hartong, J. M., and Dixon, R. S. "Monitoring Resuscitation of the Injured Patient," *JAMA*, 237:242–244, 1977.

Schroeder, J. S., and Dailey, E. K. "Techniques in Bedside Hemodynamic Monitoring," St. Louis, MO: The C. V. Mosby Company, 1976.

Weil, M. H. *The Diagnosis and Treatment of Shock*, Baltimore, MD: The Williams and Wilkins Co., 1967.

Wilson, R. F. "Shock," in *Manual of Practices and Techniques in Critical Care.* Kalamazoo, MI: Upjohn Company, 1976.

Wishard Memorial Hospital Ambulance Service, "EMT Practical Skills Manual," August, 1980.

# Chapter 12

# Descriptive Terms and Surface Anatomy

Descriptive medical terminology is used by the EMT in conjunction with the care and treatment of the patient, either in verbal or written form. To describe something to someone else over the radio is not an easy task, especially the accurate description of multiple wounds. Because the EMT will be called upon to describe for the physician or nurse the specific location(s) of wounds, it is crucial that the EMT understand and be able to communicate concisely, accurately, and calmly. Descriptive medical terminology is a universal language among the health care team. The EMT must have a fundamental understanding of the language to be able to correctly communicate medical information to the physician or nurse.

For proper orientation and description of wounds or lesions on the body, one must know the universal anatomical position (see Fig. 12–1) in which the patient:

1. Stands erect facing forward
2. Upper extremities are abducted
3. Palms face forward
4. Toes point slightly downward.

This position is used as a standard reference in medicine. By knowing the basic anatomical position, confusion lessens and terminology becomes uniform when description is necessary. When the EMT refers to right or left, he should refer to the patient's right or left, and not his own.

As one looks at the body, four basic viewpoints should be considered:

1. Body cavities
2. Body planes or sections
3. Body direction and position
4. Body movement

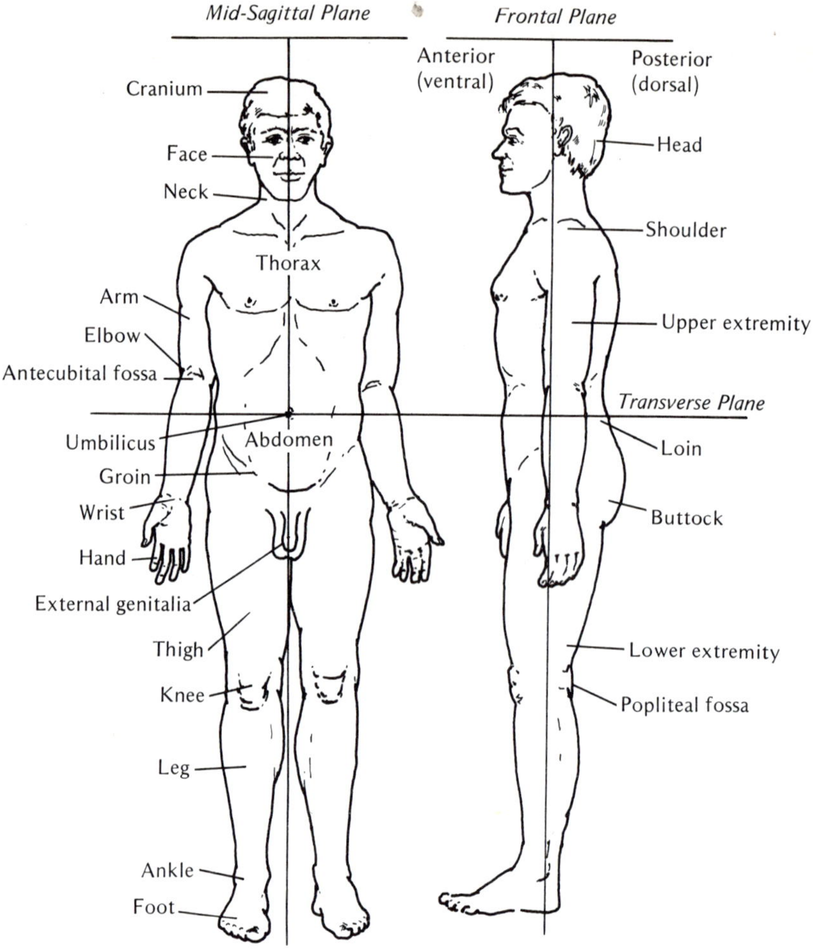


**Figure 12–1.** The universal anatomical position, body planes, and general terms of body location.

## BODY CAVITIES

The body contains a few large internal spaces or cavities within which various organs are located. There are two groups of cavities: dorsal and ventral. (See Fig. 12–2.)

### *Dorsal Cavities*

There are two dorsal cavities:

1. The cranial cavity, which contains the brain
2. The spinal canal, encasing the spinal cord

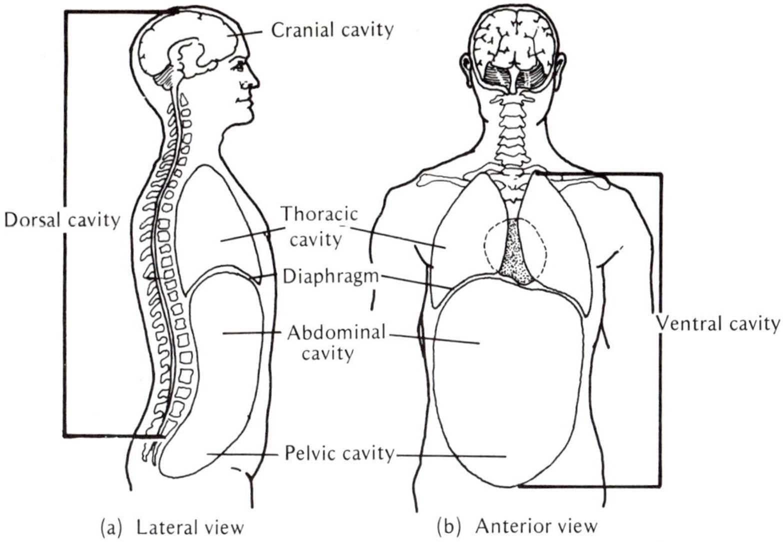


**Figure 12–2.** The dorsal and ventral cavities of the body.

Both of these cavities are connected to one another and form a continuous space.

*Ventral Cavities*

The ventral cavities are much larger than the dorsal (back) cavity. There are two ventral cavities:

1. Thoracic (chest) cavity. Contains mainly the heart, lungs, large nerves, and blood vessels

2. Abdominal cavity. Separated from the chest cavity by the diaphragm. This cavity is subdivided into two portions, one containing the stomach, kidneys, liver, gallbladder, pancreas, spleen, and most of the intestines; and a lower space called the pelvic cavity, in which are located the urinary bladder, rectum, and the internal anatomy of the reproductive system. (See Fig. 12–2.)

## BODY PLANES OR SECTIONS

The EMT will rely on imaginary lines drawn through or on the body to help identify points on the body rapidly so that description of wounds or lesions can be easily described. Three basic planes or sections divide the body (see Fig. 12–1):

1. Mid-sagittal. A vertical plane dividing the body into right and left portions.

2. Frontal. A vertical plane at right angles to the mid-sagittal section, dividing the body into front and back portions. The front portion contains the thoracic, abdominal, and pelvic cavities. The back portion contains the spinal column (back bone) and cranial cavity.

3. Transverse. A horizontal plane at the shoulders that divides the body into upper and lower portions.

## BODY DIRECTIONS AND POSITIONS

### Directions

Now that we have a start in knowing the body cavities and planes, we can begin to describe certain things on the body. We talked about the frontal plane dividing the body into a front and/or back portion. In medical terminology, when some structure is located in front of another, we say that it is *anterior* to it. If it is in back of or behind that structure, we say that it is *posterior* to it. For example, the toes are anterior to the heel of the foot and the ears are posterior to the mouth.

The mid-sagittal or mid-line plane is important because it also is used as a reference point for description. The term *medial* is used to describe something that is nearest the mid-line plane. The term *lateral* is used to describe something that is farthest from the mid-line plane. For example, the inside of the leg is called the medial side of the leg, and the outside portion of the leg is termed the lateral side of the leg. When an eye turns toward the mid-line of the body, it is deviated medially and when it turns away, looking to the sides, it is deviated laterally. (See Fig. 12–3.)

The medical term that means above or in a higher position is

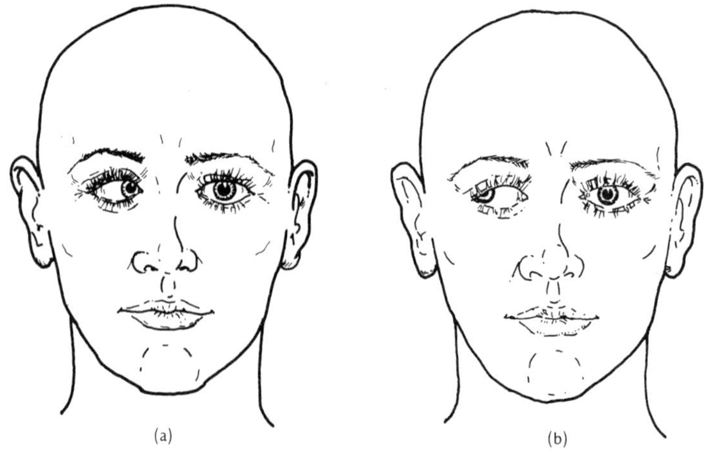

**Figure 12–3.** (a) Medial deviation of the eye; (b) lateral deviation of the eye.

*superior*, and the term meaning below or in a lower position is *inferior*. For example, the mouth is superior to the chin and the umbilicus (belly button), is inferior to the nipples. (See Fig. 12–4.)

Two terms that will be frequently be used in describing wounds or lesions are *proximal* and *distal*. Proximal means something nearest to something else. Distal means something farther away from something else. Confusion often surrounds these two terms, but if one always uses two reference points with the terms, there will be no confusion. For example, in Figure 12–4 the X can be three inches distal from the knee or twelve inches proximal to the ankle. The reference points in this case are the knee and

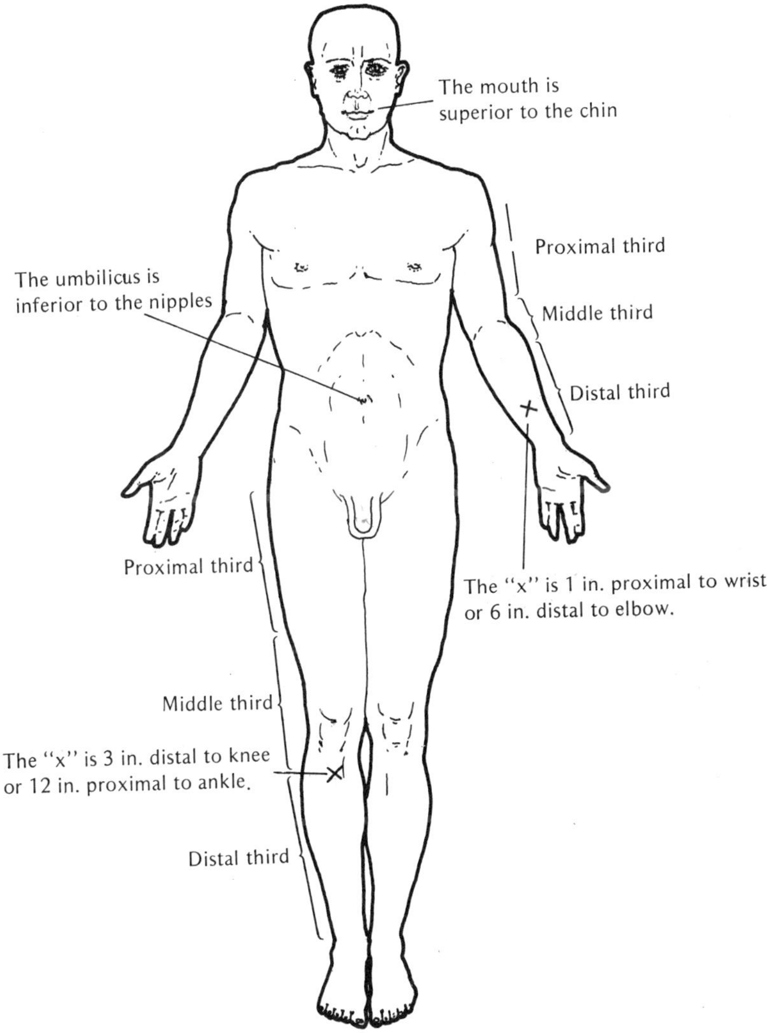


**Figure 12–4.** The medical descriptive terms superior, inferior, proximal, and distal are used to describe injury or pain location.

ankle. Remember to use two reference points. Another example in Figure 12–4, the X is one inch proximal to the wrist or six inches distal to the elbow. It's quite simple. If a wound or lesion is in the middle of an extremity, we say that the wound is on the middle one-third of the arm. This is because we can divide the limbs into three sections. (See Fig. 12–4.)

1. Proximal one-third or upper thirds
2. Middle third
3. Distal third—lower third

The term *deep* means away from the surface. The term *superficial* means near the surface. A laceration, gunshot, or stab wound, for example, may be deep or superficial.

## Positions

What concerns us here is how the patient may be positioned during field stabilization and in transport to the medical facility. The EMT must be familiar and understand these positions, so that the patient's medical problem is not aggravated. The EMT can position the patient in the following ways (See Fig. 12–5):

1. *Prone.* Placing the patient face down with the head turned to one side
2. *Supine.* Placing the patient on his back
3. *Fowler's Position.* Placing the patient in a straight-up sitting position
4. *Semi-Fowler's Position.* Placing the patient in a semisitting position at about a forty-five degree angle
5. *Left Lateral Recumbent Position.* Placing the patient on his side with head turned slightly downward. This position is recommended for all comatose patients who have not sustained trauma
6. *Shock Position.* Placing the patient in a supine position and elevating the lower extremities thirty to forty degrees
7. *Trendelenburg Position.* Placing the patient in a supine position, tilting the head down and the remainder of his body up at about thirty degrees

# BODY MOVEMENT

Description of body movement becomes important when injury has occurred and impairs body motion. We try to relate to the physician or nurse the type of movement that cannot be accomplished by using a few important descriptive terms. The terms that describe motion usually end in *-ion.*

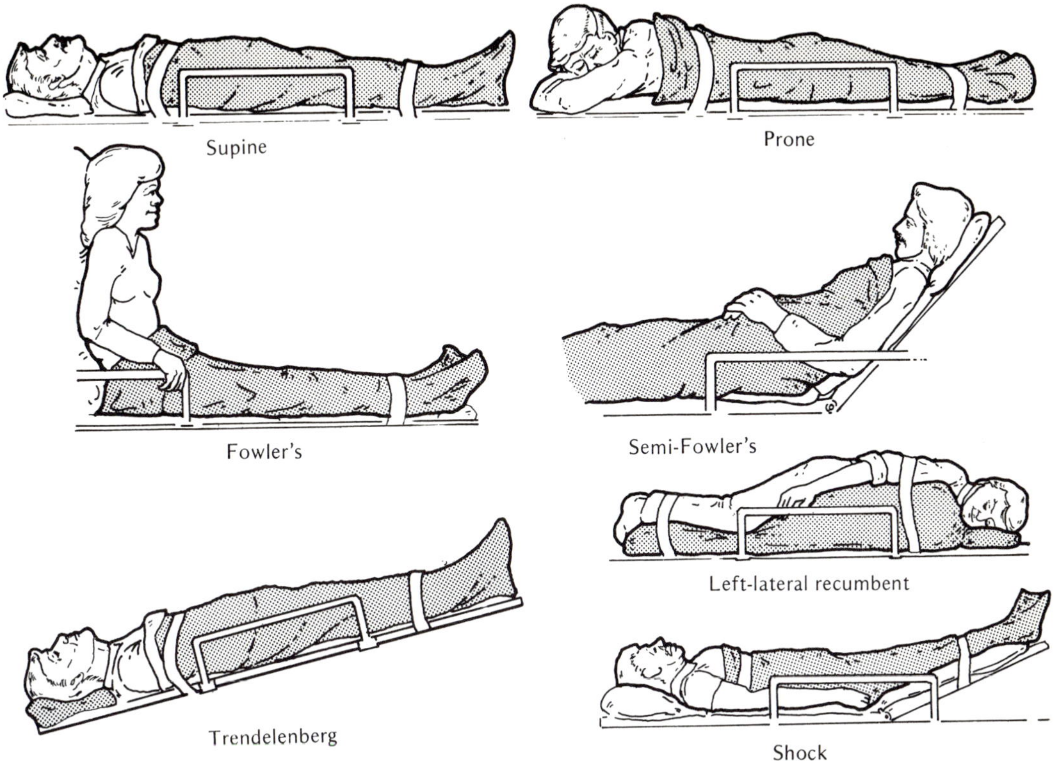


**Figure 12–5.** Various positions in which the patient may be placed depending on injury or illness.

## Abduction—Adduction

When the limbs, digits, or toes move away from the mid-line plane of the body, the motion is termed *abduction*. The prefix *ab* means away from. When these parts move toward the mid-line plane of the body, the motion is termed *adduction*. The prefix *ad* means toward the body. (See Fig. 12–6.)

## Flexion—Extension

The bending of any limb is termed *flexion*. The straightening of any limb is termed *extension*. The anterior surface of the forearm (in the anatomical position) is known as the *flexor* surface. The posterior surface of the forearm is known as the *extensor* surface. This is because flexor muscles occupy the anterior surface and extensor muscles occupy the posterior surface of the forearm. (See Fig. 12–7.)

In referring to the foot we say that when the ankle bends toward the head, it is in *dorsiflexion*. When the foot bends downward (i.e., toes

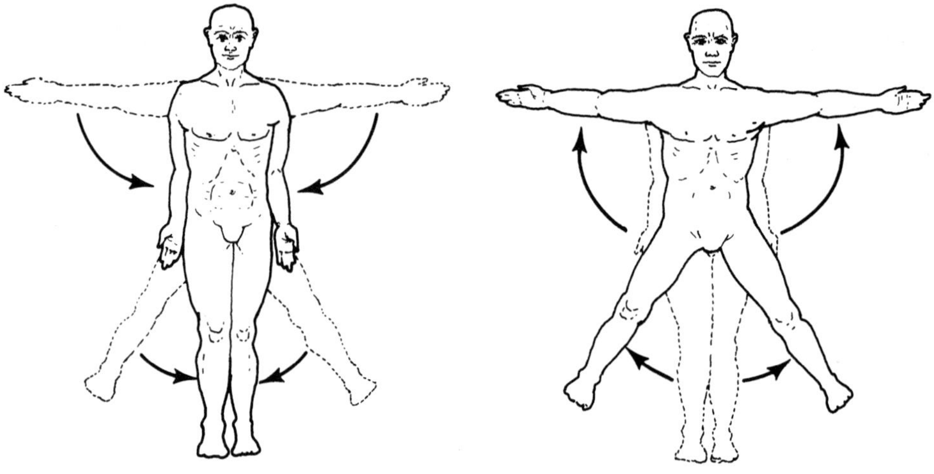

(a) Adduction

(b) Abduction

**Figure 12-6.** (a) Bringing the limbs toward the midline of the body is called adduction. (b) Taking the limbs away from the midline of the body is called abduction.

pointed downward) it is in *plantar flexion* (The sole of the foot is known as the plantar surface.) (See Fig. 12-8.)

In referring to the neck, when the neck bends forward with the chin towards the chest we say the neck is in *flexion* (lateral flexion occurs when the head is bent toward either shoulder). When the neck is bent backwards with the head and eyes pointed toward the sky, we say the neck is in *extension.* One opens the airway by hyperextending the neck, so that the tongue is lifted forward and off the air passage.

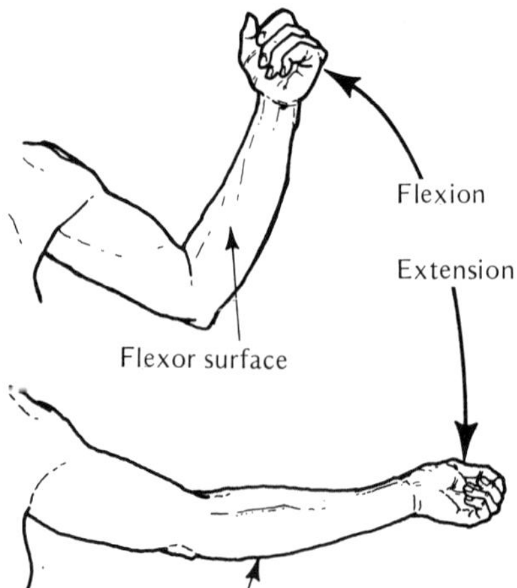


**Figure 12-7.** The action of flexion and extension.

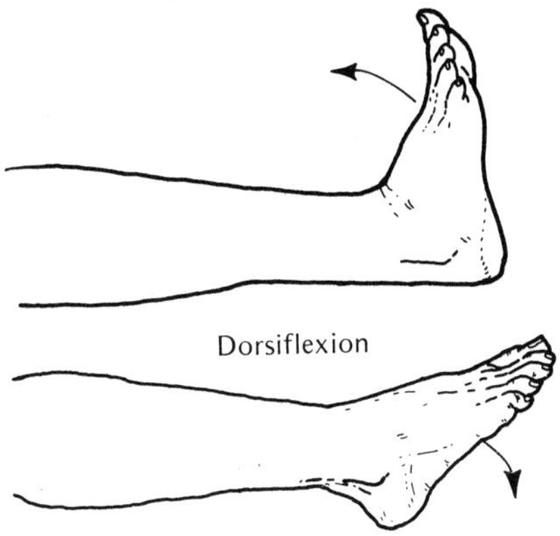


**Figure 12-8.** Dorsiflexion and plantar flexion of the foot.

## Rotation

*Rotation* occurs when any body part moves around a point. The act of shaking the head from side to side is rotation. When referring to the extremities we say that they are turned *outward* (away from the mid-line of the body) or *inward* (toward the mid-line of the body).

Outward rotation is called *external rotation* and inward rotation is called *internal rotation.* If one points his foot outward, the leg becomes externally rotated. If one points his toes inward, the leg becomes internally rotated. (See Fig. 12-9.) Some injuries produce rotation. For example,

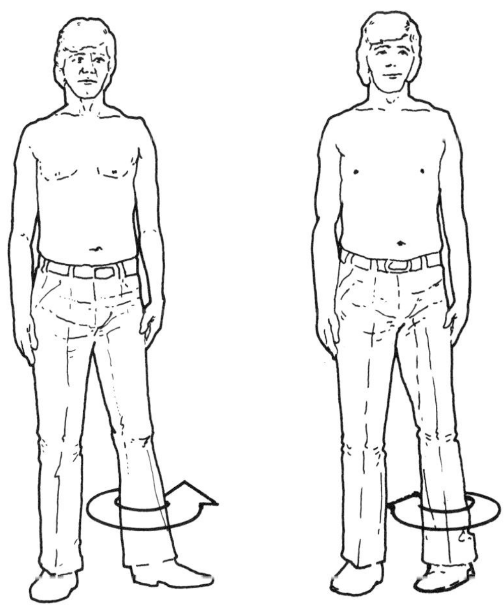


**Figure 12-9.** The movements of external and internal rotation.

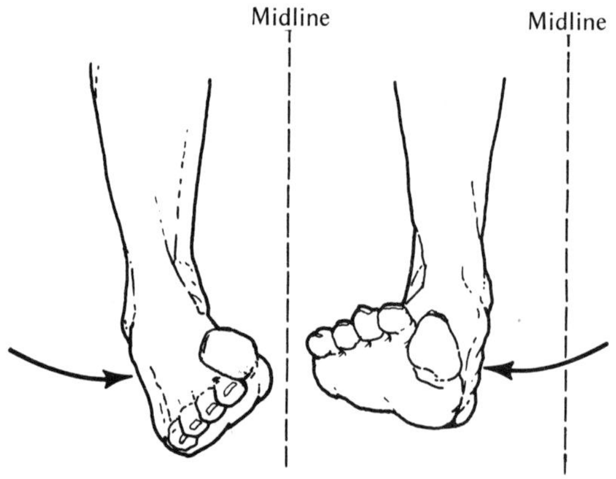


**Figure 12–10.** The movements of eversion and inversion of the foot.

oftentimes a fractured hip causes shortening and external rotation of the leg, and an anterior dislocation of the hip usually causes internal rotation of the thigh. Two other terms related to foot movement are *eversion* and *inversion.* Eversion is the outward turning of the foot, while inversion is the inward turning of the foot. Inadvertent motion of either eversion or inversion is often the cause of ankle injury. (See Fig. 12–10.)

Rotation of the forearm produces two positions related to the hand: *supination* and *pronation.* Supination results when the palm of the hand is facing anteriorly and the radius and ulna bones of the forearm are parallel. Pronation results when the palm of the hand is facing downward with the radius crossed over the ulnar bone. (See Fig. 12–11.)

These movements become important in describing what the patient can or cannot do when injured and also how you may describe the position you find the patient in. For example, the patient may be found in a supine position with the left leg externally rotated and the neck in flexion. These terms will be used often. Know and use them correctly.

## SURFACE ANATOMY

The external surface of the body is like a topographical map. Just as in reading a map, one must be able to read the surface anatomy of the body and be able to describe locations of wounds, pain, and injury. Bony prominences, muscle contour, blood vessels, lumps, depressions, and imaginary lines will allow the EMT to inspect and interpret surface anatomy and use these landmarks as reference points.

By knowing the body's surface anatomy, movements, planes of direction, position, and landmark terminology, the EMT will be able to assess, treat, and accurately report pertinent medical information regarding the patient's condition. There is no special skill required to inspect the surface

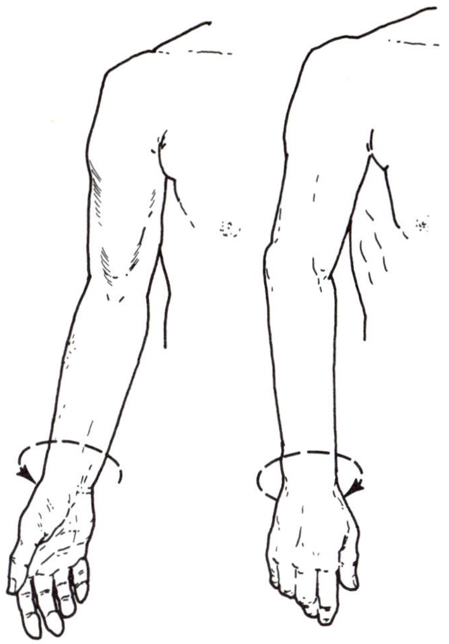


**Figure 12-11.** The action of supination and pronation.

anatomy of the patient, and it should be done on every patient. However, inspection of surface anatomy, combined with performing a primary and secondary survey, are among regular responsibilities of the EMT working in the prehospital setting. Remember, every patient must be inspected for injury, especially a patient with trauma, and the EMT must know what he is observing in order to interpret and report his findings accurately.

A logical way to study surface anatomy is to begin with the head and move toward the toes, just as when performing a primary and secondary survey of the patient.

## Skull or Cranium

The skull or cranium is made up of fused bone that protectively encases the brain and provides a cavity for sense organs (hearing, sight, equilibrium, smell, and taste.) Surface anatomy that the EMT should know includes that listed below. (See Fig. 12-12.)

1. *Vertex:* Center top of the skull.

2. *Frontal bone:* Forms the skeleton of the forehead; the anterior portion of the skull.

3. *Parietal bone:* There are two of them, one on each side of the skull.

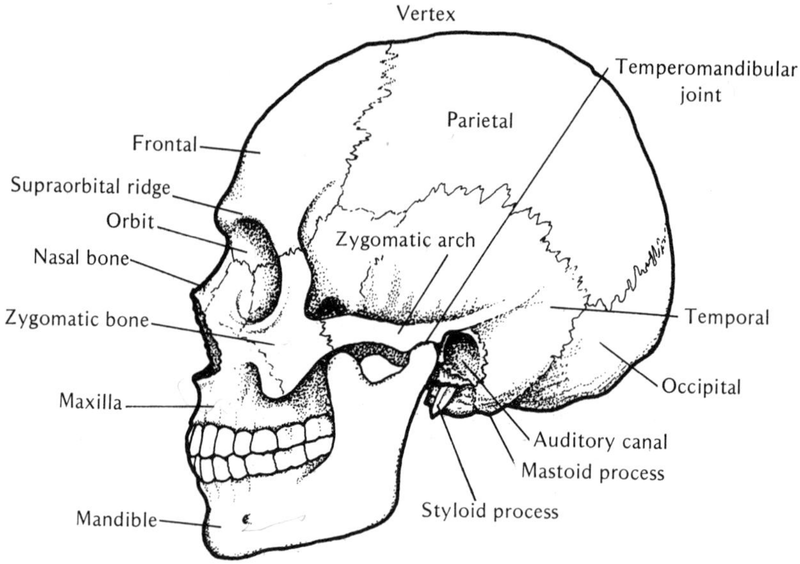


**Figure 12–12.** Bones of the skull and face: a lateral view.

4. *Temporal bones:* There are two of them; on the portion of the skull where the ears are located.

5. *Mastoid process:* The bony prominence located behind the ear. It is part of the temporal bone. Ecchymoses (bruises) of this area suggest a posterior skull fracture, and thus this area should be checked on every unconscious patient.

6. *Occipital bone:* The posterior portion of the skull.

## Face

The face presents many prominent features in the form of bumps, ridges, and depressions that can easily be described. The EMT should know these. (See Fig. 12–12.)

1. *Orbits:* The bony sockets that encase the eyes.

2. *Supraorbital ridges:* The bony prominence where the eyebrows are located. Feel this ridge above each eye. It is part of the frontal bone of the skull. Most impact forces to the face occur at these points.

3. *Zygomatic bone:* This easily palpated prominence is the cheek bone. It rests on the maxilla or the upper jaw.

4. *Zygomatic arch:* This bone on the side of the face that bridges the cheek bone, just anterior to the ear, with the temporal bone.

5. *Mandible:* The lower jaw; the only movable bone of the face.

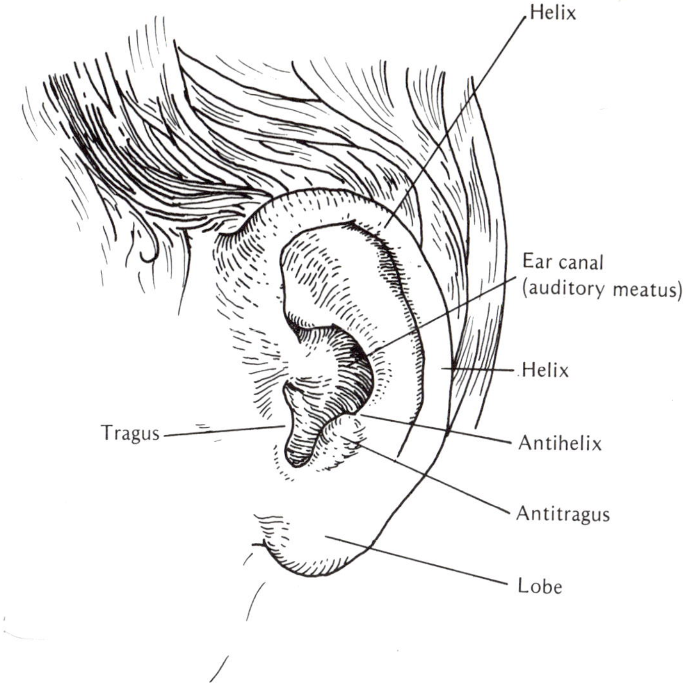


**Figure 12-13.** The anatomical parts of the ear.

6. *Temperomandibular joint:* This joint allows movement of the mandible. It can easily be felt by depressing just in front of the hole of the ear with the finger while opening and closing the mouth. This joint is infrequently dislocated. (See Fig. 12-12.)

7. *Nose:* The bridge or proximal one-third of the nose is composed of bone and the distal two-thirds of cartilage.

8. *Ear:* This cartilagenous appendage, called the pinnae (pin′nah), has several prominent ridges and bumps. (See Fig. 12-13.)

a. Helix—the lateral ridge of the ear
b. Antihelix—the medical ridge of the ear
c. Tragus—the bump just in front of the ear canal
d. Antitragus—the bump just in back of the ear canal
e. Lobe—the bottom fleshy part of the ear
f. Auditory meatus—the canal of the ear

9. *Lips:* The lips are very vascular and therefore have a distinctive vermillion color to them. The definitive color line between the lips and surrounding skin is termed the *vermillion border.* When one refers to something around the mouth it is termed *perioral.* (See Fig. 12-14.)

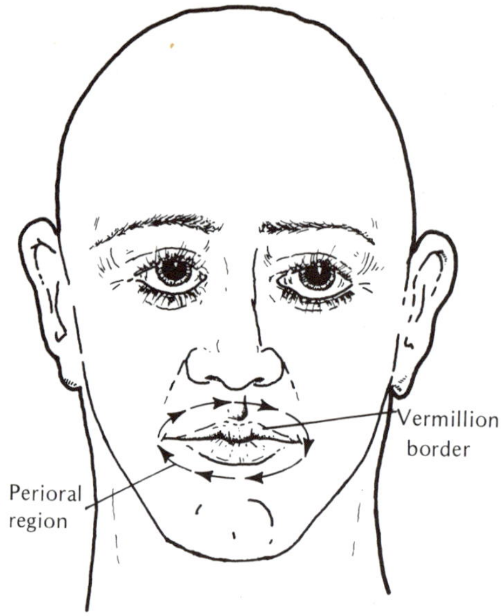


**Figure 12–14.** The vermillion border. Note region referred to as perioral.

## Neck—Anterior

The neck contains many important landmarks that the EMT should know and be able to locate. (See Fig. 12–15.)

The anterior muscles of the neck are easily visible and can aid the EMT in referring to reference points. Muscles that should be known include:

1. *Sternocleidomastoid Muscle.* Sterno (sternum) cleido (clavicle) mastoid (mastoid process). This muscle has two origins, one on the sternum and one on the clavicle, and inserts on the mastoid bone behind the ear. This muscle splits to form a triangle. At the apex of the triangle is a depression called the jugular or suprasternal notch.
2. *Trapezius Muscle.* This muscle forms the top of the shoulders.

On the anterior aspect of the neck one can feel a bump. This noticeable prominence is called the *Adam's Apple* and is more pronounced in men than women. This prominence is the thyroid cartilage. The vocal cords lie within its walls. Because in men it is larger than in women, their voices are deeper in pitch. Approximately two centimeters inferior to the thyroid cartilage is the cricoid cartilage. Between the two cartilages lies a thin membranous sheet of tissue called the *cricothyroid membrane.* This is an important landmark. Feel the slight depression between the cartilages to find this membrane. It is not uncommon that this membrane is opened surgically or by inserting a large bore needle through it to create an airway, should an upper airway obstruction exist and the patient cannot breathe. This emergency procedure is called a *cricothyrotomy* (kri″ko-thi″rot′o-me).

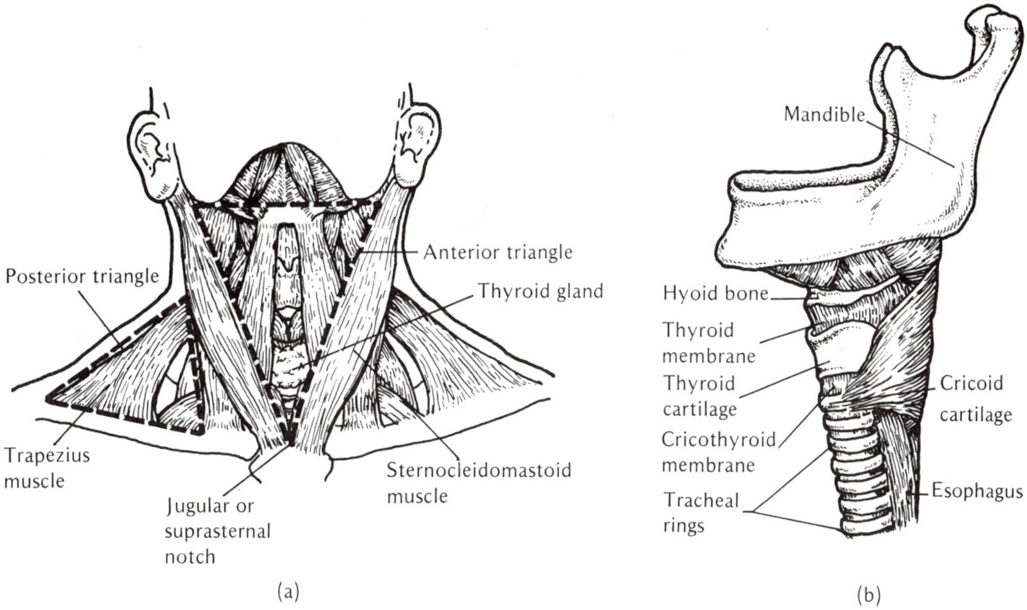


**Figure 12–15.** (a) The muscular landmarks of the anterior neck; (b) landmarks of the neck from a lateral view.

The thyroid and cricoid cartilages together form the larynx (voice box). One of the most important arteries of the body lies just lateral and deep into the thyroid prominence. Locate it and feel your pulse. This is one of the major arteries the EMT will palpate when assessing every unconscious patient. Below the cricoid cartilage one may feel the trachea (windpipe). It has anterior cartilagenous rings which give the trachea structure and stabilization, so it will not collapse when one bends the neck. If the anterior rings were not present, the effect would be much like that of bending a straw, and the trachea would be sealed off to incoming air. The trachea connects the larynx with the bronchi of the lungs. Situated on either side of the lower larynx and upper trachea is the thyroid gland. It produces a hormone called *thyroxin* that, when secreted in the bloodstream, increases tissue metabolism. Anatomically, the larynx lies just anterior to the fifth and sixth cervical vertebrae, as does the thyroid gland. The trachea extends from about the sixth cervical vertebra to about the sixth thoracic vertebra.

## Neck—Posterior

The posterior aspect of the neck has seven cervical vertebrae. One may palpate down the back of the neck and feel a very prominent bump. This seventh cervical vertebra can be used as a landmark to start the count of the thoracic vertebrae. Feel the prominence.

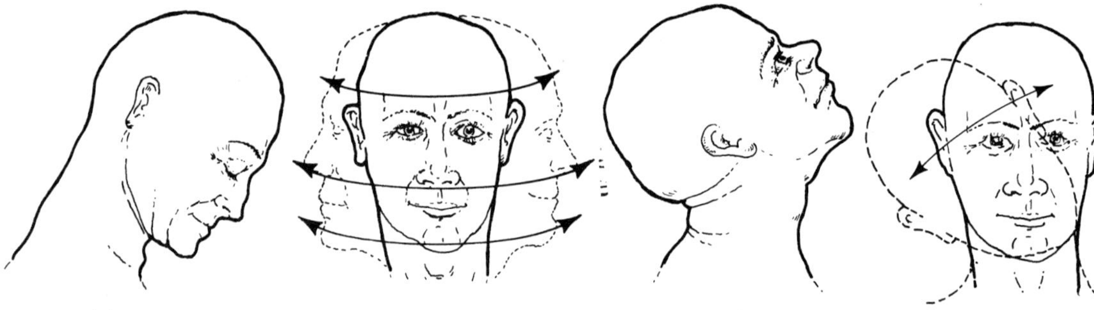

**Figure 12–16.** (a) The head in anterior flexion; (b) rotation movement of the head; (c) the head in an extension position; (d) the head in lateral flexion.

As we have previously discussed, the neck can move in four major ways (See Fig. 12–16):

1. *Anterior Flexion.* Bending the head down toward the chest.
2. *Rotation.* The motion of shaking the head in a "no" fashion.
3. *Extension.* Bending the head back as one would look to the sky.
4. *Lateral Flexion.* Bending the head to either side of the shoulders.

## Chest or Thorax—Anterior

The chest cavity or thorax is a cone-shaped bony cage that is narrow at the top and broad at the base. Twelve pairs of ribs form the bars of this cage, assisted by the sternum anteriorly and the twelve thoracic vertebrae posteriorly. The thorax is bounded superiorly by the clavicles and inferiorly by the diaphragm and costal arches. The thorax is the most continuously active part of the skeleton. (See Fig. 12–17a.)

Surface anatomy of the chest is probably the most important to know, because of the vital structures that lie beneath it and because the EMT must be able to describe injuries sustained to it quickly and accurately.

As one views the thorax anteriorly, imaginary lines can be drawn vertically for reference points. The ribs will serve as constant reference points horizontally.

Since the sternum sits in the middle of the thorax, an imaginary line can be drawn down its center for our first reference point. This line is called the mid-sternal line. As previously mentioned, the upper border of the sternum is marked by the jugular or suprasternal notch (*supra* means *above*). The sternum is composed of three parts, the manubrium or the top part is about five centimeters in length, the body or middle part is about ten centimeters in length, and the xiphoid (zif′oid) process, the last part, is very

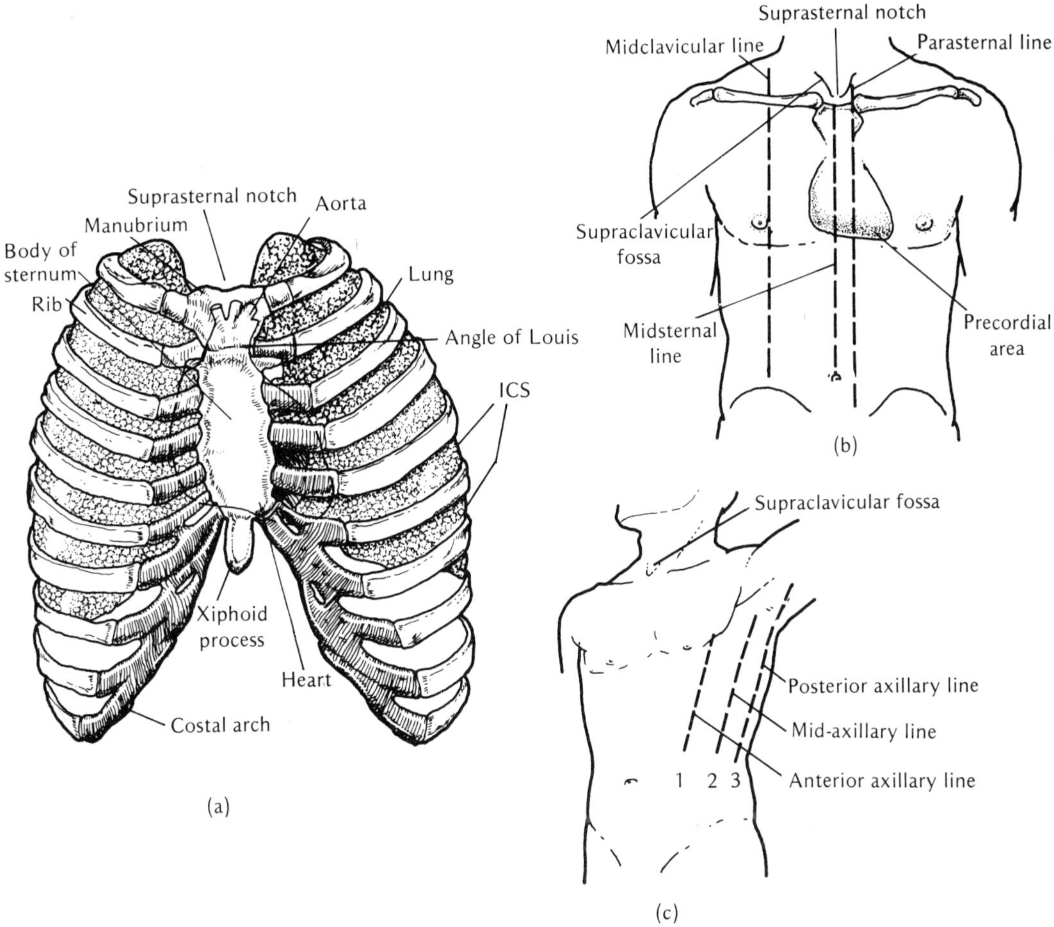


**Figure 12-17.** (a) Anatomy of the anterior chest; (b) surface reference lines of the anterior chest; (c) surface reference lines of the lateral chest.

short. As one palpates down the sternum, one should be able to feel a prominent ridge between the manubrium and body. This union site of the sternum is called the *angle of Louis* or *sternal angle.* Palpate this ridge on yourself. This is an important landmark, since the second rib articulates with the sternum at this point. Therefore, one has a reference point to count the ribs downward with accuracy, once this site is found. The angle of Louis is also important because:

1. It is the point where the right and left pleural sacs (lungs) come together.
2. It is the level of bifurcation of the trachea.
3. It is the point where the arch of the aorta begins and ends.

4. It marks the level of the lower border of the fourth thoracic vertebra.

As previously mentioned, the clavicles form the superior border of the chest cavity. The depression above each clavicle is called the *supraclavicular fossa* (*fossa* [fos′ah] is a Latin term for ditch). The apex or top of the lung sits just beneath this area.

Lines drawn vertically at the edge of either side of the sternum are called the *lateral* or *parasternal lines.* (See Fig. 12–17b,c.) A line drawn vertically from the middle of the clavicle to the bottom of the rib cage (costal arch) is called the *mid-clavicular line.* As we move laterally, we can draw three more imaginary vertical lines for surface reference. They are:

1. *Anterior Axillary Line:* A line drawn just anterior to the axillary crease of the armpit to the end of the rib cage.

2. *Mid-Axillary Line:* A line drawn from the center of the armpit down to the end of the rib cage.

3. *Posterior Axillary Line:* A line drawn from the center of the armpit to the end of the rib.

These vertical imaginary lines are all common points of reference that the EMT will use often.

The ribs serve as constant horizontal reference lines once one has located the sternal angle where the second rib articulates with the sternum. The depression between each rib is called the *intercostal space (ICS).*

The body has twenty-four ribs, twelve on each side of the thoracic cavity. All of the ribs are attached posteriorly to the twelve thoracic vertebrae, two ribs attaching to each of the twelve vertebrae.

The anterior attachment of the ribs to the sternum varies. None of the ribs actually join the sternum. Instead, there are resilient bars of cartilage called the *costal cartilages,* that extend forward from the ends of the ribs (except the last two) toward the sternum.

The first seven pairs of ribs are referred to as true ribs, since their costal cartilages actually reach the sternum. The next three pairs of ribs are called false ribs because their costal cartilages turn upward to join the cartilage of the rib above. The seventh rib has the largest costal cartilage and the last cartilage to articulate directly with the sternum. Below the seventh rib, the cartilages of the false ribs (ribs 8, 9, and 10) ascend upward to fuse with the costal cartilage of the rib above. (See Fig. 12–18.)

The last two pairs of ribs have no anterior attachment and are referred to as the floating ribs. Remember that the spaces between the ribs are known as the intercostal spaces (ICS).

The male nipples are important landmarks because they lie approximately over the fourth intercostal space. The position of female nipples varies and they are not constant landmarks.

Now that we have vertical and horizontal reference lines, description and location of injury should not be difficult. It is extremely important to

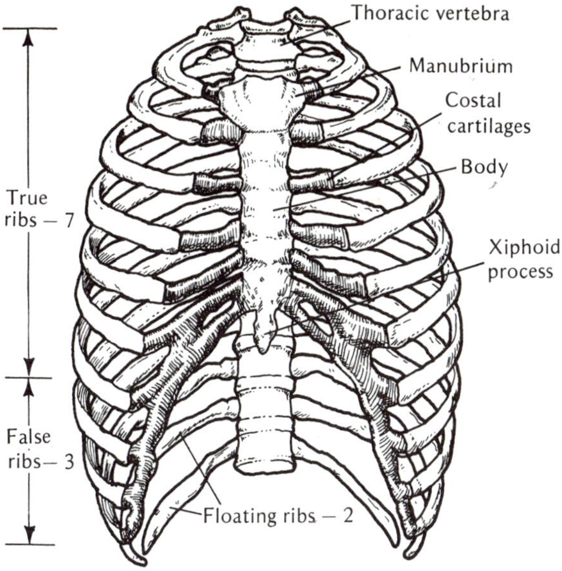


**Figure 12–18.** The anterior chest and the various types of ribs.

know what organs lie beneath these lines and landmarks so that the EMT has an idea of what may be injured when observing a wound(s).

The heart is situated on the left side of the chest between the second and sixth rib in the mid-clavicular line at the fifth ICS on the approximate level of the fifth through the eighth thoracic vertebrae.

The xiphoid process overlies a portion of the liver and sits at the approximate level of the ninth and tenth thoracic vertebrae.

The lungs fill the chest cavity from the first rib to the tenth rib anteriorly and from the first thoracic vertebra to the twelfth thoracic vertebra posteriorly.

## Chest or Thorax—Posterior

The surface anatomy of the posterior thorax includes structures such as the scapula, thoracic spine, and posterior rib cage.

The scapula is a triangular bone buried in muscle which sits on the posterior rib cage from the level of the first thoracic vertebra to the eighth thoracic vertebra. The scapula is a useful landmark because one can draw an imaginary vertical line from the top middle of the bone to its inferior edge. This line is called the *mid-scapular line.* The inferior edge of the scapula is called the *inferior angle of the scapula.* One may also use the spine as a reference by drawing imaginary lines on either side of the posterior spine. These lines are called the *paravertebral lines* or the *paravertebral area.* (See Fig. 12–19.)

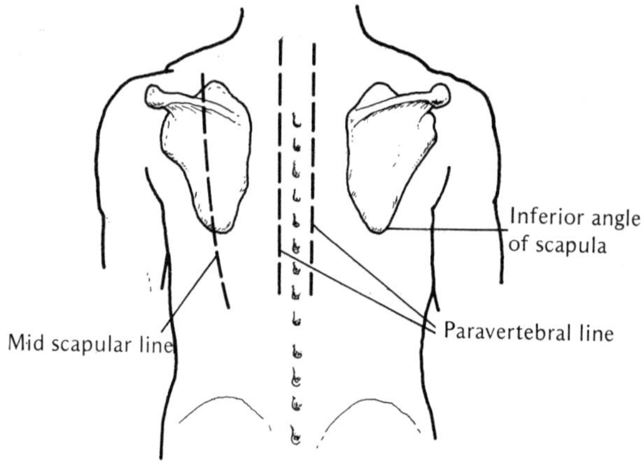


**Figure 12–19.** Surface reference lines of the posterior chest.

The EMT now has definite reference lines and landmarks on the posterior thorax, since one can now locate the seventh cervical vertebra and since we already know that the inferior angle of the scapula sits at the level of the eighth thoracic vertebra. Also, each vertebral body is about two fingerbreadths in length. Therefore, once the seventh cervical vertebra is found, one can count down using the two fingerbreaths in length to estimate roughly the location of injury, pain, and wounds to the posterior thorax.

The angle where the twelfth rib joins the twelfth thoracic vertebra is called the *costovertebral angle* and is a useful landmark.

Reference points and landmarks now exist to count with some accuracy all twelve thoracic vertebrae. The next area of the spine below the thoracic spine is the lumbar spine. It has five vertebrae. A reference for counting and locating them is simple. The iliac crests or top of the hips of the pelvis sit approximately at the level of the third and fourth lumbar vertebrae. By using the two fingerbreadth rule of approximation, one can count upward or downward to locate the first and fifth lumbar vertebrae. Another useful landmark in locating the lumbar vertebra is the umbilicus (navel) of the abdomen. It sits on the same horizontal level as the fourth lumbar vertebra.

The thorax has many lines of reference and landmarks. The EMT should know all of them for quick description of wounds, injury, and pain.

## Abdomen

It is also extremely important to be able to describe the abdomen for injury and pain. Like the chest cavity, organs that lie beneath the abdominal cavity should be known by the EMT. This is easy once reference lines and landmarks have been established.

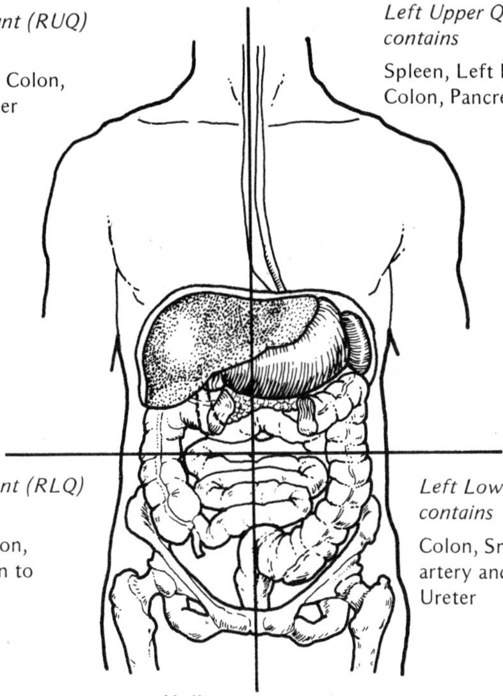


**Figure 12–20.** Surface reference lines of the abdomen dividing it into four quadrants, and the organ structures that lie beneath each quadrant.

The abdomen is bounded superiorly by the diaphragm and costal margins and inferiorly by the pubic bone. For reference, a vertical line is drawn from the xiphoid process through the umbilicus (navel) to the pubic bone and a horizontal line is drawn across the abdomen at the level of the navel. (See Fig. 12–20.) We now have divided the abdomen into four quadrants called:

1. upper-right quadrant (URQ)
2. upper-left quadrant (ULQ)
3. lower-right quadrant (LRQ)
4. lower-left quadrant (LLQ)

The EMT must know the organs and other structures that lie beneath each of the four quadrants. (See Fig. 12–20.)

The umbilicus (navel) is a useful landmark, as previously mentioned, because it is a constant structure. The umbilicus sits on the same horizontal

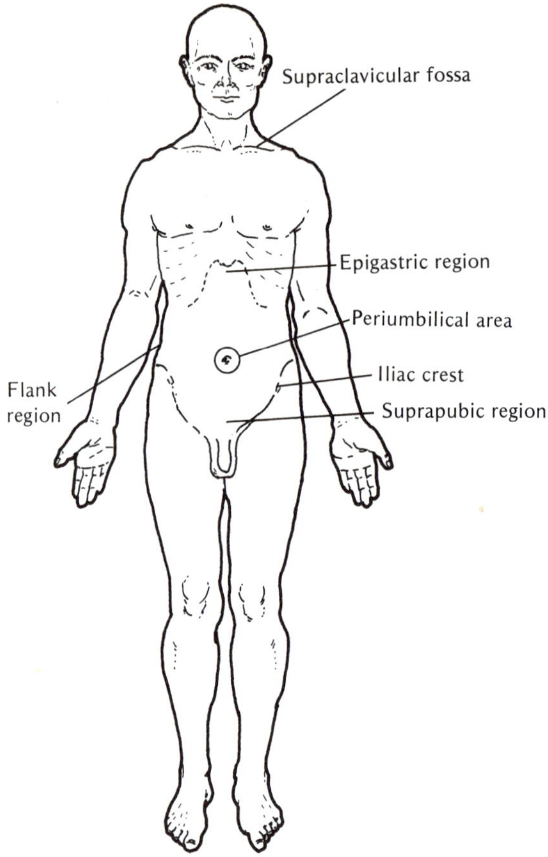


**Figure 12–21.** Regions of the abdomen and other anterior body landmarks.

plane as the fourth lumbar vertebrae and the superior edge of the iliac crests. It also overlies the division of the abdominal aorta into the two common iliac arteries. The area around the umbilicus is called the *periumbilical area* (around the umbilicus).

Other areas commonly referred to when describing wounds, pain, and injury are the epigastric region, flank region, and suprapubic region. (See Fig. 12–21.)

## Pelvis

The pelvis is an irregular bony ring that connects the upper torso to the lower torso. The pelvis consists of three pairs of bones (ilium, ischium, and pubis) all fused together. The two iliac bones form the wings (hips) of the pelvis. The iliac bones have two important landmarks. The superior edges of the iliac bones are called the *iliac crests.* They are on the same level as the third and fourth lumbar vertebrae. The anterior superior iliac spine

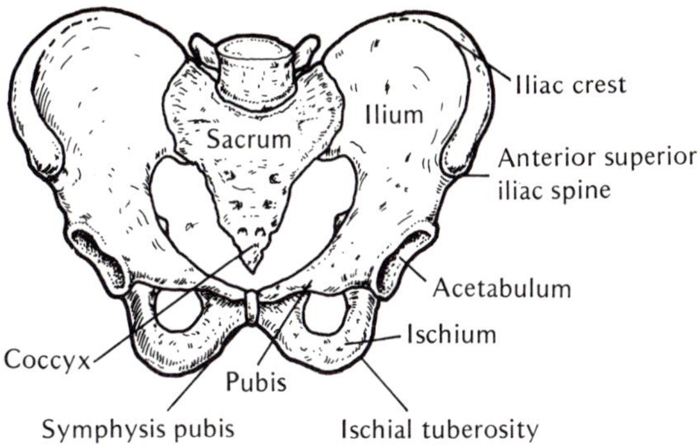


**Figure 12–22.**
Anatomy of the pelvis.

(ASIS) lies just below the horizontal level of the umbilicus. Find and palpate both of these landmarks on yourself. (See Fig. 12–22.)

The two ischial bones form the posterior portion of the pelvis. When we sit we rest on our ischial bones. A bony protuberance can be palpated through the gluteal muscles (buttock muscles) on the ischial bones. This protuberance is called the *ischial tuberosity.* The ischial bones are also important because this is where countertraction is applied when applying a traction splint.

The pelvis also has two pubic bones situated anteroposteriorly on the pelvis. The point where these two bones are fused together is called the *symphysis pubis.* Just above the symphysis pubis is the suprapubic region. An important constant structure just lateral to the symphysis pubis is the inguinal ligament. This ligament is stretched between the anterior superior iliac spine and the symphysis pubis. Just deep to the middle of this ligament is the femoral artery, a major large artery of the body that can easily be palpated. (See Fig. 12–23.) Find and palpate this artery for pulsation. (See Fig. 12–26a.)

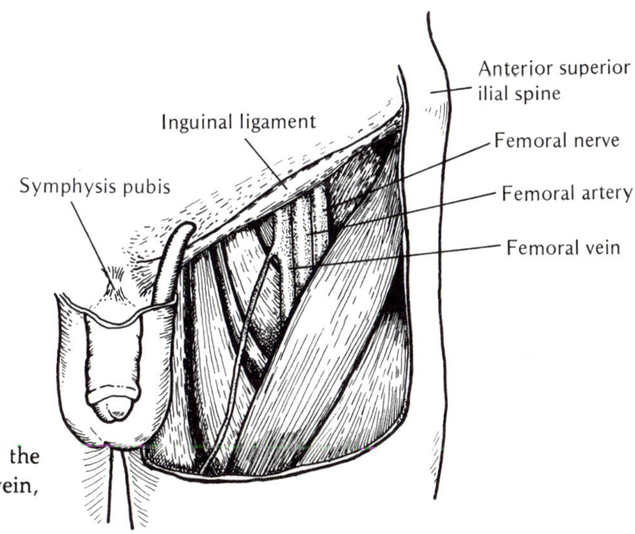


**Figure 12–23.** Anatomical location of the femoral nerve, artery, vein, and inguinal ligament.

## The Upper Extremity

The upper extremity is divided into three areas: the arm (humerus), forearm (radius and ulna), and hand. When referring to landmarks and reference points of the upper extremity, the EMT should keep in mind the anatomical position of the body.

The arm and forearm can be divided into three sections for easy reference: the proximal third, middle third, and distal third. (See Fig. 12–4.)

In the anatomical position, the anterior aspect of the forearm is called the *flexor surface.* The posterior aspect of the forearm is called the *extensor surface.* This is because of the flexor and extensor muscles in the forearm. The area on the anterior surface at the bend of the elbow is called the *antecubital fossa.* (See Fig. 12–24.)

This is the location where the patient's blood pressure is obtained. It is also at this location where large superficial veins (cephalic and basilic) course the arm and forearm. Intravenous therapy is often initiated here because large amounts of fluids can be given to the patient. The bony protuberance on the posterior aspect of the elbow is called the *olecranon* (o-lek′rah-non) *process.* This protuberance is the proximal end of the ulna. Feel it. Just medial to the olecranon process is the often self-injured ulnar nerve. When one hits this nerve, one gets an electrifying feeling of the arm

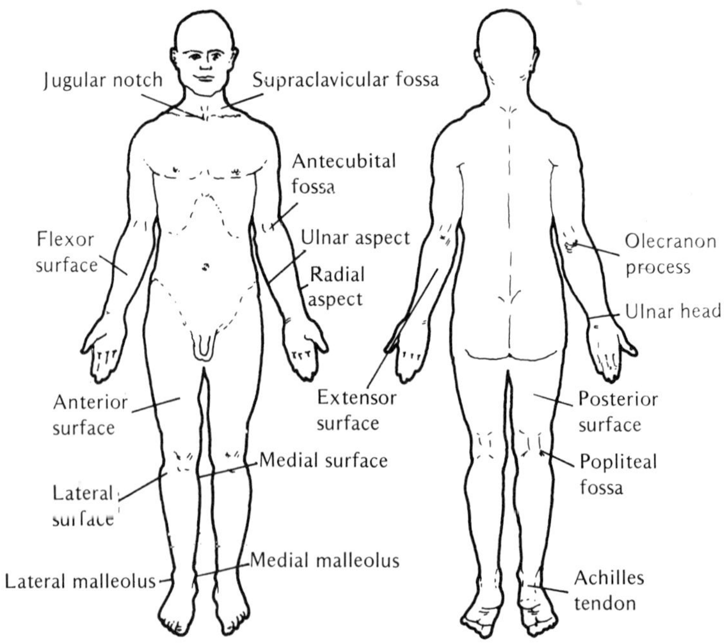


**Figure 12–24.** Descriptive terms and anatomical landmarks of the anterior and posterior aspects of the extremities.

and forearm. This is what is called hitting the "funny bone." (See Fig. 12–24.)

In referring to the side of the forearm we say that the thumb side of the forearm is the radial aspect and the little finger side is the ulnar aspect. The bump at the wrist on the little finger side is called the *ulnar head*. This is the distal end of the ulna. Another important landmark of the forearm is the flexor ligaments, on the anterior (flexor) surface at the wrist. Just lateral to the ligaments is the radial artery, the most frequently palpated artery in medicine. Feel for it. Just medial and deep to the ligaments is the ulnar artery. It is infrequently palpated because it is so deep and is sometimes difficult to find. A patient who cuts his wrist at this location may sever one or both of these arteries. Try to locate your ulnar artery.

The hand has two surfaces, the anterior or palmar surface, and posterior or dorsal surface. The dorsal surface is also called the *dorsum*. (See Fig. 12–25.)

The surface anatomy of the fingers or phalanges is simple. We name the fingers as to exactly what they are, that is, the thumb, index finger, middle finger, ring finger, and little finger. We name them this way to avoid confusion. Medicine is too confusing as it is!

## The Lower Extremity

The lower extremity can be divided into three parts: the femur (thigh), the leg (tibia and fibula), and the foot. The thigh and leg can be divided into thirds, just as we did with the arm and forearm, to locate and describe wounds quickly. (See Fig. 12–4.)

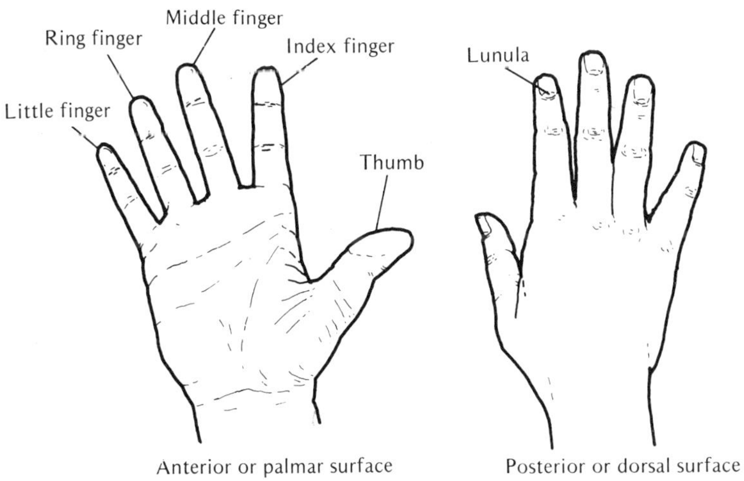


**Figure 12–25.** Palmar and dorsal surface of the hand and specific names of the fingers.

The thigh and leg have an anterior and posterior surface, a lateral surface (outside aspect), and a medial surface (inner aspect). (See Fig. 12–24.)

The patella or kneecap can be felt on the anterior surface between the thigh and leg. The posterior aspect at the bend of the knee is called the *popliteal fossa.* The popliteal artery runs down the thigh at this point. It can be palpated (although very difficult) deeply about three centimeters proximal to the center of the popliteal fossa. (See Fig. 12–26b.)

The shinbone or tibia is anteriorly positioned in the leg and is extremely superficial. It may be felt very easily, since it is only covered by skin at its most superficial location.

At the ankle on the medial and lateral aspects are two bony protuberances. The lateral (outside) bump is called the *lateral malleolus* and the medial (inside) bump is called the *medial malleolus.* The medial malleolus is created by the distal end of the tibia and the lateral malleolus by the distal end of the fibula. A large artery of the lower leg and foot can be palpated in the depression between the medial malleolus and achilles ten-

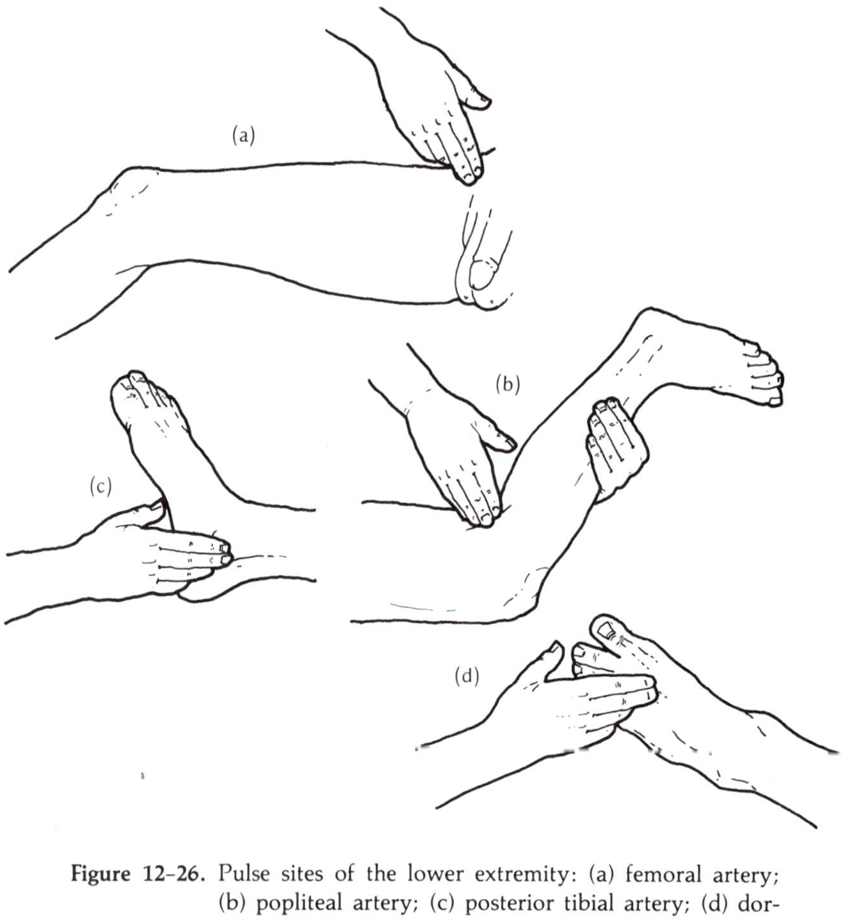


**Figure 12–26.** Pulse sites of the lower extremity: (a) femoral artery; (b) popliteal artery; (c) posterior tibial artery; (d) dorsalis pedis artery.

don. This is the posterior tibial artery. Feel it. (See Fig. 12-26c.) This artery is important to know and find when checking the circulatory status of the lower extremity.

The foot has two aspects, as does the hand. The sole of the foot is called the *plantar surface* and the top of the foot is called the *dorsal surface.* An important artery is located on the dorsal aspect of the foot. This is the dorsalis pedis artery. It may be palpated just lateral to the long extensor tendon of the great toe, in the middle of the foot between the great and second toe. This artery is not present in all people and is difficult to palpate while traveling in a moving vehicle. If the circulatory status is to be checked in the lower extremity, the posterior tibial pulse should always be palpated if possible. However, it is advisable to check and palpate for the dorsalis pedis pulse, too. (See Fig. 12-26d.) The toes are numbered from one through five; the great or big toe is number one and the little toe number five.

The EMT must be able to describe wounds, injuries, and pain on every patient. Surface anatomy should not be a guessing game. The EMT has to know what he is looking at and how to describe the location to the nurse or physician when necessary.

## *References*

American Academy of Orthopedic Surgeons, Committee on Allied Health. *Emergency Care of the Sick and Injured.* 2nd ed. Chicago, IL: American Academy of Orthopedic Surgeons, 1977.

Caroline, Nancy L. *Emergency Care in the Streets.* Boston, MA: Little, Brown & Co., 1979.

Gardner, Ernest; Gray, Donald J.; O'Rahilly, Ronan. *Anatomy.* Philadelphia, PA: W. B. Saunders Company, 1975.

Grant, J. C. Boileau. *An Atlas of Anatomy,* 6th ed. Baltimore, MD: The Williams & Wilkins Co., 1972.

Grant, H. D., and Murray, R. H., Jr. *Emergency Care,* 2nd ed. Bowie, MD: Robert J. Brady, Co., 1978.

Lankford, T. R. *Integrated Science for Health Students.* Reston, VA: Reston Publishing Co., Inc., 1979.

Stewart, Ronald D. "An Introduction to Surface Anatomy for Paramedics," *Paramedics International,* Winter 1977, pp. 27-39.

Stewart, Ronald D. "An Introduction to Surface Anatomy for Paramedics, Part II," *Paramedics International,* Spring 1977, pp. 16-19.

# Chapter 13

# Initial Assessments and Field Management of Trauma

Trauma is the leading cause of death in young children and adults up to the age of forty. Head injuries are the most common results of automobile accidents. It is estimated that four out of five accident victims have head injuries; two out of five have leg injuries; one out of four have chest injuries; and one out of seven have serious abdominal injuries. When all causes of trauma-related deaths are considered, head injury and hemorrhage lead the list. It is crucial for the EMT to provide basic life support and make initial assessments of organ systems. In order to set priorities for field management and transportation, there must be a well-established system of assessments which guides the sequence of activities. For example, a well-trained EMT must know when field assessments and stabilization procedures ought to be abandoned for immediate transport, called a "scoop and run." Although each organ system will be discussed in detail in later chapters, the purpose here is to outline the principles that are important to multiple trauma.

## BASIC LIFE SUPPORT

Basic life support is always the first consideration! An airway must be assured and anything that interferes with breathing must be dealt with at once.

Proper positioning, suctioning, the use of artificial airways, and oxygen administration should be employed as indicated. Remember to assess the carotid and femoral pulses to determine if there is good circulation. Cervical spine precautions should be exercised when positioning the head or selecting and inserting airway devices. *A cervical spine injury is assumed in all trauma patients.* A cervical collar, sandbags, and appropriate backboards should be used. (See Chapter 15.) Careful positioning is important to protect against aspiration of emesis, which is common after traumatic episodes. Particular attention should be given to an airway which is threatened by facial trauma, especially fractures of the nose and jaw and soft tissue injuries creating bleeding in the mouth or throat.

If CPR is not required, the EMT can proceed to assessment of vital signs. (See Chapter 9.)

## CONTROL OF HEMORRHAGE AND SHOCK

Bleeding should be controlled by direct pressure if feasible, based on the location of the bleeding. Using pressure points (see Fig. 11–3) to arrest severe arterial blood loss may be indicated in certain instances. Tourniquets are a last resort; however, if there is life-threatening blood loss, the EMT may apply one. (See page 260.) It should be recalled that prolonged use of a tourniquet could lead to circulatory complications which eventually may result in the loss of a limb. But once the decision is made to use one, the pressure should not be released until the patient has arrived at the hospital and a physician has taken command.

The application of antishock trousers or the initiation of IV fluids may be accomplished in the field by advanced EMTs. These measures tend to result promptly in the patient's improvement if he is in shock.

Each existing wound with related arterial bleeding must be scrutinized. Is there associated pain, pallor, loss of sensation, or inability to move the part? Pulses should be palpated (as described earlier) to ensure that arterial flow is adequate.

The presence of restlessness in a patient is one of the earliest signs of inadequate oxygenation and, depending on the situation and injury, should be looked at with a critical eye. The presence of cyanosis is a late finding of inadequate oxygenation. The EMT must stay ahead of inadequate oxygenation and anticipate respiratory difficulties by prudently administering supplemental oxygen when necessary.

## CHEST INJURIES

Chest injuries are high priority in the multiple trauma examination because of the chest's role in ventilation and circulation. A quick determination of the nature of the accident and pertinent medical history should be made. Vital signs, skin color and temperature, and the presence of movement, distended neck veins, tracheal deviation, retractions, subcutaneous (sub″ku-ta′ne-us) emphysema (em″fĭ-se′mah) and sucking sounds must be interpreted as indices of serious chest injury. (See Fig. 13–1.) A survey of respiratory function and the detection of signs and symptoms of acute distress must be performed.

Stridor (stri′dor), use of accessory (ak-ses′o-re) muscles, and nasal flaring indicate increased effort of breathing. Any open chest wound should be covered and flail segments controlled. If time permits, listen over

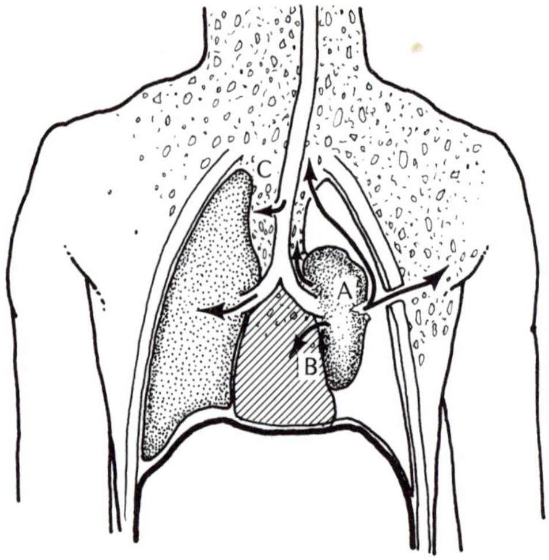


**Figure 13-1.** Subcutaneous emphysema. Air can escape into tissue from rupture of the major airway structures. The presence of crepitus (a crackling sound upon palpation that is similar to that made by compressing coarse styrofoam) should alert the EMT to a life-threatening underlying injury.

the apical pulse for distant heart sounds, which could indicate heart damage. When there is a history of a severe impact to the sternum, then the heart, large surrounding blood vessels, and major airway structures can be injured. These mid-chest impact traumas are likely to be accompanied by rapidly developing shock as well as respiratory distress. (See Chapter 17 for details of chest injury assessment and management.)

## ABDOMEN AND GENITOURINARY SYSTEM

The abdomen should be checked for wounds, rigidity, or other obvious clues to injury. Consider the presence of urinary tract trauma, particularly if there is blood on or around the genitalia (jen″ĭ-ta′le-ah), or if there is an associated fracture of the pelvis. (See Chapter 19 for details of abdominal trauma.)

## NEUROLOGICAL CHECKS

This initial neurological assessment should include levels of consciousness and pupillary responses. If time permits, check the head for lacerations (las″er-a′shunz) and fractures, inspect the ears and nose for bleeding or leaking cerebrospinal fluid (CSF), and evaluate the neurological status of limbs. The ability of the patient to move all extremities and have feeling in them as well is important to note after injury. (See Chapter 15 for details of head, neck and spinal cord injuries.)

## FRACTURE CARE

Obvious limb fractures should be promptly splinted. Be sure to assess peripheral pulses below the fracture site and cover open wounds. Depending upon local protocol, traction may be reserved for a mid-shaft femur fracture or for fractures with a distal neurovascular (nu″ro-vas′ku-lar) loss, i.e., feeling and blood supply are impaired.

A lack of feeling in an extremity distal to a fracture site may be caused by compression or damage to nerves. In such cases, feeling may return when the fracture is stabilized. (See Chapter 20 for details of assessment and management of fractures)

## SPECIAL TYPES OF WOUNDS

### Trauma Considerations

There are numerous types of trauma that require special consideration, mostly due to a more complex and subtle mechanism of injury and severe injury potential. Cases involving stab wounds, or penetrating wounds from knives, sticks, and flying objects can involve severe injury and yet look quite minor. Often external bleeding is minimal or nonexistent, but internal bleeding may be significant. Appearances can be deceiving. Often such a wound even upon close inspection will appear to be shallow, involving only the skin and subcutaneous fat. However, hospital surgical exploration very often reveals penetration into a main body cavity. As with fractures, any wound that may possibly have entered a major body cavity (head, chest, or abdomen) must be treated seriously. The EMT has the knowledge and skill to determine that a serious injury may exist, but he cannot determine that it does not exist! Among the important information that the EMT should gather is a description of the weapon or object that caused the wound, the situation in which it occurred, the location of the external wounds (*all* of them), and the approximate angle of wound entry. This information can provide clues as to what internal damage may have occurred.

Gunshot wounds require special attention due to the possible severe damage that can be inflicted. The EMT must locate all entry and exit wounds. This may not be simple. Areas often missed upon inspection of the patient include entry wounds to the head, behind the ear, back, axillary regions, scrotum, and rectal area. A small caliber weapon (a .22 or a .32) will often have a small entrance wound and small exit wound. Due to its low velocity, it often does not travel in a straight line when entering the body and may actually "bounce around" inside body cavities before exiting, if it does exit.

A large caliber weapon (.38, 357, .44), because of its high velocity, generally travels in a straight line upon entering the body, leaving a small entry wound and a large exit wound. Because of its high velocity, the projectile may damage a larger area of tissue and organs or miss vital organs altogether. This is because the higher velocity projectile does not "bounce around" upon entry.

The damage inflicted by shotgun wounds, unlike gunshot wounds, depends largely on the distance from the gun to the body. Close-range wounds may involve extremely large areas of soft tissue damage and destruction. Long-range wounds, however, often consist of a showering of pellets over a large area, any one of which could pierce a body cavity and cause damage.

The assessment of a gunshot wound should include establishing the location of entrance and exit wounds, the type of weapon used, the number of wounds, the range of fire, and the angle of entry. Often the entrance and exit wounds may be confusing; one missile may have entered, exited, and re-entered, causing three wounds. Powder burns around one wound on the skin or clothing indicate an entrance wound and that it occurred at close range. In situations with no apparent exit wound, the missile may be able to be palpated just under the skin around the entrance wound or close by. The assessment of all patients with gunshot wounds must involve a total inspection of the entire body. Many serious and even fatal wounds have gone undetected, hidden in skin folds, underclothing, or simply because other wounds distracted the rescuers who simply forgot to look for additional wounds. In any situation where the patient has multiple injuries, it is imperative that the EMT not allow himself to be overly distracted by the most obvious injury, but continue to systematically examine the entire patient thoroughly and locate all injuries. It is often easy for instance, to spend too much time and attention to an open fracture of a femur and forget to notice the more subtle but more serious chest or abdominal injury.

## MULTIPLE PATIENTS

The multiple-patient situation is perhaps the most difficult situation that the EMT will have to face. It can be extremely difficult or nearly impossible to properly assess and treat more than two serious patients with two EMTs. More than two serious patients requires the EMT to decide how many additional emergency units will be needed. Depending on the situation, the EMT must rapidly scan the scene and logically request additional special services (EMS, police, fire, utility personnel) to prevent further injury or damage. In most instances, the initial situation will seem worse than it actually is, but it is far better to request too much help than to request too little. Depending on the situation and the resources available, the EMT must decide if a moving or stationary triage (tre-ahzh') system is appropriate. Triage is a method of sorting patients according to types of injuries and priority of treatment. Mobile triage is effective for up to twelve to fifteen patients in a relatively small area. This is the most common type of multiple-patient situation that the EMT will encounter. The EMT must then move rapidly from patient to patient, pausing only long enough to perform a primary survey and rapid assessment of injuries. Seldom should more than thirty seconds be spent on any one patient. If possible, the EMT should appoint a single rescuer (hopefully an EMT, but a first-aider policeman or fire fighter would suffice) to each patient or to each small group of patients. The EMT then coordinates the care of each patient, by his appointees, rechecking their findings and treatment. The EMT must decide which patients have the highest priority and assign to them the most skilled people or treat them himself until additional medical personnel arrive. The priorities should be numbered such that the Priority One group are those with a compromise of the ABCs that can be corrected by immediate care. (Such cases may include chest injuries, severe abdominal injuries, suspected rapid internal bleeding, airway obstruction, and penetrating neck wounds.) Patients triaged into the Priority number One category should always receive primary attention and the most expert care that is available, and should be the group of patients evacuated to the nearest hospital capable of providing appropriate treatment.

The second group, or Priority Two patients, are those that may have sustained significant injuries, but are stable enough for delayed transportation to the hospital. This group would include patients with fractures, lacerations with controlled bleeding, major burns (greater than 20 percent total body surface), and abdominal pain with stable vital signs. The EMT must realize that although many injuries are quite serious, if the patient's condition is not likely to deteriorate rapidly, then treatment and transportation can be delayed.

The third group consists of those patients with minor burns, and fractures, and soft tissue injuries. Some of these patients may be able to stand and walk around and fairly well care for themselves. This group can often be utilized to provide reassurance and keep a watchful eye over the Priority Two group. This group combined with those people who were not injured, tend to be the ones that are the most severely affected by the present situation in the form of hysteria, panic, or anger. Giving them some direction or a task to perform, no matter how minor, may help keep order and calm them.

The Priority Four group consists of the obviously dead victims or those requiring CPR. It is important to understand that in disaster situations, CPR is one of the first treatments to be eliminated. The philosophy of administering the best care to benefit the most patients must be followed. It is unfair and illogical to tie up two or three rescuers trying to resuscitate one patient (with a statistically low chance of survival), when other patients can benefit by their treatment and care. It is extremely important for the EMT, who in other circumstances might expend every effort to try to care for patients like those in Priority Four to simply provide for their basic comfort and then turn his attention to other patients.

The decisions of triage are difficult and sometimes controversial, but the EMT must realize that as a medical technician, his responsibility rests with those patients who have a reasonable chance of survival because of early treatment and hospital transport. In most cases the EMT will be quickly relieved of the triage responsibility by a higher medical authority (paramedics, physicians, etc.).

One of the most common mistakes made in the management of multiple-patient incidents is that of inadequate documentation of basic information. While initial care and triage can usually take place at the scene with little or no written communication, basic information must be gathered to avoid long delays and possible errors once the patients are transported to area hospitals. Many systems of documentation exist, most incorporating the use of a simple note or tag that is attached to each patient indicating name, basic problem, priority group, and destination hospital. In the usual small-scale multi-patient incident, however, such tags are rarely available or necessary. Often it is just as effective to designate one rescuer or first aider to act as a recorder next to the triage EMT and document the number of patients, names, problems, priority, vital signs, and destinations. This information can then be pinned or placed on the patient. Regardless of the system, documentation must take place.

## *Summary*

The EMT who is dealing with the trauma patient should be familiar with the priorities of care:

1. Basic life support
2. Control of hemorrhage and shock
3. Assessment and management of specific injuries
   —Chest
   —Abdomen and genito-urinary system
   —Neurological
   —Fractures

Any injury which is threatening airway patency and breathing is cause for prompt transport to a hospital. These include fractures of the cervical spine, facial bones, ribs and sternum, bleeding into the airways, and other types of chest injuries which interfere with breathing.

If time and circumstances permit, the EMT may further assess various organ systems, but careful monitoring of the airway, breathing, and circulation must not be ignored to accomplish any detailed field examination.

TABLE 13–1. ASSESSMENT OF MULTIPLE TRAUMA

Step 1 *Primary Survey: Diagnose and Treat
- a. Inadequate ventilation
- b. Circulatory insufficiency
- c. Hemorrhage

*Remember always to suspect C-spine injuries

Step 2 Obtain and Record Pertinent Injury History

Step 3 Identify Injured Areas: Perform Systematic Review

a. Head
1. Calculate *Glasgow Coma Scale*
2. Inspect *head* and *scalp*
3. Explore *nasal* and *auditory* canals for blood, CSF.
4. Inspect *eyes* (movement, pupils, visual acuity)
5. Search the *mouth* (malocclusion, lacerations, missing teeth)
6. Inspect *face* for fractures (nose, zygoma, mandible)

b. Neck
1. Inspect for tracheal deviation, vein distention, ecchymosis.
2. Palpate for subcutaneous emphysema, bony abnormalities, tenderness.

c. Chest
1. Inspect for wounds, symmetry in breath excursions, rate and rhythm of breathing
2. Listen for breath sounds, heart sounds
3. Paplate stability of thoracic cage, for masses and tenderness

d. Abdomen
1. Inspect for wounds, ecchymosis, old surgical scars
2. Listen for bowel sounds, bruits
3. Palpate for masses, tenderness, pelvic stability, subcutaneous emphysema

e. Musculoskeletal System
1. Inspect for pathological posturing; spastic hemiplegia, appearance and function of extremities.
2. Palpate for pulses, sensation, tenderness, deformities, muscle strength

f. Perineum and Genitalia

Inspect for blood at meatus, ecchymosis of scrotum and perineum, open wounds.

g. Back and Buttocks
1. *Logroll patient* and inspect for ecchymosis, hematoma, wounds
2. Palpate vertebrae, ribs and pelvis for deformities, fractures, swelling, tenderness.

---

Vital signs should be taken at least every five to ten minutes at the scene and en route to detect trends which could indicate additional complications. (See Table 13–1.)

In multiple patient situations, or in disaster, triage of patients should be done to ensure that the *best care* can be provided for the *greatest number of patients.*

*References*

Barber, Janet M., and Budassi, Susan A. *Mosby's Manual of Emergency Care.* St. Louis, MO: The C. V. Mosby Co., 1979.

Dagnone E. E. "A Plan For Resuscitation of the Acutely Injured Patient," *JACEP,* 3:241–244, July-August 1974.

Larkin, I., and Moylan, J. "Priorities in Management of Trauma Victims," *Critical Care Medicine,* 3:192–195, 1975.

Matthewson, C. "Initial Evaluation and Treatment of Multiply Injured Patients," *Western Journal of Medicine,* 126:421–425, May 1977.

# Chapter 14

# Soft Tissue Injuries

Soft tissue injuries are injuries to the layers of the skin, subcutaneous tissue, fascia (membranes that join the skin to underlying tissue and also cover, separate, and give support to muscles), muscles, arteries, veins, and nerves. Soft tissue injuries are classified like fractures—they can be open or closed. Closed injuries are those in which the skin has not been broken. Open injuries are those in which the skin or mucous membranes have been broken. We usually do not think of the mucous membranes as being included in soft tissue because of their less obvious locations. They include the lining of the body's openings such as the anus, vagina, urethra, and oral cavity.

## CLOSED SOFT TISSUE INJURIES

When a forceful impact occurs to the body from any object, soft tissue can be damaged. This is known as *blunt trauma.* Because our body's soft tissue has resilient and elastic properties, the surface skin may not break after blunt trauma. However, in blunt trauma what we want to consider is not only surface damage, but also structural damage that may occur to organs and major vessels that lie beneath the area of impact. This is one of many reasons why the EMT must know anatomy. (See Fig. 14–1.)

In a closed soft tissue injury, the skin is not broken, but the vessels and tissue below may be crushed or ruptured. When this happens, tissue fluid and blood leak out into the surrounding tissue, which causes ecchymosis (ek″ĭ-mo′sis) (bruising). Because of the chemical breakdown of the escaped blood, it discolors and appears black and blue. This type of soft tissue injury is known as a *contusion* (kon-tu′zhun). The injured area swells and there is pain caused by the increased fluid pressure on surrounding nerve ends. The surrounding tissue eventually absorbs the escaped tissue fluid and blood, and the bruising disappears. If the blunt trauma is severe enough to cause considerable vessel and tissue damage, large

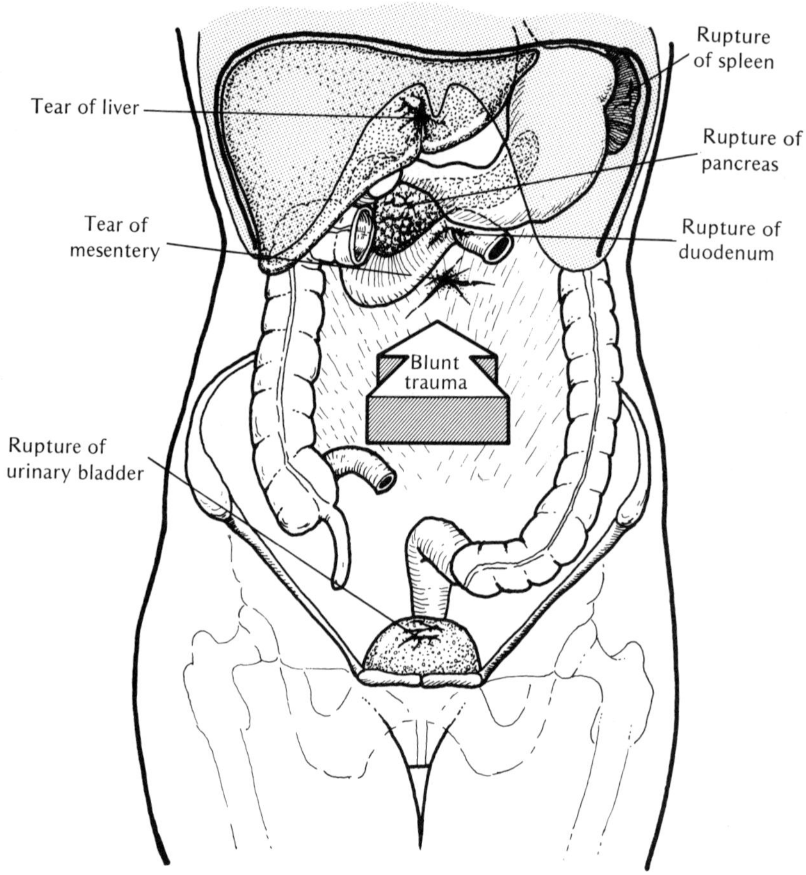


**Figure 14-1.** Blunt trauma may cause hidden internal bleeding. The EMT-A should always be alert to the signs and symptoms of hypovolemic shock.

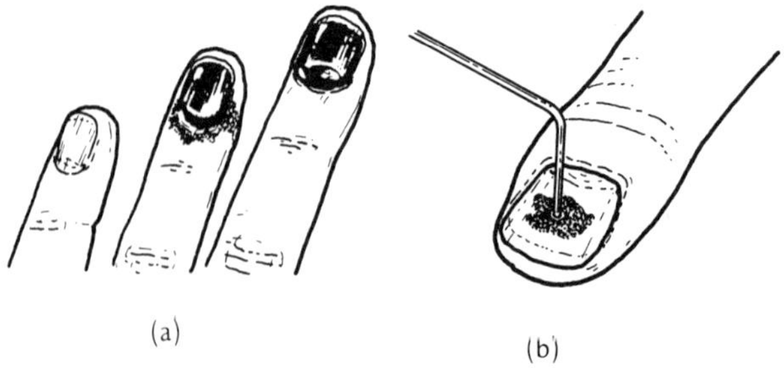


**Figure 14-2.** (a) A subungual hematoma, treated at the hospital by (b) releasing the blood causing painful pressure by heating a paperclip and boring a hole through the fingernail so blood can escape. The procedure is painless.

amounts of blood and tissue fluid will be pocketed rapidly under the contused area. This is known as a *hematoma* (hem″ah-to′mah) or blood tumor (*hemat*—blood, *oma*—tumor). Hematomas occur frequently with trauma that is sufficient enough to fracture bones. Blood is pocketed around the broken bone ends and losses of 500 cc or more is not uncommon, especially with fractures of the pelvis, femur, and hip. Another type of hematoma may occur when a solid object impacts on the top of the fingernail or toenail, causing blood to pool underneath the nail. This type of injury is called *subungual* (sub-ung′gwal) hematoma (*sub*—under, *ungual*—nail).

### Treatment

Contusions require no special emergency treatment. However, the EMT should be suspicious as to the possible damage that may have occurred to organs and other structures that lie beneath the bruised area.

Hematomas may be treated by the application of a pressure dressing, wrapped chemical cold pack, or ice pack. It is important to keep in mind the possible blood loss associated with certain fractures (especially those of the femur), and that hemorrhagic shock could ensue due to the fluid loss. Monitor the patient's vital signs. Shock trousers should be considered, not only to combat blood loss but also to stabilize the fracture site.

Subungual hematomas are not serious, but they do cause a great deal of pain. Applying a chemical cold or ice pack and keeping the extremity elevated is all that the EMT can do. Once the patient is seen in the emergency department, the hematoma will be relieved by boring through the nail with a scalpal or with a red-hot paperclip. The pressure is reduced once the blood escapes and pain is greatly diminished. Once the red-hot paperclip goes through the nail, it is immediately cooled by the pocketed blood. Both types of treatment are relatively painless. (See Fig. 14–2.)

## OPEN SOFT TISSUE INJURIES

Open injuries to soft tissue cause bleeding, environmental contamination, and possible infection to the wound. There are four types of open soft tissue injuries that the EMT should recognize and be able to describe when necessary: abrasions, lacerations, punctures, and avulsions.

### Abrasions

An abrasion occurs when the surface skin (epidermis) is scraped away. There is little or no capillary bleeding, but the injury is painful—similar to the pain from a second-degree burn. Therefore, abrasions are also known as mat burns, friction burns, and brush burns. Almost any

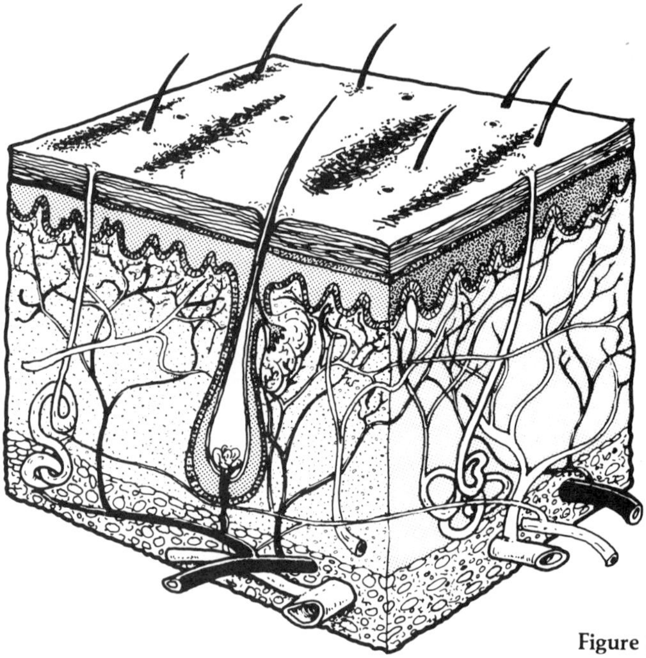

**Figure 14–3.** An abrasion.

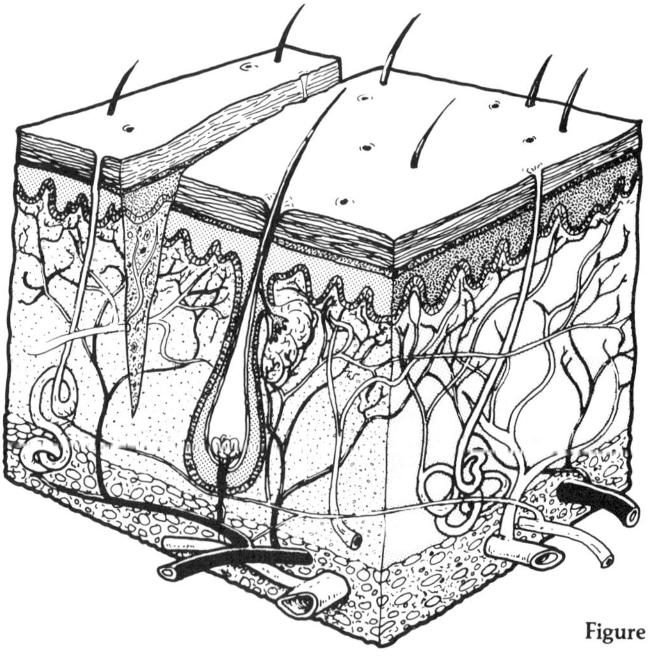

**Figure 14–4.** A laceration.

type of hard sliding on the skin could cause an abrasion. This is a very common athletic injury. (See Fig. 14-3.)

## Lacerations

Lacerations (see Fig. 14-4) can occur from any sharp edged object (knives, tin cans, glass, etc.) or from blunt trauma (fist to lip, head to windshield, etc.). Sharp-edged objects lacerate the skin, leaving fairly smooth and tidy edges. Blunt trauma due to pressure impact bursts the skin, leaving the skin edges jagged and untidy. Lacerations—cuts—may injure the dermal subcutaneous tissue and muscle. Depending on location and depth, lacerations may cause minimal or major damage to arteries or nerves and blood loss can be life threatening. Lacerations, from whatever reason, that occur to body areas in which large arteries or veins run close to the skin surface may be life threatening, especially to the neck, wrist, groin, and temporal regions of the head. This danger is another reason why knowing anatomy is important to the EMT.

## Punctures

Puncture wounds (See Fig. 14-5) result from any object that penetrates the skin. The wound is usually a small hole or slit and bleeding is minimal. Puncture injuries are usually caused by nails, ice picks, splinters, pencils, or other sharp pointed objects. Like blunt trauma, the underlying

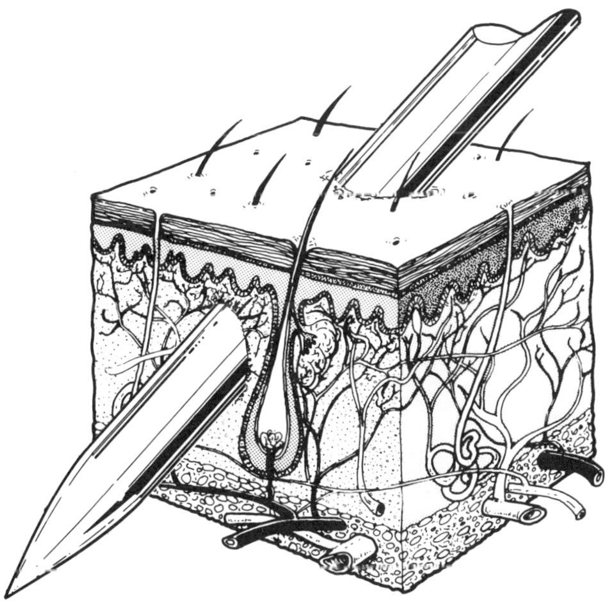

**Figure 14-5.** A puncture wound resulting in an impaled object.

anatomic structures are an important consideration. The EMT cannot see structural damage from these injuries, but he can assess the signs and symptoms of impending shock that may arise from such wounds.

With all gunshot wounds, the EMT should look for entrance and exit wounds. This sometimes is not as easy as it sounds, especially gunshot wounds from small-caliber weapons (a .22 and a .32). Areas which are frequently overlooked include the axilla, groin, rectum, and behind the ears. All patients with puncture wounds to the chest or abdomen should be watched for signs and symptoms of hemorrhagic shock.

## Avulsions

An avulsion (See Fig. 14–6) is an injury in which the skin, subcutaneous tissue, or muscle is torn away and remains as a flap or is completely "scooped" out and remains at the accident scene. When an avulsion occurs, the tissue is usually pulled away at the plane that separates it from different tissue (i.e., skin from subcutneous tissue or subcutaneous tissue from muscle).

In a *degloving* avulsion injury, the layers of the skin or deeper structures are stripped away. This injury is common when a ring on a finger is caught on an obstruction and the ring causes the skin to be pulled off. The hand is like a glove in which the skin acts as the glove covering. Just as you pull a glove off, the hand turning it inside out, so the skin does when a

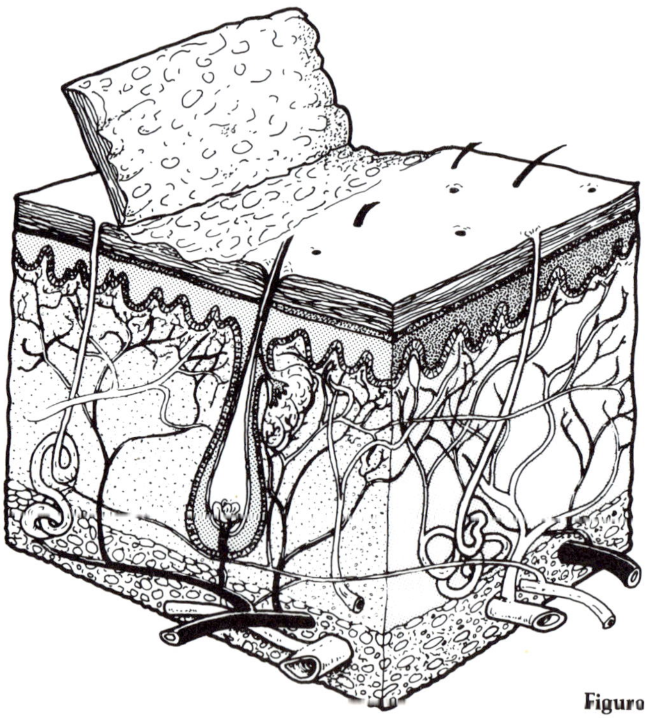

**Figure 14-6.** An avulsion.

degloving injury takes place. The EMT should try to locate any avulsed flap of tissue or limb and transport the parts to the emergency department with the patient. The parts should be wrapped in a moist sterile dressing and placed in a plastic bag and put on ice. If ice is not available, a chemical cold pack or cold water will suffice. These parts can possibly be reattached or used for skin grafting.

## TREATMENT FOR OPEN WOUNDS

The EMT's major concern with open soft tissue injuries is to control bleeding. This can be accomplished in almost all cases by (see Fig. 14-7):

1. Direct pressure (either with a pressure dressing or a hand placed directly on the wound if necessary)
2. Elevation
3. Pulse point pressure

If the injury is to the lower extremities, antishock trousers may be utilized. The EMT must be alert to other more severe injuries such as cervical trauma, fractures, and other wounds that take precedence over soft tissue injuries. Open soft tissue injuries should be covered with a sterile dressing. Very rarely is bleeding not stopped by the above measures. If

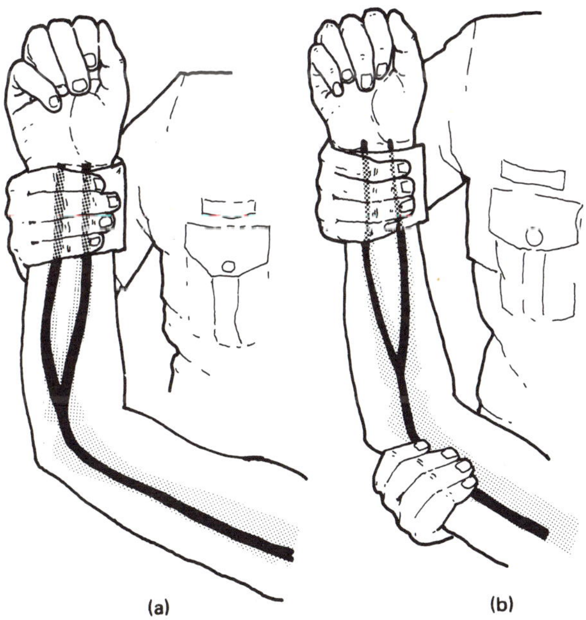

(a) (b)

**Figure 14-7.** (a) The EMT-A can control most bleeding by direct pressure and elevation. (b) If bleeding continues, pulse point pressure may be used to control the hemorrhage.

severe bleeding does persist, as on occasions it may with crushing injuries, a tourniquet should be properly applied. All fractures must be immobilized before field wound management is accomplished.

The injury must be exposed for proper inspection. The EMT can cut around the wound or cut the clothing at the seam. Large identifiable foreign material may be removed (metal with chunks of dirt, etc.), but the EMT should not debride or pick out ground in dirt and glass fragments. These items can result in mechanical tattooing (see Fig. 14–8) and should be surgically removed.

Candidates for tourniquet placement are those patients who have vascular injury not controllable by direct pressure, elevation, and pulse point pressure. The blood pressure cuff can be used to control bleeding effectively in the upper extremity. It should be placed above the elbow as one would do in taking blood pressure, and inflated above the patient's systolic blood pressure so that arterial as well as venous blood is stopped. (See Fig. 14–9a.) Profuse bleeding of the lower extremity can be controlled by shock trousers. Vascular injury to the abdomen and thorax can be managed by shock trousers as well. In situations where a blood pressure cuff or shock trousers are not available and uncontrollable bleeding is from the extremities, a simple cravat bandage may be used, as shown in Figure 14–9b. When using the cravat bandage or other wide material or a tourniquet, it should be placed above the elbow or knee to avoid neurovascular injury. Once a tourniquet is secured, it should be left in plain view. The EMT-A should always document on the patient report his treatment concerning tourniquet placement, and should relay this information to the triage nurse or attending medical practitioner upon hospital arrival. The EMT-A should never use wire or other thin material as a tourniquet, since these may cause neurovascular damage.

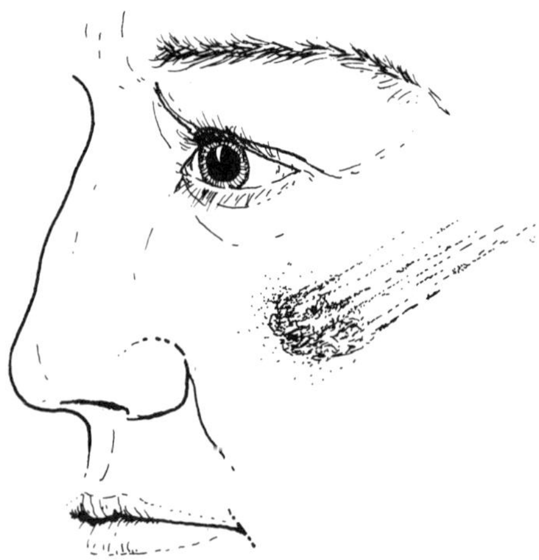

**Figure 14–8.** A mechanical tattoo produced from sliding across the road surface and grinding dirt and debris into the wound. This is commonly associated with motorcycle injury.

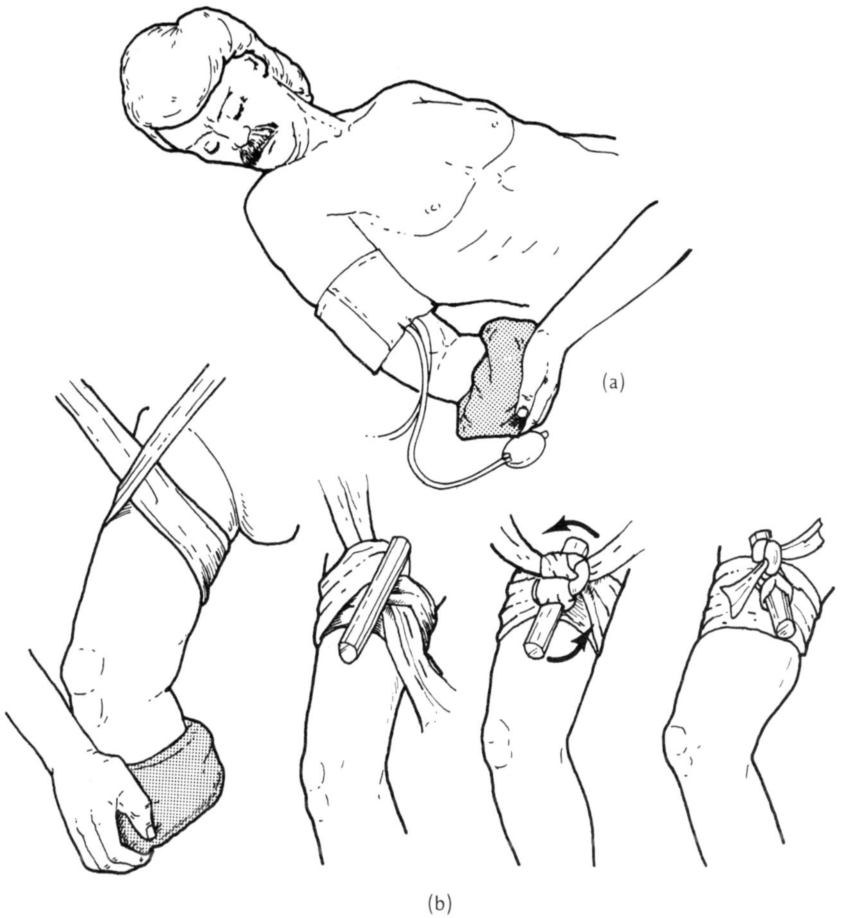


**Figure 14–9.** (a) A blood pressure cuff may be used effectively to stop uncontrollable bleeding in the upper extremity. Note direct pressure being applied to the bleeding site until the blood pressure cuff has been inflated. (b) A cravat bandage can be used to control bleeding in the lower extremity as shown using a windlass to apply the tourniquet effect.

## OTHER TYPES OF SOFT TISSUE INJURIES

### Crushing Injuries

Crush injuries are hard to forget for the experienced EMT. Because of the grotesqueness and deformity of the body produced by such an injury, the skill, knowledge, and psychological sense of the novice EMT will be taxed when caring for such a patient. By definition, a crush injury occurs when a heavy or solid object collides with the body in a short time period during which the greatest force is applied to the body.

Crushing trauma can be produced by "run over" accidents from the wheels or parts of tractors, cars, buses and trains, hydraulic equipment; falls from great heights; machine presses; and situations where the body is in the way of heavy or solid objects that collide with one another. Multiple open soft and hard (bone) tissue injuries usually occur, frequently with partial or complete amputations. Bleeding is usually (but not always) minimal because of the body's protective nervous system mechanisms that reduce the diameter of blood vessels when severed, therefore saving blood volume. This mechanism of the blood vessel to clamp down and reduce blood loss is called *vasospasm* (vas'o-spazm). (see Fig. 14-10.) This protective mechanism does not last long, so the EMT must dress wounds, immobilize fractures, and guard against potential shock by giving oxygen and transporting the patient in the shock position. The use of antishock trousers may be called for.

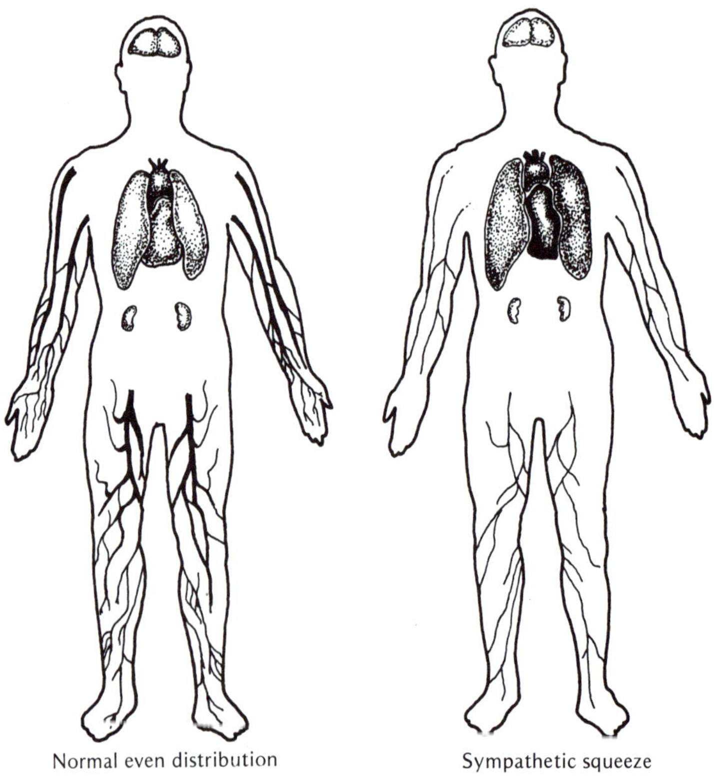


**Figure 14-10.** The body's initial response to shock constricts or "clamps down" on the vascular system to protect itself from further blood loss.

## Impaled Objects

Objects that penetrate the skin and underlying tissues and remain embedded are called *impaled objects.* Commonly, the EMT may see knives, ice picks, metal rods, scissors, pins, pencils, and splinters that have been impaled. Impaled objects must *not* be removed. Even though these objects may rupture blood vessels, the impaled object may act as a barrier that blocks or retards further bleeding. If the object is pulled out or is harshly disturbed, fatal hemorrhage could occur.

The EMT should use common sense in dealing with impaled objects. If there is bleeding from around the object, it can usually be stopped by a pressure dressing applied around it. For small impaled objects such as knives, ice picks, and rods, precut IV 4 × 4 gauze pads are ideal. For larger impaled objects trauma dressings can be cut to fit around the object to stop bleeding. There may be instances in which impaled objects may seem impossible to deal with and may have to be cut off for patient transport. In these cases, the EMT may be able to cut off the stabilized end, leaving the embedded end of the object in place. The EMT must remember that vibrations from saws and pneumatic tools may promote active bleeding. Movement should be kept at a minimum. Retrievable small impaled objects such as thorns and splinters, especially in the hands and feet, may be removed to decrease the patient's pain. Common sense should rule in these instances. As a general rule, impaled objects that obstruct the airway should be removed. This would include the throat or cheek. If the airway is clear, the EMT may still remove an impaled object from the cheek with relative safety.

## Accidental or Mechanical Tattoo

Tattooing injuries may occur along with soft tissue injuries when foreign material (grease, dirt, asphalt, and gunpowder) is ground into the skin layers and subcutaneous tissue. This commonly occurs to victims of motorcycle or skateboard accidents when the patient slides along the pavement or ground. Since this injury accompanies abrasions, the EMT should treat it as if it were the same thing. The EMT should remove large pieces of foreign material that are easily retrievable, but definitive removal of small pieces of ground-in substance is a hospital surgical procedure, performed under local or general anesthesia (an″es-the′ze-ah).

## Amputations

There may be times when you will have to manage traumatic amputation in the field. As grotesque as this may seem, your swift medical response to priorities is mandatory. Pressure dressings or antishock trousers will stop lower extremity bleeding in almost all cases. Very rarely will a tourniquet be indicated. Remember to retrieve all amputated parts and put them in a plastic bag and keep them on ice or a chemical cold pack to bring with the patient to the emergency department.

## Clamping Injuries

Children are commonly the victims of clamping or pinching injuries. These are situations in which fingers, toes, arms, legs, and head are caught between solid objects. Frequent causes are getting fingers caught in toys and poking one's head through iron railings and getting stuck. The distal part of the trapped limb swells rapidly, causing the inability to gain freedom. The EMT should apply petroleum jelly or green soap to the trapped body part and try to remove the object. If the finger or hand is caught in a small object, elevate the arm above the head to reduce swelling and transport the patient in this manner until arrival at the emergency department. Degloving injuries are possible with clamping injuries and should be guarded against. These situations are very frightening to small children and calm assurance in dealing with them is necessary. If possible, transport the child's father or mother with him.

## Harvesting Injuries

Serious agricultural injuries are usually from harvesting machinery. In the midwestern United States—"the corn belt"—extensive soft and hard tissue injuries from corn pickers and other machinery are serious and many end in amputation. Injuries are usually sustained to the extremities which cause crushing, tearing, and avulsing of soft tissues with associated multiple open or closed fractures. Farm equipment extrication knowledge is a must for those EMTs working in areas where these injuries are likely to occur. Because of the intricacy of such equipment, it would be wise for these EMTs to acquaint themselves with such equipment by taking a course in farm equipment extrication.

## Washing Machine Wringer Injuries

Injuries of this kind occur some 200,000 times each year. Body areas commonly affected are the dorsum of the hand, wrist, and forearm. Wounds produced by these accidents include a variety of forces due to compression, contusion, heat from friction, and avulsions. Information that the EMT should gather about the accident includes:

1. Age of the machine
2. Condition of the wringer
3. Extent to which the extremity entered the wringer
4. Duration of exposure
5. Measures taken to extricate the trapped extremity

The EMT should treat injuries as he would any other type of soft or hard tissue accident. He should stop the bleeding, dress wounds, immobilize fractures, and check neurovascular status. All avulsed tissue should be brought to the emergency department with the patient.

### Straddle Injuries

These injuries occur when trauma is sustained to the area of the perineum. This commonly occurs to young boys or girls who fall on the cross bar of boys bicycles or fall on objects with the legs spread apart. Contusion, hematoma, ischial fractures, and urethral tears are the more common kinds of injury. The EMT should examine the injured area for bleeding or impaled objects. The patient should be stabilized by placing him in a semisitting position to neutralize muscle pull on the possibly fractured ischium.

### High-Pressure Injection Injuries

These injuries usually occur from paint guns, grease guns, and other high-pressure hydraulic equipment. The wound produced by this type of injury is either puncturing or lacerating in nature. The injury is most often incurred to the hands, legs, or feet. The injured extremity swells rapidly from edema, and there is usually extensive tissue destruction caused from the foreign material injected under high pressure traveling along fascial planes of the body. It is difficult to estimate how much of the product has been injected; we usually underestimate. Bleeding is usually minimal. The EMT should cover the wound in dry bulky dressing and bandage the injured area in the position of function prior to transport to the hospital.

## WOUND CARE—THE DRESSING AND BANDAGE

Any material used for the purpose of covering a wound is called a *dressing*. The initial pad of material placed on the wound is called a *compress*. Dressings should be sterile if possible. A bandage is used to hold or secure the dressing in place. Bandages need not be sterile because they usually are not applied directly to open wounds. (see Fig. 14–11.)

### Dressings

Dressings have several purposes. They help control bleeding, stabilize objects, protect wounds, and prevent further contamination.

All first aid units and kits should carry assorted sizes of sterile dressings. Even though the field treatment of open wounds does not lend itself to contamination control, EMTs can minimize the chance of further contamination of open wounds by aseptically tending to wound care by the

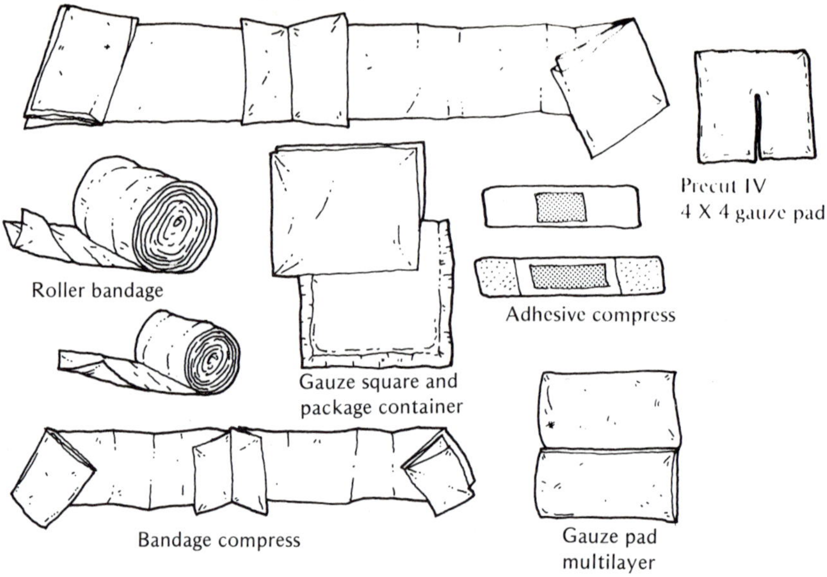


**Figure 14–11.** Types of dressings and bandage supplies.

proper use of sterile dressing material. Sterile dressings are commercially available in a variety of sizes and materials designed for just about all types of soft tissue injuries. Sterile prepacked 4 × 4s and 5 × 9s are probably used more often in the field than any other type of dressing for small wound care. The sterile prepackaged 9 × 36 trauma or universal dressing is used effectively for larger wounds encountered in multiple trauma. Other dressing materials that should be considered as part of the supply list include sanitary napkins, assorted sizes of Band-Aids®, eye patches, aluminum foil, petroleum-impregnated gauze pads and precut IV 4 × 4 gauze pads.

Even though a fairly large quantity of different size dressings will be available to the EMT, situations will arise in which sterile supplies will be exhausted. This will be common in multiple patient injuries as encountered in vehicular accidents, explosions, and mass transit accidents. In these situations, any material may be substituted for a dressing to cover wounds and control bleeding. Clean handkerchiefs, towels, wash cloths, sheets, pillow cases, and bandaging material can be utilized to cover wounds. Even your hand can be utilized if bleeding is severe.

### *Preparation*

All wounds should be exposed so that you may properly attend to the injury. Clothing should be cut or torn widely enough around the injury so that it does not interfere with your procedures. As with all responses to an emergency, all necessary supplies should be at hand when you are at the patient's side. Trips back to the emergency unit should not have to take place unless there are multiple patient injuries. Your kit should contain enough dressing materials for at least two patients. All dressing material should hold its form when wet or blood soaked. The use of tissue or cotton is not indicated in wound care since these fibers will come apart and adhere to the wound. The attending physicians will then have to clean and debride this material, making their job more difficult. Sterile dressings should be touched only at the corners and not on the site where they will make direct contact on the wound.

### *Bleeding Control—Pressure Dressing*

Any type of dressing material can be used as a pressure dressing to control hemorrhage. Sterile dressings are preferable. As stated earlier, sterile prepackaged 4 × 4 and 5 × 9 gauze pads are used more often for this purpose than any other type of dressing for small wounds. The 9 × 36 sterile prepackaged trauma or universal dressing is more convenient for larger wounds. If once applied, blood soaks through the dressing, do not take it off and inspect the injury. This may induce more bleeding. Inspection should have taken place at the onset of treatment. Reapply another dressing to the already blood-soaked one and add more pressure either by your hand or bandaging material. Elevate the limb if necessary to help control bleeding.

### *Impaled Objects—Stabilizing Dressings*

Bleeding control and stabilization of impaled objects can be very challenging, depending on the object impaled. Usually such a wound will not produce great hemorrhage. Seepage of blood from around the object will be more the rule than the exception. It is the stabilization of the object that will be important in these cases, for if the object is disturbed harshly, extensive bleeding could be a greater factor. For bleeding control and stabilization the commercially available sterile precut IV 4 × 4 gauze pads are ideal. Small impaled objects such as pocket knives, ice picks, pencils, and the like are readily stabilized by guiding the slit of the 4 × 4 around the object and stacking additional pads as needed to secure the object. Adhesive tape or other types of bandage material can then be placed over the 4 × 4s to hold them in place.

Larger impaled objects can be stabilized by cutting a hole in the middle of the trauma dressings, conforming to the diameter of the object and again stacking the dressings on one another to secure the object. Minimal movement of the object should take place during the procedure. This will decrease the chance of active bleeding. (See Fig. 14–12.)

### *Chest and Neck Wounds—Occlusive Dressings*

Occlusive dressings are those that seal open wounds hermetically. Wounds of special importance are sucking chest wounds and neck wounds

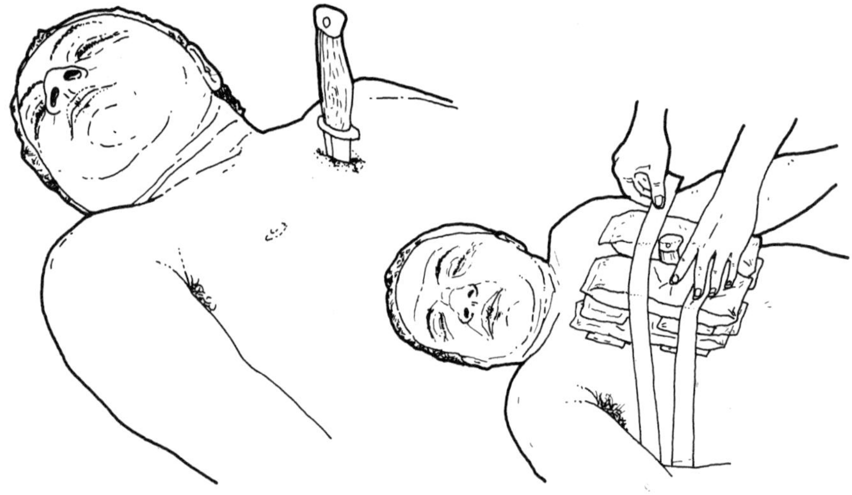

**Figure 14–12.** Impaled objects should not be removed, but should be stabilized before transportation to the hospital.

that sever jugular veins. The best type of dressing for both injuries is the sterile prepackaged petroleum-impregnated gauze pad. This dressing readily adheres to dry skin and helps seal the dressing. A bandage should be placed over the dressing, however, to insure its position and air-tight seal. Neck wounds, for obvious reasons of airway patency and circulation, should not be bandaged tightly. However, the EMT must ensure an air-tight seal to protect the patient against an air embolism as well as to control hemorrhage.

*Eviscerations—Protective Moistened Dressings*

With eviscerations (e-vis″er-a′shunz), or exposed abdominal organs, particular dressing care is required. This type of wound is best treated by applying a sterile trauma dressing moistened with sterile water or saline over the exposed organs. No attempt should be made to push the organs back into the wound. To conserve heat a strip of aluminim foil may be placed over the moistened dressing. The dressing and foil can be fixed by adhesive tape or other bandaging material. The securing bandage should only be on the sides of the dressing, not in contact with the organs. Remember that the sterile moistened dressing should be loosely laid over the exposed organs and that bandaging material should not be wrapped tightly over the exposed organs. (see Fig. 14–13.)

## Bandages

Bandages can be improvised to serve several purposes. They can:

1. Hold dressings, splints, and impaled objects in place

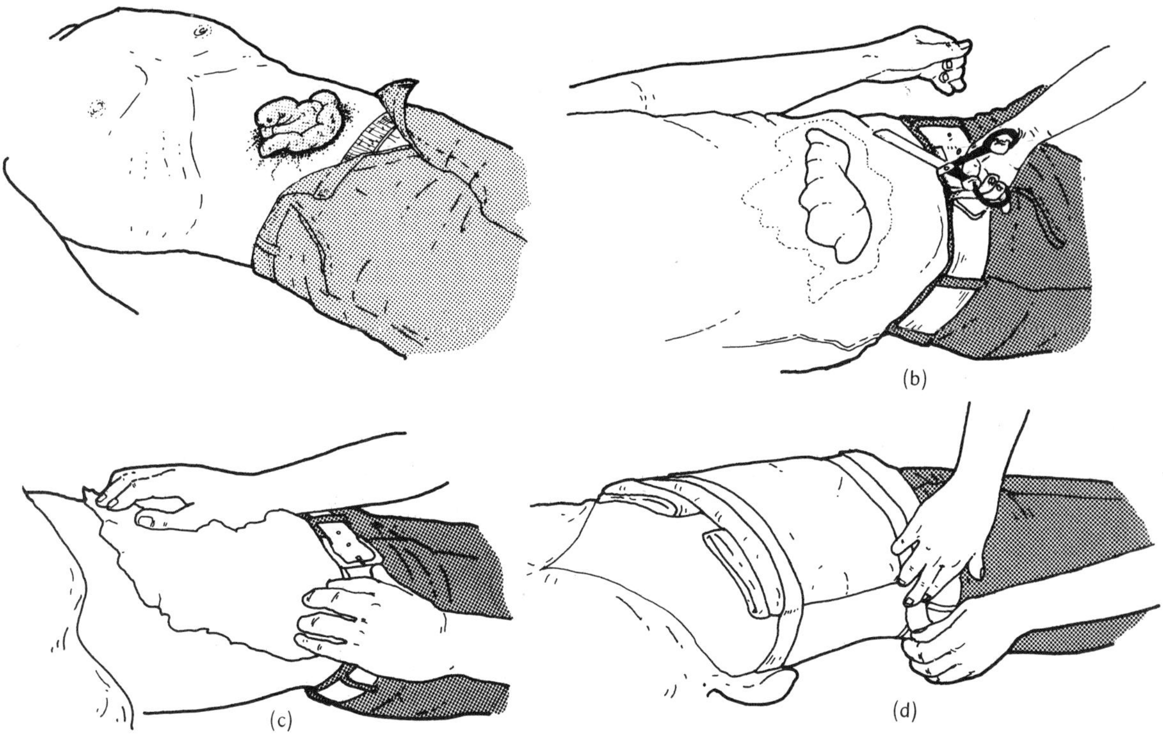


**Figure 14–13.** (a) An evisceration. (b) The EMT-A should cut away all clothing from around the wound, covering the exposed organs with a moistened sterile dressing. (c) Body heat should be conserved by covering the dressing with aluminum foil and (d) a lightly wrapped bandage should stabilize the dressing in place.

2. Prevent further wound contamination
3. Support and protect injured body parts
4. Help control hemorrhage by applying circumferential pressure
5. Aid in the comfort of the patient

In the field, the triangular and roller bandage and adhesive tape are used more often than any other items to hold and secure dressings in place.

*Triangular Bandage*

The top of the triangular bandage is called the *apex*, the bottom is called the *base* and each end of the base is called the *ends*.

With fracture and dislocations of the upper extremity it is primarily used as a sling. With open wounds, the bandage is made into a cravat to secure dressings and control hemorrhage. The cravat is made by simply

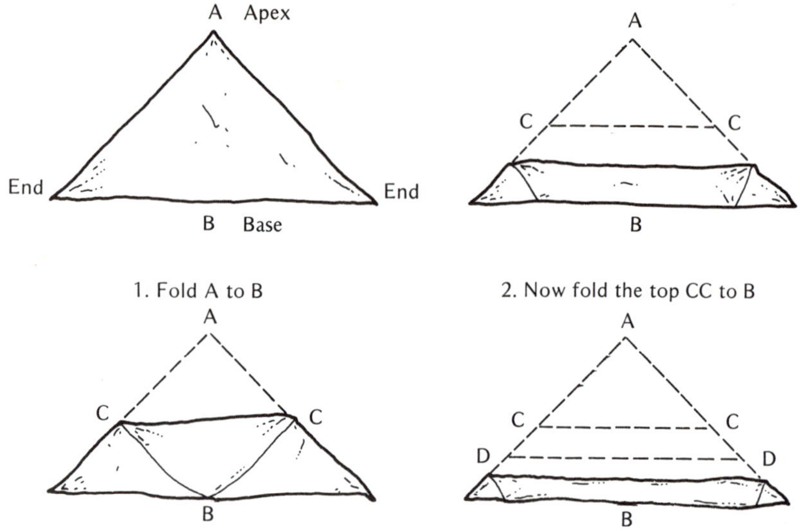


**Figure 14–14.** A cravat made from a triangular bandage.

folding the apex upon itself down toward the base of the bandage until the desired width is satisfied. (See Fig. 14–14.)

*Rolled Gauze Bandage*

The rolled gauze bandage is used in the field more often than the triangular bandage to secure dressings. As the name implies, this bandage is wound in a cylindrical shape. Rolled gauze bandages come in gauze and muslin materials, sterilized and nonsterilized, packaged and nonpackaged. It is convenient for prehospital purposes to have them sterile and prepackaged, but non-sterile bandages can be placed in a small paper bag and sterilized at the hospital. This is usually a less expensive process.

*Application:* Take the roll in the hand you favor, letting the end of the roll hang loose on the bottom. The innermost surface is then applied to the injured area and secured there by the other hand. Pass the roll around the injured part, adjusting the tension and pressure. After winding the bandage two or three times around the injured part, the bandage should be anchored. (See Fig. 14–15.) It may be necessary when winding the bandage around the injury to switch the roll from one hand to the other. The EMT should make certain that the roller bandage is:

1. Snug but not too tight. Too much pressure will impair circulation.

2. Encircling all the desired skin area. Bulging skin folds between

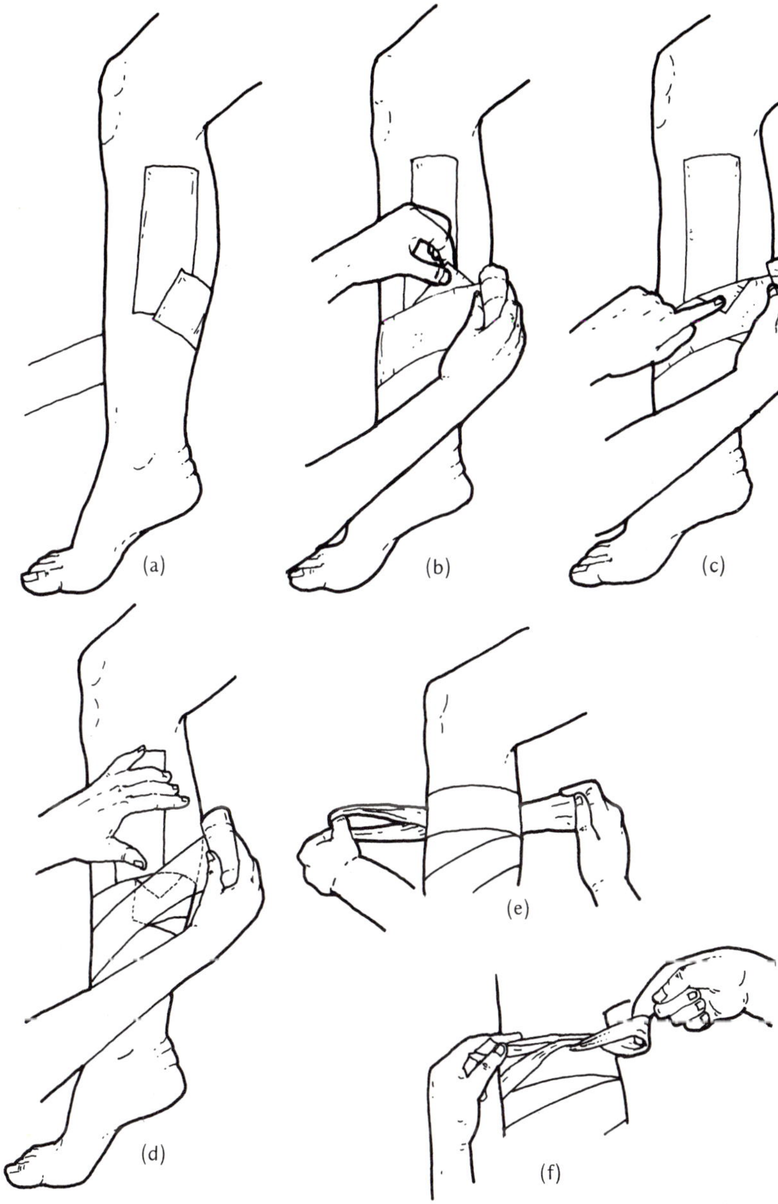


**Figure 14–15.** (a) The EMT-A anchors a bandage by first selecting a starting point, (b) allowing a corner of the bandage to protrude, then encircling the part. (c) Once encircled, the protruding corner is turned down and (d) the part is again encircled, covering the protruding end, and thereby stabilizing the bandage. (e) The bandage is secured by cutting the end, making two separate but attached pieces of material, and (f) tying a square knot.

bandage wraps may pinch the skin, causing additional irritation to the patient.

*Securing the Bandage*

Once the bandage is in place it can be secured by applying adhesive tape or safety pins. At the desired end of the roller bandage, the EMT may elect to cut the middle of the bandage several inches developing two separate but attached material pieces. These cut ends can then encircle the bandage once again and be tied off in a square knot to secure the bandage.

*Adhesive Tape:* Tape is used more often than both the triangular or rolled gauze bandage in the field to secure dressings. The reason for this is that adhesive tape is quick and simple to apply. The EMT should carry one roll each of one-half inch, one-inch, two-inch, and three-inch tape.

Some patients are allergic to cloth tape, so a roll of hypoallergic tape should be carried in the first aid kit. It is also sometimes very difficult to secure a dressing with adhesive tape, especially if the patient is diaphoretic, has blood around the injured site, or is wet for whatever reason. In these cases the EMT should try and wipe the area dry with a sterile pad and apply the adhesive tape, although at times even this fails. In these cases you may want to spray a solution called benzoin (ben′zoin) around but not on the wound. This solution promotes adhesiveness, and tape will usually stick immediately.

## GENERAL CONSIDERATIONS IN APPLYING DRESSINGS AND BANDAGES

1. The injured area must be exposed for inspection.

2. Sterile dressings and other materials should only be touched at their corners and not the surface area to be applied directly on the wound.

3. Circulatory status should be monitored after bandaging. Too tight a bandage will impair circulation. If a pulse cannot be felt, loosen the bandage. If after the bandage is loosened and a pulse is still absent, the artery may be severed.

4. In the field, once a dressing has been applied to a bleeding wound, it should not be removed. If blood soaks completely through the dressing or bandage, reapply another dressing or bandage on top of the blood-soaked one, and apply more pressure to the wound area to control bleeding. Elevate the limb if necessary.

5. Toes and fingers should be left visible if possible to monitor adequacy of circulation and nerve status.

6. The patient should be questioned as to allergies. Some patients have reactions to adhesive tape and or benzoin solutions.

The EMT will find many innovative ways to apply dressings and bandages to certain injuries. In the field you will not always have time to do a perfect job. However, the dressing or bandage should accomplish its intended purpose. With practice, the EMT should be able to dress and bandage every type of open wound neatly. As a professional, the job you do is a reflection on your ability to treat patients appropriately.

*References*

American Academy of Orthopedic Surgeons, Committee on Allied Health. *Emergency Care of the Sick and Injured,* 2nd ed. Chicago, IL: American Academy of Orthopedic Surgeons, 1977.

Barber, Janet M., and Budassi, S. A. *Manual of Emergency Care.* St. Louis, MO: The C. V. Mosby Company, 1979.

Cardany, C. R.; Rodeheaver, G. *et. al.* "The Crush Injury: A High Risk Wound," *JACEP,* Vol. 5, December 1976.

Entin, M. A. "Roller and Wringer Injuries: Clinical and Experimental Studies," *Plastic Reconstructive Surgery,* 15:290, 1955.

Erven, Lawrence W. *Handbook of Emergency Care and Rescue.* Beverly Hills, CA: Glencoe Press, 1978.

Flatt, A. E. *The Care of Minor Hand Injuries.* St. Louis, MO: The C. V. Mosby Company, 1976.

Grant, H. D., and Murray, R. H., Jr. *Emergency Care,* 2nd ed. Bowie, MD: Robert J. Brady Company, 1978.

Henderson, J. *Emergency Medical Guide.* St. Louis, MO: McGraw-Hill Book Company, 1977.

Leidelmeyer, R. "Soft Tissue Injuries by Foreign Bodies," *Emergency Product News.*

Press, E. "Wringer Washing Machine Injuries," *American Journal of Public Health,* 54:812, 1964.

# Chapter 15

# Head, Neck, and Spinal Cord Injuries

Acute injuries to the head, neck, and spinal cord pose an important responsibility for the EMT. The initial management and protection of the patient after trauma is a large determinant of the patient's eventual recovery. In this chapter, essential information regarding assessment of neurological injuries will be presented along with field management appropriate to EMT functioning.

## REVIEW OF ANATOMY AND PHYSIOLOGY OF THE CENTRAL NERVOUS SYSTEM

The central nervous system comprises the brain and the spinal cord. Although the skull bones and vertebral column provide some protection, the delicate structures are also bathed in shock-absorbing fluid called cerebrospinal fluid (CSF).

The central nervous system has three levels of operation: (1) the higher brain, where memory and reaction patterns reside; (2) the lower brain, which controls subconscious processes and vital organ activity; and (3) the spinal cord, which governs automatic motor responses and reflexes. The three levels are interrelated, and disturbances in one area of functioning affects the other two.

### Brain

The brain can be described according to three distinct sections: (1) cerebrum, (2) cerebellum, and (3) brain stem.

The *cerebrum* is the largest and most conspicuous portion of the brain, and is divided into two hemispheres. The outer gray covering of this structure is called the *cerebral cortex.* There are five lobes in each hemisphere: frontal, parietal, temporal, occipital, and insula. (The insula is not visible on the brain's surface.)

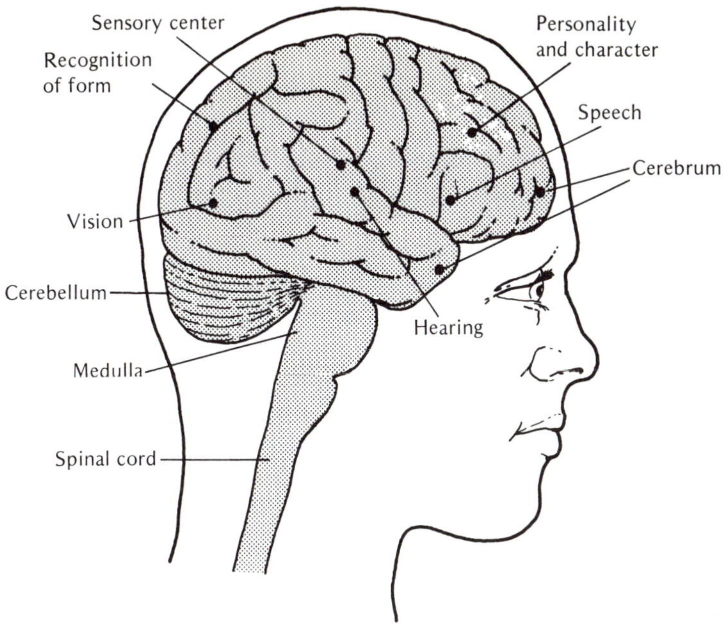


**Figure 15-1.** Major areas of brain indicating function.

There are distinct functions located in various regions of the cerebral cortex. (See Fig. 15-1.) The motor areas and the centers for vision, speech, hearing, and smell are well defined. The cerebrum is also fundamental in conditioned responses of human beings. The thalamus and hypothalamus (regulatory centers) are also located in the upper brain.

The *cerebellum* lies posteriorly in the cranium and is covered by a tent-like structure called the *tentorium.* This "roof" separates it from the back portion of the cerebrum. Activities of the cerebellum are largely "unconscious." Included are refinement and coordination of muscular movements, changes in tone and strength of extremities, and maintenance of posture and equilibrium.

The *brain stem* comprises the midbrain, pons, and medulla. The midbrain is a short part of the brain stem that lies just above the pons. These structures are important links to the spinal cord and serve as conducting pathways for nerve fibers that relay impulses to and from the cerebrum. The medulla is the vital center of the brain; it controls cardiac and respiratory function and governs vascular tone throughout the body.

A series of twelve pairs of cranial nerves exist. These are attached to the brain and supply structures in the head, neck, and abdomen. Cranial Nerve III (the oculomotor nerve) plays an important role in the EMT's assessment of pupillary responses, since it controls dilation and constriction of the pupil.

## ASSESSING HEAD, NECK, AND SPINAL CORD INJURIES

All trauma victims and patients rendered unconscious as a result of an accident should be considered to have acute neurological injury until proven otherwise. Airway management and stabilization of the neck and vertebral column should reflect concern for head and spinal cord trauma.

### Airway

The airway of a patient with suspected cervical spine injury must be managed without hyperextension. The jaw thrust and chin lift maneuvers are the recommended means of establishing an airway. The use of oropharyngeal and esophageal obturator airways and bag-valve-mask ventilation are often indicated.

Careful maintenance of the airway is crucial, since any oxygen deprivation contributes to brain swelling, or "cerebral edema." The brain stores only a ten-second supply of oxygen. Any injury that allows plasma to escape into tissues around blood vessels or one that causes venous congestion will cause an acceleration of blood flow, thus aggravating swelling. An open airway, good ventilation, and administration of oxygen can minimize these adverse circumstances. The individual with central nervous system trauma should be hyperventilated at twenty-four breaths per minute using a bag-valve-mask with supplemental oxygen at 10–12 *l*/min. The threat of vomiting and aspiration is always present post-trauma, and the EMT should be prepared to deal with this complication.

Considerations for airway management in trauma patients should include protection of the cervical spine. The EMT's role in extrication and initial field care can markedly influence the eventual outcome of a serious spinal cord injury. The use of a cervical collar, backboard, and sandbags or cravats is crucial. (See page 285.)

### Circulation

In addition to performing CPR, the EMT may be called upon to cope with hypotension, especially in the event of multiple trauma with chest or abdominal bleeding, or if the spinal cord is severed, creating peripheral vascular collapse.

If shock is apparent with head injury, suspect a cause other than the head for the occurrence. Weakness, restlessness, confusion, dilated pupils, and deterioration in the level of consciousness may be due to shock. (See Chapter 11.) Since these signs and symptoms are also indicative of head injury, the EMT may not be able to identify the underlying reason for their occurrence, but should take steps to minimize their adverse side effects.

Placing the patient in the shock position is indicated for severe hypotension, but Trendelenburg (head-down) positioning is contraindicated in head injury, since it would contribute to brain edema. Antishock trousers may be useful, but only when the patient is hypotensive and hypovolemic. Advanced EMTs are usually instructed to initiate intravenous fluids for resuscitation and for the purpose of delivering emergency drugs if needed.

Vital signs should be measured every ten to fifteen minutes. Bradycardia, hypertension, and hypoventilation suggest brain swelling due to injury. The EMT should be aware of respiratory patterns that are characteristic of various levels of injury to the brain or spinal cord. See Table 15–1.

## Level of Consciousness

The level of consciousness must be assessed early and periodically throughout the EMT's encounter with a trauma patient. The most important question to answer throughout the evaluation is: Is the level of consciousness stable, improving, or deteriorating?

TABLE 15–1. CNS SIGNS ACCORDING TO LEVEL OF DYSFUNCTION.

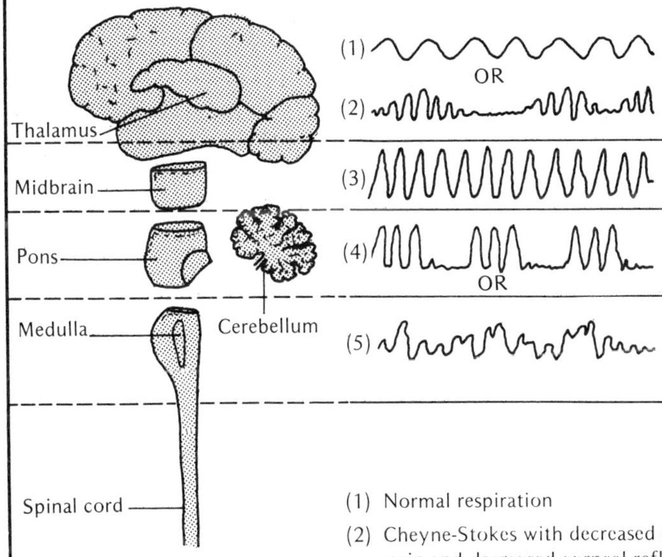


| CNS Level Affected | Respiratory Pattern | LOC | Pupils | Posture |
|---|---|---|---|---|
| Thalamus | (1) OR (2) | Stupor<br>Semi-coma | Small<br>Reactive | Decorticate |
| Midbrain | (3) | Coma | Mid-position<br>Nonreactive | Decerebrate |
| Pons | (4) OR | Coma | Mid-position<br>Nonreactive | Flaccid |
| Medulla | (5) | Coma | Mid-position<br>Nonreactive | Flaccid |
| Spinal cord | | | | |

(1) Normal respiration

(2) Cheyne-Stokes with decreased response to pain and decreased corneal reflexes

(3) Neurogenic hyperventilation; not responsive to $O_2$ and "patterned"

(4) Biot's respiration with regular periods of hyperventilation and irregular periods of apnea

(5) "Apneistic" respiration with ataxic, gasping, shallow pattern

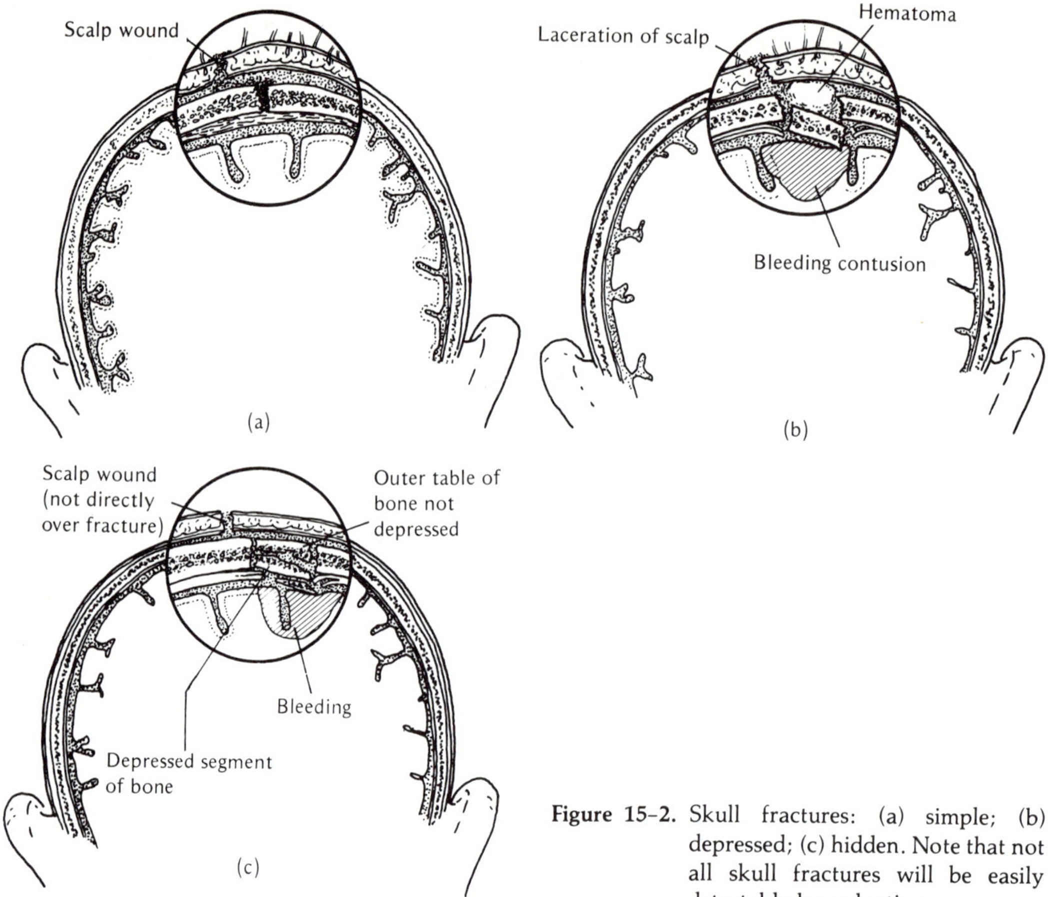


**Figure 15–2.** Skull fractures: (a) simple; (b) depressed; (c) hidden. Note that not all skull fractures will be easily detectable by palpation.

Be sure to note any evidence of drug or alcohol ingestion or other injuries that could influence neurological findings. Note rhinorrhea (ri″no-re′ah) (CSF fluid leaking from the nose), otorrhea (o″to-re′ah) (CSF fluid draining from the ear), or other clues of CSF fluid leakage such as the patient complaining of a "salty" taste in his mouth. If there is leakage of CSF from either the nose or ear, do not restrict its free flow, since "damming it up" could cause intracranial pressure to rise or allow infection to be introduced by a "wick" effect. Remember, the fluid bath of the brain is in direct communication with the outside. If the patient requires suctioning, do not suction the nose if there is any evidence of CSF leakage!. Since suctioning forces contribute to a rise in intracranial pressure, it should be done only as absolutely necessary to facilitate breathing.

The EMT should carefully search for scalp wounds or evidence of skull fractures. (See Fig. 15–2.) Any impaled object or foreign body should be left in place and covered with a sterile dressing. Lacerations of the scalp

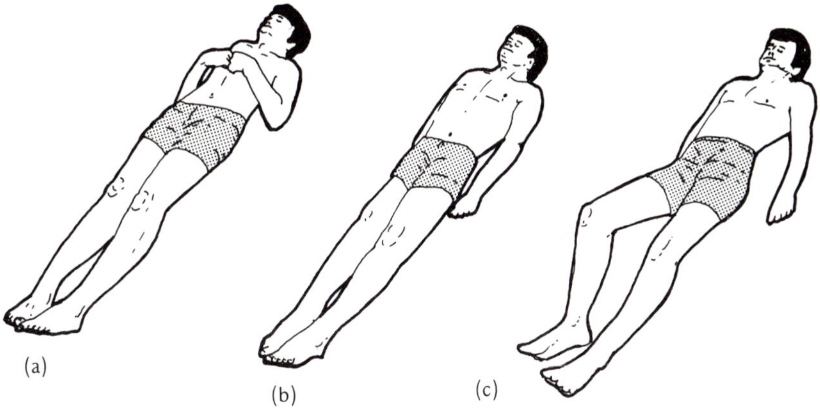

**Figure 15-3.** Abnormal posturing in CNS injury: (a) decorticate; (b) decerebrate; (c) flaccid.

tend to bleed profusely and should be managed by the application of direct pressure. Failure to control the bleeding can result in shock. Since some lacerations are not easy to detect, search the scalp carefully, parting the hair to facilitate inspection. Palpate (feel) the skull and note any indentations or obvious fractures. Do not put any pressure on unstable skull bone or brain tissue if a fracture is evident, since brain tissue and its surrounding blood vessels could be injured further. Any open fracture should be loosely covered with a sterile dressing. Look for bluish discoloration behind the ears ("Battle's sign") or under the eyes ("raccoon's eyes"). In certain skull fractures, blood leaks into tissue spaces in these regions, creating a bruised appearance.

As the motor assessments continue, both sides should be tested and compared. Abnormal posturing should be noted, and the EMT ought to determine whether or not such posturing is exaggerated by stimulation. (See Fig. 15-3.)

Seizure activity is not uncommon in severe head injury. Seizure precautions and care should be according to the guidelines outlined on pages 520–521.

## SPECIFIC TYPES OF BRAIN INJURY

### Contusion

A contusion (kon-tu'zhun) is a local brain injury characterized by bruising, hemorrhage, and edema. In response to a direct blow, or indirectly from mechanical forces, the brain can be set in motion. Since the brain is surrounded by bony irregularities, sudden jarring will cause it to rake

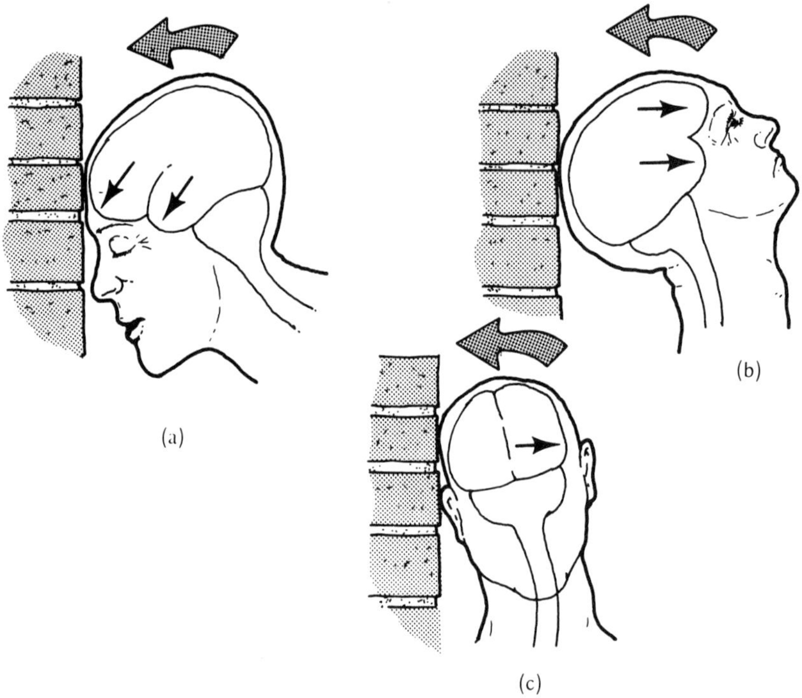


**Figure 15–4.** The type and direction of physical force determines the resultant injuries. Note that the bleeding may occur on the side opposite impact. (See b and c)

against these rough bone projections. Blood vessels and other tissues are thus damaged and bruising of the brain occurs as a result. (See Fig. 15–4.)

Signs and symptoms of a cerebral contusion will depend upon the area of the brain that is affected by the bruising.

## Concussion

A concussion (kon-kush′un) is a transient episode of unconsciousness, e.g., "being knocked out." The unconsciousness is due to a temporary interruption of neural transmissions to the center of consciousness (the reticular [rĕ-tik′u-lar] activating system, or RAS). This is thought to occur when the brain is set in motion, twisting the brain stem, and interrupting the flow of messages to the RAS. Immediate unconsciousness after head injury is always due to concussion, since blood could not collect within the head so promptly to effect unconsciousness. It is identified by history only, since there are no specific neurologic findings. The victim will report a period of amnesia varying from a few seconds to several minutes. Generally, longer periods of unconsciousness represent the more serious injuries. The EMT should always determine what the individual remembers just prior to the accident, and the first thing recalled after the accident, so the extent of transient unconsciousness can be properly estimated. Concussions themselves are not serious. Headache, dizziness, and fatigue may occur afterwards, but otherwise, recovery is complete.

## Cerebral Hemorrhage and Hematoma

A patient who has a concussion or a contusion remains stable or improves. However, a cerebral hemorrhage that involves the actual rupture of blood vessels can be life threatening. Injury to large vessels, especially arteries, can cause severe bleeding. As blood collects it can displace brain tissue and elevate intracranial pressure, thus affecting the level of consciousness. Deterioration of the level of consciousness will progress more rapidly, of course, if the hemorrhage is arterial and not contained within a confined section of the cranial vault.

If the brainstem is involved, the reticular activating system RAS will be dysfunctional and there may be coma, dyspnea, decerebrate posturing, and other abnormal neurological findings.

Occasionally when arterial injury occurs, there may be a rapidly developing hemorrhagic condition that is life threatening due to compression of brain tissue. This injury should be expected if there is a loss of consciousness followed by an interval of consciousness, and then later, a deterioration of the level of consciousness. This characteristic sequence of coma, consciousness, and deterioration demands prompt attention by medical personnel especially when there is:

1. A spontaneously dilating pupil
2. Slow pulse
3. Rising blood pressure
4. Respiratory difficulty

Rapid transport to a treatment facility is imperative since surgery will be necessary to remove the blood and control the bleeding.

## Subdural Hematoma

A subdural hematoma (hem″ah-to′mah) is caused by bleeding between dura and arachnoid membranes. (See Fig. 15–5.) It is caused by a ruptured blood vessel. Patients who have sustained trauma, who are taking anticoagulants or who have bleeding disorders are the most likely victims. The condition can be acute with rapid deterioration or may occur insidiously over days or weeks. In the slowly developing, chronic subdural hematomas, the EMT may encounter a patient with confusion and a decreasing level of consciousness with no related history of recent injury. At best, there may be a history of a fall or blow to the skull several days or

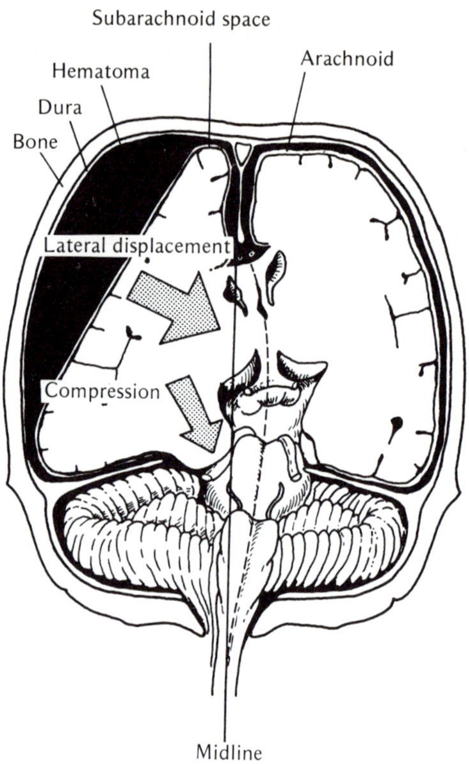


**Figure 15-5.** Subdural hematoma. Note the displacement and compression of brain tissue.

weeks ago. Chronic alcoholics who stumble, fall, and are confused or disoriented are particularly difficult to assess because there is much similarity between a head injury and alcohol-related phenomena. Transportation to a hospital is imperative for these individuals with vague signs and symptoms so that a careful medical examination can be undertaken.

## SPINAL CORD INJURY

The most common mechanism responsible for serious spinal cord injury is a flexion-rotation injury. When the cervical spinal cord is involved, death can ensue from respiratory failure. (See Fig. 15-6.) The EMT should handle all potential cervical spinal cord injuries with extreme caution, and should be skilled in immobilization of the neck for field care and transport.

The most frequent causes of spinal fracture and instability are: automobile and motorcycle crashes, cave-ins, falls from heights, and diving injuries.

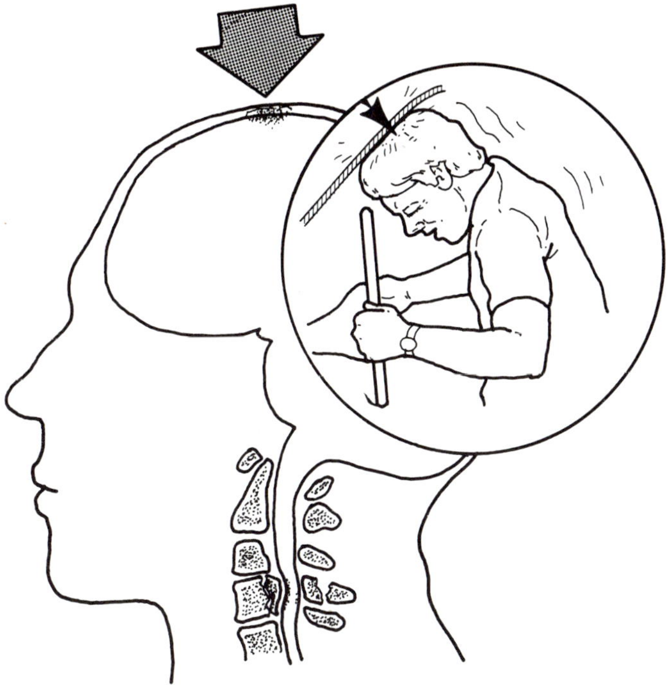

**Figure 15-6.** Head injury may be accompanied by cervical spine injury.

*The absence of neurological deficits should not cause the EMT to rule out fractures. Fractures may be present but may not impinge on the cord until the head and neck are moved.* Therefore, whenever there is a possibility of spinal cord injury, manage the patient as if one were already present! A field examination may identify spinal injury and neurological deficits, but only x-ray can *rule out* cervical spine fractures.

*Signs and Symptoms* Spinal cord injury should be suspected whenever there are any indications of the following:

1. Unusual sensations in the arms or legs, such as numbness or tingling
2. Inability to move arms or legs
3. Unexplained shock, especially with bradycardia
4. Wounds of the head, face, neck, or shoulders
5. Pain, tenderness, deformities, or muscle spasms adjacent to the spinal column
6. Unconsciousness accompanied by
   a. flaccid (flas'sid) muscles
   b. abdominal breathing
   c. priapism [pri'ah-pizm] (erection of the penis)

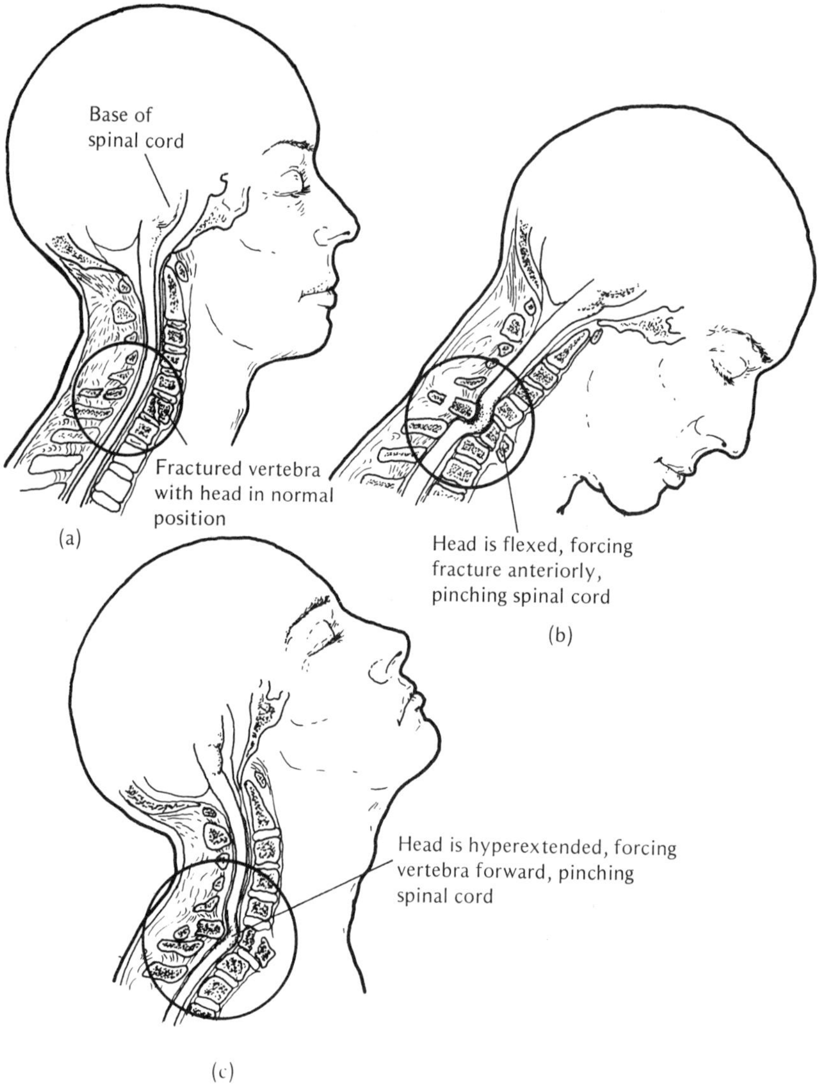


**Figure 15–7.** Examples of cord compression from unstable fracture when head is flexed or hyperextended.

### *Field Management*

*Assess Breathing* The EMT should not hyperextend the neck in an attempt to open the airway. (See Fig. 15–7.) Instead, use the alternate techniques, e.g., jaw thrust or chin lift. Maintain gentle traction, avoiding deviation from the midline. Insert an airway and assist with ventilations as indicated. Note whether or not the respirations are diaphragmatic. In certain higher spinal cord injuries there may be a paralysis of chest wall

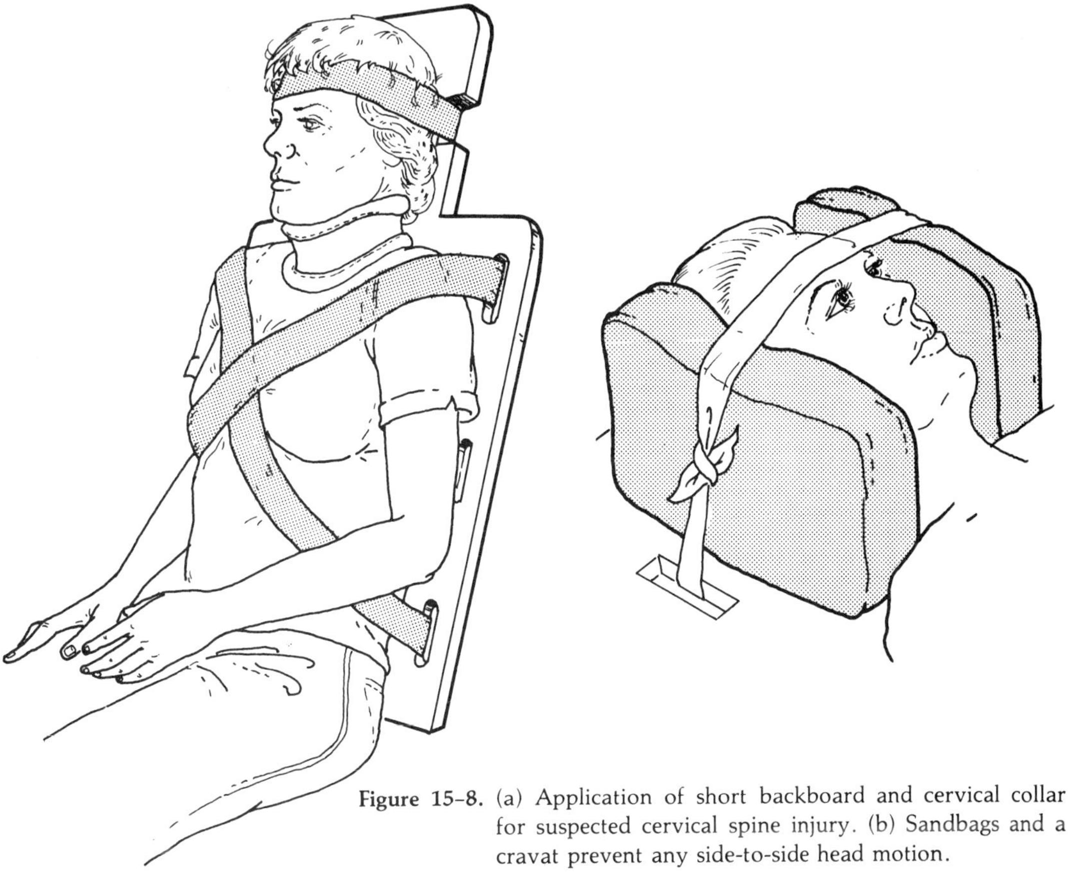

Figure 15-8. (a) Application of short backboard and cervical collar for suspected cervical spine injury. (b) Sandbags and a cravat prevent any side-to-side head motion.

muscles, making all respiratory effort dependent upon the diaphragm. Injury above the fourth cervical vertebra also paralyzes the diaphragm, and assisted ventilation is imperative! Use a bag-valve-mask with oxygen at 10–12 *l*/minute.

Extrication and cervical spine stabilization are important elements in the management of cervical spine injury. The spine should be kept in a neutral position; that is, no flexion, extension, rotation, or lateral deviation during movement of the patient. A short spine board will be required to ensure support and alignment, as the body must be moved as a unit. If the victim is wearing a helmet, do not remove it since it provides protection to the neck, and the manipulation necessary to take if off could result in further injury. Avoid any jarring or "rough handling," since these insults could cause an aggravation of cord hemorrhage and edema or even result in further compression or tearing of the delicate spinal cord tissue. Apply a cervical collar and sandbag to the head as illustrated in Fig. 15-8. (See also Chapter 34.)

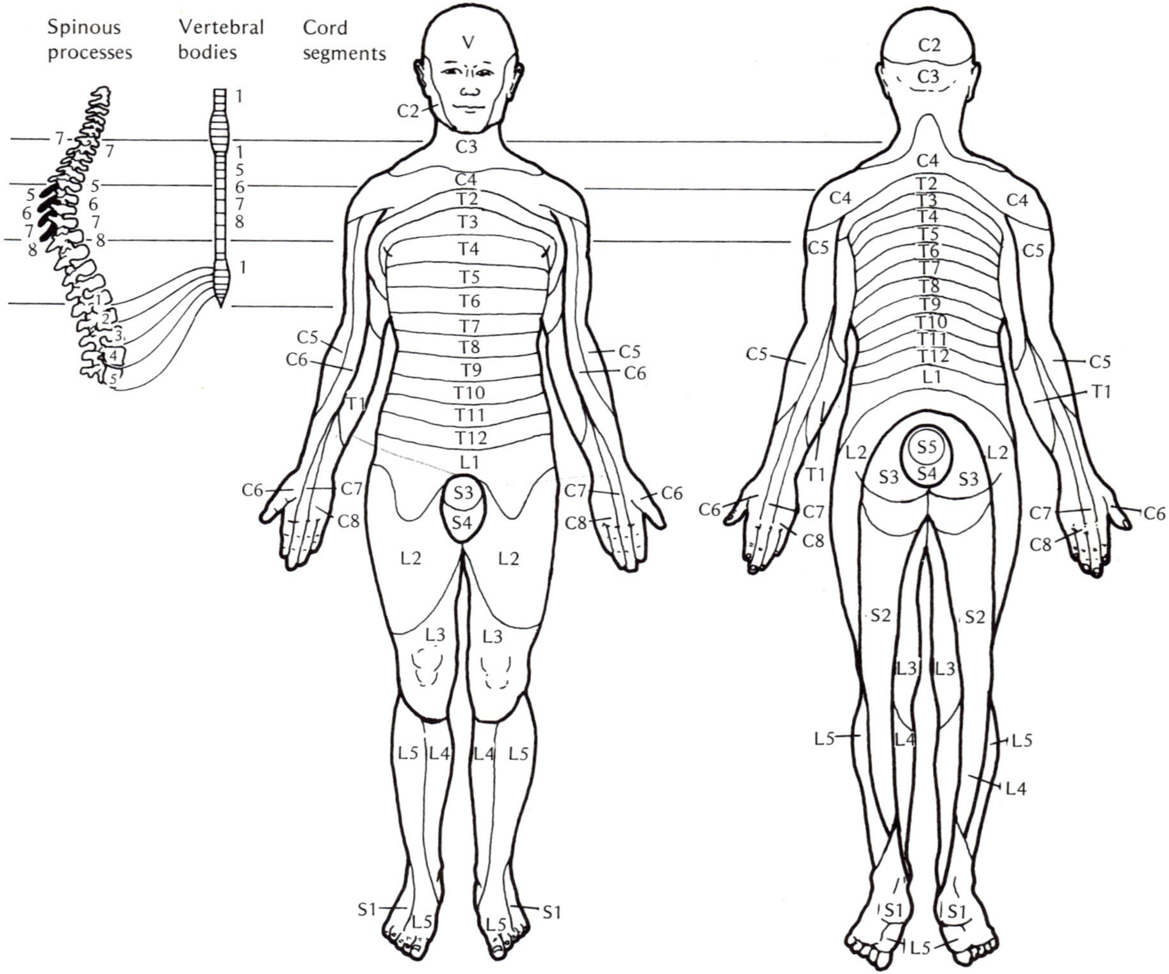


**Figure 15–9.** Body zones affected by various levels of spinal cord functioning. Note that spinal cord segments do not correspond with vertebral bodies that encase them.

## Other Spinal Cord Injuries

The outcome of any spinal cord injury will be largely dependent upon the level of impairment. Most typically, cord injuries affect all functions at or below the level of damage. For example, if the cord is injured in the thoracic region, the arms will be largely unaffected, but the trunk below the shoulders will be impaired. Lumbar spine injuries alter only functions below the waist. The outcome of a permanent transection or injury of the cord is a function of the remaining intact cord segments and the tissues they control. (See Fig. 15–9.)

EMTs should be alert to signals of cord injury at *all* levels of the spine, not just the cervical region! The selection and use of the short or long spine boards and techniques of extrication should take into account all levels of the vertebral column.

## Ruptured Disk

A ruptured disk is a vertebral injury that results from lifting a heavy object or direct injury to the back from a fall or blow. Delicate nerves are compressed and the victim may experience pain radiating down the back of the leg, difficulty in walking, or disorders of sensation. High-cord-level disk injury may affect the neck, causing nuchal rigidity (stiff neck), or the arms, with radiating pain or abnormal sensations.

EMTs should manage a suspected ruptured disk in the same manner as other spinal cord injuries, since less apparent but more serious injury could be present.

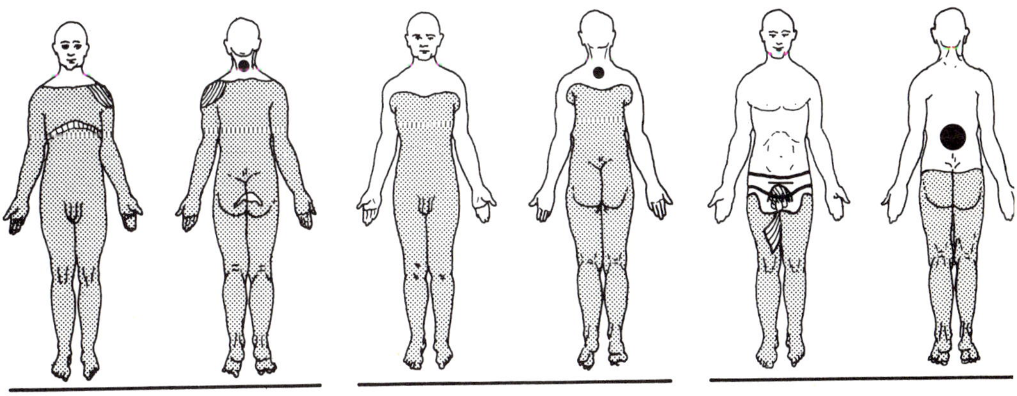

(a) Cervical cord injury (b) Thoracic cord injry (c) Lumbar cord injury

**Figure 15–10.** Approximate area of loss with (a) cervical, (b) thoracic, and (c) lumbar spine injuries. Anterior and posterior views.

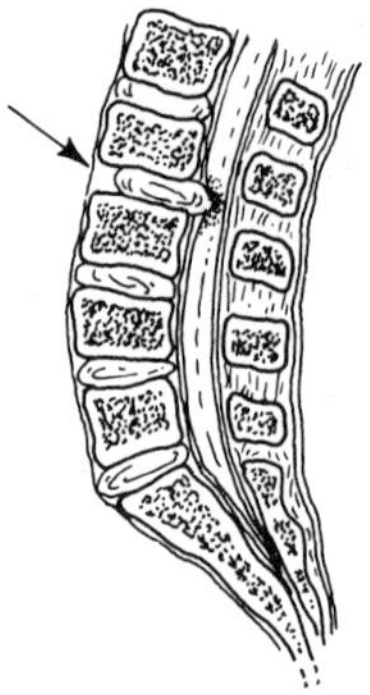

**Figure 15–11.** Ruptured disk. The cord is compressed by herniation of vertebral "cushioning" material called *nucleus pulposus* (pul-paw'sus).

### Whiplash

Violent hyperextension and flexion of the neck can result in a cervical spine injury characterized by weakness, dizziness, disturbances in walking, and other vague symptoms. There is no loss of consciousness, but muscle spasms, radiating pain, and nuchal rigidity may be noted. Rear-end collisions often result in this injury. Field care is the same as for other suspected cervical injuries.

If head rotation occurs in conjunction with the hyperextension and flexion of the neck, concussion and intracranial hemmorhage should be suspected, too.

*Care En Route to Hospital*

Airway and breathing should be monitored constantly during transport. The airway may be suctioned if necessary, but deep suctioning or prolonged aspiration should be avoided, since these stimulate gagging and vomiting as well as create elevations of intracranial pressure. If vomiting requires changing the patient's position, a log-rolling technique is imperative while the head and neck are still well stabilized.

If shock ensues, a Trendelenburg position may be used. This can be accomplished by elevating the long spine board about twelve inches or adjusting the cot if using a short spine board. A standard shock position (see Fig. 15–10) should be used in the event of head injury to avoid aggravating brain swelling. If hypovolemia and hypotension are present, anti-shock trousers may be employed.

## PSYCHOLOGICAL IMPACT OF NEUROLOGICAL INJURIES

Acute head, neck, and spinal cord injuries may result in abrupt and permanent impairment, including paraplegia, hemiplegia, and quadriplegia. The patient may ask the EMT if the apparent neurological deficit (motor or sensory) will be permanent. It is difficult for even medical specialists to predict the eventual outcome of certain injuries in the early post-trauma interval. Therefore, the EMT should reassure the patient that everything possible is being done to protect his brain and spinal cord, and that several days or even weeks may elapse before the eventual recovery can be estimated. In the meantime, gentle and careful movement, and transfer techniques that ensure the stability and alignment of the vertebral column will contribute to the patient's welfare.

## *References*

Ansbaugh, P. "Emergency Management of Intoxicated Patients With Head Injuries," *JEN* 3:9–12, May/June 1977.

Bouzarth, W. F. "Trauma at the Top," *Emergency Medicine, 7:71–84, 1975.*

Celesia, G. "Modern Concepts of Status Epilepticus," *JAMA*, 235:1571–1574, 1976.

Fishman, R. A. "Brain Edema," *New England Journal of Medicine* 293:706–711, 1975.

Guyton, A. C. *Textbook of Medical Physiology*, 5th ed. Philadelphia: W. B. Saunders Co. 1976.

Plum, F., and Posner, J. B. *Diagnosis of Stupor and Coma*, 2nd ed., Contemporary Neurology Series. Philadelphia: F. A. Davis Co., 1972.

Ransohoff, J., and Fleischer, A. "Insult and Injury—Head Injuries," *Emergency Medicine* 8:147–150, April 1976.

Weiss, M. H. "Head Trauma and Spinal Cord Injuries: Diagnostic and Therapeutic Criteria," *Critical Care Medicine* 2:311–316, 1974.

Young, J. F. "How The Brain Recognizes and Responds to Shock," *J. Neurosurg. Nurs.* 8:37–44, July 1976.

Chapter 16

# Eye, Ear, Nose, Throat, and Dental Emergencies

The EMT may encounter injury or acute medical problems related to the eye, ear, nose and throat, or even the teeth. Although these problems are usually not life threatening, prompt and appropriate care by the EMT can often relieve pain and even reduce the possibility of permanent damage to certain structures.

## ANATOMY OF THE EYE

EMTs may be able to prevent the loss of a patient's sight if they have a clear understanding of the eye structures and how to protect them if they are injured.

The human visual apparatus consists of the eyeball, the optic nerve, and the visual center of the brain. In addition, there are accessory structures to protect the eye such as the eyebrows, eyelids, tear (lacrimal [lak′rĭ-mal]) ducts, eyelashes, and the conjunctiva (kon″junk-ti′vah) mucous membrane that lines the eyelids. Six muscles control the movement of the eyeball within its bony cavity referred to as an *orbit*.

The eyeball (globe) itself is comprised of three coats: fibrous (fi′brus), vascular, and nervous tissue. The *sclera* (skle′rah), or white of the eye, forms the majority of fibrous covering of the eye. It helps to maintain the shape of the eye, as well as to protect it. The *cornea* (kor′ne-ah) is the clear fibrous covering for the "window" of the eye, and envelopes the anterior central portion of the eyeball. The vascular coat contains the iris (i′ris), the colored portion of the eye, and a hole called the *pupil* which admits light.

The *retina* (ret′ĭ-nah) is the nervous tissue which receives and transfers light rays to the brain's "sight" center.

There are two humors (fluid refracting substances) that fill the anterior and posterior chambers of the eye. These fluid humors help to maintain the shape of the eye as well as serving as refractors of light. (See Fig. 16–1.)

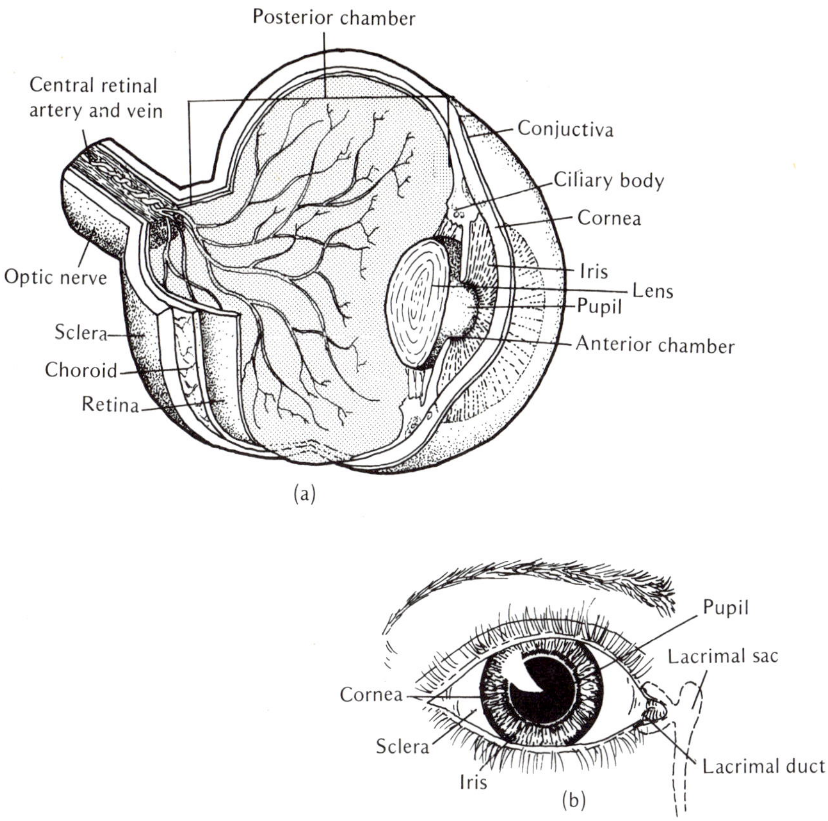


**Figure 16–1.** Anatomy of the eye: (a) cutaway of eye structures; (b) frontal view of eye.

## EYE EMERGENCIES

The *true* emergencies of the eye are: chemical burns, sudden visual loss, and penetrating injuries to the globe (eyeball). Damage to the eye should always be suspected if there is head or facial trauma. Each eye of an injured patient should be systematically inspected. Is the globe intact? Is there fluid leakage or a change in the shape of either eye? Are there visible foreign objects? Are there hemorrhages? lacerations? contusions? Are there any visible or palpable changes in the facial bones of the eye orbit? Are there any visual changes such as loss of visual acuity (ah-ku′ĭ-te) or diplopia (dĭ-plo′pe-ah) (double vision)? Are pupils equal and reactive to light? These represent important questions that can help the EMT to identify injuries, and thus institute prompt, appropriate treatment.

## Chemical Burns

The severity of a chemical burn to the eye is determined by the type and concentration of a chemical, the duration of contact, and whether it is a liquid or powdered substance. As a rule, alkalis are more dangerous than acids since they can rapidly penetrate the anterior chamber. Acids, on the other hand, combine with tissue proteins and cannot penetrate the barrier.

Immediate and copious (ko′pē-us) irrigation of the eye is the initial treatment. Normal saline should be "flooded" continuously over the eye using a contrived irrigation set-up such as noted in Fig. 16–2. A plastic IV of normal saline with administration tubing provides an ideal system.

The patient should be positioned to facilitate irrigation from the inner to the outer corners of the eye. The lids and conjunctiva (kon″junk-ti′vah) should be retracted manually to ensure thorough flushing of "pockets," which could resist the flushing procedure. A receptacle such as a wash or emesis basin is useful to have on board the ambulance to catch the irrigating fluid.

The EMT should reassure the patient as much as possible and explain the importance of the continuous irrigation, since most individuals experience great anxiety as well as pain with such chemical burns.

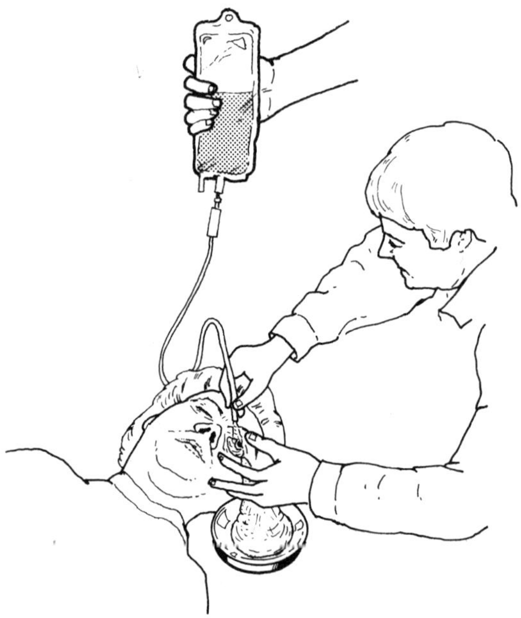

**Figure 16–2.** Emergency eye irrigation. Note the fluid is flowing from the medial aspect of the eye to the lateral aspect. This can be facilitated by turning the patient's head to the side.

## Sudden Visual Loss

Sudden loss of vision in one eye is usually due to interruption of blood supply or hemorrhage, or a detachment of the retina. An ophthalmologist (of″thal-mol′o-jist) must be secured at once if permanent visual loss is to be prevented. The EMT should ensure that the victim is promptly transported to a medical facility for this specialized attention. It is advisable to alert the hospital en route so that the ophthalmologist is at hand when the patient arrives, since even a few minutes could be crucial in the attempt to prevent permanent visual loss in the affected eye.

## Traumatic Injuries

Penetrating injuries to the globe can be caused by a wide variety of foreign objects. When the globe has been penetrated, there is little the EMT can do except to stabilize the impaled object or put a protective shield over both eyes. (Since the injured eye would normally move in response to the uninjured eye's movement, both eyes are patched.) Do not put any pressure on the eye. Notify the hospital at once, so that an ophthalmologist can be summoned, since immediate intervention is imperative. (See Fig. 16–3.)

The patient should be placed on his back for transport.

A patient with patched eyes will be frightened and will need much reassurance from the EMT. Be certain to explain why both eyes are covered to prevent the individual from fearing that he has injury to both eyes!

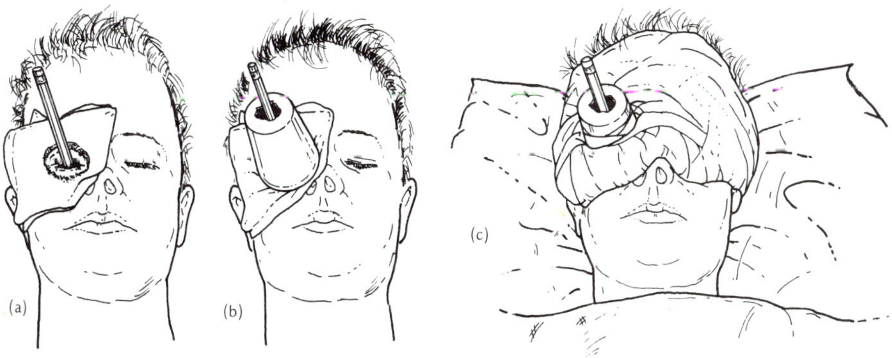


**Figure 16–3.** Management of impaled foreign object in the eye. (a) Create foundation around object with bulky pads. (b) Place plastic cup (or similar device) over object. (Cut out bottom of cup if necessary to allow object to protrude.) (c) Secure apparatus with tape. Note that both eyes are patched to prevent mobilization of affected eye by opposite eye movements.

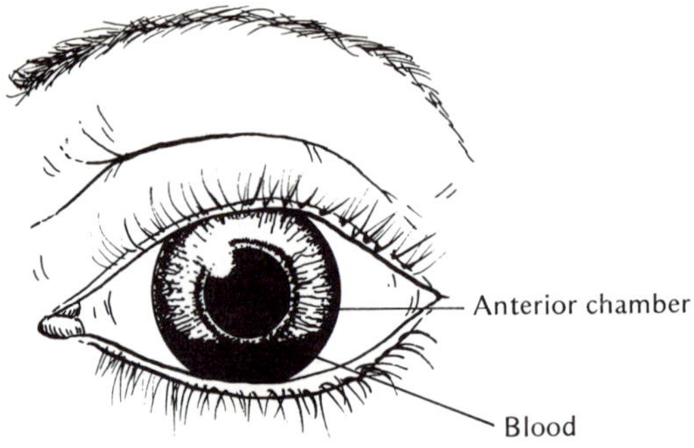


**Figure 16-4.** Hyphema. Note collection of blood in the anterior chamber.

## Blunt Trauma to the Eye

Other eye injuries the EMT should promptly recognize are a *hyphema* (hi-fe'mah) and *blow-out fracture.*

A *hyphema* is a hemorrhage into the anterior chamber of the eye, usually resulting from a missile such as a BB or blunt trauma. (See Fig. 16-4.) There is no field treatment for a hyphema except to patch both of the eyes and transport.

A *blow-out fracture* is a fracture of the floor of the bony eye orbit due to blunt trauma involving large objects, e.g., baseballs, fists. When the eye receives the blow, the intraorbital pressure is increased and the relatively weak lower portion of the orbital wall gives way into the adjacent max-

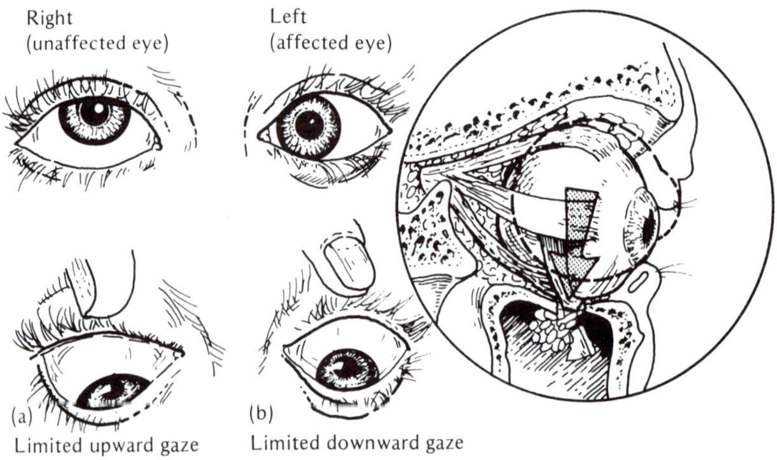


**Figure 16-5.** Blow-out fracture. Fracture of orbital floor creates limited upward and downward gaze of the affected (left) eye. Inset shows anatomical defect characterizing the injury. Dotted line represents normal position of eyeball.

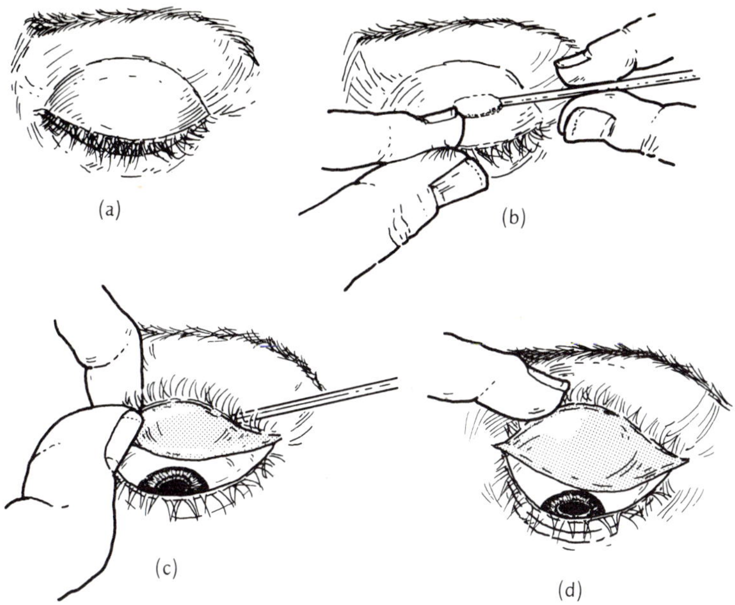


**Figure 16–6.** Steps in everting eyelid. (a) Patient looks downward. (b) Lid pulled down with fingers. (c) Eyelid pulled over rod (applicator stick or wood match, for example). (d) Everted lid facilitates removal of foreign body using *moistened* cotton applicator.

illary sinus cavity. The inferior rectus muscle often becomes entrapped in the fracture site, resulting in restricted eye movement and *diplopia* (double vision). Diplopia is created by dysconjugate eye motion, i.e., eyes do not move together.

The patient with a blow-out fracture should be made comfortable with bilateral eye patches and transported for further medical care. (See Fig. 16–5.)

## Foreign Body Removal

The EMT may occasionally be called upon to remove a small foreign body from an eye. Fig. 16–6 explains this process.

## Soft Tissue Injuries of the Eye

Lacerations and contusions of the eye are not uncommon, as a result of trauma to the face. Bleeding around the eye or eyelids can be controlled with direct pressure as long as no pressure is exerted on the eyeball itself. Pressure to the eyeball can cause permanent loss of vision due to the injury of delicate visual structures. If eyelids are lacerated, they should be gently covered with a loose dressing. Any detached tissue should be preserved in a moist dressing for possible reattachment.

Although rare, an eyeball can "pop out" of the orbit (socket) as a result of high impact injury. The EMT should cover the eye with a paper cup (or similar device) for transport, as with an impaled foreign object. No attempt should be made to replace the eye within the orbit! Cover the uninjured eye with a patch to prevent its movement from affecting the injured eye. Encourage the patient to remain quiet.

## Contact Lenses and Prostheses

One of the early steps in any trauma examination is to check for and remove contact lenses that could create injury to the eye by remaining in place during assessment and early trauma management. Figures 16-7 through 16-9 illustrate the methods for removal of the various types of lenses.

Artificial eyes (prostheses [pros-the'sez] may be left in place without harm.

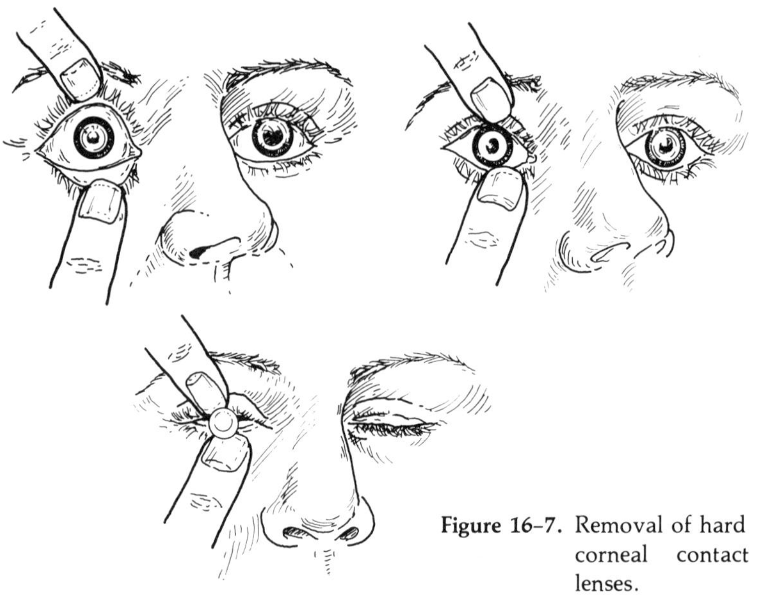

**Figure 16-7.** Removal of hard corneal contact lenses.

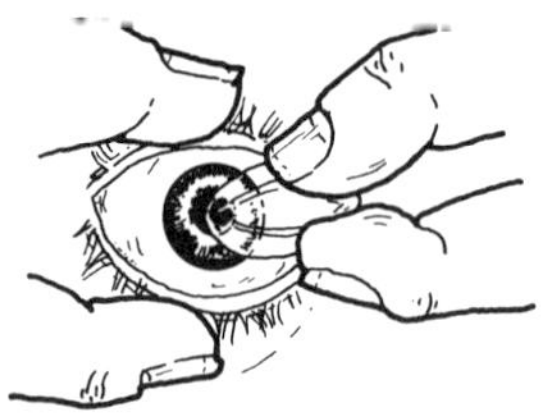

**Figure 16-8.** Soft lens removal.

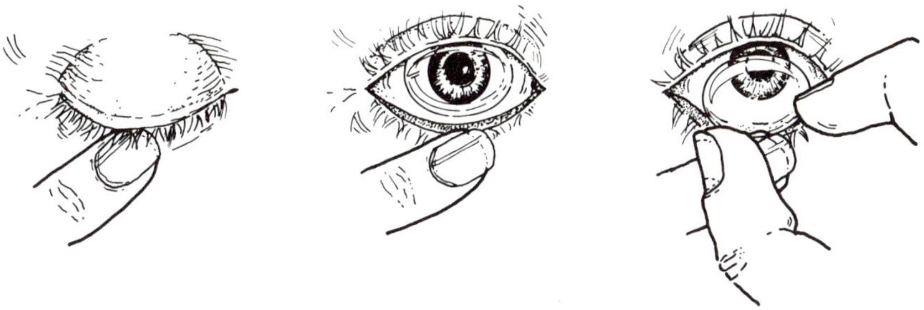

**Figure 16–9** Scleral lens removal.

## EAR EMERGENCIES

The most common ear emergency encountered in the field is partial or complete amputation of the outer ear from trauma. Management consists of placing a moist dressing over the site and preserving any amputated tissue in a moist dressing for reimplantation by a specialized surgical team. (See page 263.)

Blood or fluid draining from the ear (otorrhea [o"to-re'ah] should be considered as it potentially relates to head injury. (See page 278.) It may be due to infection or local trauma to the ear, too, however. Diving injuries, a slap over the ear, or sudden altitude changes can result in the rupture of the eardrum due to sudden pressure changes. The patient will complain of pain, dizziness, ringing in the ear, and possibly hearing impairment.

No field treatment is indicated other than making the patient as comfortable as possible while en route to a hospital.

## NOSE EMERGENCIES

Epistaxis (ep'ĭ-stak'sis) (nosebleed) is the most common nose emergency and can be either a minor problem or a life-threatening emergency since the hemorrhage can be extensive. It is especially hazardous for individuals with bleeding disorders, hypertension (high blood pressure), or for those on anticoagulant (an"tĭ-ko-ag'u-lant) ("blood-thinner") therapy.

If there is a head-injury (i.e., fractured skull, facial fractures) *do not* attempt to apply pressure to stop the nosebleed, since it could block off the free flow of CSF, and thus elevate intracranial pressure. (See page 278.) For nosebleeds of other causation, apply pressure by pinching off the nostrils. Pressure should be applied for at least 10 minutes in order to stop normal bleeding. Encourage the patient not to blow his nose. A gauze square placed between the upper lip and the gum, or the application of ice, may slow down some bleeding.

The patient should be permitted to sit up to avoid accidental aspiration of blood. Provide a basin for the patient to expell blood that has collected in the mouth, since swallowing blood can produce nausea and vomiting.

Vital signs should be assessed en route for patients with epistaxis, since blood loss can contribute to shock. Furthermore, any elevation in blood pressure may denote a hypertensive cause for the bleeding episode.

## THROAT EMERGENCIES

Most throat emergencies involve penetrating, obstructing, or aspirated foreign bodies. The procedure for managing those which obstruct the airway is discussed thoroughly in Chapter 10 in relation to basic life support.

Occasionally trauma results in a fractured larynx (voicebox). A direct blow to the neck by a fist, a steering wheel, or baseball can injure this structure, producing edema, subcutaneous emphysema, hemorrhage (see page 245), and airway obstruction. Such severe neck injuries may be accompanied by cervical spine trauma, too, so careful immobilization is imperative. Signs and symptoms of laryngeal fracture may be easily overlooked during the basic examination since other traumatic injuries may be more obvious. However, the EMT should observe and palpate the neck for edema and be cognizant of subjective complaints. Shortness of breath, voice changes, or respiratory stridor (see page 305) suggest laryngeal (lah-rin'je-al) injury. A surgical airway is usually required to ensure ventilation, so rapid transport of the patient to a hospital is imperative. Suction the airway as needed and provide supplemental oxygenation. Avoid positive-pressure ventilation since it may exaggerate or extend subcutaneous emphysema.

Injuries to major blood vessels in the neck can create fatal hemorrhage or air embolism (em'bo-lizm). (See page 268.) Use the usual pressure method to control the bleeding and insist that the victim remain in a head down position with the feet elevated (Trendelenburg position) since sitting upright encourages embolization. (See Fig. 11–2, page 212.)

## DENTAL EMERGENCIES

Teeth being displaced from the gums as a result of trauma is the most common dental problem faced by the EMT. The tooth (or teeth) should be saved for reimplant by placing it in a saline solution. If the victim is alert and having no breathing or swallowing problems, the tooth may be placed under the tongue or between the gum and jaw lining for preservation. There is some evidence that the chance for successful reimplantation is heightened by keeping the tooth warm and in its natural chemical environment.

The EMT should always search the mouth for teeth or dentures as a part of the basic trauma exam, since broken partial plates, broken teeth, or displaced dentures can obstruct the airway.

## FACIAL LACERATIONS AND FRACTURES

Facial trauma may involve lacerations to the cheek, which is richly supplied with blood. Pressure may need to be applied on both internal and external surfaces by a gauze pad to successfully control bleeding. Foreign bodies may require removal if they contribute to hemorrhage or make it difficult to retard bleeding. This is the only site from which an impaled object can be removed without fear of additional structural damage. Airway patency is paramount, and if a foreign body is blocking it, remove the object!

Facial trauma may create airway problems, shock from profuse bleeding, intracranial injury, and even damage to the cervical spine. As the EMT approaches a patient with obvious or suspected trauma to the face, initial attention should be given to the airway. Do not tilt the head or hyperextend the neck. Observe the precautions outlined in Chapter 15 for suspected cervical spine injury. (See page 282.)

The oral cavity should be assessed regularly for blood, secretions, CSF drainage (see page 278), and foreign objects such as teeth that have been displaced. Suction the airway as necessary *unless* there is evidence of CSF leakage. In the latter case, avoid any suctioning, since there may be a direct communication from the nose or mouth to the base of the brain. Airway devices and supplemental oxygen, as well as assisted ventilation, may be required to maintain oxygenation. (See Chapter 10.)

The EMT should appreciate the fact that facial fractures may not be obvious. Careful inspection and palpation are required to discover certain injuries. Bleeding; loss of teeth or malocclusion; increased salivation; or the inability to talk, swallow, or open and close the mouth suggest facial trauma. CSF leaks from the nose or ears, the presence of a blow-out fracture (see page 294), or asymmetry of facial structures are other clues to such injuries. A neurological evaluation including assessment of the level of consciousness is in order to detect the presence of a serious intracranial injury which often accompanies facial trauma. Special attention should be given to victims of fist fights, football, basketball, and other sports where considerable force may have been used to create the injury.

The position for transport will be determined by the considerations attending other injuries to the head, neck, chest, and abdomen and the status of the vital signs. If feasible, the mouth should be dependent (in a downward position) to permit the gravity drainage of blood and saliva from the mouth.

*References*

Charles, R., and Corrigan, E. "Epistaxis and Hypertension," *Postgrad. Med.*, 53:260–261, 1977.

DeWeese, D. D.; Liebman, E. P.; Norman, F. W.; and Saski, C. T. "From A to Z in Nosebleed Control," *Patient Care*, 12:66, 1978.

Havener, W. H., and Makley, T. A. "Emergency Management of Ocular Injury," *Ohio State Med. J.*, 71(16):776–779, November 1975.

Hyndiuk, R. A. "What Is an Eye Emergency?" *Wis. Med. J.*, 75(9):S80–81, September 1976.

Schindler, R. A. "The Bloody Nose," *Emerg. Med.*, 10:34, 1978.

Stephenson, H. E., Sr. "Dental Emergencies," in Stephenson, H. E., Jr., ed, *Immediate Care of the Acutely Ill and Injured*. St. Louis, MO: The C. V. Mosby Co., 1978.

Taugher, P. J. "Practical Concepts in Management of Ocular Trauma," *Wis. Med. J.*, 75:86, September 1976.

Ziter, W. D. "Dental Emergencies" in Cosgriff, J. H., Jr., and Anderson, D. L. *The Practice of Emergency Nursing*. Philadelphia, PA: J. B. Lippincott Co., 1975.

Chapter 17

# Respiratory and Chest Emergencies

## MECHANISMS OF BREATHING

The chest or thoracic cavity extends from the shoulders to the diaphragm and includes twelve pairs of ribs. It contains the lower airways, the heart, lungs, inferior and superior vena cavae (ve'nah ka've), the aorta, and the esophagus.

Lungs are elastic and they expand and collapse by a mechanism of pressure exchanges which are facilitated by the muscles of respiration. The intercostals and the diaphragm are the main muscles which are important to breathing, but there are accessory muscles in the chest wall, neck and abdominal wall which also facilitate the processes of ventilation.

The lungs are maintained in a functional state and are prevented from collapsing by a negative pressure which is maintained in the pleural space, between the lungs and the chest wall. When one expands the chest wall during inhalation, and the diaphragm descends, the negative pressure increases and the lungs fill with air. On exhalation, the lungs recoil as negative pressure falls, by a relaxation of intercostal muscles and an elevation of the diaphragm.

The diaphragm not only aids in chest motion essential to breathing, but it serves as a barrier separating the contents of the chest and abdomen. Its relative position is quite variable though. It descends to the fourth lumbar spine on inspiration and ascends to the sixth intercostal space on expiration. This fact is important for the EMT to appreciate. For instance, one tends to think of the abdomen as the portion of the trunk below the rib cage, but as the diaphragm ascends, the abdominal cavity actually extends upward to near the nipple line. Any injury below the nipples should essentially be viewed as an abdominal injury, too. (See Fig. 17-1.)

The need for oxygen is the most essential basic human need since living cells cannot function and survive without it. The respiratory system,

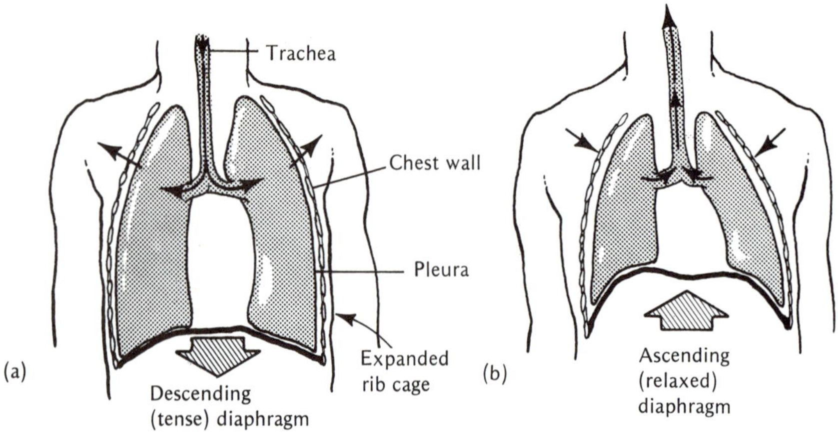


**Figure 17-1.** Motion of respiratory structures on (a) inhalation and (b) exhalation.

acting also with the heart and its circulatory pathways, is responsible for ensuring that the body has a constant and ample supply of this vital gas.

In alert and conscious patients, you know that enough oxygen is getting to the brain for at least the moment. In unconscious patients, you will have to engage in an in-depth data-gathering routine to determine whether or not there is adequate oxygenation of vital organs, and if not, what might be contributing to interferences in cellular respiration.

Several factors are crucial in the maintenance of oxygenation to cells, and they represent various neurological, endocrine, chemical, and mechanical interfaces with the heart and lungs. The involved brain centers must be intact and communicate to the respiratory system the stimulus to breathe when the level of carbon dioxide in the arterial blood reaches an excessive level. Since the nerve energy reaches the chest by travelling along the spinal cord, this structure, too, plays a crucial role in breathing. Of course, the airway structures, diaphragm, and chest wall muscles must work together in order to carry oxygen from the environment and eventually into the blood stream for transportation to cells throughout the body. Certain hormones, chemicals, and other substances constantly interact to ensure a balanced respiratory exchange of oxygen and carbon dioxide. Nature's complex process by which cells receive oxygen and dispose of carbon dioxide is called *respiration*. The parts of the process include *ventilation*, *diffusion*, and *circulation*.

*Ventilation* refers to *inspiration* (inhaling) and *expiration* (exhaling). Diffusion is the movement of gases across membranes; in the case of respiration, the movement of oxygen from the lungs into the blood stream, and carbon dioxide from the blood stream back into the lungs for exhalation. *Circulation* is the transportation of diffused gases in the blood to and from cells where oxygen is taken up and carbon dioxide is given off.

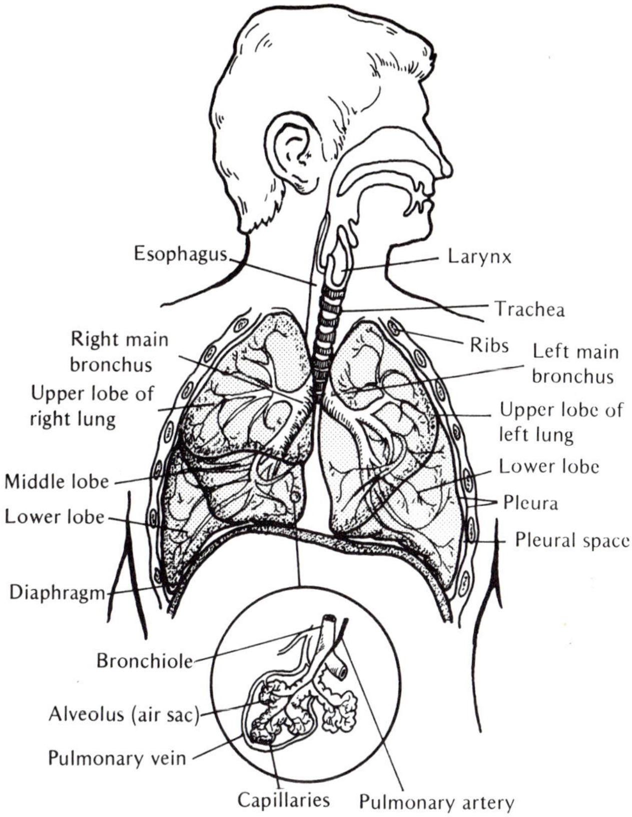


**Figure 17-2.** Anatomy of respiratory tract.

The continuous process of respiration involves an upper respiratory tract and a lower respiratory tract. It is helpful to briefly consider the components of each.

The upper respiratory tract is comprised of the nose, pharynx, larynx, and the top portion of the trachea. These structures filter, warm, and humidify air before it reaches the lungs. Upper airway structures are richly supplied with blood and mucous membranes that bring air to body temperature and condition it prior to its entry into the more delicate linings of the lower tract.

The lower respiratory tract is comprised of the lower portion of the trachea, bronchi, bronchioles, and the alveoli. (see Fig. 17-2.) These structures further the conditioning of air, as well as eventually transporting it at the alveolar level into the blood.

The stimulus to breathe is derived from the level of carbon dioxide in the blood. When it reaches an excessive amount, breathing is stimulated. When it reaches an unusually low level, the respiratory response will be a slower rate of breathing, which is also more shallow in nature. Carbon dioxide will thus build up in the blood, once again and trigger the stimulus to breathe. If excessive carbon dioxide builds up, breathing will deepen and accelerate to "blow off" the excess.

As the level of gases adjust with each breath, and with each breath being stimulated or repressed by the level of gases, there is a vital balance maintained in the normal individual.

## BREATHING DIFFICULTIES

One of the most challenging patients that the EMT will manage is the individual who is experiencing breathing difficulty. Since *airway* is the first priority in supporting life, the EMT will need to be prompt in assessment and treatment of several types of breathing difficulties which may be due to airway obstruction (see page 171), longstanding medical problems, and acute illness or injury which involves respiratory structures, (e.g., nose and upper airway structures, as well as the trachea, bronchi, and lungs which lie within the chest). In addition to degenerative disease and infection of these respiratory structures, emotions, drug reactions, inhalation accidents, and spinal cord injury also are implicated in episodes of breathing problems.

The patient in respiratory distress is truly frightened and is struggling for the "breath of life." It is essential that the EMT be sensitive to the needs for help and reassurance expressed by the individual while continuing to collect data regarding the episode and beginning treatment. It is crucial, of course, that the EMT promptly rule out correctable causes of dyspnea, such as an obstructed airway, before proceeding with further assessment and management.

### Assessment

Initially the ABCs of basic life support should be ascertained—airway, breathing, and circulation. When these have been assured, further data collection can be undertaken.

#### *Look at the Patient*

A careful inspection of the patient will tell you a great many things about the seriousness of his breathing problem. Is there cyanosis? How hard is the patient working to breathe?

*Cyanosis* is a bluish-gray skin discoloration due to oxygen compromise in the tissue. It is easily noted by looking at the nailbeds, earlobes, lips, and the area around the mouth, since there are many superficial blood vessels in these areas. It is important to have good lighting (preferably natural) to ensure that skin color is not distorted by artificial means.

Normal breathing is characterized by an inspiration which is about twice as long as the expiration. If the *inspiration* is labored and prolonged, upper airway obstruction is probable. If the *expiration* is prolonged, lower airway obstruction is to be suspected.

There are several other factors which provide clues to how hard the patient is working to breathe. Patient positioning is usually characteristically affected by breathing difficulties. Some individuals sit or stand up to aid their chest muscles in the effort to inhale and exhale. Individuals with long-term respiratory problems, or those with acute episodes of dyspnea may sit in a chair and lean over with their elbows or hands on their knees to increase respiratory volume. (See Fig. 17–3a.) Others may purse their lips to aid in air exchange. (See Fig. 17–3b.)

*Orthopnea* (or″thop-ne′ah) is a term used to denote that the individual must assume an upright position to overcome difficult breathing. The number of pillows that a patient uses in order to breathe effectively is essential for the EMT to determine since there generally is a more serious problem if considerable "propping up" is needed. A patient who requires two pillows is said to have "two-pillow orthopnea;" one who requires three pillows, "three-pillow orthopnea," and so on.

The EMT should observe the patient's face, neck, and chest as he is breathing and note unusual muscular activity that is evident and aiding in inhalation and exhalation. Accessory muscles between the ribs (inter-

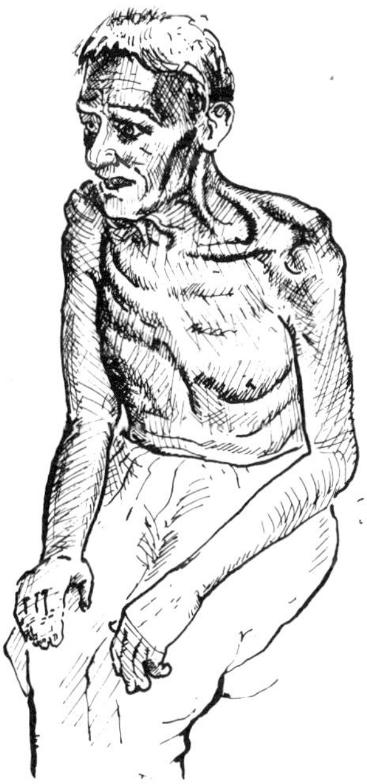

(a)

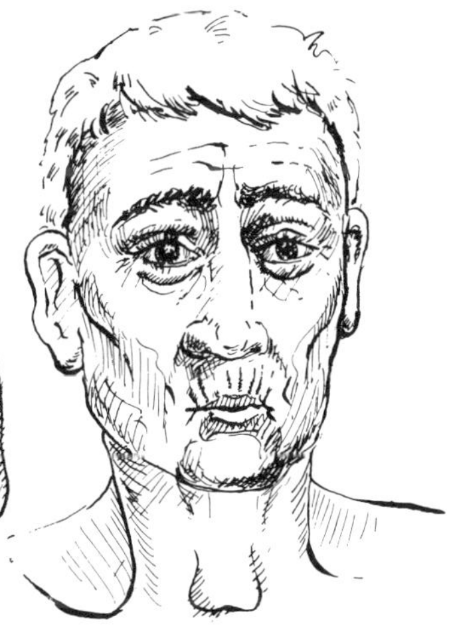

(b)

**Figure 17–3.** (a) Characteristic breathing effort associated with chronic obstructive lung disease. Note the elevation of shoulders and the use of accessory muscles. (b) Pursed lip breathing of chronic obstructive lung disease.

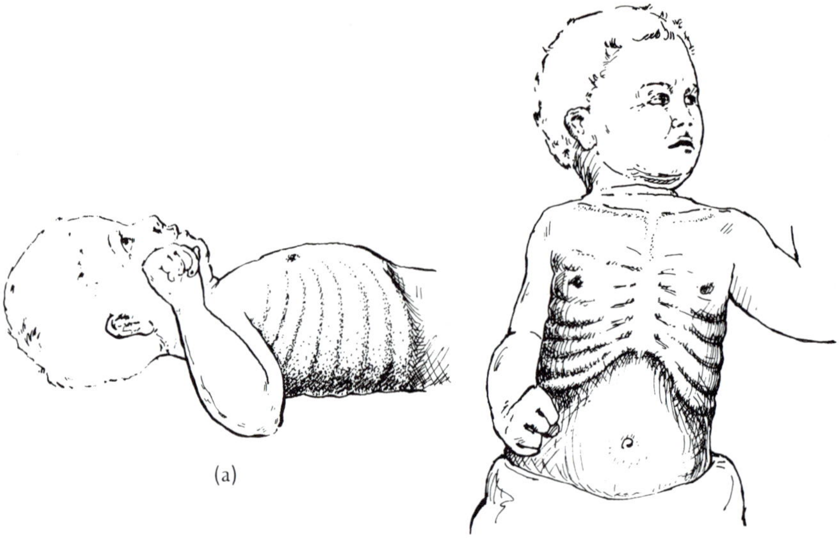

(a)

(b)

**Figure 17-4.** (a) Lateral view of rib cage retractions indicating respiratory distress. (b) Anterior view of rib cage demonstrating retractions.

costals) are sometimes used excessively in air exchange. When they forcefully contract, there is a "pulling inward" called *"retractions."* These retractions are quite evident in young children with dyspnea. (See Fig. 17-4.) There may be a "pulling in" at the neck, just above the sternum (breastbone) during retractions, a struggle to take in air. This particular retraction is referred to as a "tracheal tug," and is indicative of an obstructed airway.

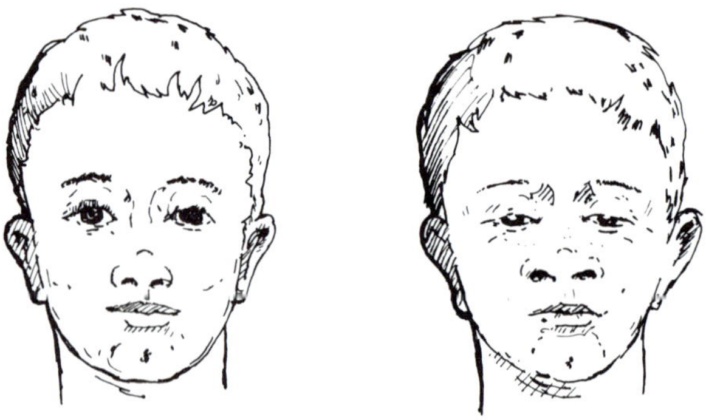

(a) (b)

**Figure 17-5.** (a) Normal nose; (b) marked nasal flaring.

Flaring of the nostrils also is a characteristic observation relating to respiratory distress. The widening of these nasal air passages is quite evident in infants who are experiencing dyspnea. (See Fig. 17–5.) Flaring is usually accompanied by intercostal retractions and paradoxical respiratory movement.

*Paradoxical* (par″ah-dok′se-kal) *respiratory movement* is characterized by a "retraction" of the epigastrium upon inhalation. (Normally, the chest and upper abdomen expand or rise with inspiration and fall with expiration.) This paradoxical respiratory movement is to be carefully distinguished from paradoxical chest wall motion which accompanies a flail chest. (See page 314.) (See Fig. 17–6.)

Extreme respiratory effort, like most hard work, is accompanied by considerable *diaphoresis* (sweating). The individual who has struggled in breathing for a prolonged period will look exhausted, and be unable to focus on anything else. Avoid asking questions which require complex answers (over a word or two). Speaking requires air and this patient has none to spare!

### *Listen to the Patient*

The EMT should listen carefully to what the patient says as well as listening for the sounds that accompany breathing.

The patient will be able to provide much information about his breathing. If the patient feels that he is having trouble "getting his breath,"

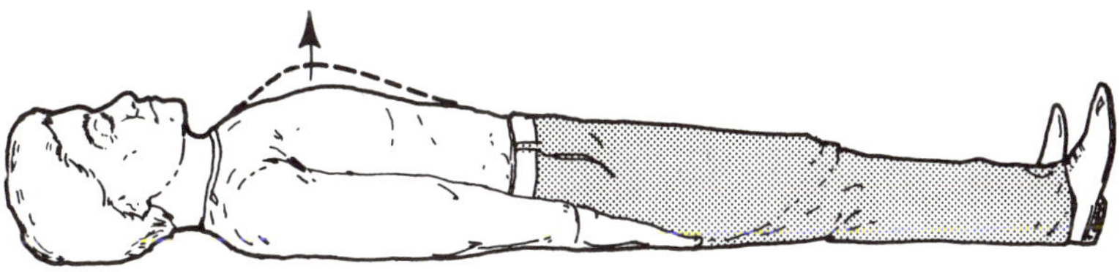

(a) Normal chest and abdominal rise during inhalation.

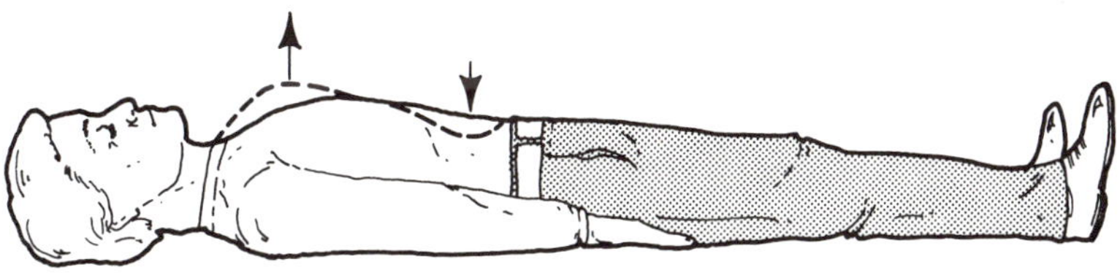

(b) "Paradoxical" indrawing of the stomach area during inhalation. Indicative of labored respirations.

**Figure 17–6.** (a) Normal chest and abdominal rise during inhalation. (b) "Paradoxical" indrawing of the stomach area during inhalation; indicative of labored respirations.

or is consciously aware of "shortness of breath," then the patient is *dyspneic* or has *dyspnea.* Dyspnea is a term which is used to refer only to the patient's own subjective feeling of difficulty in breathing or "air hunger."

Some patients with chronic problems in respiration have become used to their breathing difficulty and no longer experience *dyspnea,* but are objectively "short of breath" as you observe them. When such individuals do complain of *dyspnea,* they are usually extremely ill and require prompt emergency care. It is essential that the EMT realize that patients with chronic respiratory problems (e.g., emphysema and asthma) are accustomed to treating themselves for breathing problems, using a variety of medications, nebulizers, and other devices, so when they *do* call for emergency asistance, they consider their problem "out of control" and thus demand your prompt attention in assessment and management.

The EMT can learn a lot about how effective the patient is breathing by listening to the chest with the stethoscope. There is a series of anatomical points on the anterior and posterior thorax which contribute to a thorough chest assessment. (See Fig. 17–7.)

With the diaphragm of the stethoscope, the EMT should listen (auscultate) over the apex of one lung, just below the mid-clavicle, and then on the opposite side in the same place to compare sounds. Next,

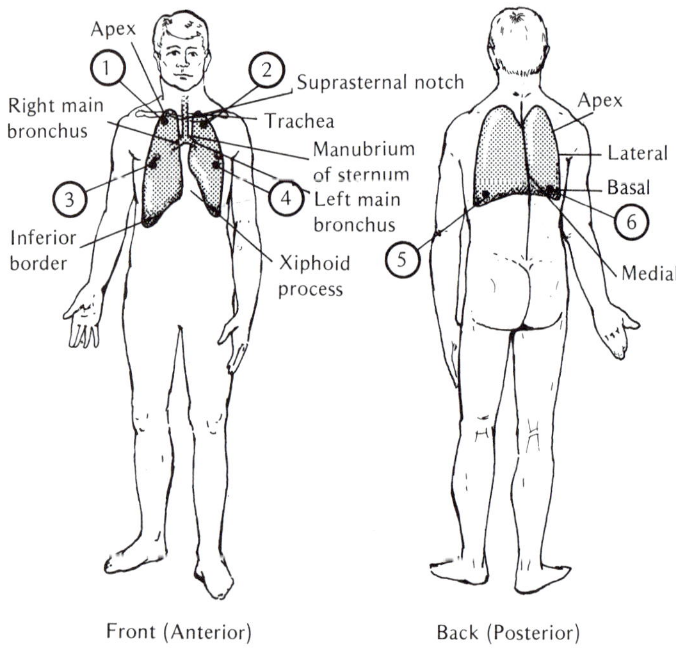


**Figure 17–7.** Anterior and posterior sites for listening to breath sounds. Numbers suggest sequence for listening and stethoscope placement.

auscultate just below the nipple and about two inches laterally. Finally, listen over the base of both lungs by placing the stethoscope over the posterior thorax at the level of the eighth and ninth ribs. Be certain to carefully compare both sides. It is helpful to ask the patient to breathe deeply with his mouth open to accentuate the sounds of air moving in and out of the lungs. Normal breath sounds are fairly loud, free flowing, and even on both sides in all areas. If you doubt that the patient is moving enough air, he is not! It is possible for the chest to be going through the motions of ventilation without air being moved.

Abnormal sounds which you may hear in listening to the chest include: rales, rhonchi, and wheezing. The EMT should bear in mind that *noisy breathing implies some obstruction.*

*Rales* (rahlz) are vibrating, disconnected breath sounds heard during inspiration. They indicate that air is passing by secretions in the lower airways. *Fine* rales sound like the "fizz" heard over the bottleneck of a "just opened" carbonated beverage or the crackling sound which occurs when several hairs in a strand are rolled back and forth between the fingertips as they are held near the ear. These abnormal breath sounds may also be louder and coarser if larger airways are affected by secretions. *Medium* rales are prominent and sound like sand being dropped into an empty tin can. *Coarse* rales are "gurgling" sounds, sometimes like bubbles being blown under water.

*Rhonchi* (rong'ki) are musical, vibratory sounds (fine popping noises) which are heard more easily during expiration. They are usually the result of narrowed larger airways and are of longer duration than rales. In the asthmatic patient, (see page 310), rhonchi can be heard on inspiration as well as on expiration.

*Wheezing* is a high-pitched or whistlelike noise usually noted on exhalation. It is caused by constriction or obstruction in the lower airways in conditions such as asthma.

Another term which the EMT should know is *stridor.* Stridor is a high-pitched crowing or "seal-bark" sound, classically caused by obstruction of the larynx. A stethoscope is not necessary to hear this sound. It may be apparent during inspiration or expiration, or both. *When* stridor occurs in the breathing cycle is important for the EMT to note. (Since stridor is common in children with certain upper respiratory tract infections and is also a symptom of a foreign body in the respiratory tract, it is considered in more detail on page 494 in relation to childhood emergencies.) Coughing and shortness of breath may be associated.

A *cough* is also important to note and record. Is it raspylike or barklike? Is it productive, i.e., does it produce sputum? If it is productive, the EMT should note content, color, characteristics, and odor of the sputum. Thick yellowish or greenish sputum which is foul smelling is common in lung infections. Pink frothy sputum is indicative of pulmonary edema. (See page 325.) Blood-tinged sputum may suggest tuberculosis or lung injury. Is pain associated with the coughing episode? Does any particular activity make it better or worse? Answers to these questions may be helpful in determinng the nature of the underlying problem.

The EMT should also try to determine if there is any history of breathing disorders and if the shortness of breath had a sudden or gradual onset. Also, note if the patient has ever had the same problem in the past. Certain types of heart disease, as well as lung problems, can cause dyspnea. Find out, too, what the victim was doing when the problem had its onset. One kind of heart failure classically presents by a patient's becoming "short of breath" after he lies down at night. (See page 325.)

Other factors seemingly unrelated to breathing also should be assessed since they may provide valuable clues about cardiovascular activity.

Are the *neck veins* full and pulsating while the patient is in a semisitting (not lying or sitting up)? Is there edema (swelling) of the feet and ankles? Either of these, when found, may indicate a cardiac cause for the breathing problem.

### Other Assessments

Vital signs are important to assess for all patients, but are extremely valuable in the data gathering related to breathing disturbances. (Review Chapter 9.) If breathing difficulty is accompanied by a rapid pulse or a drop in blood pressure, for example, shock may be the underlying cause. Rapid breathing associated with an elevated temperature could point to infection. Irregular or unusual respiratory patterns with a rise in blood pressure and a slow pulse could indicate a brain disturbance. (See page 277.)

## CHRONIC BREATHING PROBLEMS

The EMT will often encounter patients who have chronic respiratory problems and who are in acute distress. As mentioned earlier, most are used to treating minor flare-ups of their disease and their calling for medical assistance indicates that they feel "out-of-control." Chronic conditions that are commonly found include: asthma (az'mah), bronchitis, and emphysema. These problems, sometimes, are referred to as "chronic obstructive lung disease" (COLD), or "chronic obstructive pulmonary disease" (COPD). These conditions have *increased resistance to air flow* as a common finding.

### Asthma

Asthma is basically an allergy which irritates the bronchi, triggering wheezing and dyspnea. A typical attack begins when the individual is exposed to an allergen, which can be quite different for each patient. Smoke, smog, cold air, weather changes, dust, fumes, certain drugs, and even emotions can precipitate an acute asthmatic attack. At first, there is a dramatic effort of breathing with hyperventilation (see page 312), dyspnea, and diaphoresis (sweating). Some patients experience coughing, wheezing, rapid breathing, and an accelerated heart rate.

The irritated air passages become swollen and begin to secrete a sticky substance which plugs the surrounding airways, with small ones being affected first. At this point, patients begin to cough in an attempt to raise the mucus, but it is not uncommon for the cough to be nonproductive. When airway obstruction extends to larger airways, there is considerable distress with noticeable retractions, nasal flaring, and extreme "air hunger." Of course, the patient is restless and anxious. The EMT will have little difficulty detecting the asthmatic in crisis, due to obvious distress and characteristic expiratory wheezing which can usually be heard without a stethoscope. The oxygen is getting into the lungs without resistance, but there is considerable labor involved in pushing out the carbon dioxide which quickly will "wear out" the patient, in addition to depressing the respiratory drive.

When the basic assessments are made, they should include routine vital signs and a careful history of the onset of this attack and previous ones. During chest auscultation, (aws″kul-ta′shun) note how well air is moving, since extensive air trapping at obstruction sites can significantly interfere with free air passage in and out of the lower tract. Eventually, if the problem is not corrected, the carbon dioxide level will rise to a level which will depress any stimulus to breathe and respiratory failure will ensue.

On-the-scene management should include the administration of oxygen and considerable encouragement and reassurance since the condition is a frightening one for the patient to experience. Some patients will fight the administration of oxygen by mask, since it increases their feeling of suffocation. A nasal cannula is recommended with a low liter flow—1-2-3 *l*/min. High flow oxygen would, of course, tend to further depress the carbon-dioxide stimulus to breathe.

Intravenous therapy and specific drugs are essential in managing the acute attack, so rapid transportation to the hospital is vital.

## Bronchitis

*Bronchitis* (brong-ki′tis) is an inflammation of the bronchial tree due to either infection or chronic irritation from smoke or fumes. Coughing and spitting are prominent symptoms. Chronic bronchitis is complicated by respiratory insufficiency and ultimately emphysema.

## Emphysema

*Emphysema* (em″fĭ-se′mah) is characterized by an overdistention of the alveoli [al-ve′o-li] (air sacs) in the lungs. After a prolonged period of respiratory irritation and resistance to expiration ensues, the alveoli do not

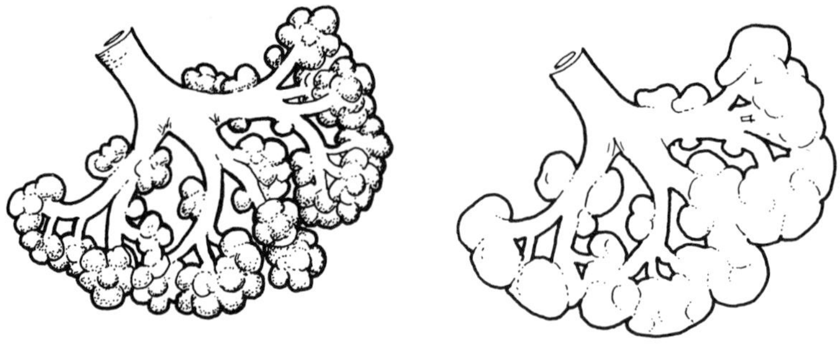


**Figure 17–8.** (a) Normal respiratory structures; (b) effects of emphysema on respiratory structures. Note the blister-like ruptured air sacs that trap air.

empty upon expiration and eventually rupture from the overdistention. As the walls of tiny air sacs are ruptured, they become blisterlike pockets of air which are stagnant. The body tends to wall off these useless air pockets by scar tissue. (See Fig. 17–8.)

The patient with an acute bout of emphysema has the classic signs and symptoms of respiratory distress including: coughing, dyspnea, retractions, nasal flaring, and so forth. Since the problem is a long-term one, the rib cage tends to be elevated giving the chest a "barrel-like" appearance. Abdominal wall tone is lost, too, so the abdomen may protrude as well.

Oxygen therapy is crucial and should be given by nasal cannula at low flow rates, 1–2 *l*/min. to avoid depressing the respiratory drive.

### Complications in the Management of Chronic Obstructive Respiratory Problems

It is crucial that the EMT observe the patient most carefully during oxygen administration, since the normal respiratory drive is depressed. If slow, shallow respirations occur, the patient may be experiencing a complication known as "carbon dioxide narcosis" (*Narcosis* [nar-ko′sis] means a sleep-like state.) Other evidence of this complication includes: flushed skin, flaccid or twitching of the extremities, mental confusion, and falling blood pressure. If the patient fails to move air on his own in amounts sufficient to meet baseline needs, assisted breathing by mechanical means is indicated.

## HYPERVENTILATION SYNDROME

Occasionally, individuals "hyperventilate" when they are extremely anxious or otherwise emotionally upset. As a result, there is an increase in the amount of air entering the lungs and a blowing off of too much carbon dioxide. This causes the blood to become too alkaline and consequently creates some characteristic signs and symptoms including dizziness, faintness, numbness and tingling of the hands, feet and around the mouth, and even chest pain. The patient feels considerable "air hunger." Vital signs will ordinarily reveal both a rapid heart and respiratory rate, but the blood pressure will be normal.

Listen carefully to the chest to check for overall air movement and determine if there are any abnormal breath sounds which could indicate that there is something wrong in the respiratory tract, such as a pulmonary embolus (see page 328.) Ask too if the patient is a diabetic, since a diabetic complication can be manifested by hyperventilation. Finally, check with the patient to determine if he has ingested any drugs or inhaled any substances which could give rise to an abnormal breathing episode. Remember, too, that the hypotension of shock can stimulate rapid respirations. (See page 205.)

It is imperative that the EMT understand that the individual who is hyperventilating is scared, even though there may be nothing seriously wrong. Having the patient breathe into a paper bag and rebreathe his own expired air will alleviate the symptoms by readjusting nature's balance of oxygen and carbon dioxide. Explain *before* the process what you are doing and continue to reassure the patient as he attempts to slow down and control his breathing. In a few minutes the annoying, but benign symptoms will disappear and the patient may resume breathing room air.

It is advisable to transport the individual who hyperventilates to be certain that there is no underlying serious problem that triggered the current episode.

## CHEST TRAUMA

Chest trauma is a leading cause of accidental death. Crimes of violence and steering wheel injuries account for the majority of penetrating and nonpenetrating chest wounds which are death producing.

Chest injuries cause serious respiratory difficulty whether the wound is open or closed. Initial attention should be given to the presence of dyspnea and breath sounds. The progressive worsening of dyspnea or the diminishing of breath sounds may indicate that there is serious injury.

All chest injuries, whether or not there are immediate indications of breathing problems, should alert the EMT to complete a thorough assessment including a detailed history of the accident, as well as a systematic survey of respiratory functioning. Pulses in all extremities should be checked to note any loss of arterial blood flow, which could indicate serious vascular injury.

### Closed Chest Injuries

Closed chest injuries occur without any break in the skin over the chest wall. The heart and blood vessels, as well as the lungs, may be bruised or lacerated by fractured ribs.

## Fractures of Ribs or the Sternum

Chest trauma may produce fractures of the ribs or the sternum. They occur quite commonly in the elderly trauma victim.

Upper ribs are seldom fractured since they tend to be well protected by the shoulder girdle. The sternum is prone to severe injury by steering wheel impact in vehicular collisions. Fractures of the ribs or the sternum seldom are major problems for field EMTs, unless they contribute to a flail chest, (see below) or if underlying soft tissue has been contused. Hemoptysis (coughing up blood) or the presence of subcutaneous emphysema indicates serious injury to the lungs, blood vessels, or airway structures. Cardiac tamponade is a distinct possibility, too, with impact-related sternal trauma, so the EMT should be alert to the potential for shock due to a declining cardiac output. (See Chapter 11.) Hemoptysis, subcutaneous emphysema, or developing shock requires prompt transport to a hospital.

The history of the accident, localized pain (especially with coughing or deep inspiration,) dyspnea, and the presence of crepitus (crackling sound produced by rubbing together of bone fragments) are important clues to fractures of the chest wall. In some instances the fractures may be quite apparent upon palpation, or there may be bruising or chest wall deformity. However, x-rays are essential for confirmation of these injuries.

The patient will have much pain, especially on deep inspiration or coughing. A conscious patient may be able to pinpoint the exact fracture site on the rib cage. Reassurance is in order for this individual, as you search for clues to associated soft tissue injury, primarily of the heart, lungs and large blood vessels. The major problem is *not* the fracture, but the hidden damage that may lie underneath the bony thoracic wall.

Taping of rib fractures or the fractured sternum should not be done unless they are contributing to flail (flāl) chest, since this practice limits chest motion and decreases ventilatory efficiency. Deep breathing should be encouraged en route to the hospital.

## Flail Chest

A *flail chest* is the result of a loss of integrity of the chest wall, which allows a portion of the chest wall to move independently of surrounding segments. When two or more ribs are fractured in more than one place, or if the sternum is broken away from the rib structures, a *flail* or floating segment of the chest exists.

The effect of any chest wall movement that represents independent activity of one chest portion results in disturbance of breathing pressures associated with inspiration and expiration. Rather than aiding in breathing, the free-floating portion actually interferes with normal respiration. For example, when one inhales, the chest wall normally pushes out to permit lung expansion, and falls as exhalation occurs. When a flail segment exists, the involved chest portion draws in on inhalation and expands on exhalation. (See Fig. 17–9.) This opposite effect experienced by the flail or free-floating section impairs normal respiratory efficiency, making breathing successively more difficult, minute by minute. Furthermore, a chest wall injury of the severity to produce a flail segment is likely to be accompanied by soft tissue damage of the heart and lungs.

If a flail chest is noted, the EMT should place the patient on the affected side on a spine board to stabilize the flail portion by using body weight. If this approach is not feasible, the flail segment can be immobilized with sandbags or a pillow splint. Direct hand pressure can be applied over the flail portion during exhalation to stabilize the wall and prevent paradoxical motion. A semi-Fowler's position should be employed if the patient is not in shock.

Respirations must be assisted if there is poor ventilation. A bag-valve-mask unit is recommended in the prehospital care phase. Of course, the patient should be positioned on the affected side and rapidly transported to a hospital emergency department for definitive management of the injury.

## Pneumothorax

A pneumothorax (nu″mo-tho′raks) is an increase of air pressure within the chest cavity (pleural space), which reduces lung volume expan-

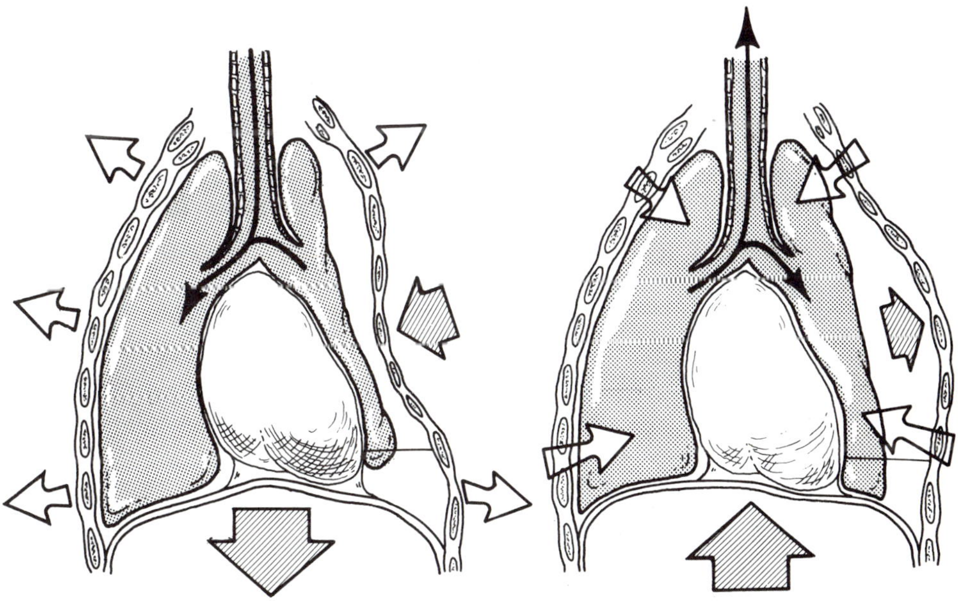

(a) (b)

**Figure 17–9.** Flail chest: (a) on inspiration the flail segment moves inward; (b) on expiration the flail segment moves outward.

sion. If there is a considerable amount of air in the chest, it may contribute to a collapsed lung, producing a *pneumothorax*.

A *spontaneous* pneumothorax can occur without injury due to a rupture in a weakened portion of lung tissue. Sharp chest pain and dyspnea are experienced by the patient when the lung collapses. Breath sounds will be absent. Respiratory support (oxygen at 8 *l*/min.) and rapid transportation to a treatment facility is necessary. If the air continues to leak into the cavity with each respiration, a tension pneumothorax follows, endangering the great vessels, the heart, and the opposite lung.

## Tension Pneumothorax

A tension pneumothorax causes a lung to collapse by trapping air within the chest cavity on inspiration which cannot escape on expiration (Fig. 17–10). With each breath, the pressure within the chest cavity increases and eventually the lung will collapse due to pressure build-up. When the pleural space on one side is completely filled with air, the mediastinum (containing the heart and large blood vessels) begins to shift toward the uninvolved side. Of course, this interferes with the normal functioning of the remaining lung, and air exchange is reduced resulting in severe hypoxia. The vena cava becomes kinked and obstructed, which prevents blood from flowing freely into the right side of the heart for reoxygenation. Veins in the neck may be quite distended and the trachea may deviate to the side as pressure builds from the back up of blood that cannot enter the heart and lungs. The chest will be silent, and heart sounds may be

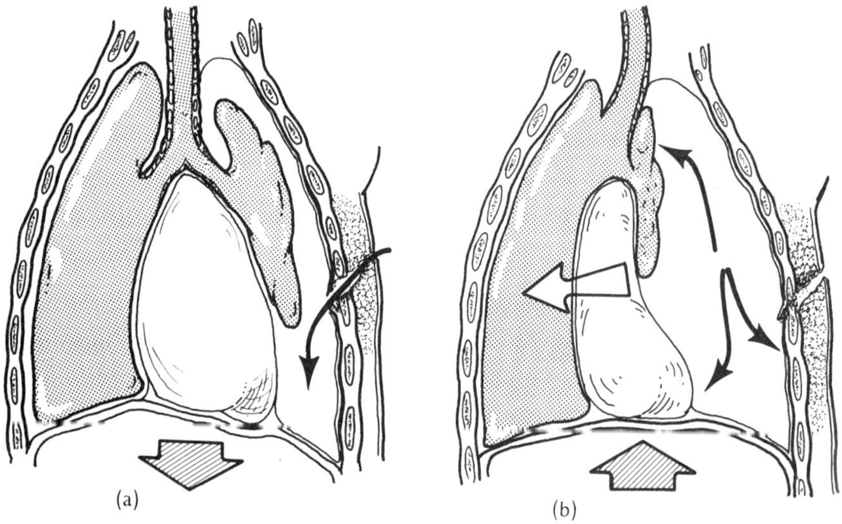


**Figure 17–10.** Tension pneumothorax: (a) air enters cavity on inspiration; (b) on expiration, air cannot escape and pressure (tension) builds, eventually compressing the opposite lung.

difficult to hear. The trachea will deviate away from the side with absent breath sounds. Paradoxical chest movement will usually be obvious and cyanosis will be quite apparent. If blood is also collecting in the chest, due to vessel rupture, the condition is termed a *hemothorax*. If considerable blood is lost, signs of shock may be present as well. The EMT should remember that ineffective oxygenation, as well as blood loss, can cause a rapid weak pulse and a low blood pressure.

If a tension pneumothorax is developing, the accumulating air must be given a chance to escape. One method used by paramedics or physicians is to insert a needle into the chest cavity at the second intercostal space, four finger-breadths from the sternum (with the patient sitting up), to allow air to escape (air rises!) and thus release the pressure. (See Fig. 17-11.) The end of the needle is covered (using a fingertip) during inspiration and uncovered during expiration. (Removing an occlusive dressing may create a dramatic improvement for some patients.) A finger cot or a finger from a rubber glove (with a slit) is used with a needle. The hole is small and the finger device long in order to advantageously use external air pressure to close the valve on inspiration. A commercial device or a contrived flutter valve is used. A tension pneumothorax can be easily confused with cardiac tamponade. If the EMT recognizes a tension pneumothorax, the patient must be quickly transported to the hospital for treatment described above.

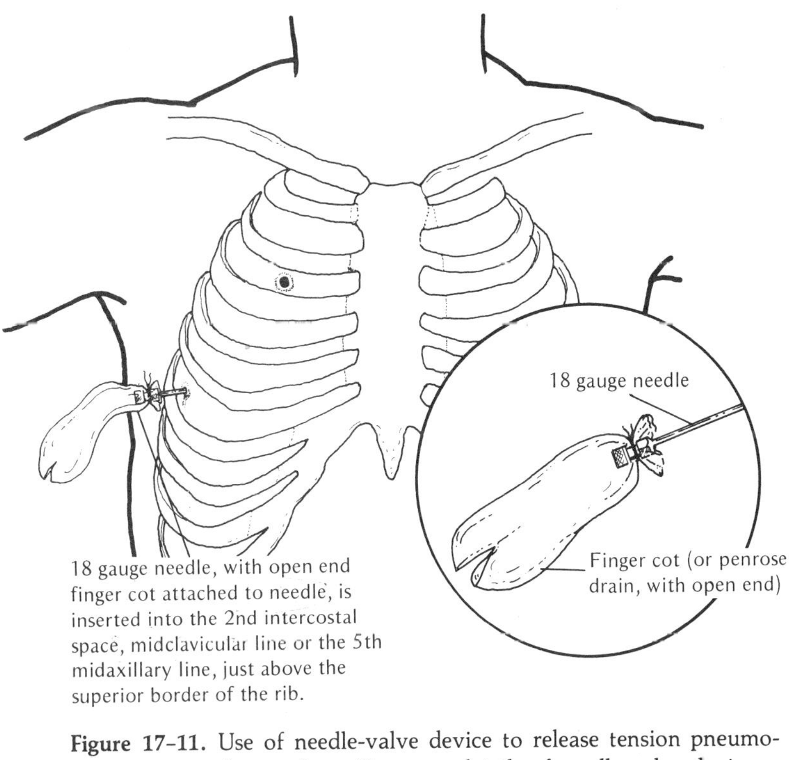


**Figure 17-11.** Use of needle-valve device to release tension pneumothorax. Inset illustrates details of needle-valve device.

## Cardiac Tamponade

Chest injuries can produce bleeding into the pericardial sac which envelops the heart. As the sac fills with blood, the heart is compressed and chambers cannot fill completely during the filling cycle of the heart beat (diastole) and therefore, there is a limited amount of blood available for circulation to the body organs and parts.

The EMT should suspect cardiac tamponade if there is chest trauma, especially over the sternal area. Distended neck veins, a drop in blood pressure, cyanosis, and distant (hard to hear) heart sounds are common indicators of the condition. The patient should be promptly transported to a treatment facility in high Fowler's position receiving oxygen en route.

The patient will usually show prompt improvement when the pericardial sac is aspirated, removing the blood, and permitting the heart to expand and fill normally.

The EMT should remember that it is crucial to make a thorough assessment of apparent chest injuries with primary attention directed to establishment and maintenance of a patent airway. Open chest wounds should be covered and a tension pneumothorax promptly identified. Flail segments should be controlled by splinting the floating portion of the rib cage with the patient's own weight or with sandbags or pillow splints. Vital signs, including a careful check for air movement and breath sounds, should be a high priority during transportation to a hospital for definitive care. Shock, if present, should be treated in the usual manner with application of antishock trousers and IV fluid therapy utilized according to local protocols.

## Open Chest Injuries

Open chest injuries imply a penetration of the chest wall. Gunshot wounds and stabbings often result in such injuries. A pneumothorax or hemothorax often coexists, with injury to the heart and great blood vessels also a distinct possibility. Dyspnea is prominent, and a shock state from severe blood loss is a likely occurrence. Ventilatory assistance and rapid transport to a hospital is mandatory. (See Fig. 17–12.)

A "sucking" chest wound describes a penetrating injury that permits outside air to enter the pleural space when the patient inhales. The volume of this air trapped outside the lung within the chest expands with every breath, eventually limiting the expansion of the lung. The "sucking" sound of air passing in and out of the wound gives the injury its name.

The EMT should promptly bandage the wounds with an airtight dressing. Petroleum-impregnated gauze, plastic food wrap or aluminum foil may be used. Merely placing the heel of the hand over the wound is better than no attempt to stop the abnormal "sucking" in of air. The EMT must realize that such action can convert a "sucking" wound into a tension pneumothorax if the lung tissue has been damaged, especially if the patient has been intubated, and is being "bagged." In such cases, the dressing *should not be occlusive,* but should permit air passage. The clue for the

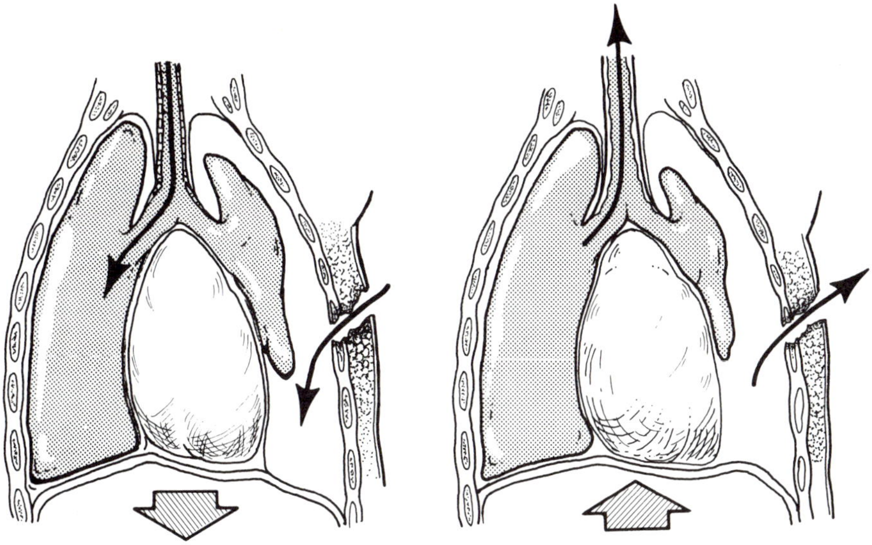


**Figure 17–12.** Open pneumothorax: (a) inspiratory airflow; (b) expiratory airflow.

EMT to remove an occlusive dressing is merely the patient's worsening condition after its application. An open pneumothorax is considerably more tolerable than a tension pneumothorax.

### *Impaled Foreign Objects*

An impaled foreign object should be stabilized using a bulky dressing. (See page 267 for detailed discussion of impaled objects.)

## Other Chest Trauma

### *Tracheal-Bronchial Injuries*

The larger airways (trachea, bronchial tree) can be ruptured due to blunt or penetrating chest trauma. Dyspnea, hemoptysis (he-mop′tĭ-sis), (spitting up blood), subcutaneous emphysema, and a pneumothorax are among classic signs and symptoms of such an injury. The EMT should place the patient in a semi-Fowler's position and promptly transport to a hospital, administering high flow oxygen en route.

### *Ruptured Diaphragm*

The diaphragm can be injured by blunt or penetrating trauma, resulting in bowel being pushed into the chest. The conscious patient will complain of severe shoulder pain and the EMT will note lung displacement upward as breath sounds are auscultated. The EMT should support the patient's respiration during transport by giving high flow oxygen (8 *l*/min.)

and assisting ventilatory efforts as necessary. At the hospital (or occasionally in the field if EMT-Ps are present), a nasogastric tube will be inserted to decompress the stomach and aid in the breathing effort.

*Traumatic Asphyxia* (as-fik′ se-ah)

This chest injury is due to compression or crushing injuries. The sternum is pushed in and, thus, it places considerable pressure on the heart and the surrounding blood vessels. The heart's chambers cannot fill and empty in the normal manner and blood is backed up into the veins of the head and neck, causing them to enlarge. With increasing pressure building with the back-up of blood, there is hemorrhage into the surrounding tissue, resulting in bluish discoloration and swelling. The tongue, lips, and eyes may be affected, causing swelling and discoloration.

The EMT should transport the patient at once, giving 100 percent oxygen and assisting ventilation as necessary.

*Chest Injury and Shock*

A serious and life-threatening complication of chest injury is shock due to damage of large arteries and veins which enter and leave the heart. Rapid, developing shock post-chest trauma should cause the EMT to suspect damage to great vessels in the chest.

The administration of oxygen and the use of antishock trousers may forestall catastrophe long enough for transport to a hospital capable of immediate chest surgery to repair the hemorrhagic vessels. Death is not uncommon in such injuries due to respiratory as well as circulatory compromise.

*References*

Cordell, A. R. "Evaluation of Major Cardiac and Vascular Injury to the Chest," *Emerg. Med. Serv.*, pp. 11–16, July/August 1977.

Jackson, D. H.; and Murphy, G. W. "Non-Penetrating Cardiac Trauma," *Mod. Concepts Cardiovasc. Dis.* 45:123–128, 1976.

Naclerio, E. "CIBA Symposium on Chest Trauma," Vol. 22, No. 3, Summit, N. J.: The CIBA Corp., 1970.

Pories, W. J.; and Gaudiani, V. A. "Cardiac Tamponade," *Surg. Clin. North Am.* 55:573, 1975.

Symbas, P. N., *et al.* "Penetrating Cardiac Wounds: A Comparison of Different Therapeutic Methods," *Ann. Surg.* 183:377–381, 1976.

Trunkey, D. "Invasive Chest Procedures: How and When." Lecture at the Annual ACEP/EDNA Scientific Assembly, New Orleans, November 1976.

# Chapter 18

# Cardiovascular Emergencies

## CHEST PAIN

One of the most frightening symptoms that the EMT will face is "chest pain." Chest pain can range from an annoying symptom to a life-threatening factor. The initial approach to the patient with this problem is to provide supportive care while attempting to systematically determine the nature of the pain. Chest pain may be due to a wide variety of cardiac, respiratory, vascular, or other phenomena which involves structures and organs in and around the chest. Ordinarily, when an individual calls the EMTs for assistance, the pain is either acute or "out of control," thus representing a true emergency.

The patient should first be assessed for the ABCs of basic life support, airway, breathing and circulation. Once these have been assured, the EMT should assist in making him comfortable, probably supporting him in an upright sitting position. It is important, of course, to reassure the patient that you are there to help him become more comfortable. Administering oxygen at 2–4 *l*/min. by nasal cannula usually aids in relieving anxiety as well as reduces the potential hazards from hypoxia. In the meantime, it is important to determine if the chest pain is of a traumatic or nontraumatic origin.

If there has been recent injury to the chest, the assessment will focus on the accident and the resultant symptoms that it produced relating to the chest, giving special attention to soft tissue injury of the heart and lungs. (See Chapter 17.)

Chest pain of nontraumatic origin must be carefully assessed in a systematic manner, giving primary attention to the related history of its onset and its characteristics.

Determine *when* the pain started. Did it have a gradual or sudden onset? Does the pain come and go, or is it constant? Find out whether or not the individual was engaged in activity or was resting when the pain began or worsened. Does anything make it better or worse—such as lying down, sitting up, eating, activity, or breathing deeply?

Ask the patient to explain *where* the pain is. Is it in the chest or upper abdomen? Does it confine itself to the area under the sternum or does it seem generalized over the anterior chest wall? Does it radiate to the arms, neck, shoulders, jaw, or back?

Many times the EMT will get excellent data merely by asking the patient to tell about his pain. Often this approach will give you more accurate information since it is fairly easy to "put words into the patient's mouth." If the EMT says, "Does the pain feel like a vise? Does it radiate? Is it crushing?" the patient is apt to affirm everything, assuming that "yes" answers will get the right response. Remember that most patients will suspect that chest pain automatically means a "heart attack."

A careful physical examination will reveal additional information that is helpful. Look carefully at the characteristics of respirations, and assess the skin color. Are the neck veins distended? Are there any signs of chronic pulmonary problems (barrel-shaped chest, scars from previous chest surgery, etc.)?

When vital signs are taken, special care should be given to the characteristics of the respiratory effort. Breath sounds should be assessed as previously described in Chapter 17.

## CHEST PAIN OF CARDIAC ORIGIN

Although the EMT will not be diagnosing the underlying cause of chest pain, it is important that he understand the nature of the pain to determine whether or not it represents a serious or immediate threat to life. One of the most common types of pain that the EMT must thoroughly assess is angina pectoris.

### Angina Pectoris

*Angina Pectoris* (or merely *angina* [an-ji′nah]) is a term used to describe chest pain that is retrosternal (re″tro-ster′nal) (behind the sternum or breastbone). The pain originates from the oxygen-deficient myocardium (mi″o-kar′de-um) and it is nature's way of signaling that "something is wrong." In order to understand angina, it is important to know the underlying reasons for its occurrence.

The myocardium is supplied with oxygen derived from the blood supplied by the right and left coronary arteries. The left coronary artery has two major branches. The coronary arteries fill during *diastole* (di-as′to-le), the relaxation part of the cardiac cycle that occurs after the pumping or contraction force, *systole* (sis′to-le). The proper filling of coronary arteries depends upon an efficient and regular cardiac rhythm, an adequate volume of circulating blood and to a large degree upon their elasticity and patency. For example, unusually rapid or irregular cardiac rhythms do not permit adequate filling of the coronary arteries during diastole, and when blood volume is drastically reduced, perhaps by hemorrhage, the supply is not sufficient to fill the coronary arteries, and thus, a portion of the myocardium may be deprived of oxygen. If there is a degenerative disease of the vessels, such as atherosclerosis (ath″er-o″skle-ro′sis) (or hardening of the arteries,) or a blood clot (thrombus [throm′bus]) the resistance to filling is increased and, therefore, the coronary arteries may not receive the amount of blood flow needed to nourish the heart itself. One of these factors, or a combination of several, often contribute to a poor blood supply for the myocardium and it becomes *ischemic* (is-kem′ik) (oxygen-starved).

The body responds to ischemia by altering its method of producing energy for cellular life processes. This adaptation to oxygen deprivation is termed *anaerobic* (an″a-er-o′bik) (without oxygen) *metabolism.* The chemical by-products of this modified energy production cycle are largely acid substances which irritate the tissue causing pain. Therefore, when a patient complains of chest pain, the EMT must think about the possibility of the pain being caused by inadequate oxygenation of the myocardium.

The supply of oxygen that the heart requires is dependent upon the demands that are being placed upon it to meet tissue needs. For instance, when the patient is stressed by unusual physical exertion, considerably more oxygen is required than when the patient is resting. Most individuals initially will experience chest pain of cardiac origin, after exercise or while under extreme stress.

Chest pain from angina can usually be relieved by rest or by drugs known as *vasodilators* (vas″o-di-lāt′orz). One of the most popular vasodilating agents is nitroglycerin (ni-tro-glis′er-in) which promotes relaxation of the coronary arteries and thus improves their filling. The EMT may encounter patients with chest pain who regularly use nitroglycerin to control their symptoms, since it provides a prompt response, within a minute or two. Nitroglycerin is a tiny white pill which patients place under their tongue where it is readily dissolved and absorbed into circulation. It achieves its pain-relieving effects in several ways, but primarily, it dilates (enlarges and relaxes) the coronary arteries so that they fill more readily and completely. Some patients will experience side effects of headache and a flushed face and neck soon after using nitroglycerin, but these are short-lived. Occasionally the EMT will be in a situation to administer this agent on the scene, using a fresh supply from the vehicle since some forms of nitroglycerin deteriorate with improper storage that permits exposure to air, light, or heat, thus making the drug ineffective. If a patient has taken his own nitroglycerin and no results have been noted, (especially after an additional dose five minutes later), he is likely to call for emergency medical assistance since nonresponsiveness to this agent may suggest preinfarction or myocardial infarction angina.

## Myocardial Infarction

Preinfarction (pre″in-fark′shun) angina or chest pain of myocardial infarction reflects actual cellular destruction of a myocardial area due to loss of coronary artery blood flow. A *thrombus* (blood clot) that blocks arterial circulation is the most common cause of this condition. Other causes are hypovolemic shock from hemorrhage or dehydration, or occlusion due to inflammatory processes caused by infections. Angina of this more severe type may be accompanied by sweating and weakness, too. If any relief is obtained by nitroglycerin or Isordil (another vasodilating drug prescribed for angina) the relief is only temporary and usually is not complete relief. The consequences (size and location) of a myocardial infarction, of course, depend upon the site of coronary artery occlusion and whether or not there are any additional blood vessels in or near the involved area to take over some of the burden of nourishing the heart.

A *myocardial infarction* or *coronary occlusion* represents incurred damage to the heart muscle. In simple angina, no permanent damage has been done to cardiac tissue.

### *Signs and Symptoms of a Myocardial Infarction*

The patient who has suffered a myocardial infarction may exhibit a variety of signs and symptoms. The location and extent of the damage to the heart's circulation will determine the severity of the "heart attack" and influences the patient's response.

Chest pain is the primary symptom of the infarction and usually is of sudden onset at the occurrence of circulatory interference. It may be tolerated for several weeks by some patients if it is not perceived as *severe* pain. Others will seek emergency medical assistance at once. The EMT must remember that pain is a highly subjective phenomenon and each individual has a unique response.

It is not uncommon for patients who have a myocardial infarction to experience "indigestion." Nausea, vomiting, and hiccoughing are results of an irritation to certain nerves which lie close to the heart and are influenced by its circulatory status.

Other signs and symptoms occur when the body recognizes the crisis and the nervous system responds. Sweating and anxiety are typical reactions to the pain and, of course, somewhat reflect the fears of the patient.

Vital signs reveal a drop in blood pressure due to poor pumping efficiency of the heart, and the pulse rate quickens in response to the reduced cardiac output, as well as the patient's apprehension that a life-threatening emergency may exist.

Cyanosis, distended neck veins, edema, and changes in heart sounds are also noted in certain individuals who have suffered a myocardial infarction. The EMT should be alert to these signs, as well as the classic chest pain, and be prepared to intervene.

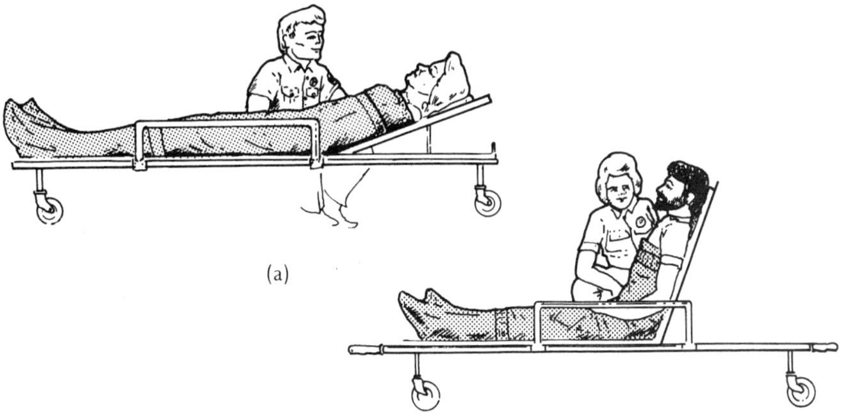

(a)

(b)

**Figure 18–1.** (a) Semi-Fowler's position; (b) High-Fowler's position.

*Management*

Any patient who is suspected as having a "heart attack" should be managed as if one were known to exist. Allow the individual to sit in a semi Fowler's position; then loosen clothing around the neck and provide oxygen by nasal cannula at 6–8 *l*/minute. (See Fig. 18–1.)

EMTs who have advanced training may apply monitoring electrodes, initiate an intravenous infusion, and administer specific medications for dysrhythmias [dis-rith′me-ahz] (abnormalities of heart rhythm).

## Acute Pulmonary Edema

Patients who have damage to the heart muscle may develop what is called *congestive heart failure.* This complication arises when the heart muscle is unable to contract forcefully enough to empty the various chambers during the cardiac cycle. Blood then backs up into the lungs and systemic circulation, creating an emergency demanding prompt management.

When blood becomes "congested" in the heart and lungs the blood pressure rises in an effort to force circulation by increased contractions. As blood pressure rises, fluid leaks out of the vessels into surrounding tissue spaces or air spaces. When the air spaces or sacs are saturated with fluid from the blood stream, the condition is termed *pulmonary edema.*

The lungs ordinarily can handle the venous blood returning to the right atrium from the systemic circulation, but when there is pulmonary edema, and the lungs are engorged or congested, blood backs up into the systemic (body) veins. The neck veins, for example, become quite full or distended and this sign should alert the EMT to a heart failure condition. Position the patient in semi Fowler's and turn the head to observe the neck veins. If they are distended more than two inches above the sternal notch, right heart failure is evident.

The feet, legs, and hands may also be swollen, indicating a congestion of venous blood which is unable to be accepted by the heart.

*Management*

Since pulmonary edema is aggravated by lying down, most patients will be unable to tolerate any position except sitting in high Fowler's; (see Fig. 18–1) in fact, the majority of pulmonary edema onsets are at night, occurring shortly after the individual goes to bed. Patients will insist on sitting up "to breathe" since this not only reduces the work of breathing, but reduces the blood flow to the heart.

The EMT who suspects this complication should check vital signs carefully while taking a history. The heart rate will probably be quite rapid and the blood pressure markedly elevated. Oxygen should be provided by nasal cannula at 6–8 *l*/min. in the field.

Advanced EMTs will initiate an intravenous line for medication delivery only, taking precautions to restrict the volume delivered. High fluid volumes would tend, of course, to only aggravate the problem. The hospital physician may direct the team to give diuretics (di″u-ret′iks) to reduce the body water content, digitalis (dij″ĭ-tal′is) to strengthen the heart, or morphine to cause venous pooling and relieve anxiety, thus easing the respiratory effort. Some authorities recommend that the patient be transported with the head at the back of the vehicle to lessen the impact of venous blood entering the heart as the vehicle decelerates.

*Rotating tourniquets* are another useful mode of temporarily reducing blood flow to the heart. EMTs may be directed to apply a series of three tourniquets (see Fig. 18–2) to trap venous blood in the legs and arms until the heart can "catch up" in its emptying process. Initially both legs (due to their high venous blood volume) and one arm are used as venous blood traps. *The EMT should insure that an arterial pulse is still present in each leg and arm!* Every fifteen minutes one tourniquet is removed and applied to the extremity without a tourniquet. No tourniquet is left in place longer than forty-five minutes. When tourniquets are eventually removed, they are removed at fifteen-minute intervals—*not all at once!* If they were, the heart would be overwhelmed with venous blood returning to the right heart and it would decompensate very quickly in its weakened state.

*Procedure for Rotating Tourniquets*

1. Explain the procedure to the patient; tell him how it will help him.

2. Place the patient in a high Fowler's position and continue to administer oxygen by nasal cannula at 6–8 *l*/min.

3. Check distal pulses in all four extremities.

4. Apply a wide venous tourniquet on both thighs and the left arm, as close to the trunk as possible. Be certain that the arterial pulse is still

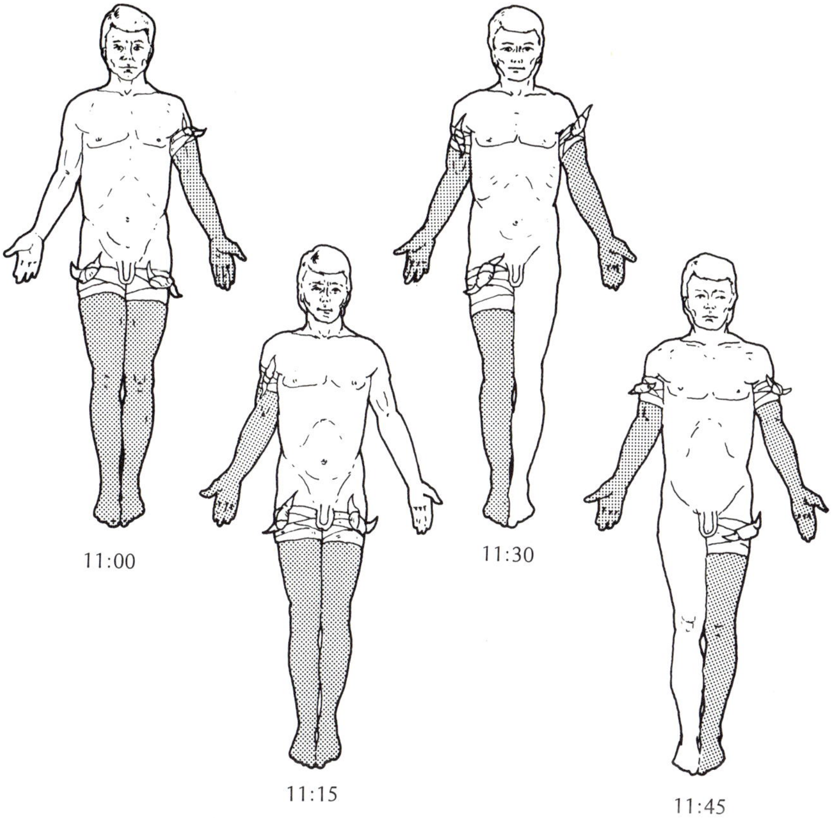


**Figure 18–2.** Plan for application of rotating tourniquets. Note that initially one arm and two legs are occluded with venous tourniquets to maximize early effects of procedure.

palpable after application. (Record the time of application.) (See Fig. 18–2)

5. Beginning clockwise, remove one tourniquet every fifteen minutes and apply to the free extremity. Start with the left arm; move it to the right arm. After fifteen minutes, remove the left leg tourniquet and transfer it to the left arm, and so forth. Never have tourniquets on all extremities at the same time!

6. When the procedure is discontinued, remove the tourniquets one by one at fifteen minute intervals in a counterclockwise fashion, using the established plan of rotation.

## Dissecting Aortic Aneurysm

The aorta is the largest vessel in the body that transports arterial blood. It is composed of several layers of tissue, which permits its elasticity and strength to respond to changing pressures of blood flow on exit from the left ventricle.

During the process of aging, the aorta, like other vessels, begins to lose its elasticity as mineral deposits build up and blood flow becomes impaired. "Hardening" of arteries, weakened cardiac function, and hypertension (high blood pressure) create both structural weaknesses and enlargement of the aorta, resulting in the formation of an aneurysm. Blood may also leak between the layers of the vessel and cause a tearing or dissection of the wall. (See Fig. 18–3.) As pressure builds within the aorta, the patient experiences severe, constant chest pain that is "agonizing." It characteristically radiates to the back and may also radiate to the abdomen. Nothing will alter the pain—neither rest, nitroglycerin, nor changes in movement or position. Blood pressure may be elevated and often varies from limb to limb due to blood flow disturbances. One or more peripheral pulses may be absent.

The danger of aneurysms and dissection, of course, is rupture of the vessel with profound hemorrhage. Without an aorta to supply arterial blood for other body parts, the patient will soon die.

If the EMT assesses a patient and finds that the chest pain is characteristic of a dissecting aortic aneurysm, prompt transportation to a hospital is imperative. Most patients will be sweating, pale, and apprehensive; and some may have signs of a cerebrovascular accident (stroke) such as hemiplegia (hem"e-ple'je-ah) or paraplegia. (See page 330.) A High-Fowler's position should be employed with oxygen administered per nasal cannula at 6–8 *l*/min.

Advanced EMTs may be instructed to initiate intravenous fluids as a route for emergency drugs and to combat shock in the event of a rupture or "blow-out" of the aneurysm.

En route, the hospital should be notified of the patient's impending arrival and a full account of the history, signs and symptoms, and response to treatment should be provided. It is also essential to support and reassure the anxious patient, and to provide as much comfort as possible since the intense pain is unrelenting.

## Pulmonary Embolism

A pulmonary embolus is an obstruction to blood flow within a branch of the pulmonary artery. It usually results from a free-flowing thrombus (clot) that has formed elsewhere in the body (legs, pelvis, etc.) and is carried by the bloodstream into the major circulatory network. Embolus formation can involve substances other than blood. For example, bone fragments and fat can be released from fracture sites into circulation; or air can be introduced into circulation by various mechanisms, including scuba diving, medication injection, or even douching. Rarely, amniotic fluid can be transported into circulation during pregnancy or early labor, creating a pulmonary embolism.

When the pulmonary circulation is obstructed, chest pain is common. It is sharp, is accompanied by dyspnea, and worsens with deep inspiration.

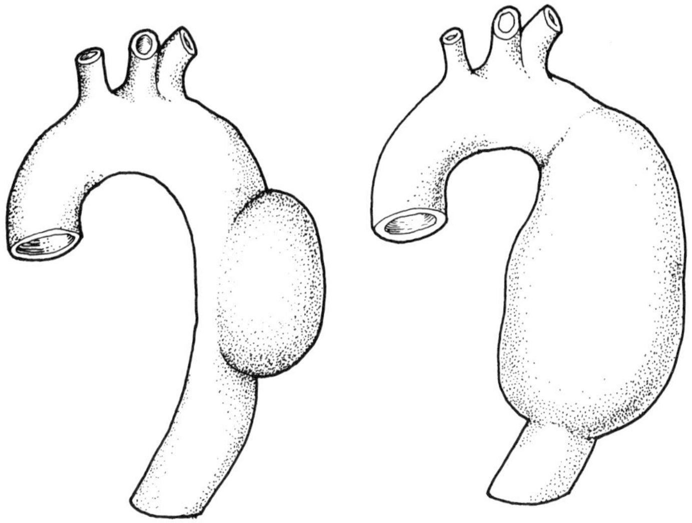

(a) Aortic aneurysms

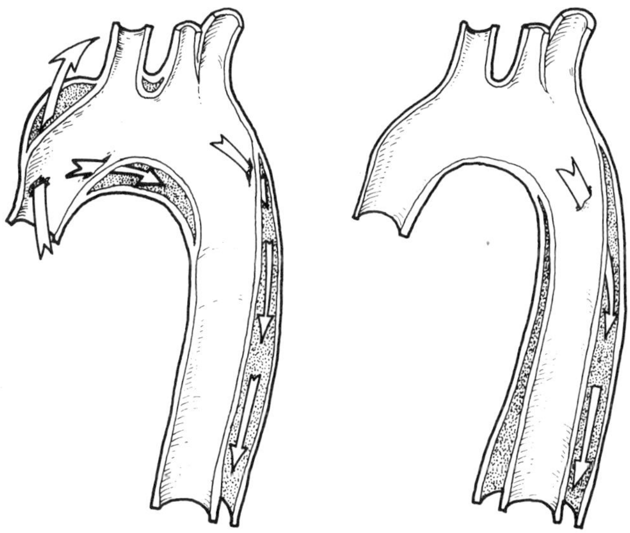

(b) Dissections of aorta. Note blood flow between vessel walls.

**Figure 18–3.** (a) Aortic aneurysms; (b) dissections of aorta. Note blood flow between vessel walls.

Tachycardia, pale skin, lowered blood pressure, wheezing, and anxiety are also commonly noted.

If a pulmonary embolus impairs only a small portion of the pulmonary circulation, symptoms may be mild or vague. However, if a major obstruction to flow is created, a life-threatening condition exists.

The EMT should be alert to the possibility of pulmonary embolism, especially in patients with a history of recent pelvic or abdominal surgery, poor circulation, prolonged bed rest, blood disorders, tumors, and heart disease. Young women who take oral contraceptives are also likely candidates for this emergency.

The care of a patient with suspected pulmonary embolism is the same as for other acute chest pain emergencies previously described.

### Pericarditis

Pericarditis is an inflammation of the sac that surrounds the heart. Trauma, infection, heart disease, and tumors commonly precede its development.

Chest pain is deep and constant and is often described as "knife-like." Onset of the pain is typically gradual, and the patient may report that it is reduced by leaning over and increased by swallowing or deep breathing. Radiation to the neck and left arm is also common.

The patient with suspected pericarditis should be transported to the hospital for care, observing the care regimen described earlier for patients with acute chest pain.

## SUSPECTED CEREBROVASCULAR ACCIDENT (CVA—STROKE)

A cerebrovascular accident results from an interruption to blood flow to the brain. This may be caused by a clot within a vessel, a vasospasm (intense constriction (narrowing) of a blood vessel which slows or occludes flow), or hemorrhage from an aneurysm or ruptured vessel. The cells which depend upon the blood flow by the particular vessel quickly become anoxic and begin to die in less than four minutes. Furthermore, all body functions controlled or influenced by the affected area are impaired or lost. For example, if the speech area is involved, the individual may be unable to talk; if visual centers are involved, blindness may result. The usual causes of CVAs are the same as those cerebrovascular causes responsible for the unconscious state.

The signs and symptoms of a CVA are, of course, dependent upon the area of the brain involved, and include sensory disturbances and motor dysfunction. Speech difficulties, blindness, confusion, paralysis of one side of the body, incontinence, seizures, and changes in vital signs are among the most common. Certain strokes can be readily identified due to the unilateral (u″ne-lat′er-al) (one-sided) facial weakness that results. There may be severe pain in one eye (with eyelid drooping.) The involved cheek may droop and there will be a distinct puckering of that cheek on expiration. Headache and forehead pain on one side may be intense. As the airway is assessed, the EMT may note that the tongue deviates to one side with resultant drooling from the corner of the mouth. In certain kinds of brain hemorrhage, nuchal (nu′kal) rigidity (stiff neck) and vomiting may

Table 18–1. Differentiation of Chest Pain

| | *Characteristics* | *Onset* | *Location* | *Factors which alter it (↑ makes it worse) (↓ decreases it)* |
|---|---|---|---|---|
| Angina | Aching, heavy, burning, choking | Sudden; lasts a few minutes | Retrosternal or may radiate to arms, jaw, teeth, and neck | ↑ by activity, eating, cold weather, stress, lying down<br>↓ Nitroglycerin, rest |
| Myocardial infarction | Viselike, crushing, constricting, severe | Sudden; lasts 30 minutes to one hour or more | Retrosternal or left chest; may radiate to arms, jaw, teeth, neck | ↑ Movement, anxiety, exertion *not relieved* by Nitroglycerin or rest |
| Dissecting aortic aneurysm | Severe, tearing pain; constant; agonizing | Sudden | Mid-chest; radiates to back or possibly to abdomen | Nothing ↑ or ↓ |
| Pneumothorax (See Chapter 17) | Tearing | Sudden | Side of chest | ↑ Breathing |
| Pulmonary embolism | Severe, sharp, knifelike; accompanied by dyspnea | Sudden | Side of chest | ↑ Breathing |
| Pericarditis | Deep pain that is constant and knifelike | Usually gradual | Retrosternal; may radiate to neck and left arm | ↓ Leaning forward<br>↑ Swallowing, deep breathing |

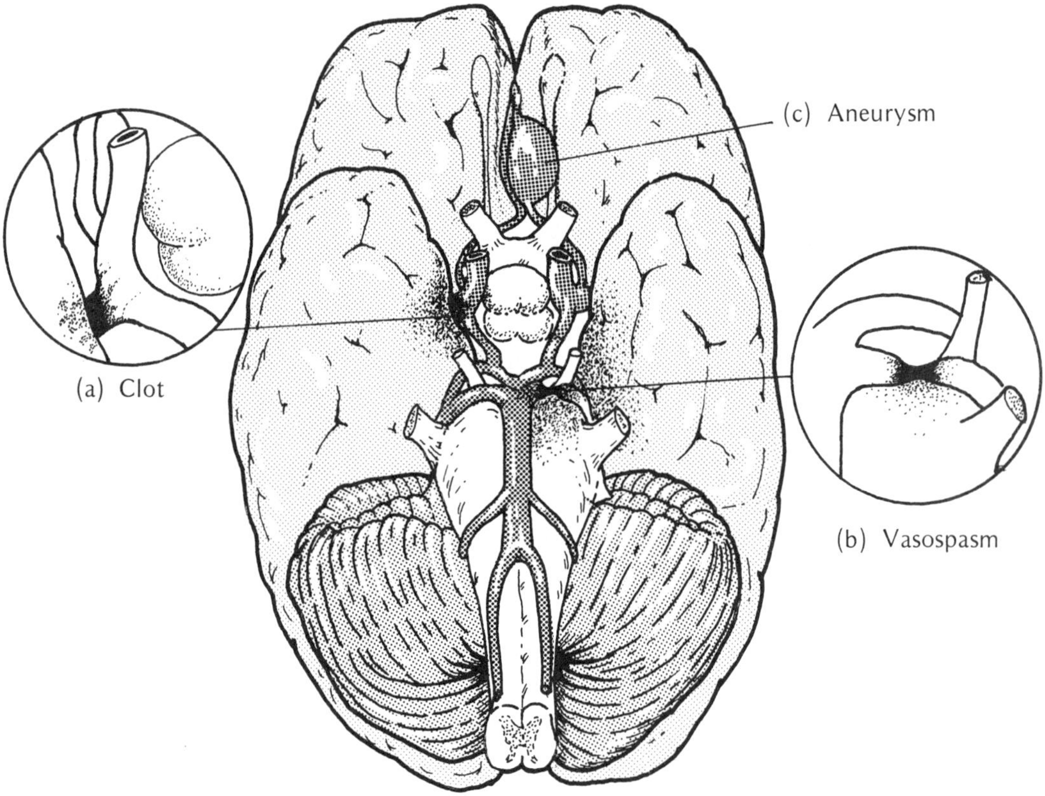


**Figure 18–4.** Causes of a cerebrovascular accident: (a) clot; (b) vasospasm; (c) aneurysm that ruptures.

be apparent. The victim of a stroke may exhibit varying levels of consciousness.

It is interesting to understand that the motor fibers from the brain, which control the lower portions of the body, cross at the level of the medulla. Therefore, if there is a CVA on the left side of the brain, the right side of the body will be affected below the head level. Brain functions which are observable and reflect activity above the medulla will be altered on the same side as the brain is injured. For example, pupillary disturbances would be noted in the left eye for a left-sided CVA.

## Transient Ischemic Attacks

Some individuals suffer transient ischemic (is-kem′ik) attacks (TIAs) or "ministrokes" before they experience a typical CVA. A TIA is indicative of a transient interruption of blood supply and oxygenation to a localized area of the brain. Since the effect is brief and localized, recovery usually occurs in twelve to twenty-four hours without any residual damage. The transient ischemic attack is thought to result from the closing of small intracranial arteries by blood clots or plaques (plaks) from "hardened arteries," a sudden drop in blood pressure or cardiac output, or from mechanical compression of a vertebral artery by head-turning.

Associated signs and symptoms are headache, light-headedness, dizziness, and fainting or a "drop attack." Some victims have a loss of tone in the involved extremities, blurred vision, speech disturbances, confusion, sensory disturbances, and even seizures. Although less dramatic than a stroke and temporary in nature, these signs and symptoms are "warnings" that a major cerebrovascular accident may be impending.

EMTs who encounter patients having a history that suggests TIAs should encourage the individual to seek medical attention at once, even though a total recovery from the transient attack seems evident. Since TIAs are caused by the same problems that eventually result in cerebrovascular accidents, they must be promptly studied by a medical specialist. Careful management of the underlying cardiac or vascular problem can be an important component in preventing a devastating stroke.

## Field Management

When a stroke seems apparent, the EMT should give primary attention to protecting the patient's airway during transport to a medical facility. Position the patient on his side semiprone with the head elevated and face dependent to permit the pooling of secretions in the cheek rather than the throat. Suction as necessary and use airway adjuncts or assisted ventilations if indicated. Oxygen should be given by nasal cannula at 6–8 *l*/minute. Anticipate vomiting since it is likely early in the poststroke period. Take special care to prevent gagging or choking since these elevate intracranial pressure and could make the condition worse.

Monitor vital signs en route since trends of pulse, blood pressure, and respiratory rate are important data in predicting the eventual course of brain injury.

Strokes, like other brain injuries, may result in behavior which is unusual for the patient. He may become combative and use abusive language or profanity. Do not reprimand, scold, or roughly treat the individual whose behavioral control is not possible due to brain tissue hypoxia or other injury. If restraints are necessary for uninvolved extremities, pad them well and check for adequate circulation on a regular basis.

If the eye has been affected by the CVA and the blink reflex is absent, protect the cornea by closing the lid and covering the eye with a sterile gauze square. Explain what you are doing, and why, to reassure the patient.

The importance of careful field management of the patient with a CVA, especially attention to the airway, can greatly influence the eventual outcome for the patient.

*References*

Barber, Janet M., and Budassi, Susan A. *Mosby's Manual of Emergency Care, Practices and Procedures.* St. Louis, MO: The C. V. Mosby Co., 1979.

Barber, Janet M.; Stokes, Lillian S.; and Billings, Diane M. *Adult and Child Care: A Client Approach to Nursing.* St. Louis, MO: The C. V. Mosby Co., 1977.

Berte, J. B. *Pulmonary Emergencies.* Philadelphia, PA: J. B. Lippincott Co., 1977.

Biddle, T. L. "Acute Pulmonary Edema," *Hosp. Med.*, pp. 56–78, December, 1977.

Dack, S. "Acute Pulmonary Edema," *Hosp. Med.*, 14:112, 1978.

Dalen, J. E., *et al.* "Dissection of the Thoracic Aorta: Medical or Surgical Therapy?" *Am. J. Cardiol*, 34:803–808, 1974.

Galant, S. P. "Status Asthmaticus," in Pascoe, D. J., and Grossman, M., editors: *Quick Reference to Pediatric Emergencies.* Philadelphia, PA: J. B. Lippincott Co., 1973.

Plum, F., and Posner, J. B. *Diagnosis of Stupor and Coma,* 2nd ed., Contemporary Neurological Series. Philadelphia, PA: F. A. Davis Co., 1972.

Shibel, E. M., and Moser, K. M. ed. *Respiratory Emergencies.* St. Louis, MO: The C. V. Mosby Co., 1977.

Shoemaker, W. C. "Algorithm For Early Recognition and Management of Cardiac Tamponade," *Crit. Care Med.*, 3:39–63, 1975.

Van Leeuwen, G. J. "Pediatric Emergencies," in Stephenson, H. E., Jr., ed: *Immediate Care of the Acutely Ill and Injured,* 2nd ed. St. Louis, MO: The C. V. Mosby Co., 1978.

# Chapter 19

# Abdominal Emergencies

## TRAUMA AND MEDICAL COMPLAINTS

Abdominal trauma is often a component of multiple trauma and requires prompt assessment and management by the EMT. Many patients with abdominal injuries have coexisting head and chest injuries, which take precedence in the initial care; however, there are also many instances in which alcohol or drug intoxication or coma complicate the evaluation of abdominal complaints. Since intra-abdominal injury may be severe without any external evidence, it is imperative that there be a systematic and thorough approach to any pain or other indications of abdominal problems.

Deaths from abdominal trauma usually occur from undetected or uncontrolled hemorrhage or peritonitis (inflammation of the lining of the abdominal cavity due to rupture of an organ, particularly the bowel). Any patient who has any severe impact involving the abdomen must be viewed with suspicion for such complications.

Organs within the abdominal cavity move freely and even change positions with activity, respirations, or displacement from surrounding distended organs. They are more vulnerable in some locations than in others, due to an enhancement or loss of anatomical protection. The vascular, solid organs such as the liver and spleen are most often injured. Hollow organs like the stomach or intestines are rarely ruptured unless highly distended. The rib cage provides a certain amount of protection for the abdominal organs when it is intact. However, if ribs become fractured, they may actually be the source of damage to the abdominal organs, particularly the liver and the spleen. (See Fig. 19–1.) Pelvic fractures may contribute to intestinal tears, rupture of the bladder, laceration of the ureters, bruising of the kidney, and so forth. The classic seat belt injury is among those resulting in such findings. (See Fig. 19–2.)

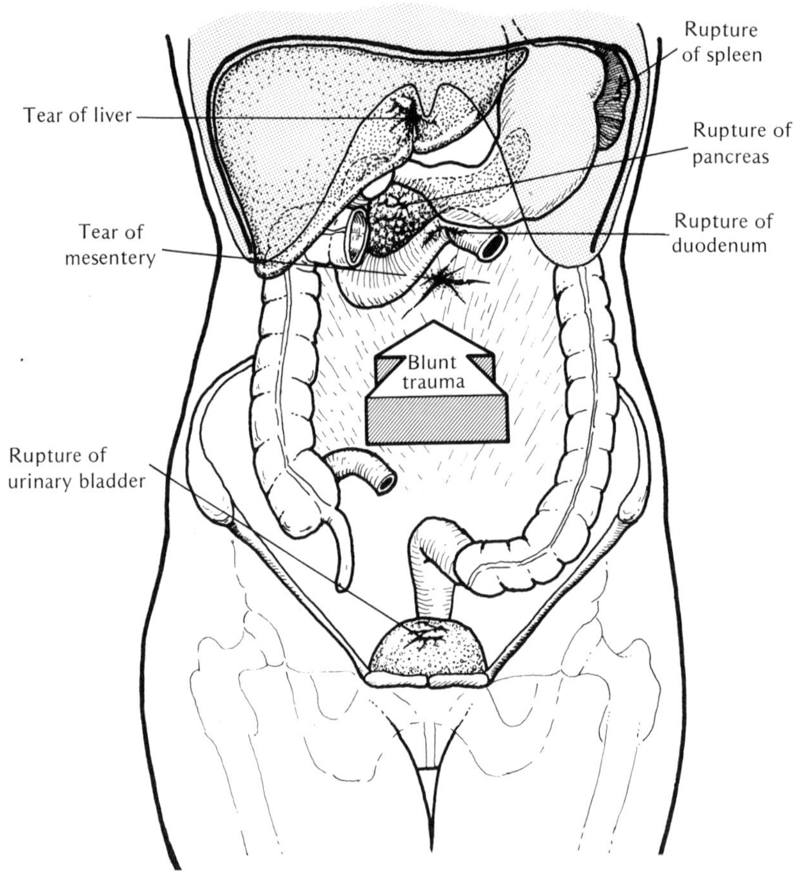


**Figure 19–1.** Organs easily damaged by blunt abdominal trauma.

The EMT should obtain a history that includes attention to details. Was the patient wearing a seat belt? Did he impact the steering wheel? How fast was the vehicle moving? When did the patient eat? Empty his bladder? Anything which can assist in evaluating the forces of trauma are useful in predicting the real nature of injuries.

## ABDOMINAL EXAMINATION

It is often difficult to differentiate important finds relating to abdominal trauma from those that reflect injury to the head, chest, and extremities. Furthermore, in many cases, effects of drugs or alcohol may complicate your examination and its interpretation. In the meantime, shock may become life-threatening.

If feasible, the patient's abdomen should be exposed completely for

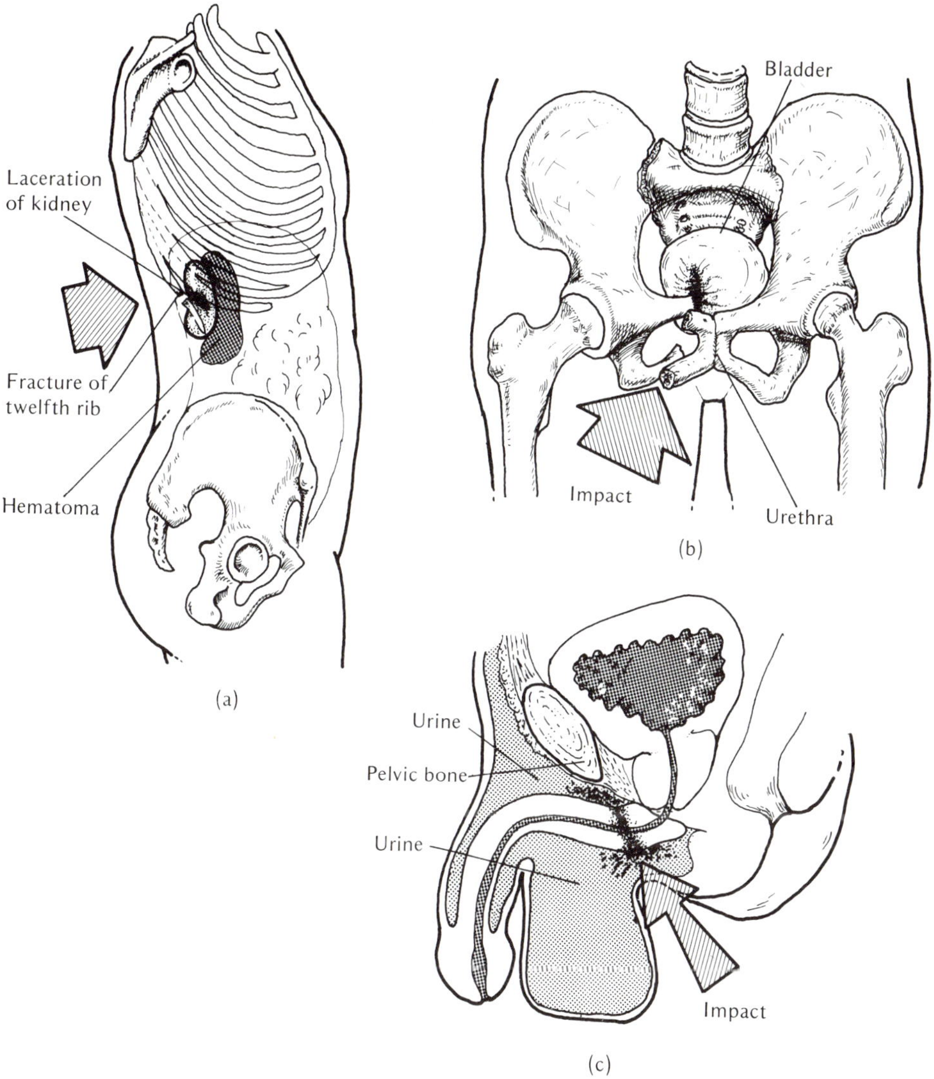


**Figure 19-2.** Trauma to the urinary tract from rib fractures and pelvic fractures. (a) Laceration of kidney from rib fracture. (b) Ruptured bladder from pelvic fracture. (c) Torn urethra from "straddle" injury. Note urine leakage into surrounding tissue.

survey and a measurement of abdominal girth. (See Fig. 19-3.) A measurement of the abdomen at the level of the umbilicus can be a valuable indicator of an enlarging abdomen due to bleeding or other organ damage. This early measurement, when compared with later ones at the hospital, can be most helpful in evaluating abdominal trauma.

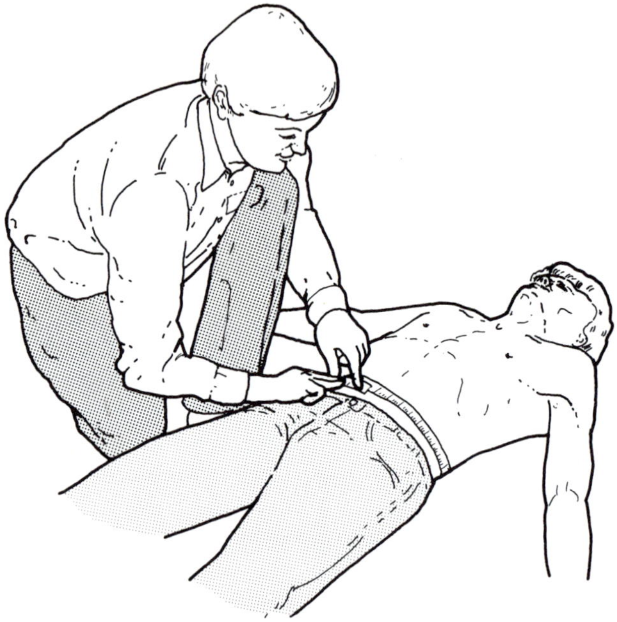

**Figure 19–3.** Measurement of abdominal girth can be a valuable indication of abdominal enlargment due to bleeding within the abdomen or other organ damage.

The patient may be in severe pain. The EMT should note whether symptoms worsen or are less evident over time and whether changes in posture or position affect the degree of discomfort. Referred pain should not be overlooked. For example, shoulder pain could reflect direct injury or might represent diaphragm irritation from blood, bile, or feces. (See Fig. 19–4.)

The abdomen should be inspected for lacerations, discoloration, bruises, or other signs of trauma. Also remember that the patient has a back side, too! Logroll the individual and search the surface for evidence of injury. Pelvic or vertebral fractures often contribute to organ damage which may be reflected by a hematoma at the level of the lumbar spine.

Patients who have ecchymosis (ek″ĭ-mo′sis) (bruising) are candidates for severe internal trauma, but with a slow blood loss. The signs of bruising do not ordinarily appear until twelve to twenty-four hours after injury. Patients who feel that they cannot afford hospital care, or those with no means of transportation are likely to not actively seek medical care after injury. Of course, some persons may have been traumatized, but do not perceive their problem as serious and thus do not elect to be examined. EMTs should be especially cognizant of the later signs of abdominal trauma when assessing a derelict (e.g., vagrant, bum, drunkard) since they sustain such injuries while being "rolled."

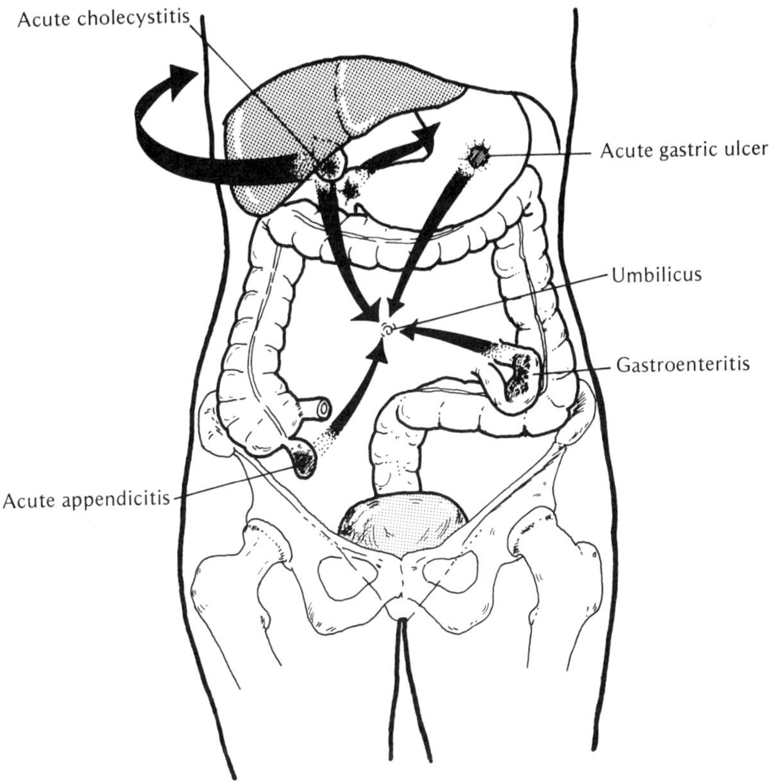


**Figure 19–4.** Pain radiation patterns from acute abdominal conditions.

Abdominal tenderness or rigidity can reflect serious traumatic injury. The EMT should gently palpate over the entire abdominal wall. Before palpating, EMTs should be certain to warm their hands, since cold hands will cause the patient to tense his abdomen. Instruct the individual to relax as much as possible and breathe deeply, which aids in relaxation. Palpation is done with the fingers of one hand, gently pressing downward an inch or two over the entire surface of the abdomen. If a pulsating or throbbing mass is felt, no further examination should be done and the patient should be rapidly transported, since this phenomenon may indicate an aortic aneurysm, which is life threatening. (See page 327.) Any points of obvious injury should be left until the last, since tenderness may cause the patient to tense his abdominal wall muscles, making the remainder of the examination more difficult. Subcutaneous emphysema may be noted. It usually represents injury of the respiratory tract with a resultant downward displacement of air. However, certain injuries of the bowel or rectum could also induce subcutaneous emphysema.

The EMT should be alert to blood on underclothing which may have escaped from the urinary tract or the rectum. Fresh blood from either site indicates internal organ hemorrhage.

Nausea and vomiting are likely when there has been any injury to the abdomen. The EMT must be cognizant of this fact and prepared to protect the airway. (See page 144.) EMT-Is or EMT-Paramedics may be instructed to insert a tube for gastric decompression.

The EMT must assume that all patients who have been traumatically injured in the abdominal region are likely to bleed internally. Since blood loss can be rapid and massive in such instances, life-threatening shock is to be anticipated.

Vital signs should be taken as soon as the basic airway, breathing, and circulatory needs are assured. If there are any signs or symptoms of shock, antishock trousers should be readied while the abdominal examination is being completed. An EMT-I or EMT-Paramedic may also plan to establish one or two IV lines for administration of fluids. It is imperative that the upper extremities be used for fluid administration in abdominal trauma.

The vena cava, a large and important blood vessel which carries blood from the lower body areas to the heart and lung, is frequently torn or occluded in abdominal trauma. Of course, in such instances, the life-sustaining IV fluid would be merely lost into the abdomen and not serve to assist in supporting the vital circulatory volume.

Antishock trousers are extremely valuable aids in controlling shock from abdominal trauma. They should be placed on the patient and inflated partially as soon as evidence of serious trauma is detected. When hypovolemia or shock is apparent (see Chapter 11), they should be inflated further to maintain a satisfactory blood pressure. The abdominal portion should not be inflated in the event that there are impaled objects in the abdomen, or if penetrating wounds have permitted the escape of abdominal organs (evisceration). (See Fig. 14–3.)

If long distance transports are required, advanced EMTs may be instructed to insert a catheter into the patient's bladder which promotes comfort and assists in monitoring urine output which serves as a helpful monitor of cardiovascular status. Furthermore, blood noted in the urine soon after trauma suggests serious damage to the kidneys or other parts of the urinary system.

The EMT who inserts a catheter should never force its advancement if resistance is met, since there may be structural problems that could be worsened by this additional manipulation. If there has been a "straddle" injury to the perineum (per″i-ne′um), no attempt at catheter placement should be made, due to a high likelihood of urethral injury.

## The Pregnant Patient

A patient who is in later pregnancy should be kept on her right side to prevent hypotension that tends to result from compression of the vena cava by the pregnant uterus. This lowered blood pressure may be thought to be from low blood volume and thus too much fluid may be inadvertently given. The right side-lying position and elevation of the legs may be sufficient to restore a low blood pressure to normal if no bleeding exists within the abdomen. Furthermore, if there is bleeding within the pelvis or lower extremities, any compression of the vena cava would obstruct circulation and actually increase hemorrhagic blood loss.

## OTHER ABDOMINAL COMPLAINTS

Acute conditions of the abdomen may result from a complication of a long-term disease process or may actually represent a suddenly developing crisis. There are many problems which can present with signs and symptoms of an "acute abdomen." Pain, tenderness, vomiting, and shock are among those most likely to be encountered by the EMT.

Appendicitis, perforated ulcers, ruptured ectopic (ek-top'ik) pregnancy, renal infections, dissecting or ruptured aneurysm (see page 327), bowel obstruction, renal stones, and infections are only representative of the many conditions that result in acute abdominal complaints.

### Assessment

The EMT should obtain a thorough history of the pain, including onset, duration, nature of any radiation, and if any position or activity makes it more or less tolerable. A history of vomiting or changes in bowel or bladder function should be noted. For women of child-bearing age, an ectopic pregnancy should be considered and, therefore, a menstrual (men'stroo-al) history is relevant.

Vital signs should be obtained and an abdominal examination completed. (See page 336.) The presence of abdominal pain, tenderness and rigidity may indicate peritoneal irritation from blood, feces, or other abdominal contents. It may be possible to distinguish abdominal wall pain from intra-abdominal pain by placing the patient in a head-up position. Pain from abdominal organs usually is lessened in an upright position, but abdominal wall pain would be unaltered.

When the peritoneum has been inflamed or irritated by leaking blood, feces, urine or gastric juices, this condition is termed *peritonitis* (per"ı-to-ni'tis).Peritonitis paralyzes the intestinal tract and results in constipation and abdominal distention, since gas and feces accumulate in the intestine. Any changes in bowel or bladder habits over a three- or four-day period must be noted.

The vomiting of blood is called *hematemesis (hem"*ah-tem'e-sis). Vomiting of bright red blood indicates bleeding in the upper gastrointestinal tract. If the emesis contains dark material that resembles coffee grounds, this suggests that there is bleeding and that the blood has been retained in the stomach long enough to be acted upon by the digestive juices.

The chemical processes of digestion create this phenomenon commonly called "coffee-ground emesis." This condition is classic with the patient who has bleeding from a peptic ulcer. Blood in the gastrointestinal tract which has not been vomited, passes through the bowel and further chemical processes act on it, producing feces that are dark and tarlike in consistency. Bright red bleeding from the rectum may occur from trauma, but typically occurs from hemorrhoids which have been irritated.

Bleeding from the urinary tract or blood in the urine may be caused by urinary tract infections, kidney stones, hypertension (see page 155), and bleeding disorders. Pain and urgency regarding voiding (urinating) may indicate the presence of venereal disease, especially when no bleeding has been evident.

The EMT should note the presence of any of these and attempt to estimate how long the problem has been present, and determine the approximate quantity of lost blood. Shock protocols should be followed.

## Renal Stones

The pain from renal stones can be excruciating when they become mobile and begin to descend through the urinary tract. The pain is "colicky" (kol′ik-e) or intermittent and may radiate to the abdomen, scrotum, or labia. (See Fig. 19–5.) The patient will appear "ashen" and diaphoretic. No position can be assumed that is comfortable and writhing or thrashing about is not uncommon. Some have compared the patient's behavior to the pregnant woman in hard labor. Nausea, vomiting, hematuria (blood in the urine), tachycardia, hypotension, and abdominal distention are likely. A feeling of bladder fullness and an urge to void frequently are often associated with urethral stones.

The EMT can do little to comfort this patient and prompt transportation to a hospital is indicated if renal stones are suspected by history or presentation. Acute appendicitis, a ruptured or dissecting aneurysm, an ectopic pregnancy, or acute gall bladder disease have some similar signs and symptoms so the assessments must be ongoing throughout the transport to promptly detect developing shock or peritonitis.

## Testicular Torsion

Testicular (test-tik′u-lar) torsion is a *dire* clinical emergency characterizd by a twisting of the spermatic cord or the testicle. Pain is intense within the back, flank, and abdomen. Nausea, vomiting, and fever are also associated. The scrotum may be "hot to touch," edematous, and reddened. Immediate surgery is indicated to untwist or remove the affected testicle, so rapid transportation to a hospital is imperative.

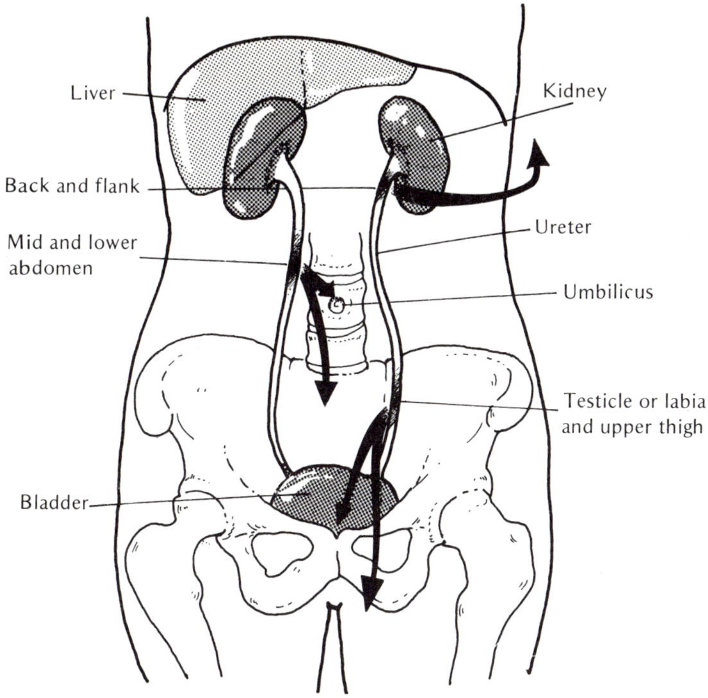


**Figure 19-5.** Characteristic patterns of pain radiating from stones in the urinary tract.

*References*

Barber, Janet M. "Blunt Abdominal Trauma," *Nursing Clinics of North America,* pp. 211–222, Vol. 13, No. 2, June 1978.

Davis, J. J.; Cohn, I.; and Nance, F. C. "Diagnosis and Management of Blunt Abdominal Trauma," *Ann. Surg.* 183:672, 1976.

Generelly, P.; Moore, T. A., III; and LeMay, J. T. "Delayed Splenic Rupture Diagnosed by Culdocentesis," *JACEP,* 6:369–371, 1977.

Jergens, M. E. "Peritoneal Lavage," *Am. J. Surg.,* 133:365–369, 1977.

Meads, G. E., *et al.* "Traumatic Rupture of the Right Hemidiaphragm," *J. Trauma* 17:797–801, 1977.

Shahinpour, N. "The Adult With Bleeding Esophageal Varices," *Nurs. Clin. North Am.,* 12:331–343, 1977.

Steele, M., and Lim, R. C. "Advances in Management of Splenic Injuries," *Am. J. Surg.,* 130:159, 1975.

Wein, A. J., *et al.* "Controversial Aspects of Blunt Renal Trauma," *J. Trauma,* 17:662–666, 1977.

# Chapter 20

# The Musculoskeletal System

The EMT will probably encounter more musculoskeletal injuries in the field than any other type of medical problem. Statistically, musculoskeletal injuries to the extremities are the most common and are seen most often in males in the twenty to forty age group. Vehicular, occupational, and athletic accidents are the major contributing sources. Extremity fractures are rarely life threatening, but may pose a risk to life if associated major blood vessels are severed. The EMT must be able to properly manage and prevent the possibility of further injury in all musculoskeletal trauma. To do this effectively, the EMT must understand the components of the musculoskeletal system and why and when prevention of further injury is necessary.

Components of the musculoskeletal system include bone, cartilage (kar′tĭ-lij), ligament (lig′ah-ment), muscle, and tendon. Each of these components have specific functions that make the musculoskeletal system operate in harmonious fashion.

## SKELETAL BONE

The human skeleton is composed of some 206 bones. It serves four major functions:

1. Locomotion for the body
2. Protection for major organs
3. Formation of specific blood cells
4. Storage and exchange of chemicals, calcium, and phosphate

The human skeleton includes the axial skeleton (bones of the head, neck, and trunk) and appendicular skeleton (bones ot the extremities). (See Fig. 20–1.)

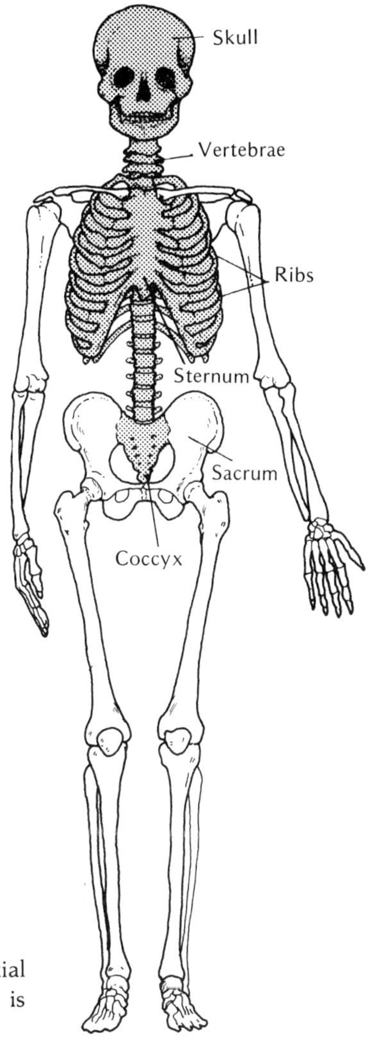


**Figure 20–1.** The appendicular and axial skeleton. The axial skeleton is shaded.

*Bone types*

Bones are classified according to their shape. We have long bones, short bones, flat bones, and irregular bones.

*Long bones* are those whose length is greater than their width. In the upper extremity they include the clavicle, humerus, radius, and ulna. In the lower extremity they include the femur, tibia, and fibula. They also include the metacarpals, metatarsals, and phalanges (fah-lan′jēz).

*Short bones* are almost equal in their dimensions. They include the bones in the hand (carpals) and feet (tarsals)

*Flat bones* come in different sizes and include the ribs, sternum, scapula, and some bones of the skull.

*Irregular bones* are different shaped bones, which include the vertebrae, pelvic bones, and some bones of the skull.

## Growth and Development

Bone is a specialized living connective tissue. It is composed of compact (hard) bone on the outside and spongy (soft) bone on the inside. Each long bone has a shaft known as the diaphysis (di-af'ĭ-sis). The end of a long bone is known as the epiphysis (e-pif'ĭ-sis). The interior shaft (diaphysis) of long bone consists of a hollowlike tube called the *medullary cavity* occupied by red or yellow bone marrow. Red marrow gives rise to red blood cells and certain white blood cells. The production of red and white blood cells starts at infancy, and production decreases with age, when there is an increase in the amount of yellow marrow (fat). In the adult, red marrow is present in the ribs, vertebrae, femur, humerus, sternum, and hip bones. Yellow marrow (fat) is contained in the shafts of the radius, ulna, tibia, and fibula. (See Fig. 20-2.)

In growing bones, their ends (epiphyses) are separated from their shafts (diaphyses) by a growth center called the *epiphyseal plate.* It is at

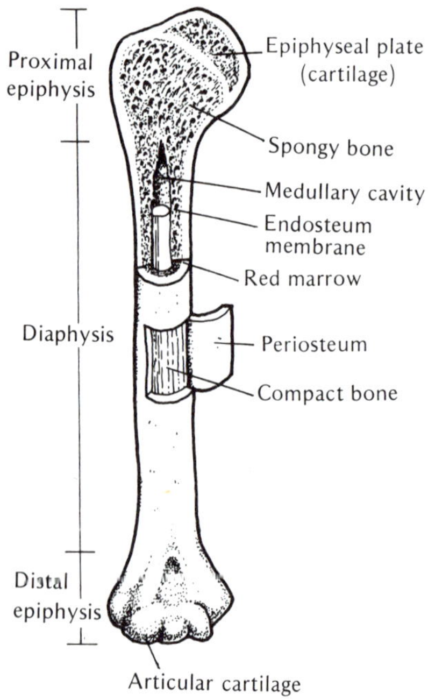


**Figure 20-2.** The internal and external anatomy of a long bone with a saggital section view of the proximal epiphysis.

this plate where bone growth occurs. Fractures in these areas during the growth years could affect the future growth of bone and retard the length. The growth plate in growing bone is composed of cartilaginous material which chemically turns to bone with age. Outside or compact bone is surrounded by a very thin special tissue called *periosteum* (per"e-os'te-um). The inside marrow cavity is lined by a tissue called *endosteum* (en-dos'-te-um). (See Fig. 20-2.) Both periosteum and endosteum have the ability to promote bone growth when disturbed, as would occur to a bone that has been fractured. Normally, when a bone does fracture, mending starts to take place very quickly. A new growth of bone cells in the fractured area is developed and encloses the injured site. This growth around the fracture site is called a bone collar. Uncomplicated fractures of long bones generally heal in six to eight weeks. (See Fig. 20-3.) Bones of growing children are very pliable and can withstand a great deal of stress because of the cartilagenous bone structure in the growing bone. Because bones are living tissue, they are richly supplied with blood vessels and nerves. Bones are supplied with a nutrient artery that pierces compact bone at the shaft and divides lengthwise into two major branches that supply the marrow and compact bone. Arteries that supply the joints pierce the compact bone and supply the spongy (soft) bone and ends of the bone. It is extremely important for growth purposes that this blood supply not be disturbed. Fractures in the arterial area are dangerous to growth of the bone. (See Fig. 20-4.)

Calcium and phosphate are two chemicals necessary for proper bone growth. Ninety-nine percent of the calcium in the body comes from bone and is responsible in aiding muscle contraction and coagulation of blood.

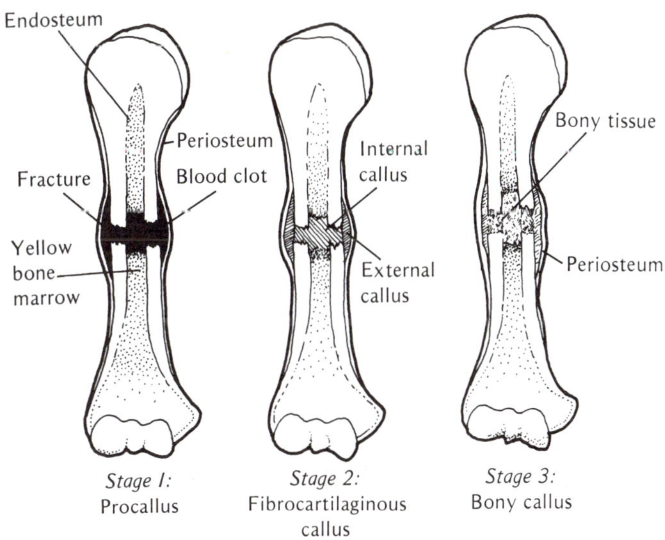


Figure 20-3. Repair stages of fractured bone.

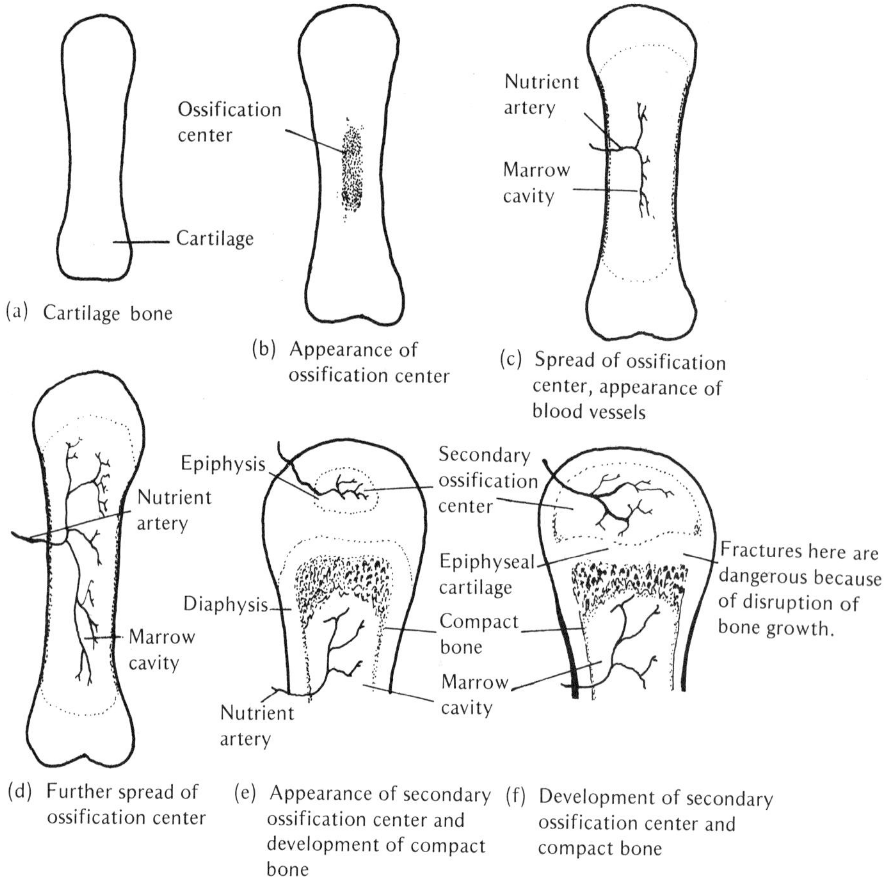


**Figure 20–4.** Stages in bone formation.

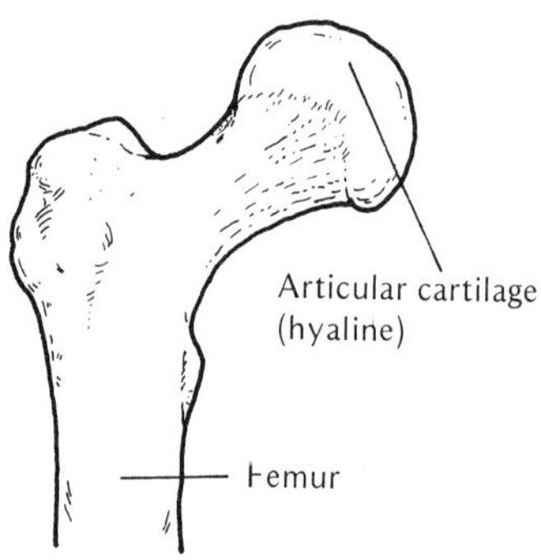


**Figure 20–5.** Articular cartilage covers bone ends for free joint movement.

## Cartilage

Cartilage is a tough resilient living connective tissue. In the human body there are three types, each with a different chemical composition.

*Hyaline or Articular Cartilage,* the most abundant, covers the articular ends of bone and aids in free movement at the joint. (See Fig. 20–5.) When the hyaline cartilage is injured, it is replaced by a weaker cartilage called *fibrotic cartilage. Elastic cartilage* contains elastic fibers and gives structure and support and is chiefly found in the ear, larynx, auditory tube, nose, and trachea. (See Fig. 20–6.)

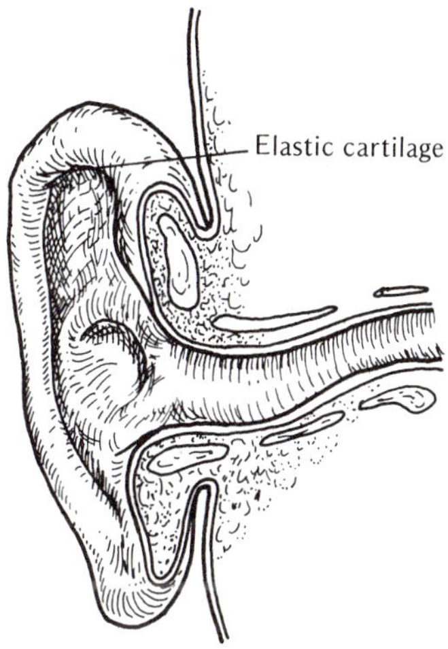


**Figure 20–6.** Elastic cartilage of the ear.

## Joints

Joints are regions in the skeleton where two or more bones meet. They are not a continuation of bones. They allow for body motion with minimum friction. Joints are usually named from the two bones that articulate or meet with one another. For example: the point where the clavicle joins the sternum is known as the sternoclavicular joint; the point where the acromion of the scapula joins the clavicle is known as the acromioclavicular joint. Movable joints are termed *synovial* (sĭ-no′ve-al) *joints* because the joint contains synovial fluid, a thick gel-like substance which lubricates the joint, allowing for friction-free movement. The synovial fluid that is deposited over the articular or hyaline cartilage creates a very slippery surface. The articular surface of the bone is covered with the hyaline cartilage and it is enclosed by what is called the *joint capsule.* The inner surface of the joint capsule is lined by a vascular synovial membrane which produces synovial fluid that fills the joint cavity and provides lubrication. (See Fig. 20–7.)

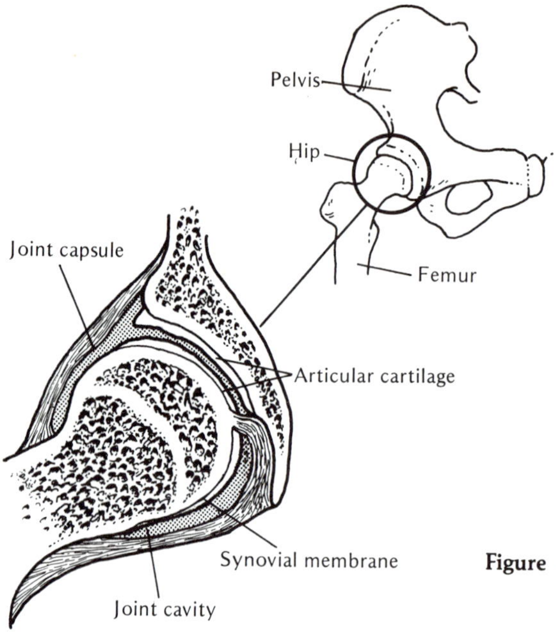


**Figure 20–7.** The joint capsule contains synovial fluid that lubricates the joint.

Other joints in the skeletal system where bones meet, such as skull bones and symphysis pubis, allow little or no motion and are termed *fused joints*. (See Fig. 20–8.)

*Types of Joints*

Synovial joints will be our main concern here, because of the importance of body motion and because there are more of them in the skeleton. The range of motion at joint sites is under the influence of muscles, ligaments, and shapes of bone. The major types of synovial joints are described below.

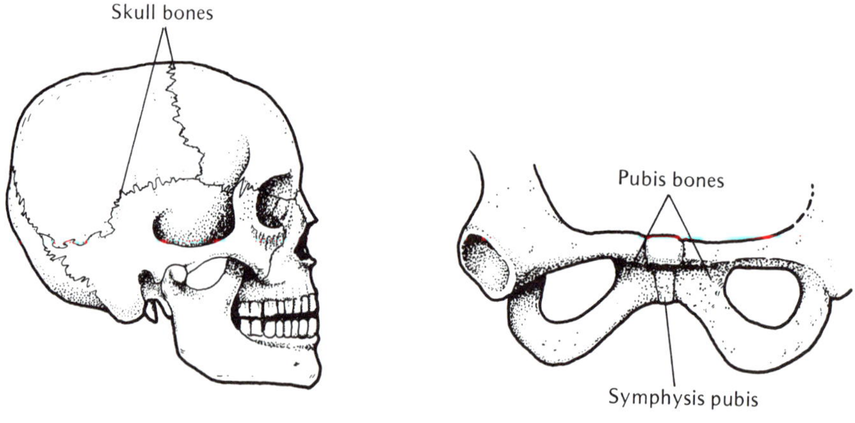


**Figure 20–8.** Fused joints allow little or no movement.

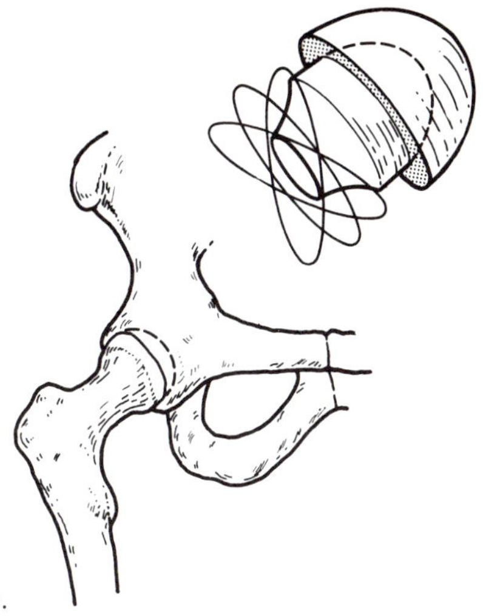

**Figure 20-9.** A ball and socket joint: the hip.

1. *Ball and socket joint (Spheroidal)*—The shoulder joint is an example. The top part of the humerus (the ball) fits into a depression of the scapula (the socket). Because of their construction, the arm has the capability of extension, flexion, adduction, abduction, and circumduction. The hip joint is another example of a ball and socket joint. (See Fig. 20-9.)

2. *Hinge joint (Ginglymus)*—As the name implies, this joint acts only as a hinge. The finger joint and knee joints are examples. They allow only for extension and flexion. (See Fig. 20-10.)

3. *Pivot joint (Trochoid)*—This joint allows bones to pivot on one another. The movement of the radius on the ulna would be an example. The joint allows the forearm to go into supination and pronation with the aid of the distal radius and ulnar joint.

4. *Saddle joint (Sellar)*—The bones of this joint act as saddles by their construction. The joints of the wrist (radiocarpal joint) and hand (carpal-metacarpal) are examples. These joints allow for flexion, extension,

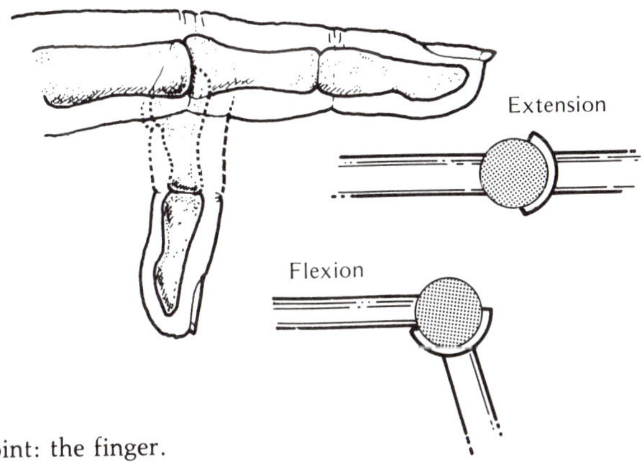


**Figure 20-10.** A hinge joint: the finger.

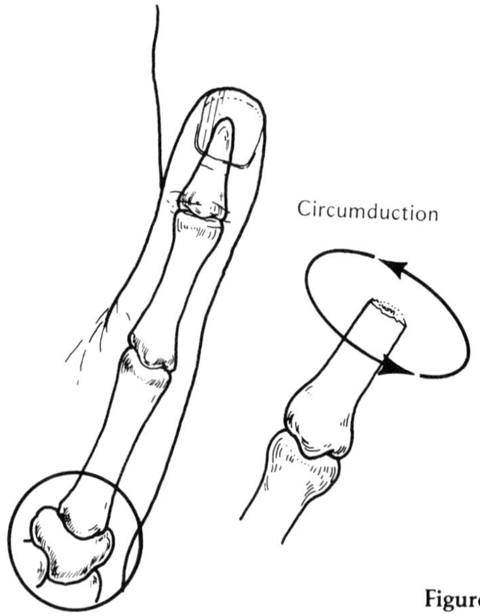


**Figure 20–11.** A saddle joint: the thumb.

abduction, adduction, and circumduction. The thumb, which is a carpal-metacarpal joint, is the most important. It permits flexion, extension, abduction, adduction, circumduction, and opposition. (See Fig. 20–11.)

If the range of motion (ROM) of a joint goes beyond its maximum allowable limits, several different types of injuries may occur:

1. Stretched or torn ligaments (sprain)
2. Stretched or torn muscles (strain)
3. Avulsion fractures
4. Dislocations (Displacement of the bone from the joint. This may be in an anterior, posterior, medial, or lateral displacement.)

## Ligaments

Ligaments help stabilize the skeleton by binding bone to bone. These "little ropes" help oppose body action by not allowing joints to move more than their allowable limits. If the motion in a joint goes too far, ligaments can be stretched. This type of injury is known as a *sprain.* (See Fig. 20–12.) Ligaments have a blood and nerve supply and help initiate protective muscular reflexes for joint motion.

## Tendons

Tendons are the terminal portions of the muscles that cross over joints and attach the muscle to bone. They are subject to injury as are

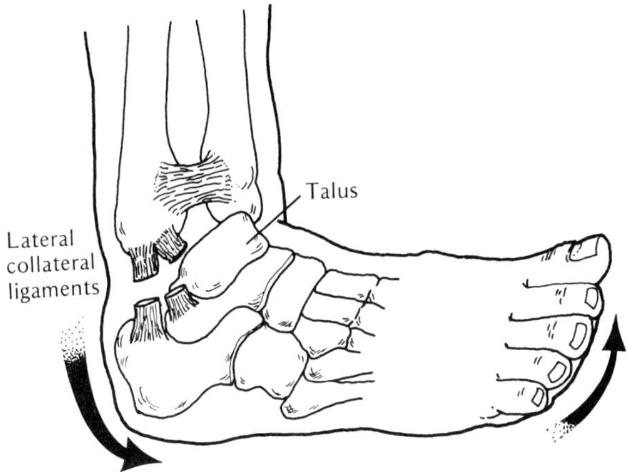


**Figure 20-12.** Sprains occur from torn or ruptured ligaments.

muscles and bones. Too much stress put on a joint can cause the tendon to stretch. Since tendons have a nerve and blood vessel supply, when injured they bleed and cause pain. A force strong enough to stretch tendons can injure other structures, such as muscles, and this results in a strain.

## Muscles

Muscles are a specialized living tissue that help maintain vital functions for life. There are three different types: skeletal, smooth, and cardiac. They are classified as being either voluntary or involuntary in nature.

### *Voluntary Muscle—Skeletal*

Skeletal muscles are attached to bone and most muscles of the body and are located in the extremities. They are termed *voluntary* because they are normally under our conscious command. Muscle cells specialize in the function of contraction (shortening) and relaxation (lengthening). (See Fig. 20-13.) The contraction and relaxation of muscle cells are created normally by chemical reactions. However, muscles may also contract by electrical (electric shock) or mechanical (trauma) stimulation.

Skeletal muscles act as levers to permit different ranges of motion in our extremities. This lever action ability occurs because most skeletal muscles cross over joints. So when the muscles are stimulated, they contract and cause movement at a joint. Skeletal muscle movement is coordinated by the central nervous system. Nerve branches from the different levels of the spinal cord penetrate every skeletal muscle. Therefore, any injury to the spinal cord which causes nerve impairment will also impair muscle function where the nerve innervates that muscle group.

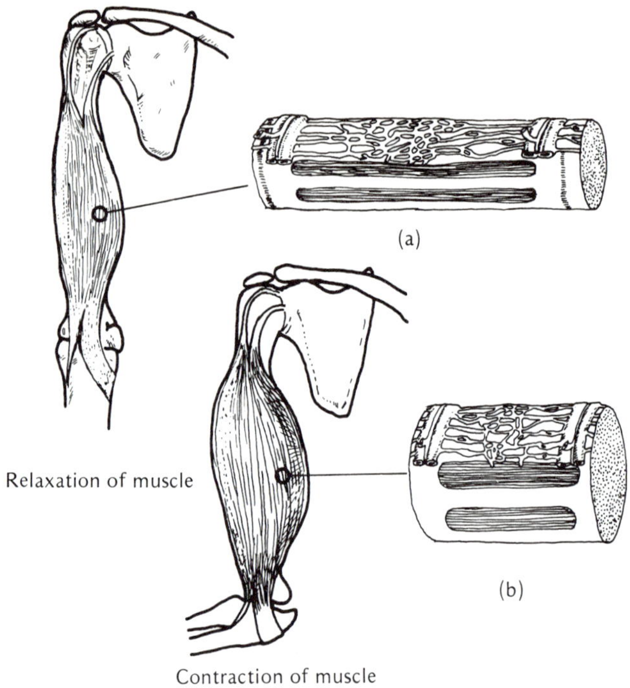


**Figure 20-13.** (a) Relaxation of muscle; (b) contraction of muscle.

*Origin and Insertion*

When a skeletal muscle contracts and shortens, one of its attachments usually remains fixed and the other one moves. The fixed attachment is called the origin of the muscle and the movable one, the insertion of the muscle. In the extremities the more distal parts are usually more mobile; therefore, the distal attachment is usually called the insertion. (See Fig. 20-14.)

*Intermuscular Septum and Blood Vessels*

Muscles are grouped together to perform specific motions such as extension or flexion of an extremity. These muscle groups are separated by a very thin transparent sheath called an intermuscular septum. This septum not only separates muscle groups but provides a frictionless surface to adjacent muscle groups and other close structures. The septum contains nerves and blood vessels that supply the muscles. The intermuscular septums are important because they act as barriers that normally prevent swelling in one area from extending into another area. If swelling is contained within the septum, pressure will increase and the circulatory status may become compromised. (See Fig. 20-15.) This can sometimes be seen in a venomous snake bite victim. So much pressure is caused by the release of body fluid

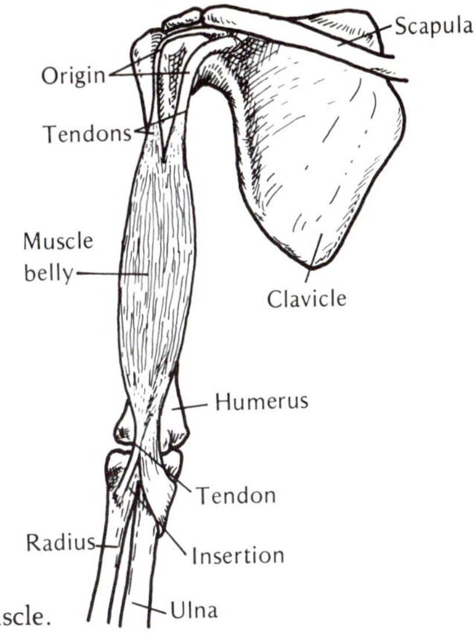


**Figure 20-14.** Origin and insertion of muscle.

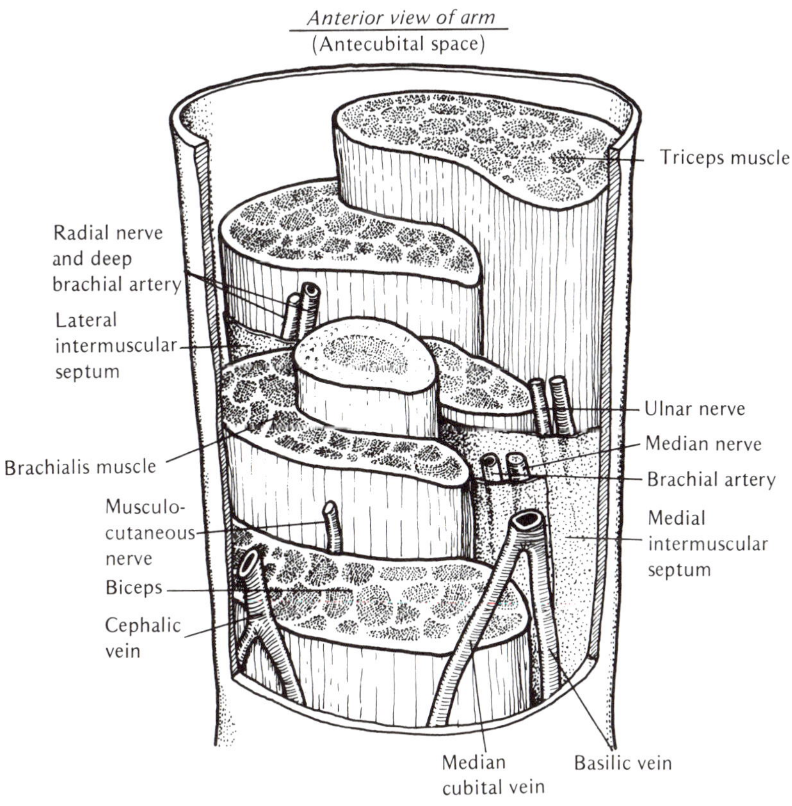


**Figure 20-15.** The intermuscular septum. Note the blood vessels and/or nerves contained in each septum.

in the extremity due to the body's reaction to the snake venom that the victim's extremity must be sliced open to decrease the fluid pressure inside (a surgical procedure called a *fasciotomy* [fash″e-ot′o-me]). *The EMT must remember that pressure in a confined space is an enemy to the body.* Other natural body barriers would include the skull, pericardium, and *pleural cavity*. Any buildup of free fluid that cannot escape will either cause great pain or death, depending on location and the injury that caused the escape of fluid.

### *Involuntary Muscle—Smooth and Cardiac*

Both smooth and cardiac muscles are richly supplied with blood vessels and nerves. They are termed *involuntary* muscle because we cannot always voluntarily command them to perform. For instance, we cannot voluntarily command our hearts to stop beating, nor can we voluntarily stop internal body secretions. The involuntary muscles are under the major control of the autonomic nervous system.

*Smooth Muscle.* Smooth muscle is contained in the blood vessels, pupils of the eyes, and most organs of the body. Contraction of smooth muscle occurs in much the same manner as in skeletal muscle, but at a slower rate. Contraction of smooth muscle is wavelike or rhythmic. *Peristalsis* (per″ĭ-stal′sis) is a term that describes the rhythmic contraction of smooth muscle as fluid or solid products pass through internal tubular structures. (See Fig. 20-16.) For instance, the rhythmic contractions of the esophagus are responsible for peristalsis that propels food to the stomach. The most important factors controlling the wavelike contractions of smooth muscle are:

1. The amount of stretch applied to the muscle
2. Local irritation
3. Effects of the autonomic nervous system

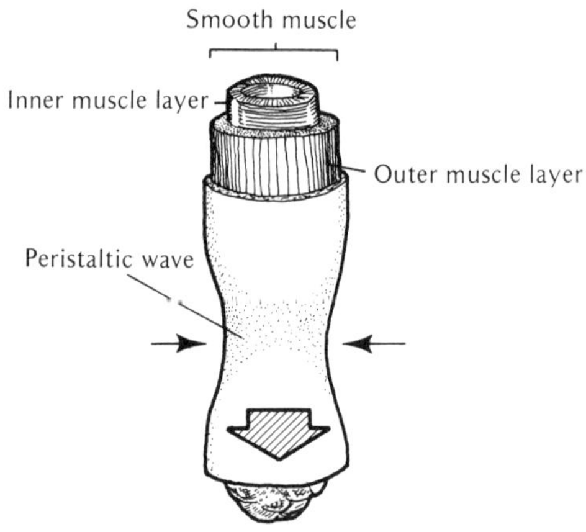


**Figure 20-16.** The anatomy of smooth muscle allows for peristalsis.

*Cardiac Muscle.* Cardiac muscle is unique to the heart. Unlike other muscle, it requires a constant supply of oxygen. (This is why it is always important to give all possible heart attack victims oxygen.) Coronary arteries feed the heart muscle with nourishment and oxygen. Any narrowing or blocking of the coronary arteries causes immediate severe pain (ischemia [is-ke'me-ah]). For instance, when a patient suffers from angina pectoris (narrowing of coronary arteries) or from a myocardial infarction (complete blocking of a coronary artery), he has severe substernal chest pain.

The cardiac muscle also has a slower contraction rate than skeletal muscle, but faster than smooth muscles. This is because the blood can be pumped out of the heart more effectively. Muscular contraction of the heart occurs rhythmically approximately seventy-two times per minute in an adult.

*Voluntary and Involuntary Muscle—The Diaphragm*

The diaphragm is a skeletal muscle attached to the sternum, lower ribs, and lumbar vertebrae. It is the most important muscle of respiration, but not essential for breathing. It separates the thoracic cavity from the abdominal cavity. (See Fig. 20-17.) The diaphragm is both voluntary and involuntary because we can consciously control our breathing rate or stop it (voluntary control). However, we cannot hold our breath for an extended period of time or we would pass out and then respirations would resume once again (involuntary control).

*Muscle Spasm*

Any local irritation factor that affects muscles, such as a severe cold, lack of blood flow, or overexercise of muscle can cause pain. This pain is

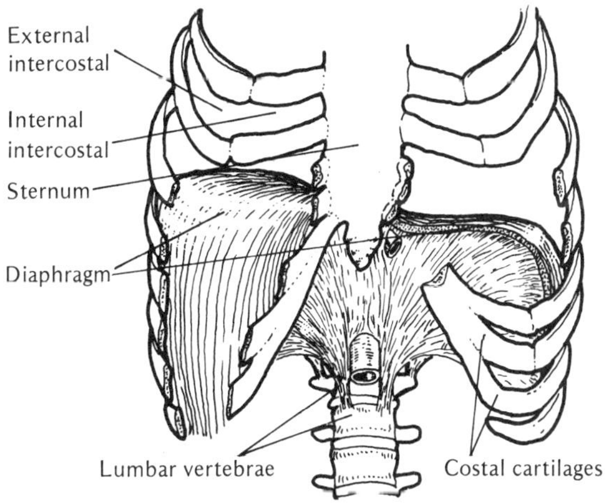


**Figure 20-17.** The diaphragm attaches to the ribs, sternum, and vertebrae.

transmitted from the muscle to the spinal cord, causing the muscle to contract (in a spasm). The muscle spasm causes pain because the contracting muscles compress the blood vessels inside the muscle and reduce or cut off blood supply.

The EMT should remember that injuries such as fractures can cause great muscle spasm to occur. Thus, we must properly splint fractures to help reduce spasm and pain.

### *Rigor Mortis*

One of the most characteristic changes that occur after death is stiffening of the body. This boardlike stiffness is known as *rigor* (stiffness) *mortis* (death). It varies how soon after death it occurs and how long it lasts.

Rigor mortis is chiefly due to the loss of a compound known as ATP (adenosine triphosphate), which gives energy to muscles.

## ANATOMY OF THE APPENDICULAR SKELETON

The appendicular skeleton consists of the upper and lower extremities. (See Fig. 20–1.)

### Upper Extremity

Skeletal bones of the upper extremity include the clavicle, scapula, humerus, ulna, radius, carpals, metacarpals, and phalanges. (See Fig. 20–18.)

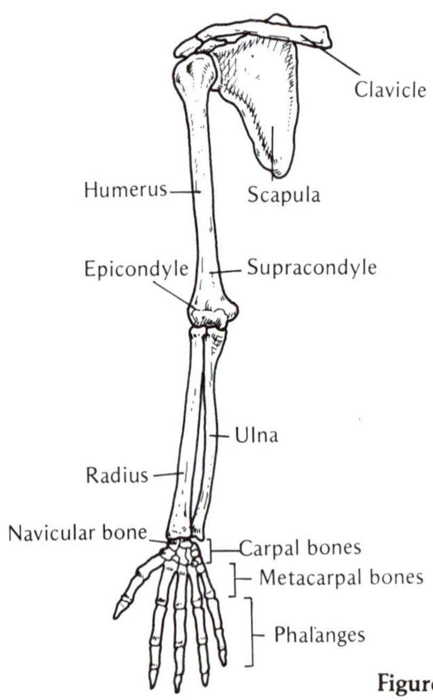


**Figure 20–18.** Anatomy of the upper extremity.

*Shoulder Girdle*

The shoulder girdle is formed by the scapula or shoulder blade and the clavicle or collarbone. (See Fig. 20–19.)

*Clavicle (Collarbone)*

The clavicle is a long bone that acts as a support for the shoulder. It has a medial or sternal end and a lateral or acromial end. The medial end articulates with the manubrium (mah-nu′bre-um) (upper part of the breast bone) to form the sternoclavicular joint. The lateral end articulates with the top of the scapula known as the acromion and forms the acromio-clavicular joint. Anatomically, the clavicle is positioned where it is subjected to frequent injury. This is due in part because of its anterior location and its very little anterior muscle protection. Clavicular injuries occur frequently in contact sports, since motion of the clavicle is limited.

*Scapula (Shoulder Blade)*

The scapula is a flat triangular bone situated on the posterior lateral thoracic rib cage. The scapula is connected to the clavicle and articulates with the humerus (upper arm) at the glenoid cavity. This connection constitutes the gleno-humeral joint (ball-and-socket joint). The scapula moves quite freely which allows for a wide range of motion for the shoulder girdle. The scapula is well protected because it is embedded in muscle. Violent direct trauma is usually required to injure this bone.

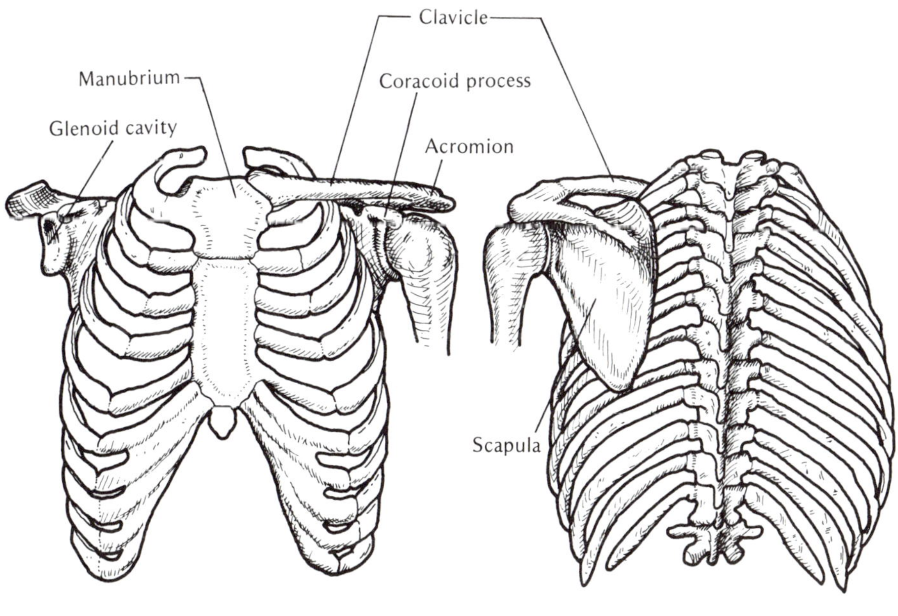


Anterior

Posterior

**Figure 20–19.** The shoulder girdle.

### *Humerus (Upper Arm)*

The humerus is a long bone. The proximal end forms part of the shoulder where it articulates with the scapula in the glenoid cavity. The distal end of the humerus articulates with the radius and ulna and forms the upper part of the elbow joint.

### *Radius and Ulna (Forearm)*

The radius and ulna are long bones. The proximal ends of the radius and ulna make up the lower part of the elbow joint. The radius and ulna at the joint articulates with the humerus. The distal portion of the radius articulates with the carpal bones of the wrist, and together they form the wrist joint. The posterior side of the ulna at its proximal end has a bony projection, the olecranon (o-lek'rah-non) process, known as the elbow or funny bone.

The radius is shorter than the ulna and is on the thumb side of the forearm. The ulna is located on the little finger side of the forearm.

### *Carpal Bones (Wrist)*

Carpal bones are short bones. There are eight of them, situated in two rows, four in each row. The top row consists of the scaphoid, lunate, triquetrum, and pisiform. The bottom row consists of the trapezium, trapezoid, capitate, and hamate. (See Fig. 20–20.) The wrist is very mobile and articulates with the metacarpals, radius, and with one another. The bone most frequently fractured in the wrist is the scaphoid.

### *Metacarpal Bones (Hand)*

Metacarpal bones are considered long bones. There are five that articulate proximally with the phalanges and distally with the wrist.

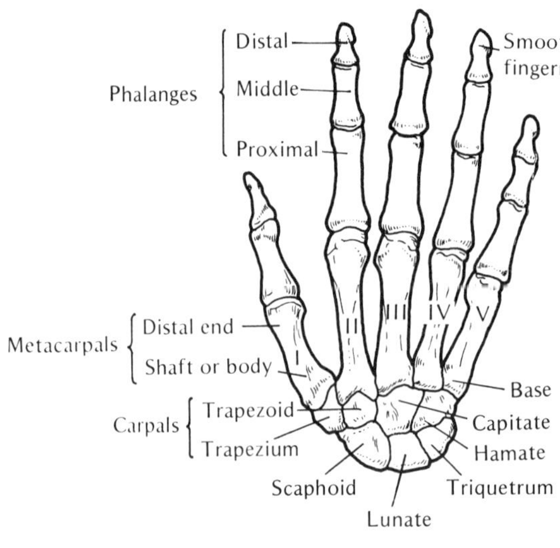


**Figure 20–20.** Bones of the wrist and hand.

*Phalanges (Fingers)*

The phalanges are short bones. There are three bones in each finger, except for the thumb, which has two bones. The finger bones are divided into three parts: distal, middle and proximal. The distal phalanges form the fingertips; the middle and proximal phalanges form the knuckles.

## Lower Extremity

Skeletal bones of the lower extremity include the pelvis, femur, patella, tibia, fibula, tarsal, metatarsal, and phalanges.

*Pelvis (Hip Bone)*

The pelvis is an irregular bone that connects the upper torso to the lower torso. The pelvis is divided into three bones which are all fused together. The ilium or innominate bones are known as the wings of the pelvis, which flare out to form the hips. The ischium is the lower posterior part of the pelvis. When we sit we rest upon our ischium. It is also here where the pressure from a traction splint is felt. The pubis is the lower anterior bone. The ilium, ischium, and pubis all fuse together at the bottom of the pelvis to form the acetabulum (as″e-tab′u-lum) (the socket) into which the head (the ball) of the femur (ball and socket joint) fits. (See Fig. 20–21.)

*Femur (Thigh)*

The femur is the longest, largest, and heaviest bone in the human skeleton. The femur has a proximal end (the head) that fits into the acetabulum, a shaft (middle part) and a distal end that forms the upper part of the knee joint. On the medial and lateral surface of the distal femur are bony bumps known as condyles. The distal femur articulates with the tibia. (See Fig. 20–22.)

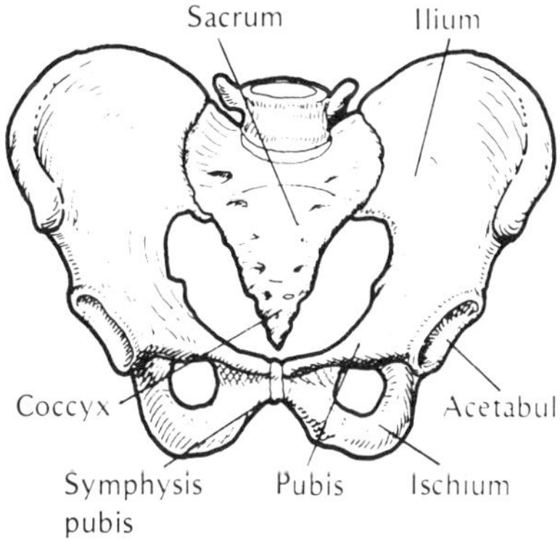


**Figure 20–21.** The pelvis.

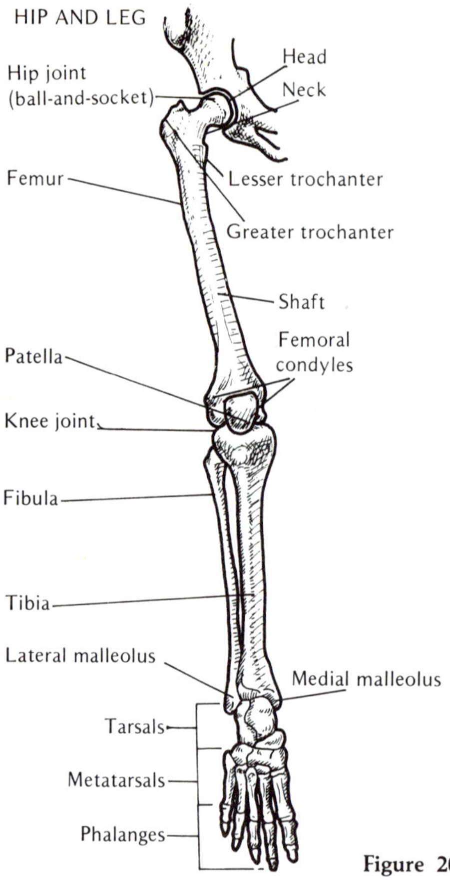


**Figure 20–22.** Anatomy of the lower extremity.

*Patella (Kneecap)*

The patella is a small triangular bone that sits just anterior to the knee joint. By its location, it affords some protection to the joint. The patella is encased in the tendon of the upper thigh muscle (quadriceps muscle). When this muscle is relaxed you can move the patella; when the muscle is tightened you cannot. Injury to the patella may occur from violent contraction of the quadricep muscle or by direct trauma.

*Tibia and Fibula (Leg Bones)*

The tibia and fibula are long bones that run parallel to one another. The tibia or shin bone is the second largest and heaviest bone in the body after the femur. The proximal end of the tibia articulates with the distal femur to form the lower part of the knee joint. The distal end of the tibia articulates with the tulus, a tarsal bone of the ankle. The tibia is on the medial side of the leg.

The fibula is formed just below the knee joint and runs distally to articulate with the talus. The fibula is on the lateral or little toe side of the

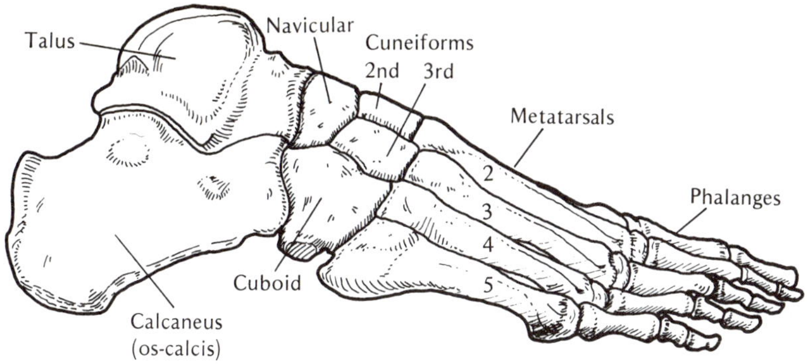


**Figure 20-23.** Bones of the foot.

leg. At the distal end of the tibia and fibula are two bony prominences known as the malleoli. (See Fig. 20-22.) The prominence on the distal tibia is known as the medial malleolus, whereas the prominence on the distal fibula is known as the lateral malleolus. Injuries to the tibia are much more common because of its anatomical closeness to the skin surface.

*Tarsal Bones (Ankle)*

There are seven short bones that form the ankle. The calcaneus or os calcis (heel bone) bears and transmits all body weight. The talus (ankle bone) articulates with the tibia and fibula to form the ankle joint. There is also the cuboid, navicular, and three cuneiform bones. The navicular, cuboid, and cuneiforms together with the metatarsal bones form the arch of the foot. (See Fig. 20-23.)

*Metatarsal Bones (Foot)*

The metatarsal bones are considered long bones. There are five metatarsal bones which are longer and thicker than the metacarpal bones. The metatarsal bones articulate with the tarsal bones to form the tarsal-metatarsal joint. The metatarsals are numbered one through five, one being on the big toe side and five on the little toe side.

*Phalanges (Toes)*

Phalanges are short bones. There are three bones in each toe except for the big and little toe, each of which has only two bones.

## INJURIES TO BONES—FRACTURES

A fracture is the disruption in the continuity of bone. Laypersons frequently use the terms *break* and *crack* to denote a specific difference in the severity of bone injury, but both terms medically mean the same as a fracture. The EMT must remember that a fracture is more than just a broken bone. Forces strong enough to break bones may also injure muscles, blood vessels, and other surrounding soft tissue.

## Categories of Fractures

Fractures are usually addressed as being:

1. *Closed (simple)*—the skin has not been penetrated by the underlying broken bone fragments.

2. *Open (compound)*—the skin has been broken, creating an open wound exposing the bone. This open wound can be created from the underlying sharp bony fragments breaking through the skin; or from external direct trauma, which first causes the open wound and then fractures the bone, exposing it.

The EMT should use the terms *closed* or *open* whenever denoting a fracture. (See Fig. 20-24.)

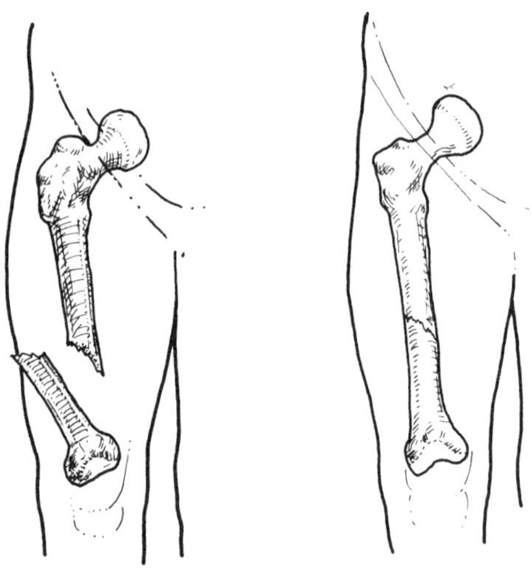

Open fracture Closed fracture

**Figure 20-24.** (a) Open or compound fracture; (b) closed or simple fracture.

## Classification of Fractures

Fractures are classified according to the direction of the fracture line. (See Fig. 20-25.) They include:

1. *Greenstick fracture*—a fracture in which the bone does not break completely. This type of fracture occurs only in children and young adolescents.

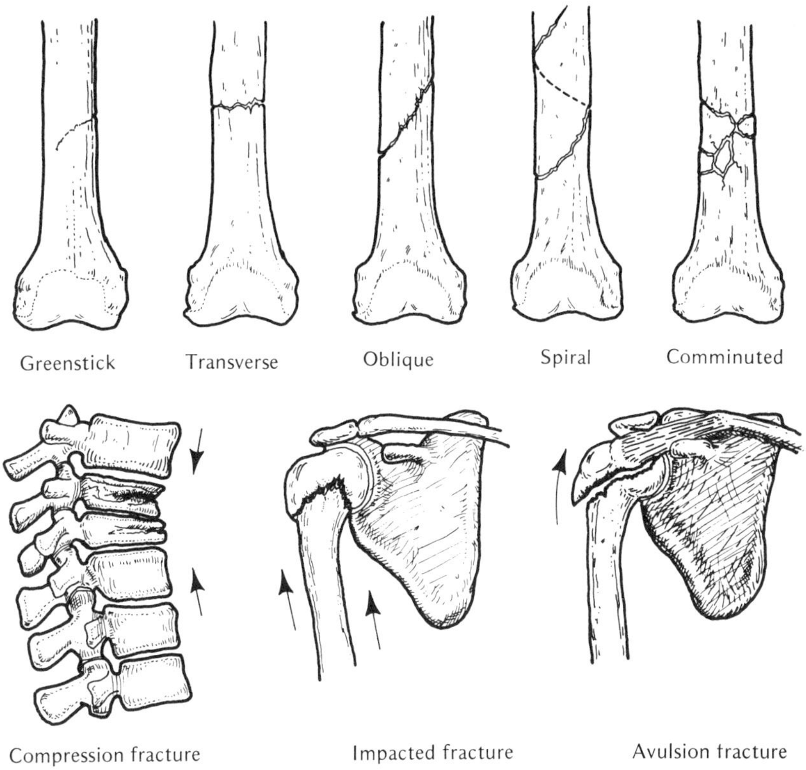


**Figure 20-25.** Classification of fractures.

2. *Transverse fracture*—a bone that is broken straight across (ninety degree angle).

3. *Oblique fracture*—a bone broken in a diagonal line (forty-five degree angle).

4. *Spiral fracture*—this line of fracture spirals around and through bone.

5. *Comminuted fracture*—a fracture in which the bone is broken into three or more fragments.

6. *Compression fracture*—This type of fracture, which compresses the vertebrae, is a common injury to the spine. It is usually due to diving accidents, falls from heights, or acceleration-deceleration accidents.

7. *Impacted fracture*—a fracture in which the bone fragments are embedded in the substance of one another.

8. *Avulsion fracture*—a piece of bone is pulled away from its primary structure. This type of fracture usually occurs when twisting injuries pull ligaments so violently that a piece of bone comes with it.

One can see that there are several ways in which bone integrity can be disrupted. Unfortunately we are not x-ray machines and we cannot see exactly what type of fractures exist. Nevertheless, the EMT should be aware of these different types of fractures because many times the way in which the injury occurs may help determine the kind of fracture that the patient could possibly have.

## Mechanism of Injury

One of the responsibilities of the EMT in the field, at the accident scene, is to note how the injury may have occurred or what the mechanism of injury was. This will aid the physician later in determining injury possibilities. When any force exceeds bone strength, musculoskeletal injuries may occur. Factors that may cause fractures include:

1. *Direct trauma*—the injury occurs at the point of impact (e.g., a broken leg caused from the bumper of a car).

2. *Indirect trauma*—the injury occurs away from the point of impact (e.g., a fractured forearm occurring when the hand is used to shield the fall).

3. *Disease process*—an illness that causes the bone to weaken or decay so that a slight bump may be all that is necessary to cause a fracture (e.g., cancer, rickets, etc.).

4. *Compressional force*—a force that flattens or presses bone into one another (e.g., a patient who jumps from a high place may incur a compression fracture of his vertebrae. Also common in acceleration-deceleration injuries). (See Fig. 20-26.)

5. *Muscle contraction*—an injury or illness that causes the muscle to contract so violently that the bone fractures (e.g., electric shock, seizures, tetany, etc.).

6. *Stress (fatigue) forces*—forces in which fractures are caused by repeated stress on the bone (e.g., army recruits who march for long periods of time may fracture bones of the feet. Also, skydivers who make many jumps frequently have compression fractures of the vertebrae).

## Assessment of Fractures

The EMT must remember that with every patient the airway, breathing, and circulatory status are the first priorities in patient assessment. After these are checked then you can proceed with further assessments.

To thoroughly assess the patient for fractures, ask him first where he hurts. Do not move him to investigate this area. If the patient has clothing over the injury, it must be removed so that you can inspect the area more closely. After investigating the patient's immediate complaints, you should very lightly palpate and compress bony areas from head to toe, asking the patient as you proceed if what you are doing hurts in any way.

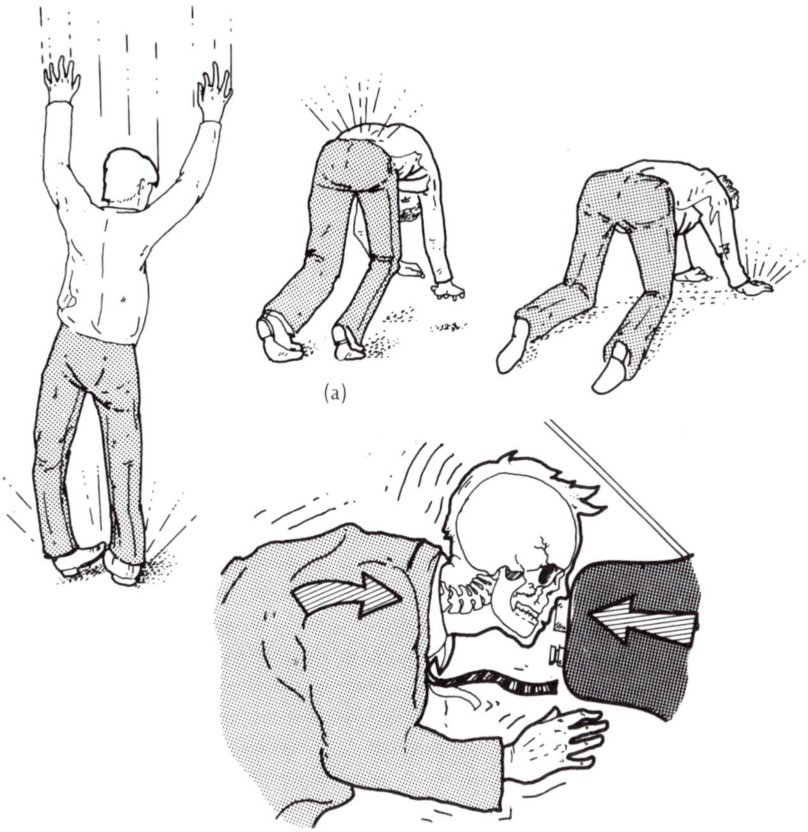

(a)

(b)

**Figure 20-26.** (a) Compression fractures may occur from jumping from heights or (b) acceleration-deceleration injuries.

While touching the patient, feel for depressions and deformities. It is not infrequent that the patient has a fracture and is not bothered by it. Make sure you palpate the entire spine and lightly compress the ribs and pelvis to elicit pain response. By investigating the patient in this manner you can determine the need for special transport using a spine board or spine immobilizer and the proper position for ambulance transport. With every patient that the EMT suspects a fracture, check for the "five Ps." These include:

1. *Pain*—pain occurs with almost every fracture. Usually there is point tenderness at the injured site and inability to move the affected area. Pain associated with a fracture is caused by tension from swelling and bone fragments that irritate nerves.

2. *Pallor*—paleness to the skin. The color of the area should be noted, as well as temperature. If there is lack of blood flow below the frac-

ture site, the limb will be cool. Remember to take into consideration the environmental conditions in which the patient is located.

3. *Paresthesia* (par″as-the′ze-ah)—a numbness or tingling sensation. This may be present distal to the fracture site if there is nerve damage from the injury.

4. *Paralysis*—inability to move a limb. This condition may be present if the nerve has been damaged. The EMT should always assess movement and feeling distal to the fracture site. Check to see if the patient can move his fingers and toes.

5. *Pulse*—Is there a pulse distal to the fracture site? The EMT should always determine the circulatory status distal to the injured site—in the upper extremity determine if brachial and radial pulses are present. In the lower extremity determine the presence of femoral, popliteal, posterior tibialis, and dorsalis pedis pulses.

The EMT should also check for the following fracture signs and symptoms during his assessment.

1. *Swelling*—Swelling may occur with fractures due to a loss of soft tissue fluid or blood escaping into the subcutaneous tissues.

2. *Deformity*—the contour of the possibly injured extremity should be noted. The EMT should check the opposite extremity to compare shape and equality. What looks abnormal to you may be quite normal to the patient.

3. *Crepitus*—crepitus (krep′ĭ-tus) is a crackling sensation that may be felt upon palpation. This is due to bony fragments moving against one another. The EMT should never purposely check for this sensation. Crepitus is usually felt when the patient moves while you are stabilizing the injured part.

4. *Ecchymosis* (ek″ĭ-mo′sis)—bruising. A blue-black discoloration to the skin. This is usually indicative of trauma to the injured area.

5. *Inability to move*—the patient will usually guard against moving the injured part.

### *Other Considerations*

Since most fractures occur to the extremities, shirts, pants, shoes, gloves, etc., must be removed or cut away to inspect the injured area and determine treatment needed. A common-sense approach to the patient and situation should be used. Depending on the situation, honor and understand the patient's modesty. This is especially true of adolescents and elderly female patients. If it is possible and medically prudent to move the patient away from onlookers, stabilize the patient and complete your assessment in a more conducive area, such as in the ambulance. If crowd control is possible, ask that it be enforced!

The upper extremity skeletal bones include:

Clavicle } shoulder
Scapula }

Humerus—upper arm

Ulna } forearm
Radius }

Carpals—wrist

Metacarpals—hand

Phalanges—fingers

## Shoulder Fractures

### *Clavicle*

Fractures to the clavicle usually occur between the inner two-thirds and outer one-third of its length. Clavicle fractures are common in children and occur frequently in contact sports and falls onto an outstretched arm.

*Signs and Symptoms:* Because of the clavicle's close proximity to the humerus, the patient will usually have his arm close to his side and not move it. There is point tenderness over the injured area upon palpation, and there may be deformity. The EMT should always lightly palpate both clavicles and compare the contour of both shoulders.

*Complications:* If the fracture occurs in the inner two-thirds of the clavicle, be alert to the possibility of a pneumothorax. Listen for breath sounds! The top of the lung can extend above the first anterior rib during inspiration, so the lung lies close to the clavicle. (See Table 20-2.)

The subclavian artery and vein, as well as the brachial plexus, lie inferior to the clavicle and could be injured. (See Table 20-1.) Check the circulatory and nerve status of the arm on the injured shoulder side. (See Fig. 20-27.)

TABLE 20-1. POSSIBLE SITES OF VASCULAR TRAUMA WITH ORTHOPEDIC INJURIES

| *Bone* | *Vessel* |
|---|---|
| Depressed clavicle fracture | Subclavian artery or vein |
| Supracondylar fracture of humerus | Brachial artery |
| Proximal tibia fracture | Popliteal artery |
| Posterior knee dislocation | Popliteal artery |
| Anterior shoulder dislocation | Axillary artery or vein |
| Posterior pelvic (ilium) fracture | Iliac artery |
| Ribs | Intercostal artery or vein |

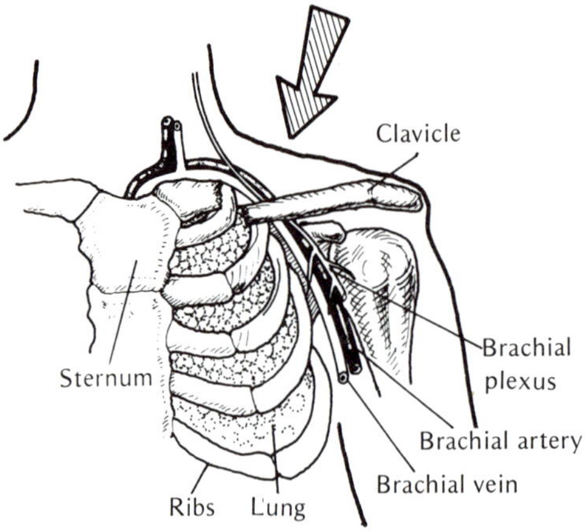


**Figure 20–27.** A depressed fractured clavicle may injure the brachial plexus and/or create a pneumothorax. The EMT-A should always check these possibilities during assessment.

*Stabilization:* The fractured clavicle can be stabilized by the sling and swath. If there is any reason to believe that pulmonary status has been compromised from the injury, do not let the patient walk to the ambulance.

*Scapula*

A fractured scapula is an uncommon injury because the bone is embedded in muscle. However, severe direct trauma could cause the scapula to fracture. (See Fig. 20–28.)

*Signs and Symptoms:* Bruising, swelling, point tenderness, and pain upon shoulder movement.

*Complications:* Since posterior ribs two through seven lie under the scapula, they could be fractured from the trauma and puncture the lung. The EMT should rule out the possibility of a pneumothorax. Auscultate (aws′kul-tāt) lung fields front and back. (See Table 20–2.)

*Stabilization:* The injured shoulder should be immobilized by applying a sling and swathe.

Table 20–2. Possible Sites of Visceral Trauma with Orthopedic Injuries

| *Bone* | *Viscera* |
|---|---|
| Depressed clavicle fracture | Lung |
| Anterior and posterior first through tenth ribs | Lung |
| Scapula | Lung |
| Xiphoid process | Liver |
| Posterior tenth through twelfth ribs | Kidneys |
| Left anterior second through fifth ribs | Heart, lung |
| Pelvis | Bladder, urethra, colon, intestine |

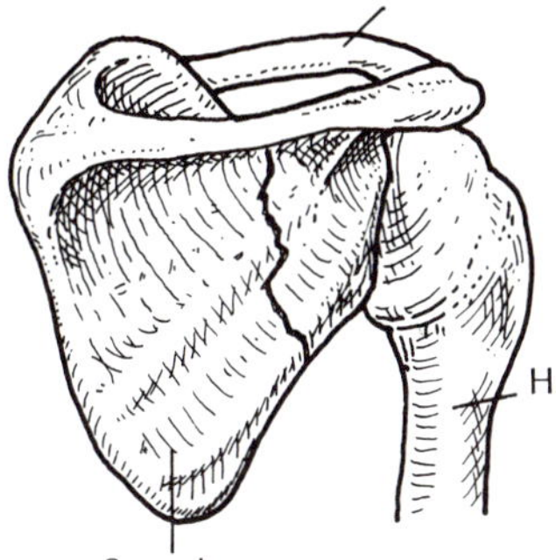


**Figure 20-28.** A fractured scapula, posterior view.

## Upper Arm

### *Humerus*

The humerus is divided into three portions to describe fracture sites. Fractures to the humerus may be proximal, midshaft, or supracondylar. The supracondylar or distal portion of the humerus is discussed in elbow fractures.

TABLE 20-3. POSSIBLE SITES OF NERVE DAMAGE WITH ORTHOPEDIC TRAUMA

| *Bone* | *Nerve* |
|---|---|
| Depressed clavicle fracture | Brachial plexus |
| Middle and distal third of humerus | Radial |
| Distal humerus, proximal, and distal radius and ulna | Median |
| Medial epicondyle of humerus | Ulnar |
| Proximal lateral fibula, dislocated knee | Peroneal |
| Ischial fractures | Sciatic |
| Posterior hip dislocation | Sciatic |
| Anterior shoulder dislocation | Brachial plexus |

TABLE 20-4.
AVERAGE BLOOD LOSS WITH FRACTURES

| *Bone* | *Blood Loss* |
|---|---|
| Pelvis (generally) | 1000-2000 |
| Posterior pelvis | 1000-3000 |
| Ribs | 125 cc per rib |
| Femoral shaft | 500-1000 cc |
| Distal femur | 500-800 cc |
| Humerus | 150-350 cc |
| Distal humerus | 250-500 cc |
| Radius and ulna | 250-500 cc |
| Tibia and fibula | 250-600 cc |

TABLE 20-5. NERVE TEST

| *Injured* | *Motor Assessment* |
|---|---|
| Brachial Plexus | Cannot raise the shoulder; cannot externally rotate arm; cannot supinate forearm or hand. |
| Radial nerve | Cannot extend wrist or fingers—"wrist drop"—cannot extend thumb. |
| Median nerve | Cannot flex wrist—"monkey hand." |
| Ulnar nerve | Pain deficit on ulnar aspect of little finger. |
| Peroneal nerve | Cannot dorsiflex or evert the ankle. |
| Tibial nerve | Cannot plantar flex ankle or flex the toes |
| Sciatic nerve | Cannot flex the leg at the knee joint. Cannot extend the hip joint. |

*Signs and Symptoms:* The EMT should be alert for swelling, crepitus, deformity, pain, point tenderness, and inability to move the arm.

*Complications:* The radial nerve passes around the mid-shaft portion of the humerus and may be injured in a mid-shaft fracture of the humerus. (See Fig. 20-29a.) The radial nerve allows for dorsiflexion of the wrist and elevation of the thumb. If the radial nerve is disrupted, the wrist hangs

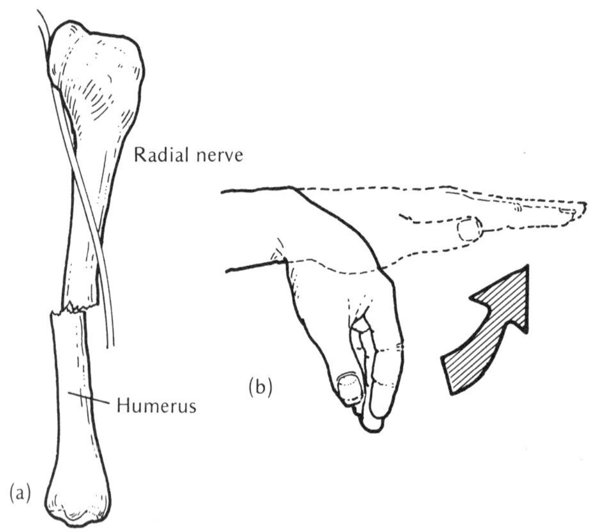


**Figure 20-29.** A midshaft fracture of the humerus could injure the radial nerve. (b) The patient with such nerve involvement will usually have a characteristic wrist drop.

limply in a flexed position. This is known as a "wrist drop." (See Fig. 20–29b.) The EMT can test radial nerve integrity in a patient with a mid-shaft fractured humerus by asking the patient to extend his thumb in a "hitch-hiker" sign position. (See Table 20–5.)

*Stabilization:* The humerus may be splinted by using any conventional rigid splint. The medial side of the humerus should rest closely to the side of the chest wall and a rigid splint applied to the lateral side of the upper arm. The splint should immobilize the shoulder joint above and the elbow joint below the fracture. With a roller bandage securing the splint, place the injured arm in a sling and complete stabilization with a swathe. Other splinting techniques can be used depending on the surrounding injury conditions, but the joint above and below the injured site should be immobilized.

## Elbow

The elbow is the most anatomically complicated joint in the upper extremity. (See Fig. 20–30.) It consists of the distal end of the humerus and proximal ends of the radius and ulna, which all articulate together to make the elbow joint.

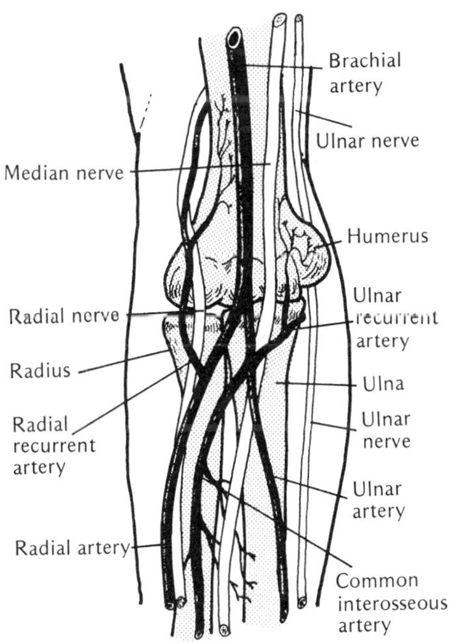


Figure 20–30. The elbow joint and its neurovascular pathways. One can see why injury to the elbow may be quite complicated.

## Supracondylar Fractures (Distal Humerus)

These are serious fractures and are common in children but uncommon in adults. Direct or indirect trauma (e.g., shielding a fall with an outstretched hand), are the usual causes.

*Signs and Symptoms:* Swelling occurs rapidly. Deformity, pain, and inability to move the arm and forearm are characteristic.

*Complications:* Rapid swelling (See Fig. 20–31a.) as bone fragments can press against the brachial artery and median nerve. An absent radial pulse in the presence of a supracondylar fracture may produce a condition that cripples the hand and forearm known as *Volkmann's Ischemic Contracture.* This condition is due to an absence of blood or oxygen supply to muscle tissue. It must be corrected within four to eight hours or muscles in the forearm and hand will shrink and harden, leaving the patient with a stiff forearm and a clawlike hand deformity. (See Fig. 20–31b.)

*Stabilization:* A supracondylar fracture can be stabilized by using any type of rigid splint. If the arm is bent at the elbow a sling and swath may be added. If the fracture is angulated, splint the arm in the position found. The splint should immobilize the shoulder joint and the wrist joint so no movement of the arm or forearm is allowed. Remember to assess the radial artery and nerve status before and after splinting.

## Proximal Radius and Ulnar Fractures

These fractures are common in adults. Indirect trauma such as shielding a fall with an outstretched hand is usually the cause.

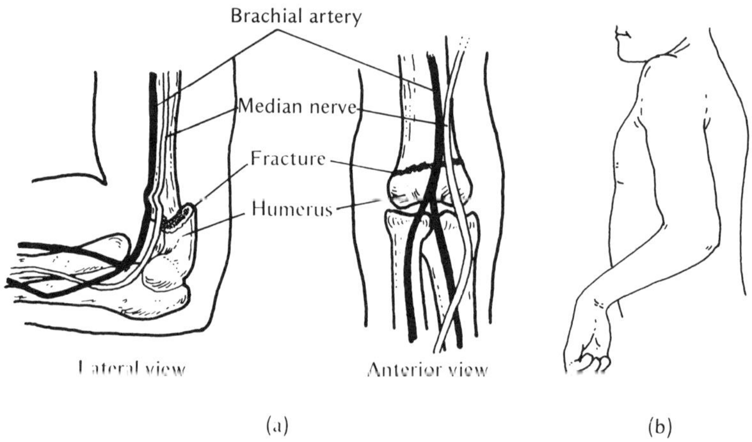


**Figure 20–31.** (a) Supracondylar fracture of the humerus impinging the brachial artery and median nerve. (b) Volkman's Ischemic Contracture due to lack of blood flow to the forearm and hand muscles.

*Signs and Symptoms:* Inability to move the arm and forearm, pain, rapid swelling, deformity, and crepitus are usually present.

*Complications:* Because of the close proximity of the brachial artery in this area, it could be occluded. Therefore, a Volkmann's contracture could occur.

*Stabilization:* As with a supracondylar fracture, splint according to presentation and monitor the neurovascular status.

## Forearm Fractures

### *Radius and Ulna*

Any force strong enough to break one bone in the forearm usually breaks the other. This is because of the close relationship of the two bones. (See Fig. 20-32.) Direct or indirect trauma is usually the cause. Again, shielding a fall with an outstretched hand is a common mechanism of injury in the adult. Greenstick fractures are common at this location in children.

*Signs and Symptoms:* Crepitus, deformity, point tenderness, swelling, and inability to move the injured area are common occurrences in the presence of these fractures.

*Complications:* Neurovascular compromise and Volkmann's Contracture.

*Stabilization:* This fracture should be stabilized with a rigid or inflatable splint, immobilizing the elbow and wrist joints.

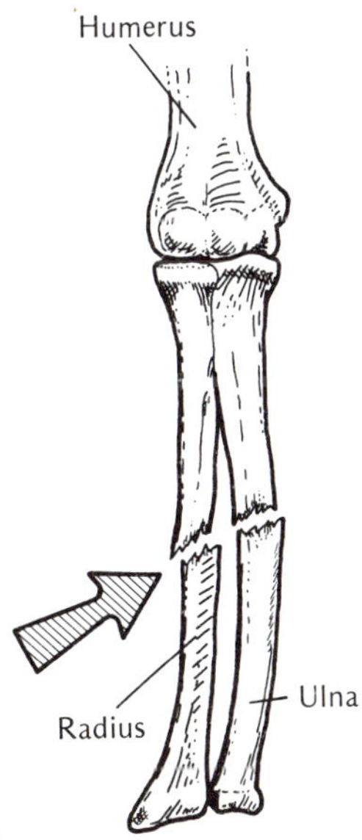


**Figure 20-32.** A midshaft fracture of the radius and ulna.

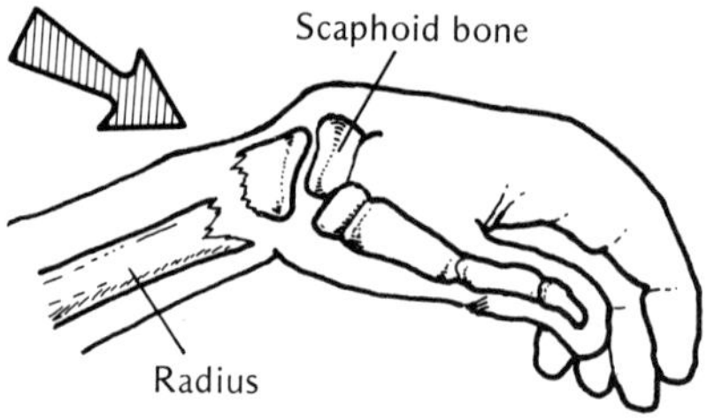


**Figure 20–33.** A Colles Fracture.

## Wrist

The wrist articulates with the hand and forearm. It consists of the distal end of the radius and ulna and the carpal bones.

## Distal Radius and Ulnar Fractures

These fractures are common in the middle and later decades of life. The most common cause is shielding a fall with an outstretched arm and hand. An associated fracture of the elbow or shoulder may accompany this fracture.

*Signs and Symptoms:* Swelling, inability to move the wrist and hand, crepitus, pain, and deformity may be present. Deformity is classic with this type of fracture and is known as a Colles Fracture or silver fork deformity. (This is because the angle of the fracture in association with the forearm and hand looks like a dinner fork.) (See Fig. 20–33.) The opposite angle fracture at this site is known as a Smith's Fracture.

*Complications:* Usually none.

*Stabilization:* This fracture should be stabilized with rigid splints, immobilizing the elbow and wrist joints. Monitor neurovascular status.

## Carpal Bones

Of the eight carpal bones, the scaphoid bone is the most commonly fractured bone in the wrist. A scaphoid fracture is sometimes associated with a Colles Fracture from breaking a fall with an outstretched hand or from hyperextension of the wrist.

*Signs and Symptoms:* Pain, limited wrist motion, swelling, and point tenderness are common findings.

*Complications:* A scaphoid fracture does not heal well because the blood supply to the bone is not evenly distributed to all parts of it.

*Stabilization:* All possible fractures of the wrist should be immobilized with the hand in the anatomical position. Patient should not be able to move either the wrist or hand once splinted and wrapped.

## Hand

The hand articulates with the carpal bones and is connected to the forearm. The hand is composed of five metacarpal bones and five phalanges.

Spiral and transverse fractures are usually more common than any other type of fracture. Direct or indirect trauma may fracture the hand. Crush injuries are common.

## Metacarpal Fractures

Injuries to the metacarpal bones usually occur from direct trauma. Contact sports (boxing) and a variety of industrial accidents are major contributors to these injuries.

Two types of fractures that may be seen with frequency include: the Boxer's fracture and Bennett's fracture.

### *Boxer's Fracture*

This fracture occurs in fighters when the fist strikes an object directly. The injury occurs to the proximal portion of the fifth metacarpal (little finger knuckle). (Fig. 20–34.)

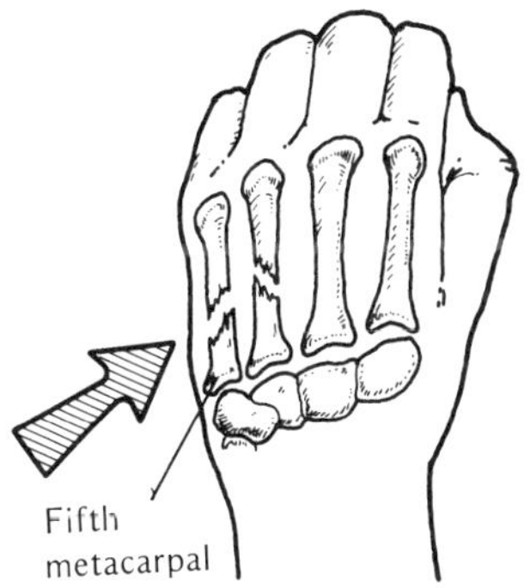


**Figure 20–34.** A Boxer's fracture.

*Signs and Symptoms:* There is loss of the fifth knuckle prominence associated with pain, inability to move the little finger side of the hand, and swelling.

*Complications:* Usually none.

*Stabilization:* The hand should be immobilized in the position of function.

### *Bennett's Fracture*

This fracture occurs at the base of the first metacarpal (thumb). The cause is usually a direct force applied to the end of the thumb. (See Fig. 20–35.)

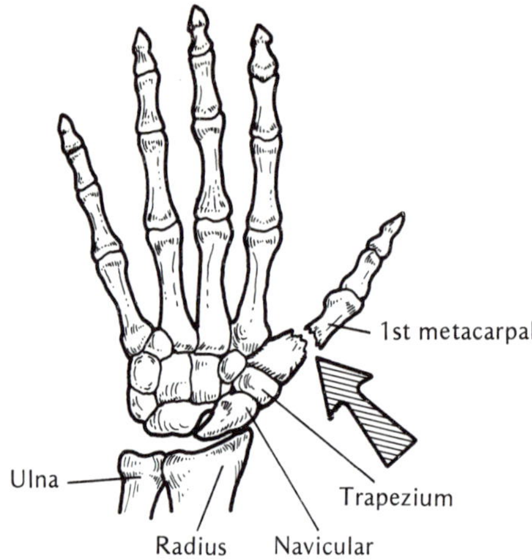


**Figure 20-35.** A Bennett's fracture

*Signs and Symptoms:* The patient usually has an inability to move the thumb side of the hand. There is pain, swelling, and point tenderness.

*Complications:* Usually none.

*Stabilization:* The hand should be immobilized in the position of function.

## Fingers (Phalanges)

The fingers of the hand take more abuse because of their location than any other anatomical structure in the body. Direct and indirect trauma are the most common causes of injury. (See Fig. 20-36.)

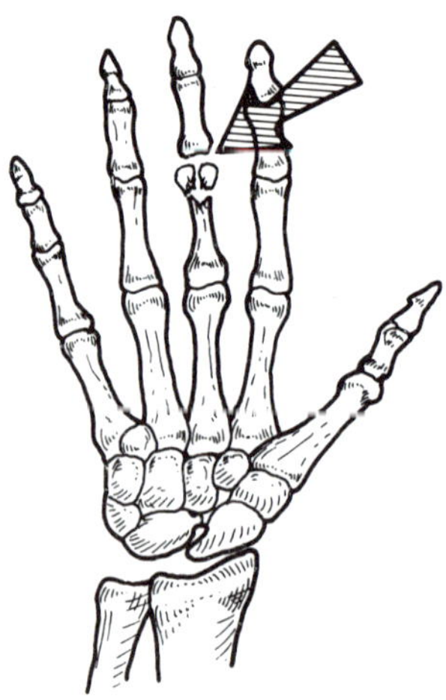

**Figure 20-36.** A fractured phalange.

*Signs and Symptoms:* Pain, swelling, deformity, and inability to move the affected finger(s) are the common findings.

*Complications:* Usually none.

*Stabilization:* The fingers can be immobilized by splinting one against the other or splinting the whole hand in the position of the function.

## DISLOCATIONS

A *dislocation* is a complete displacement of the bones from their articular surfaces that form a joint. The resultant relocation of the bone comes to lie in the soft tissue surrounding the joint. Since ligaments are localized thickenings around a joint that bind bone to bone, they are usually stretched or torn at the time of dislocation. Most dislocations result from direct trauma, indirect trauma, and violent muscle contractions. The most characteristic signs and symptoms are pain, swelling, limitation of joint movement, and gross deformity of the part. The EMT should always check the circulatory and nerve status distal to the injury for possible damage. This is extremely important because of the neurovascular complexity associated with all major joints. Recall that joints are commonly named from the bones that form them.

### Upper Extremity Dislocations

Common dislocations in the upper extremity include (see Fig. 20–37):

1. Acromioclavicular Joint }
2. Sternoclavicular Joint } shoulder
3. Glenohumeral Joint }
4. Elbow Joint
5. Radiocarpal Joint—wrist
6. Interphalangeal or Metacarpophalangeal Joint—finger

#### *Acromioclavicular Joint*

This joint is formed where the acromion and clavicle meet. A complete dislocation occurs when the ligaments (conoid and trapezoid) are ruptured. This injury is usually caused by direct trauma and is very common in contact sports, e.g., football. A complete dislocation of the acromioclavicular joint is also known as a shoulder separation. (See Fig. 20–38.)

*Signs and Symptoms:* The most characteristic sign is that the clavicle rides far above the acromion, especially when the arm hangs down. This deformity can readily be seen and palpated. Associated pain, swelling, and limited motion of the arm is also common.

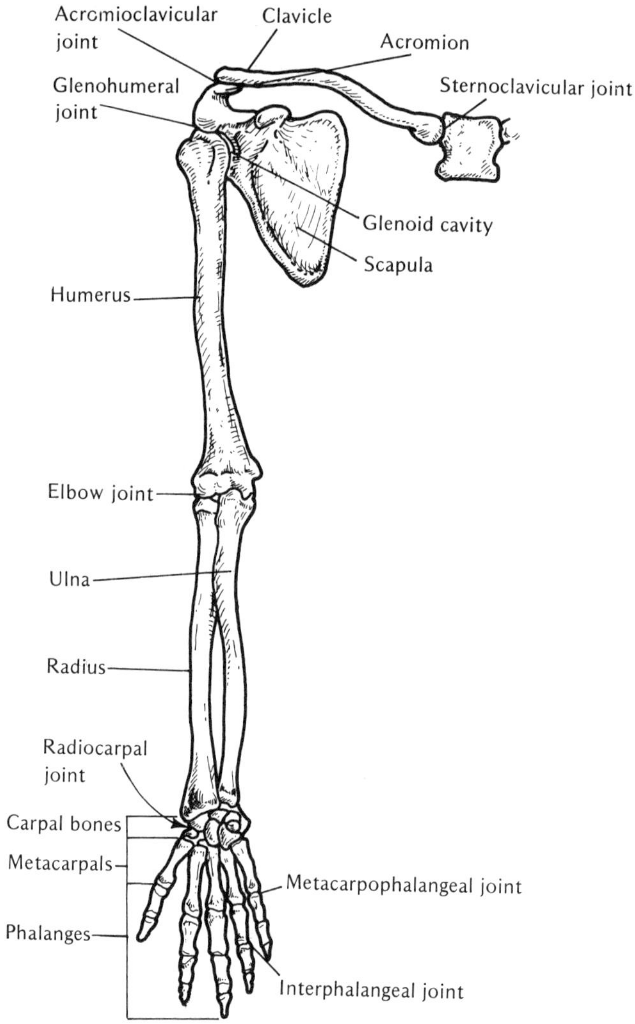


**Figure 20–37.** Joints of the upper extremity.

*Complications:* There are usually no complications, but the neurovascular status should be assessed.

*Stabilization:* By the time you arrive on the scene, the patient will probably be in the most comfortable position. However, putting the arm in a sling and swathe will provide some added comfort.

*Sternoclavicular Joint*

This joint is formed where the clavicle joins the sternum. Dislocations at this area may occur when the patient shields a fall with an outstretched

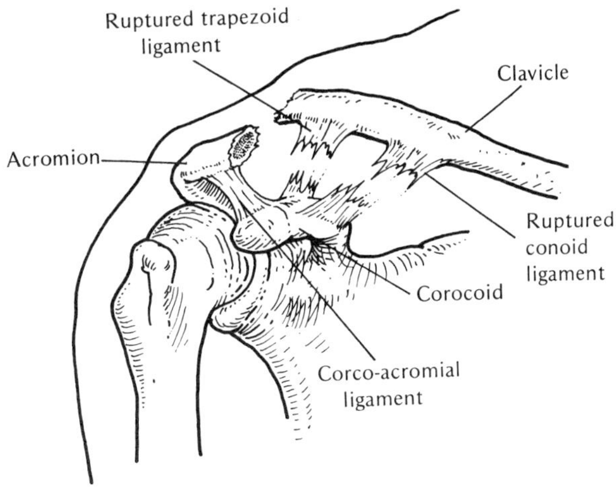


**Figure 20-38.** A complete dislocation of the shoulder.

arm and hand (indirect trauma), or experiences direct trauma. Sterno-clavicular dislocations can occur either anteriorly or posteriorly.

In an anterior dislocation the medial end of the clavicle comes to lie in front of the manubrium (top part of the breast bone). In a posterior dislocation, the clavicle lies in back of the manubrium.

*Signs and Symptoms:* Deformity is either a bulge in front of the sternum or a depression next to the sternal notch. Pain, swelling, limited motion of the shoulder, and redness are associated.

*Complications:* Anterior dislocation—usually none.

Posterior dislocation—the clavicle could impinge on the trachea, esophagus, or great vessels (subclavian artery and vein).

*Stabilization:* The EMT should keep the patient's arm close to the side of the body and apply a sling and swathe. If airway or circulatory status is jeopardized, rapid transport to the hospital with red lights and siren should take place.

### *Glenohumeral Joint*

This joint is formed where the head of the humerus (ball) fits into the glenoid cavity (socket). (It is a ball and socket joint.) A shoulder dislocation can be either anteriorly or posteriorly displaced. An anterior dislocation usually occurs by an excessive force of abduction and external rotation of the humerus. (See Fig. 20-39.) This injury is common in both children and adults and may occur during athletic sports or a fall on an extended arm and hand. A posterior dislocation to the glenohumeral joint is rare. It may occur, however, during seizure activity in which the extended arm is abducted and internally rotated.

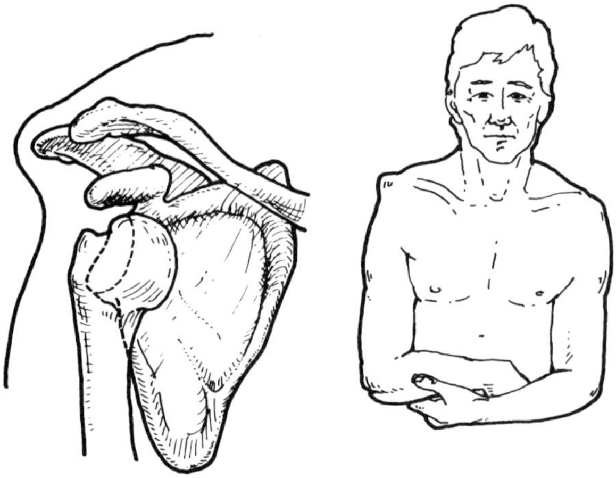

(a) (b)

**Figure 20–39.** (a) Anterior dislocation of the shoulder. (b) Patients with such an injury usually "guard" the injury by holding the injured side as shown. Note the classical protrusion of the acromion and loss of normal shoulder roundness.

*Signs and Symptoms:* Classically, the shoulder loses its normal roundness and appears to be flattened. Severe pain, swelling, and inability to move the arm are also common. The patient is often seen supporting the injured joint and arm with his other hand.

*Complications:* Check pulses distal to the injured site for circulatory status. (See Table 20–3.) Nerves that could be affected include the axillary, radial, median, and ulnar. Check for this nerve integrity distal to the dislocation.

*Stabilization:* The patient may not let you touch him because of the pain. If this is the case, let the patient guard the injury while you monitor and assess neurovascular status during transport. If the patient can tolerate some slight movement, apply a sling and swathe for comfort. This should immobilize the joint enough to give a little relief. Try to avoid quick starts and stops enroute to the hospital.

*Elbow Joint*

This joint is formed by the distal end of the humerus articulating with the proximal ulna. Dislocations in the elbow joint usually occur when a fall is shielded with an outstretched arm or hand. It is common in both children and adults and during contact sports. (See Fig. 20–40.)

Both anterior and posterior dislocations are possible. A posterior

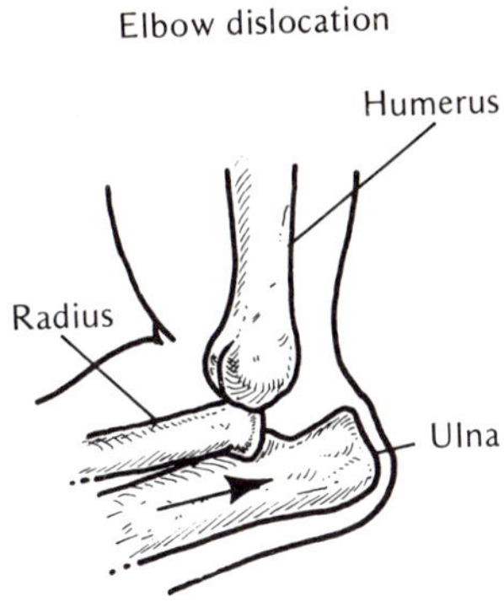


**Figure 20–40.** An elbow dislocation.

dislocation occurs when the distal humerus comes out of the joint capsule forcing the radius and ulna backwards with the ulna lodging behind the distal humerus. An anterior dislocation is very rare.

*Signs and Symptoms:* Rapid swelling, marked deformity, extreme pain, and very limited motion of the forearm.

*Complications:* Neurovascular status could be compromised; check nerve and circulatory status distal to the injury.

*Stabilization:* This patient may not let you touch him. Proceed to immobilize in the best method possible. If the elbow is straight, stabilize with a rigid splint. If the elbow is at an angle, improvise the splinting in the position of the bent elbow.

### *Wrist Joint*

This joint is formed by the distal radius and ulna articulating with the carpal bones (scaphoid, lunate, and triquetrum). This dislocation is seen in both children and adults and is common in contact sports. It may occur when the victim has fallen on the palm of the hand or is shielding a fall with an outstretched arm and hand. The dislocation usually occurs at the junction of the radius and carpal bones. (See Fig. 20–41.)

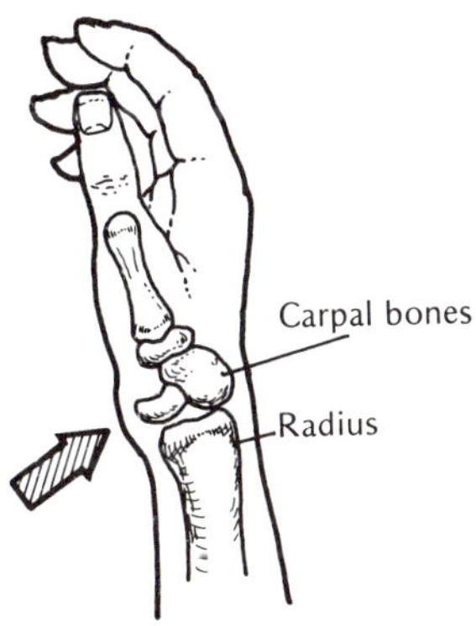


**Figure 20–41.** A wrist dislocation.

*Signs and Symptoms:* Pain, swelling, deformity, and limitation of motion at the wrist joint.

*Complications:* The median nerve could be impaired.

*Stabilization:* Immobilize the wrist by splinting, or if the patient is severely agitated by movement, let him stabilize the joint. However the joint is managed, always check the neurovascular status.

*Interphalangeal or Metacarpophalangeal Joint (Finger)*

Interphalangeal (in″ter-fah-lan′je-al) or metacarpophalangeal (met″ah-kar″po-fah-lan′ge-al) joints are those that form between the phalanges and metacarpal bones. Dislocations to these areas are usually the result of direct trauma (e.g., hitting the ends of the fingers on a hard object). Although most frequently encountered during sports activity, it is common in all age groups. (See Fig. 20–42.)

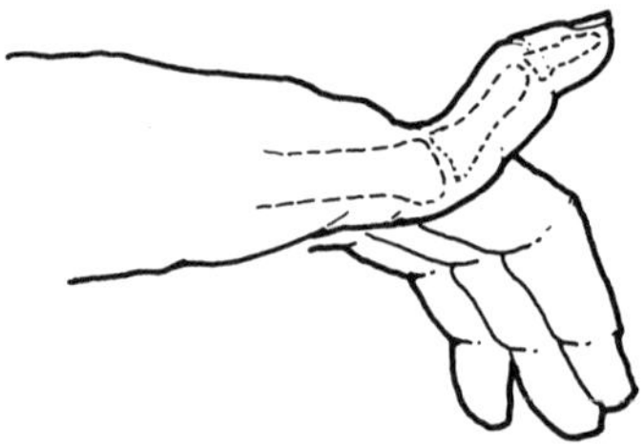

**Figure 20–42.** A finger dislocation.

*Signs and Symptoms:* Pain, swelling, deformity, and inability to move the fingers at their joints.

*Complications:* Very rare.

*Stabilization:* Splint the extremity in the most comfortable position for the patient or let him stabilize the injury with the other hand if it is too painful for him to have you manipulating it. Check for other possible injuries and monitor neurovascular status.

## LOWER EXTREMITY FRACTURES

Bones of the lower extremity include (see Fig. 20–43):

Ilium, Ischium, Pubis } pelvis
Proximal Femur—hip
Femur—thigh

Tibia, Fibula }—leg
Tarsals—ankle
Metatarsals—foot
Phalanges—toes

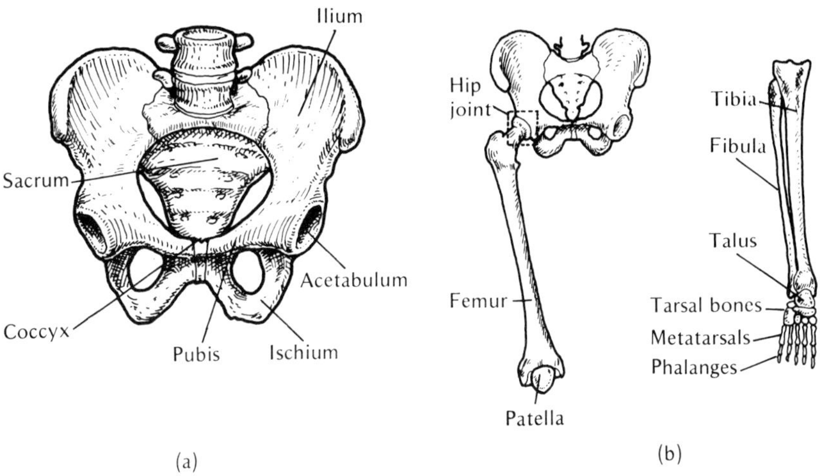


**Figure 20-43.** (a) Bones of the pelvis and (b) lower extremity.

## Pelvic Fractures

Fractures of the pelvis may involve the pubis, ilium, or ischium bones. The ilium is considered the posterior portion of the pelvis. The ischium and pubis are considered the anterior pelvis. Fractures to the pelvic bones occur frequently in direct trauma, e.g., automobile and motorcycle accidents, crushing injuries, and falls. They are more common in the adult and elderly patient. (See Fig. 20-44.)

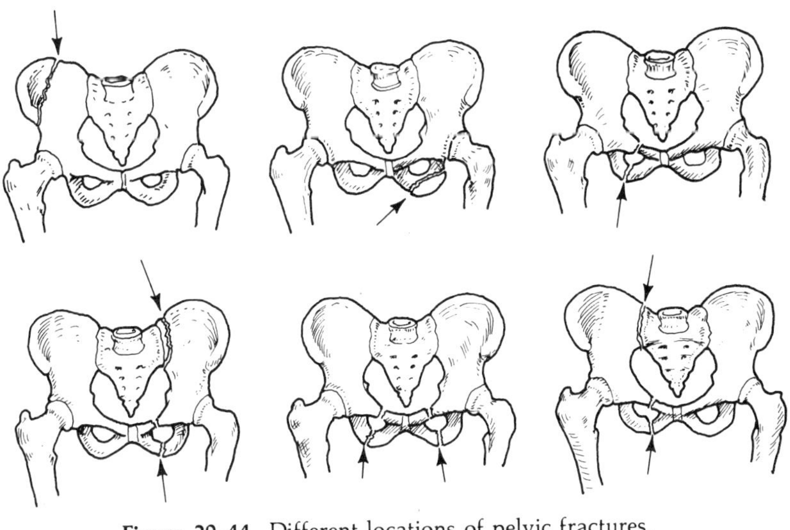

**Figure 20-44.** Different locations of pelvic fractures.

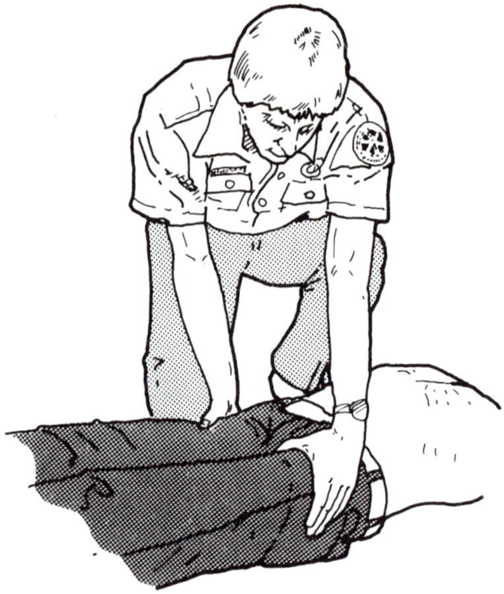

**Figure 20–45.** The pelvic compression test used to rule out the possibility of pelvic fracture.

*Signs and Symptoms:* Pain, inability to move the legs, muscle spasms in the lumbar spine, crepitus, point tenderness, and ecchymosis are common findings. The EMT should lightly compress the iliac crests to elicit a pain response when ruling out pelvic injury in all trauma patients. (See Fig. 20–45.)

*Complications:* Fractures to the posterior pelvis (ilium) may also injure large blood vessels, nerves (sciatic), and viscera (vis′er-ah) that lie close to the bone. Sixty to seventy percent of these patients will require blood transfusions averaging 7 or 8 pints of blood. Anterior pelvic fractures (ischium and pubis) are usually not accompanied by large blood vessel and nerve damage, but may injure the urethra, bladder, and other viscera that lie in close proximity to these bones. Hypovolemic shock is common with pelvic fractures. (See Table 20–4.)

*Stabilization:* These patients should be placed on a long padded spine board. A pillow may be placed under the knees to reduce muscle spasm and provide comfort. If the patient exhibits signs and symptoms of shock, antishock trousers should be applied. The trousers should be inflated to 30–40 mm Hg to stabilize the fracture. If the patient's blood pressure is not stabilized, inflate the trousers to 50–70 mm Hg. The patient's circulatory and nerve status should be monitored every five minutes.

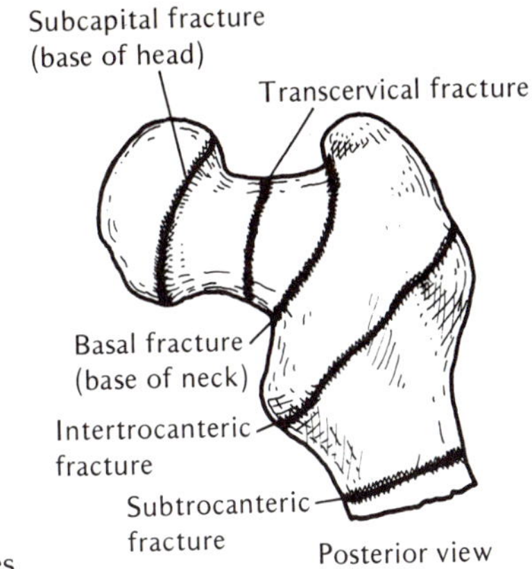


**Figure 20-46.** Types of hip fractures.

## Hip Fractures

The hip is defined as the proximal end of the femur from just below the greater trochanter (tro-kan′ter) to the head of the femur. Hip fractures are specified by x-ray and can be of five varieties. (See Fig. 20-46.) They are:

1. Subcapital—base of the femoral head
2. Transcervical—through the neck of the femur
3. Basal—base of the neck of the femur
4. Intertrochanteric—through the trochanter
5. Subtrochanteric—just below the trochanter

Hip fractures are very common in the elderly patient due to falls, and the young adult due to trauma, e.g., auto accidents or falls from high places.

*Signs and Symptoms:* The patient with a hip fracture will classically have shortening of the injured leg, with external rotation of the hip and leg. Pain with associated muscle spasm and inability to move the leg are also usually present.

*Complications:* Hypovolemic shock is common depending on the extent of injury.

*Stabilization:* Hip fractures are difficult to distinguish from pelvic fractures. The EMT should rule out a pelvic fracture by pelvic compression. If the EMT believes that only a hip fracture exists, the patient should be placed in a traction splint. If the patient may have a fractured pelvis along with the injured hip, he should be placed on a padded long spine board. Pillows should be placed under the flexed knees for comfort during transport. If signs and symptoms of shock appear, antishock trousers should be applied and inflated to stabilize the blood pressure. A traction

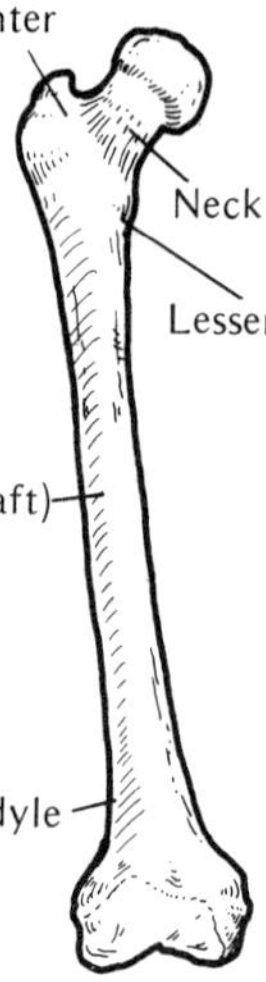


**Figure 20–47.** Anatomy of the femur bone.

splint may be placed over the trousers if indicated. Vital signs should be monitored every five minutes during transport.

## Femur Fractures

The femur is the longest, largest, and heaviest bone in the body. (See Fig. 20–47.) Therefore, injuries to this bone can be serious. Fractures to the femur are common in both children and adults and are usually the result of direct trauma.

*Signs and Symptoms:* Severe pain, deformity, angulation, muscle spasms, crepitus, inability to move the leg, and shortening of the leg are all common findings.

*Complications:* Hypovolemic shock is very common. This patient may lose up to one to two liters of blood. (See Table 20–4.) Open fractures are also common. (See Fig. 20–48.)

*Stabilization:* The fractured femur should be placed in a traction splint whenever possible. Antishock trousers may be indicated once you arrive on the scene. If signs and symptoms of shock are present, place the antishock trousers on the patient after which you may place the traction splint on the injured limb. Vital signs must be monitored every five minutes. Trauma severe enough to fracture the femur may have produced other injuries. The EMT should always check the pelvis along with the rest of the leg and foot.

## Knee Fractures

The knee joint consists of the distal femur (supracondylar area) and the proximal tibia, which articulate with one another. Fractures to the knee are common in both children and adults and usually occur from direct

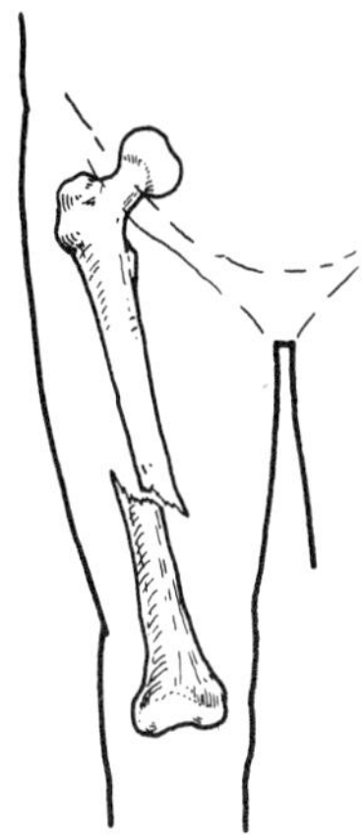

**Figure 20-48.** The patient with a fractured femur may lose 1–2 liters of blood. Shock is common with this type of injury.

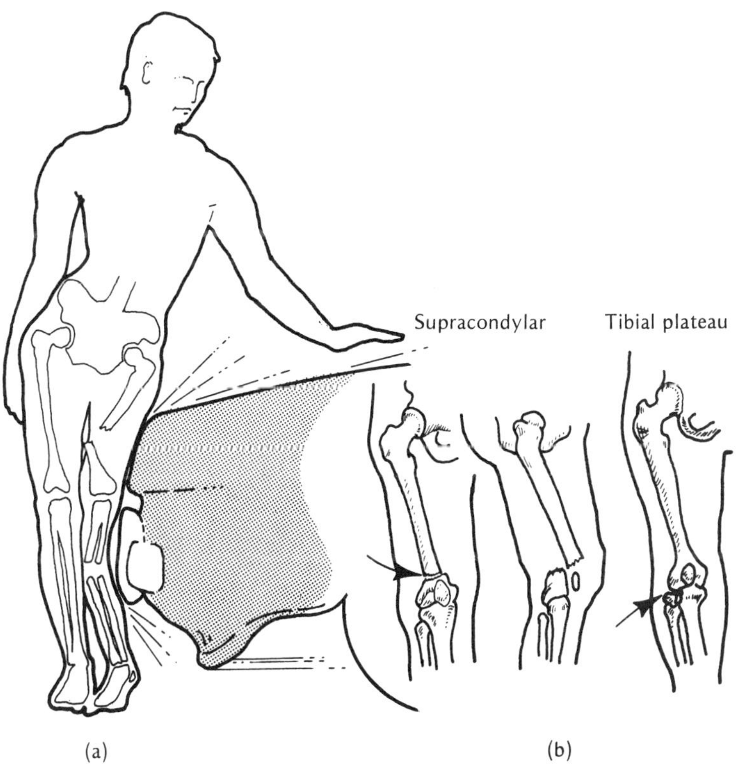


**Figure 20-49.** (a) A common pedestrian injury is the bumper fracture. (b) Creating a supracondylar fracture as well as other extremity fractures.

trauma, e.g., auto and motorcycle accidents, pedestrian-auto accidents (bumper fracture). (See Fig. 20–49.) The knee is the most anatomically complicated joint in the lower extremity.

*Signs and Symptoms*: Pain, deformity, angulation, rapid swelling, crepitus, and inability to move the injured leg are common findings.

*Complications:* The popliteal artery or peroneal nerve may be damaged. If the popliteal artery has been disrupted, the patient will not have distal pulses. If the peroneal nerve is damaged, the patient will not be able to dorsiflex or evert the ankle and sensation over the lateral surface of the foot will be lost. (See Fig. 20–50.) The EMT should check these neurovascular structures in every patient with a possible fractured knee. (See Tables 20–1 and 20–5.)

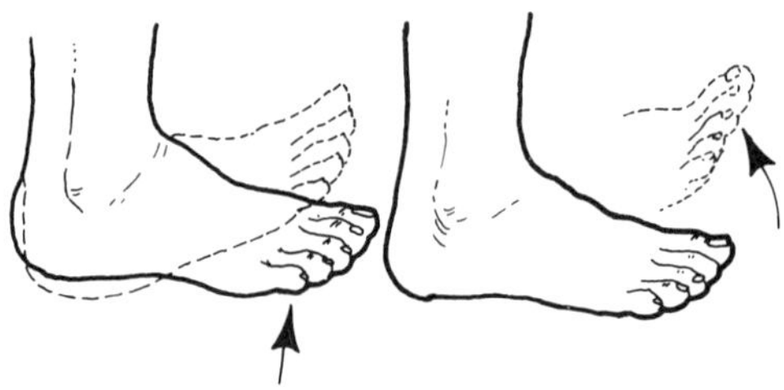

**Figure 20–50.** The inability to dorsiflex the foot as shown by the dotted lines may indicate peroneal nerve damage. The EMT-A should always check the neurovascular status in all patients with knee injury.

*Stabilization:* The injured knee should be stabilized in the position it is found. The EMT should use rigid splints to immobilize the joint area. Ingenuity is often called for with these injuries when splinting, because of the position of the patient's leg when found. Regardless of the splinting technique used, it should immobilize the entire leg if possible.

### *Fractures to the Patella*

The patella is a small triangular sesamoid bone. Direct trauma is usually the cause of injury, (e.g., the knee hits the dashboard of the car). The patella is held in place by the quadriceps femoris tendon and the bone helps protect the joint. The quadriceps femoris is the large bulky thigh muscle that extends the leg. (See Fig. 20–51.)

*Signs and Symptoms:* Swelling, deformity, pain, and point tenderness are all common. Classically, the patient will not be able to raise the leg with the knee extended.

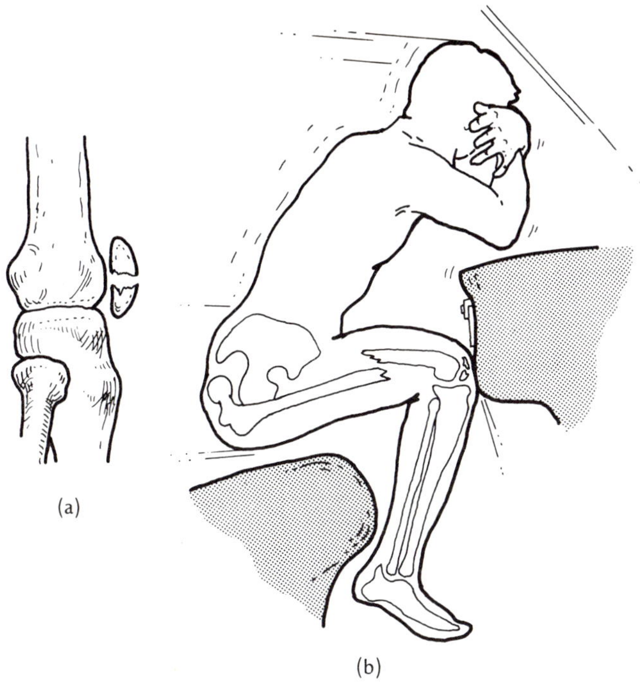

**Figure 20-51.** (a) Fractured patella; (b) a dashboard insult, a common mechanism of injury.

*Complications:* Usually none. However, forces strong enough to injure the patella may also injure the knee, pelvis, femur, and lower leg. The EMT should assess the lower extremity for all possible injury.

*Stabilization:* Splint the injured area above and below the knee joint to completely immobilize the leg. Make sure to check distal nerve and vascular status.

## Leg Fractures

The leg includes the tibia and fibula and both run parallel to one another. As in the forearm, a force strong enough to break one bone usually breaks the other.

### *Fractures to the Fibula and Tibia*

These fractures are common in both children and adults. They occur frequently from direct and indirect trauma and twisting forces (ski injuries). (See Fig. 20-52.)

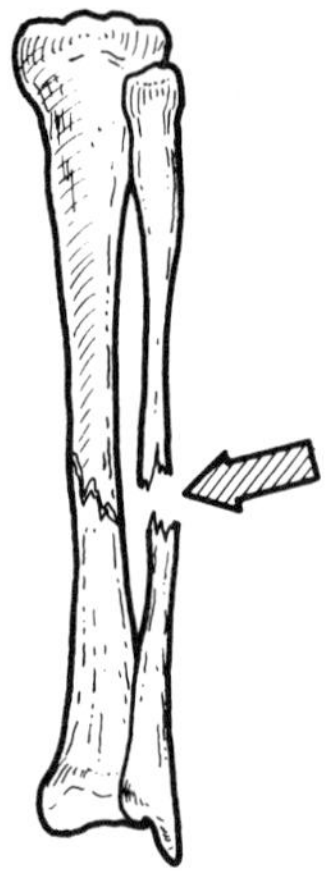

**Figure 20-52.** Midshaft fracture of the fibula and tibia.

*Signs and Symptoms:* Pain, deformity, angulation, swelling, crepitus, and inability to move the leg are common findings.

*Complications:* Because the tibia (shin bone) lies so close to the skin surface, fractures of the tibia are often open. Soft tissue damage often accompanies these fractures with angulation. Fibula fractures are rarely a problem because the fibula is buried deep in muscle.

*Stabilization:* If the tibia is severely angulated it should be straightened and put into a traction splint. Air splints work equally well. The EMT should assess the neurovascular status distal to the injured site.

## Ankle Fractures

The ankle consists of the distal portion of the tibia and fibula and tarsal bones (talus), which articulate with one another. The ankle is one of the most frequently injured areas of the skeletal system, because of the repeated stress put on it. Running, jumping, and twisting injuries, as well

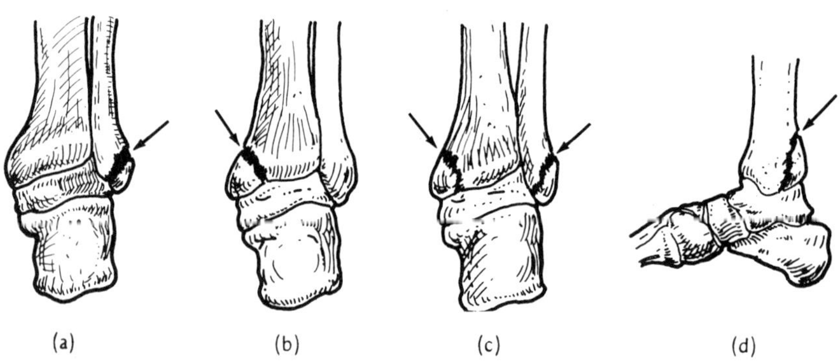


**Figure 20-53.** Various types of ankle fracture.

as direct and indirect trauma are the usual causes of injury. Fractures to the ankle are common in all age groups. (See Fig. 20-53.)

*Signs and Symptoms:* Rapid swelling, pain, point tenderness, and inability to move the foot are common findings.

*Complications:* As in all joint fractures, nerve or vascular impairment can occur.

*Stabilization:* A pillow splint is ideal for this fracture. Air or board splints may be used equally as well. The EMT should check for distal pulses and nerve status.

## Heel Bone Fractures—Os Calcis

Fractures to the heel bone are common in older children and adolescents. The fracture usually results from direct trauma, e.g., jumping from high places onto a hard surface. (See Fig. 20-54.)

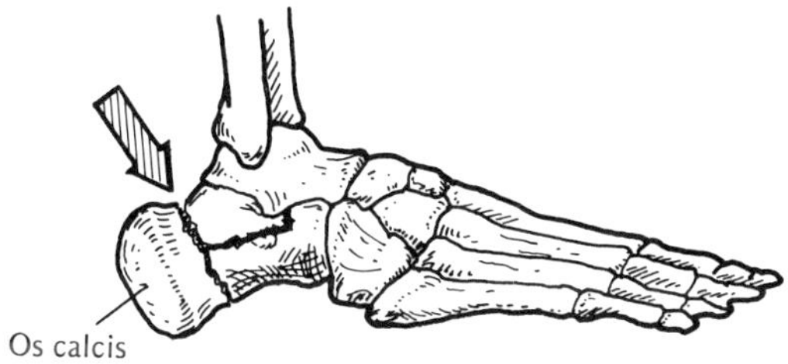


**Figure 20-54.** A heel bone (os calcis) fracture usually occurs from sudden impact after a jump.

*Signs and Symptoms:* Swelling, pain, point tenderness, and tip toe limping are common findings.

*Complications:* Compression fractures to the lumbosacral spine are often associated with the injured heel, due to the compression force of a sudden stop. The EMT should palpate the spinal column as well to rule out a possible fracture.

*Stabilization:* Pillow, air, or board splints stabilize these fractures well.

## Foot Fractures—Metatarsal

The foot consists of the five metatarsal bones. Metatarsal fractures are common in all age groups and are due to direct trauma. Fractures of the second and third metatarsal bone are usually injured from stress associated

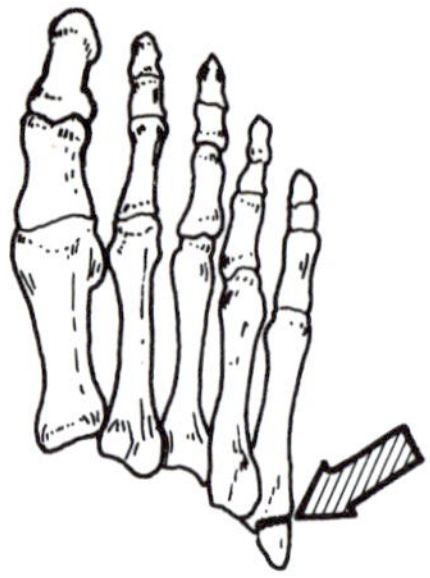

Figure 20-55. A metatarsal fracture.

with constant weight bearing after prolonged walking, hiking, or marching. This type of fracture is known as a march or fatigue fracture. (See Fig. 20-55.)

*Signs and Symptoms:* Pain, point tenderness, crepitus, swelling, and inability to bear weight on the foot are common findings.

*Complications:* Usually none.

*Stabilization:* Pillow, air, or board splints stabilize foot fractures equally well.

## Avulsion Fracture

The ankle bones are more prone to avulsion fractures than any other skeletal area. This is due to the extreme amount of stress forces that can occur to them. Usually the patient twists his ankle so violently that ligaments of the tibia and fibula are stretched enough to pull a piece of bone away from one of the ankle bones where the ligament is attached. Avulsion fractures occur mostly to the tibia and calcaneus bones. (See Fig. 20-56.)

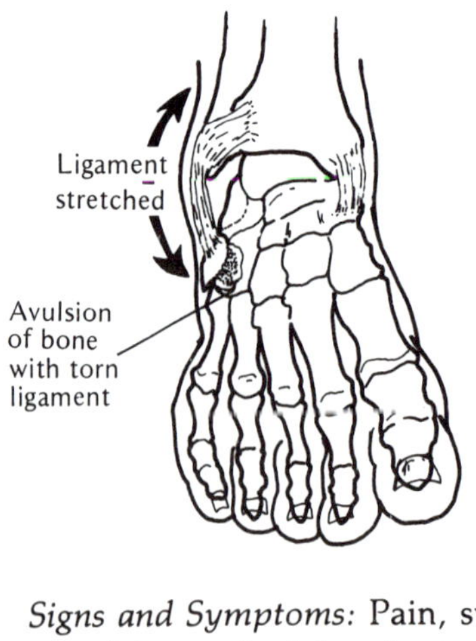


Figure 20-56. An avulsion fracture.

*Signs and Symptoms:* Pain, swelling, point tenderness, and inability to bear weight on the injured extremity are the usual findings.

*Complications:* Usually none.

*Stabilization:* These fractures can be immobilized by applying a pillow, air, or board splint and elevating the injured limb.

## Toe Fractures—Phalanges

Toe fractures are common to all age groups and, like the fingers, are subject to everyday trauma. The more common causes of injury occur from direct trauma, e.g., stubbing the toes or dropping heavy objects on them. (See Fig. 20-57.)

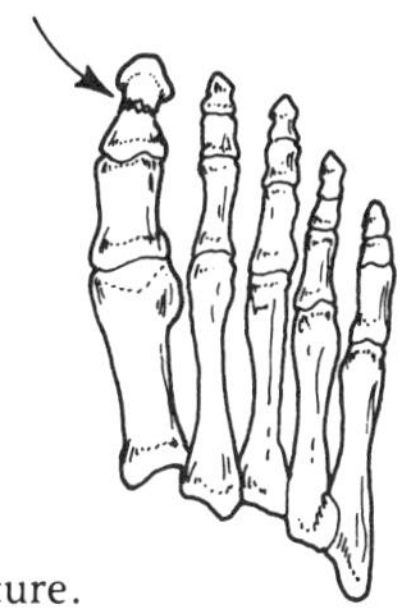

**Figure 20-57.** A phalangeal fracture.

*Signs and Symptoms:* Pain, point tenderness, swelling, deformity, ecchymosis, and inability to bend the toe are common findings.

*Complications:* Usually none.

*Stabilization:* The toe may be immobilized by taping one toe to the other or by using short padded tongue blades. If open wounds exist, wrap the foot in a sterile dressing and elevate the extremity.

# LOWER EXTREMITY DISLOCATIONS

Common dislocations in the lower extremity include:

1. Hip joint
2. Knee joint—tibiofemoral joint
3. Patella
4. Ankle joint—tibiotalas joint
5. Foot

## Hip Joint

The hip joint is formed by the head of the femur (ball) articulating within the acetabulum (socket) of the pelvis. The hip can be dislocated anteriorly or posteriorly.

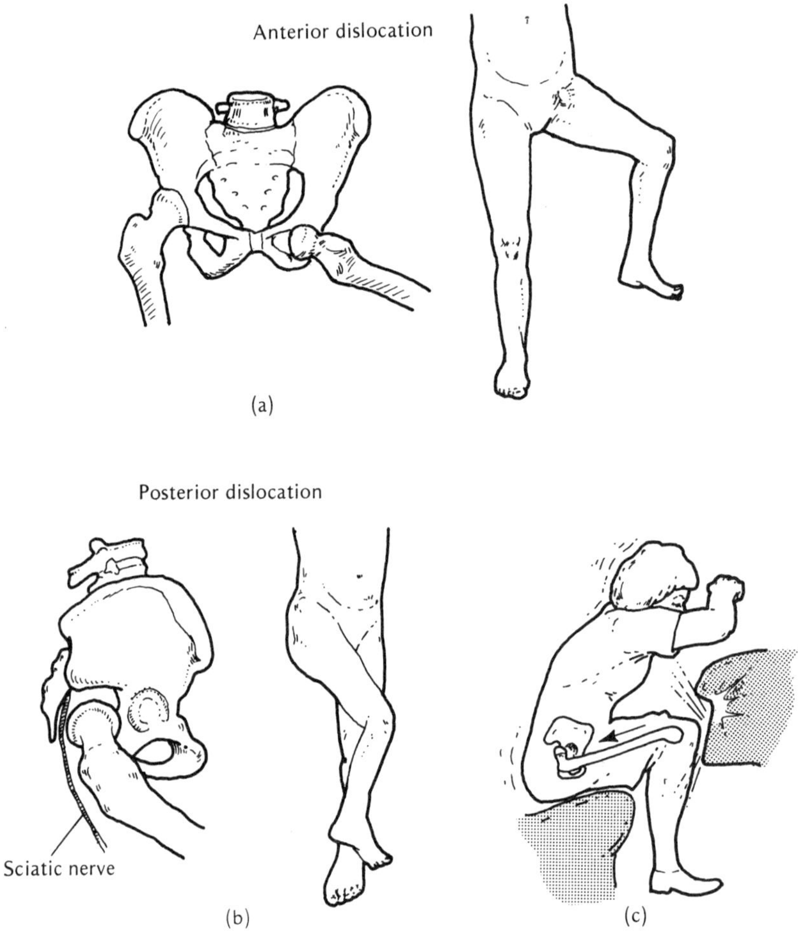


**Figure 20-58.** (a) Anterior hip dislocation; (b) posterior hip dislocation; (c) mechanism of injury resulting in a posterior hip dislocation.

*Hip Dislocation—Anterior*

An anterior dislocation is quite rare. It can be caused by a force that abducts the leg. For example, if you were standing with one of your legs on a dock and the other in a boat and the boat suddenly departed from the dock, your leg would be quickly abducted. If the force were great enough, the head of the femur could "pop" out of the acetabulum and come to lie just anterior to it. (See Fig. 20-58a.) All age groups are affected equally.

*Signs and Symptoms:* Characteristically, the patient's hip is slightly flexed, abducted, and externally rotated. Pain, deformity, swelling, muscle spasm, and limitation of motion (LOM) to the leg are seen.

*Complications:* The femoral artery and vein could be impinged —check the pulses distal to the injured site.

*Hip Dislocation—Posterior*

A posterior dislocation is more common and usually results from indirect trauma. The mechanism of injury usually occurs when the knee hits the dashboard of the car or the extended leg is stopped on impact by the floor board of the vehicle. (See Fig. 20-58c.) The posterior dislocation is more common because of the way hip stability is maintained. Three ligaments help maintain stability in the hip joint where they bind the head of the femur and the acetabulum. The three ligaments are collectively called the Y ligament, and they are extremely tight when the hip is extended (standing). This tightness causes the head of the femur to be pulled more tightly into the acetabulum. When the hip is flexed (sitting position), the ligaments relax, causing the hip joint to be less stable. Posterior dislocations are more common in adults but all age groups are affected.

*Signs and Symptoms:* The characteristic posture assumed by the injured leg is shortening, flexion of the hip, and internal rotation. (See Fig. 20-58b.) There is also marked deformity, intense muscle spasm, pain, and inability to move the leg.

*Complications:* The sciatic nerve may be impaired. The sciatic nerve essentially serves all muscles below the knee, so check for foot movement. If the nerve is affected, a characteristic foot drop could result. Check distal pulses for circulatory status.

*Stabilization:* Victims of anterior or posterior dislocations are sometimes difficult to manage because of the awkwardness of the injury and pain. The EMT should place the patient on a padded long spine board and place pillows or rolled blankets under the flexed knees to provide some added comfort. Do not move the legs from their initial position, especially in the posterior dislocation, because of the possible impingement of the sciatic nerve. Try to avoid sudden starts and stops during patient transport.

## Knee Joint (Tibiofemoral)

The knee joint is the largest joint in the body. The joint is formed by the distal femur articulating with the proximal tibia and patella.

Dislocation of the knee is one of the rarest joint dislocations in the body. Knee dislocations may occur anteriorly or posteriorly. An anterior dislocation (tibia lies anterior to the distal femur) may occur when forceful hyperextension of the knee occurs. The most common cause is direct trauma, automobile and motorcycle accidents (e.g., the distal femur strikes the dashboard or handle bars), and athletic injuries (e.g., a tackling injury in football). (See Fig. 20-59.)

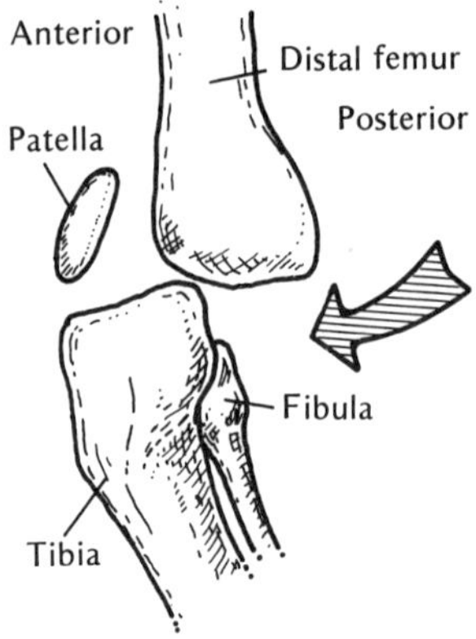


**Figure 20–59.** Anterior knee dislocation.

A posterior dislocation (tibia lies posterior to the distal femur) may also occur when direct trauma, usually automobile or motorcycle accidents, force the tibia posterior to the femur (e.g., when the proximal tibia strikes the dashboard or motorcycle handlebars). (See Fig. 20–60.) Knee dislocations are more common in young adult males, but may occur in all age groups and sexes.

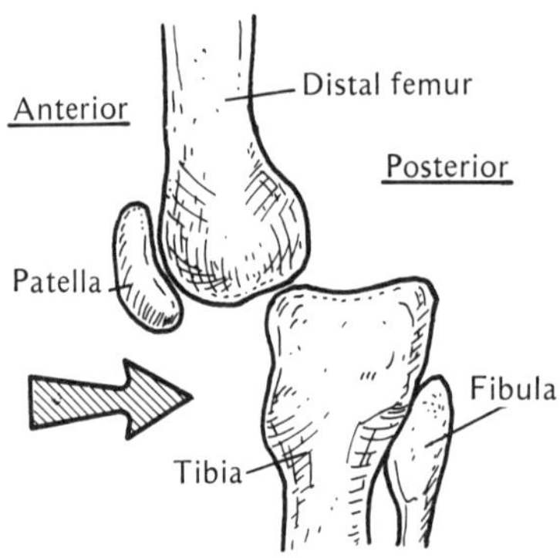


**Figure 20–60.** Posterior knee dislocation.

*Signs and Symptoms:* Rapid swelling, pain, inability to move leg, deformity, and point tenderness.

*Complications:* Approximately 50 percent of all knee dislocations involve the disruption of the popliteal (pop-lit′e-al) artery. (See Fig. 20–61.) The peroneal (per″o-ne′al) nerve, which runs on the lateral side of the knee, may also be damaged. (See Tables 20–1 and 20–3.)

*Stabilization:* The EMT must check pulses, peroneal nerve status, (e.g., can the patient extend the foot and big toe), temperature, and color distal to the injury. The injured knee should be immobilized in the same

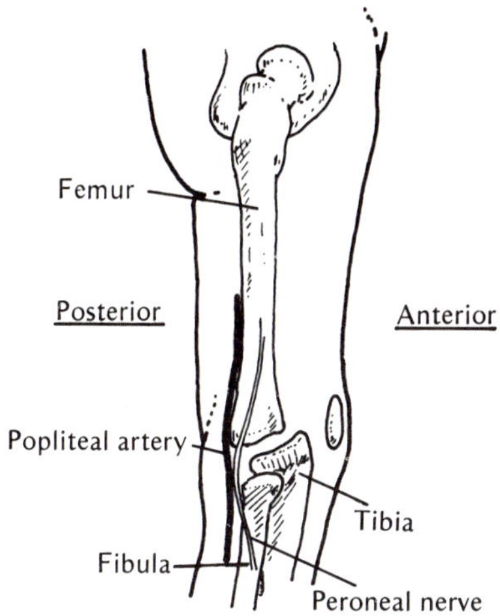


**Figure 20-61.** Neurovascular injury occurs in 50% of all patients who traumatically dislocate the knee.

position as you found it. Board splints may be applied to the injury. The EMT may be called on to improvise splinting skills with this injury. Pillows or rolled blankets may be utilized around the splinted area to provide comfort during transportation. Monitor vital signs and distal pulses. If distal pulses cannot be felt, radio to the designated hospital and inform the emergency department personnel as to the type of injury you have and the neurovascular status of the patient. Be sure to check for associated trauma, which commonly occurs with this type of injury.

## Patella Dislocation

The patella is usually dislocated when the distal quadricep tendon is ruptured. Moreover, since the patella is anchored firmly in this tendon, direct trauma to the tendon or powerful muscle contraction of the quadricep muscle may dislocate the patella. The patella usually will dislocate laterally, but it may occur on the medial side depending on the mechanism of the injury. (See Fig. 20-62.) This injury is more common in young athletes, but it may occur at any age.

*Signs and Symptoms:* Pain, point tenderness, and a palpable gap is usually felt. The patient will be unable to lift the leg with the knee extended, just as with a fractured patella.

*Stabilization:* The EMT should splint and immobilize the dislocated patella in the most comfortable position for the patient. Partial straightening of the knee, if bent, may be accomplished if it does not promote more pain to the patient.

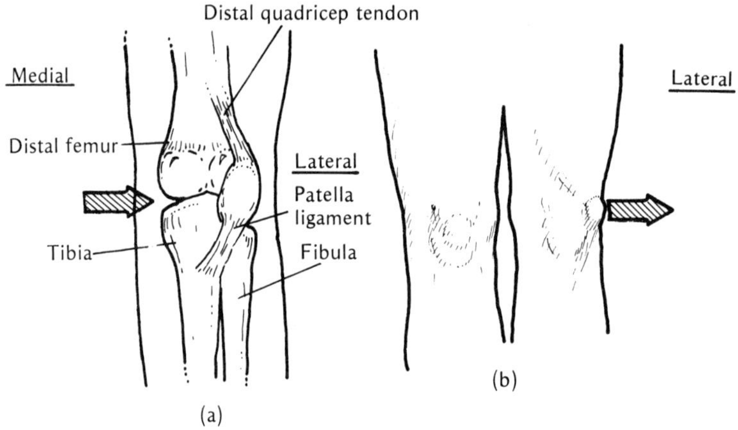


**Figure 20–62.** (a) Lateral dislocation of the patella. (b) The EMT-A will usually see an anatomical change in the dislocated patella.

## Ankle Joint (Tibiotalar Joint)

This joint is formed by the distal tibia articulating with the talus. The EMT will find difficulty in distinguishing whether or not a fracture or dislocation is present. It is not unusual to find a fracture associated with a dislocated ankle. (See Fig. 20–63.) Remember, too, that forces strong enough to fracture or dislocate any joint will usually cause injury to ligaments, muscle, and tendons. A dislocated ankle is usually the result of direct trauma—automobile accidents, athletic injuries, and twisting forces. Young adults are most often the victims.

*Signs and Symptoms:* Pain, point tenderness, rapid swelling, deformity, and inability to move the foot.

*Complications:* A true ankle dislocation without a fracture is rare. Because violent forces are required to dislocate the ankle, it is often an open dislocation. Infection and neurovascular compromise may occur.

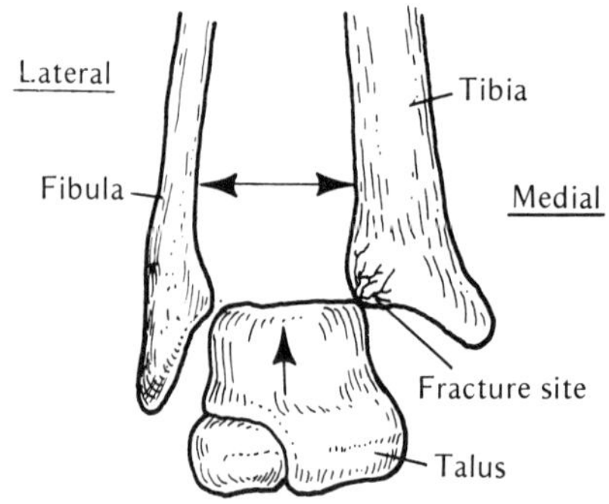


**Figure 20–63.** A fracture-dislocation of the ankle.

*Stabilization:* The victim's ankle may be stabilized by immobilizing the foot and ankle with padded board splints, pillow splints, or air splint, but only if the dislocation is closed. An open dislocation should be immobilized with padded splints and the open area covered with a sterile dressing. The neurovascular status must be monitored, and the emergency department personnel notified if the dislocation is open and/or neurovascular compromise exists.

### Foot (Tarsalmetatarsal Dislocation)

Dislocations of the foot are rare injuries. They usually occur as a result of twisting forces from automobile or motorcycle accidents. All age groups are affected. A dislocation to the foot may be through the mid-tarsal region (Chopart's Dislocation), tarsalmetatarsal region, metatarsophalangeal or interphalangeal (toes) region. (See Fig. 20–64.)

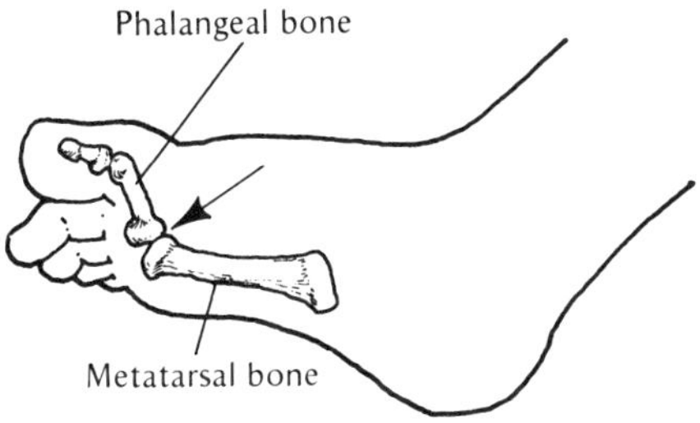


**Figure 20–64.** A metatarsophalangeal dislocation.

*Signs and Symptoms:* Severe pain, swelling, deformity, and inability to move foot or toes.

*Complications:* A mid-tarsal dislocation (Chopart's dislocation) is frequently open and circulatory status with this injury is usually compromised. Check neurovascular status, color, and temperature of foot and toes. A tarsalmetatarsal and interphalangeal dislocation is usually not complicated.

*Stabilization:* The foot can be stabilized by applying a pillow splint. Monitor vital signs, neurovascular status, and check for associated injuries.

## SUBLUXATION

A subluxation is a partial or incomplete dislocation of bones that form a joint. A subluxation may occur as a result of the same forces that occur in fractures and dislocation—direct trauma and indirect trauma. A joint area where subluxation commonly occurs is subluxation of the radial head.

## Subluxation of the Radial Head

This injury is exclusively seen in infants and young children and is known as "Nursemaid's Elbow." The injury is usually the result of pulling forcefully on a child's hand or forearm. This forces the proximal radius out of its encircling ligament. As a result, the child will not move his arm and is often seen holding the injured elbow with the opposite hand. There are usually no associated complications. The injury should be stabilized by immobilizing the elbow in a sling and swathe.

## Strains

When muscles and/or their tendons are stretched beyond normal limits, a strain occurs. Strains may occur with any type of forceful stretch, including direct and indirect trauma, twisting, and athletic injuries.

*Signs and Symptoms:* Pain, point tenderness, discoloration, swelling, and inability to move affected joint or injured area.

*Stabilization:* The injured area should be elevated and wrapped with a compression dressing. Cold packs should be applied, and the patient should be instucted to decrease use of the area for a short period of time to permit healing.

## Sprains

A sprain is a stretching or tearing of ligaments at the joint. Since ligaments are a localized thickening of the joint, a force strong enough to stretch or tear them usually causes other surrounding soft tissue injuries. This may occur from any violent force, directly or indirectly. Joints commonly affected include the shoulders, knees, and ankles. A mild sprain is usually defined as the partial disruption of the ligament(s) at the joint. A severe sprain is defined as the complete rupture of the ligament(s) at the joint. (See Fig. 20–65.)

*Signs and Symptoms:* Much the same as a strain—pain, point tenderness, swelling, discoloration, and inability to move joint area.

*Stabilization:* Sprains should be wrapped with a compression bandage and elevated; cold packs should be applied, and little or no weight should be permitted to bear on the injured joint.

# TREATMENT OF MUSCULOSKELETAL INJURIES

The role of the EMT when confronted with musculoskeletal trauma is to (1) perform a primary survey and assessment; (2) manage the patient's more serious injuries; and (3) properly immobilize the musculoskeletal in-

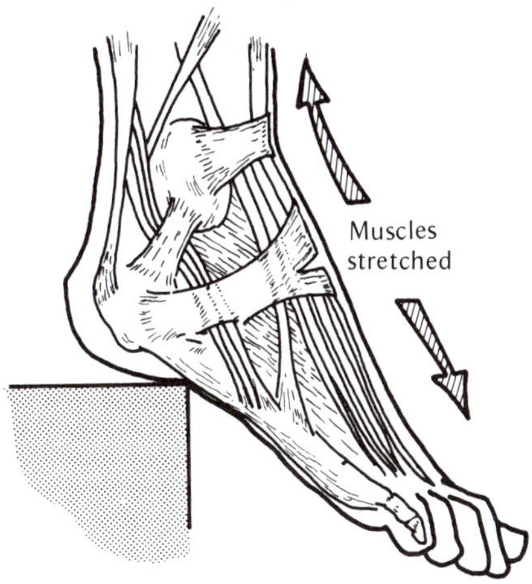


**Figure 20-65.** Strains occur from torn or stretched muscles and/or tendons.

juries. Since musculoskeletal injuries rarely pose a threat to life, a calm, unrushed systematic approach to the patient is necessary. By proceeding in this fashion, the EMT's actions may make the difference between a swift rehabilitation process and a long-term stay in the hospital with limb dysfunction. Musculoskeletal injuries are stabilized and immobilized to prevent:

1. Movement of broken bone fragment and joints
2. Neurovascular injuries
3. Additional pain
4. Additional swelling and hemorrhage
5. Muscle spasm
6. Other soft tissue injuries

In the field of medicine, there are no hard and fast rules. We have to consider the whole patient and the situation that surrounds each patient when we treat them, especially in the field! There are many right ways to treat the patient to accomplish the intended goal. The EMT must rely on his experience and common sense when treating musculoskeletal injuries, and if in doubt about the injury, splint the fracture in the position found.

## Angulated Closed Fractures

Fractures of the femur, tibia, fibula, humerus, radius, and ulna that are angulated may be straightened and splinted if: (1) joints are not involved, (2) dislocations are not involved, and (3) neurovascular compromise exists. (The EMT should contact the medical facility and report neurovascular findings and request permission to straighten the fracture.)

Again, if any doubt exists as to the extent of musculoskeletal injury, splint in the position found and monitor neurovascular status. If you do not initially straighten, and during transport the patient loses distal pulses, contact the medical facility and report findings.

## Angulated Open Fractures

Open fractures are serious injuries, especially in large bones (femur, pelvis, tibia). Besides considerable hemorrhage, environmental contamination to the wound and exposed bone pose a real threat of infection. The EMT should never try to push exposed bone back into the wound. The EMT should first stop any bleeding from the wound site by gentle pressure using a sterile dressing over the wound before splinting. Isolated angulated compound fractures should be immobilized in a traction splint if:

1. The injury does not involve a joint
2. There are no associated dislocations
3. The wound is relatively "clean" (e.g., no ground in dirt, grease, or manure)
4. In the position found, there is arterial compromise.

If there are multiple fractures along the angulated extremity associated with the open fracture, it is best to splint the extremity in the position found. These types of fractures may also be stabilized in antishock trousers, especially when a "shocky" state exists. If the EMT elects to place a traction splint on the patient, he will see that the exposed bone ends will probably go back into the wound due to the traction. That is what they should do! If neurovascular compromise is evident before or after splinting, the EMT should contact the designated hospital and report accurately and concisely the extent of injury and associated findings. The physician will then give direction as to the next step in medical management.

Management of musculoskeletal injuries differs from region to region. Check with your local medical director or training officer concerning specific field management.

### *Straightening Angulated Fractures*

Straightening means bringing the angulated fracture back into normal alignment with the rest of the limb. The EMT should have all necessary splinting equipment at hand before the straightening process begins.

To straighten an angulated fracture, the EMT should follow the steps as outlined below (See Fig. 20-66):

1. Inform the patient as to what you are going to do and why.

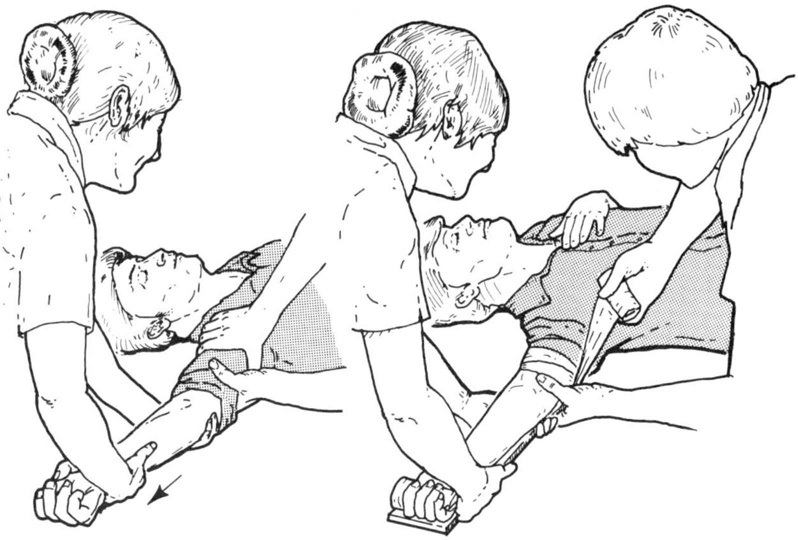

**Figure 20-66.** Procedure for straightening an angulated fracture.

2. The patient should be told that the process may be painful, but the pain should subside once straightened and immobilized.

3. With the aid of your partner, have him stabilize the limb above the injury, while you grasp the limb below the injury. With steady movement gently straighten the angulation.

4. Splint the fracture site so that the joints above and below are immobilized and monitor the neurovascular status.

5. Transport the patient with the injured limb elevated. Patients with lower limb fractures (femur or pelvis) should be placed on a padded long spine board.

## SPLINTS

Anything used to prevent movement of a joint for the purpose of bone immobilization after an injury is called a splint. There are four types of splints that the EMT may utilize to immobilize musculoskeletal injuries: (1) rigid splints, (2) soft splints, (3) traction splints, and (4) pneumatic splints. (See Fig. 20-67.) These splints may be used singly, together, or improvised, depending on the patient's injury and situation encountered. With the exception perhaps of splinting fractured fingers and toes, two EMTs are usually required to properly apply most splints. Many states regulate the types of splinting materials that must be carried on emergency transport units.

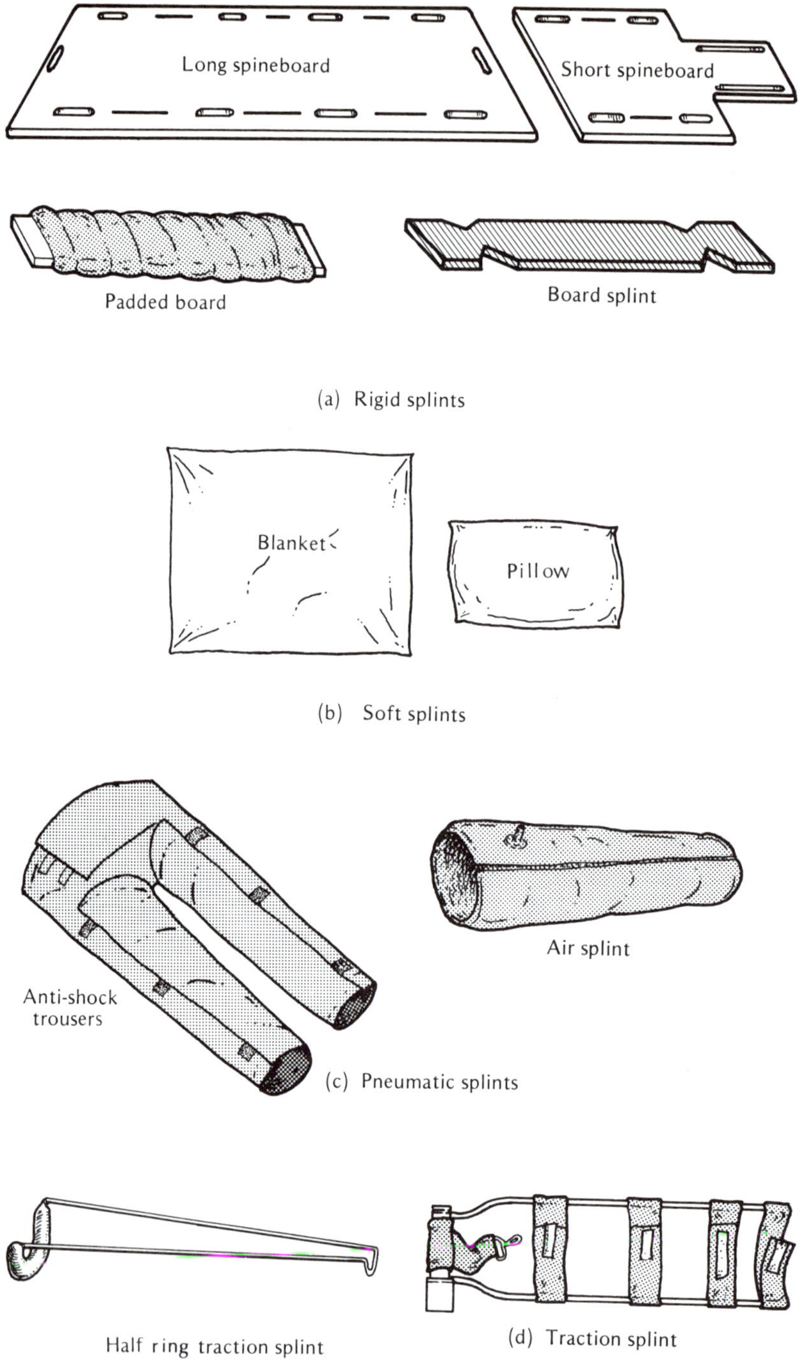


**Figure 20-67.** Various types of splints: (a) rigid splints; (b) soft splints; (c) pneumatic splints; (d) traction splints.

## Rigid Splints

Commercially available splints such as padded boards, wire ladder, premolded metal or plastic, creased cardboard, and long or short spine boards are all common types of rigid splints. Other appliances that may substitute for commercial splints in the field may include a folded newspaper, umbrellas, hockey sticks, a tree limb, a canoe paddle, boat oars, and tongue blades. Just about anything can work if need be. Because patients come in all sizes, the EMT must have available and choose a splint that is appropriate in size to immobilize the joint above and below the injured part of the patient. Unless the rigid splint is smoothly premolded to fit the extremity, all hard splints should be padded before application to aid in patient comfort. The EMT may manage a fracture with a rigid splint in the following manner (see Fig. 20–68):

1. Expose the injured area.
2. Cover all open wounds with sterile dressings.
3. Have all necessary splinting equipment at hand.
4. Explain to the patient what you will be doing and why.
5. One EMT stabilizes the limb above the injury, while the second EMT grasps the extremity below the injury and aligns angulation if need be.
6. The splint(s) is snugly applied to the extremity so that it immobilizes the joints above and below the injury after bandage materials are applied to secure the splint.
7. After splinting, monitor the neurovascular status distal to the injured site. Rigid splints can be improvised more than any other type of splint because you can fit them to immobilize almost any type of musculoskeletal injury.

## Soft Splints

The sling and swathe, folded pillows, blankets, and bandages to secure one limb to another are all considered soft splints. Although they are termed *soft*, when properly applied they immobilize joints above and below the injured site.

*Sling and Swathe:* A sling is a commercially available or handmade triangular bandage used primarily to support and immobilize injuries to the upper extremity. They are stabilized by a swathe (a wrap or binder). Injuries to the clavicle, scapula, humerus, and forearm can all be immobilized easily by a sling and swathe and rigid splints. A sling and swathe may be applied as follows (see Fig. 20–69):

1. Expose the injured area.
2. Cover all open wounds with a sterile dressing.

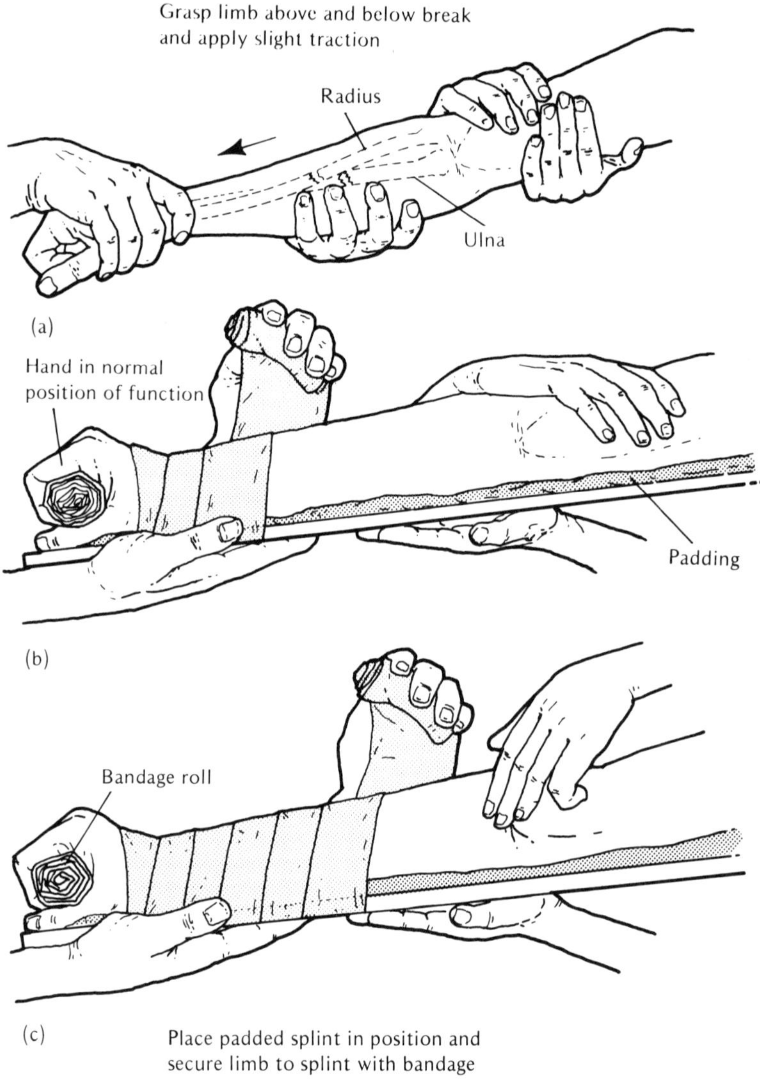


**Figure 20-68.** Procedure for applying a rigid splint.

3. Have all necessary equipment at hand.

4. Explain to the patient what you will be doing and why.

5. Bring the humerus close to the chest wall and bend the arm at the elbow (if no injury), at a ninety-degree angle, bringing the forearm across the anterior chest wall. Pad the area where the humerus will contact the side of the chest wall for comfort.

6. Apply the sling and raise the forearm within the sling, so that the patient's hands lie just below the middle line or the fourth or fifth anterior rib.

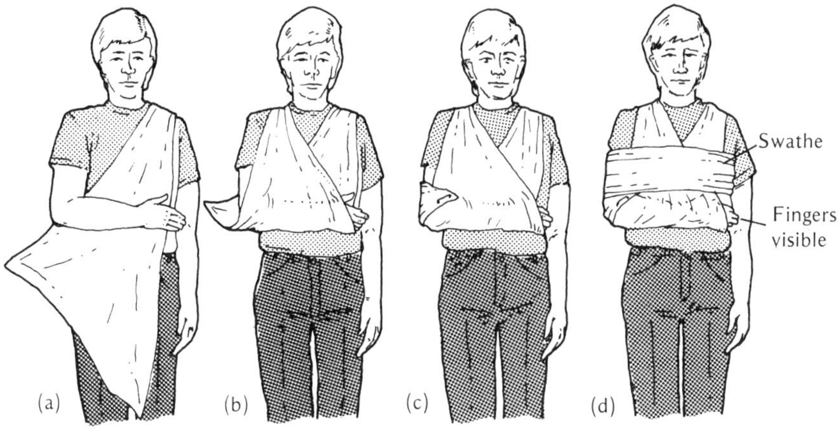


**Figure 20-69.** Procedure for applying a sling and swath.

7. Fold across the extended apex of the sling and fasten it to the sling material at the elbow. Tie off the ends of the sling at the back of the neck. For comfort, place a 4 × 4 under the knot. Do not place the knot at the side of the patient's neck. (Large vessels that run through the side of the neck may become irritated and/or blood flow may become obstructed.)

8. Leave the fingers visible so temperature, nerve, and vascular status may be monitored.

9. A swathe is then used by wrapping it around the patient's torso to immobilize the injured area. The swathe should not cross the injured area.

*Folded Pillows and Blankets:* These splints offer a lot of comfort and good immobilization to injuries of the foot and ankle. Splints of this nature should be molded around the posterior, medial, and lateral sides of the injured foot or ankle and fastened at the anterior aspect. Toes should be left exposed to monitor neurovascular status. (See Fig. 20-70.)

*Limb to Limb Splints:* Injuries, especially to the fingers and toes, may be splinted by lightly binding the injured digit or toe to the adjacent uninjured one. Hip and leg injuries may also be immobilized by lightly binding the injured extremity to the uninjured one. It is important that the EMT always place padding between one limb and the other, so that direct skin contact does not occur. This will aid in patient comfort and reduce the chance of skin irritation caused by direct skin contact. (See Fig. 20-71.)

## Pneumatic Splints

*Inflatable Air Splints:* Air splints immobilize injuries by circumferential pressure applied to the injured area and limb. There are two types: (1)

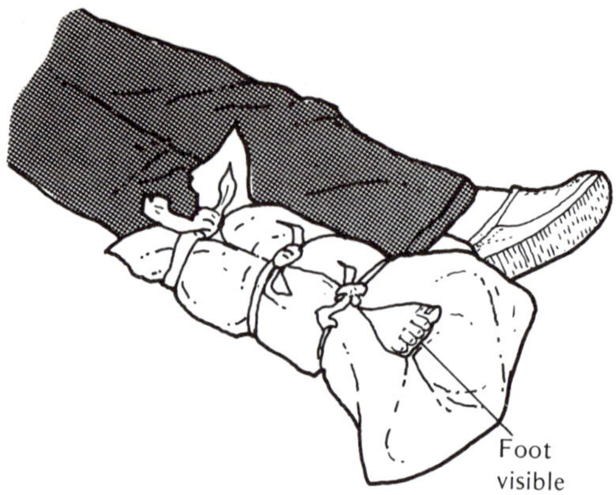


**Figure 20-70.** The pillow splint may be used effectively to immobilize injury to the ankle or foot.

plastic splints—orally inflatable, and (2) shock trousers—inflatable by foot pump.

*Plastic Air Splints:* These splints are commercially available in different sizes to accommodate upper and lower extremity injuries. They come in two varieties: (1) zipper type, and (2) "slip over" models. The zipper type can open up so that the limb may be placed in them.

The "slip over" model must be put on the arm or leg much like you would put a sock on your foot. The extremity must be guided into the splint. They are often quite cumbersome to apply. These splints should not be used for fractures to the humerus, hip, or femur because they cannot immobilize the joint above the injured site.

Important points to remember when applying plastic air splints are:

1. Do not place the zipper seam over the injured area or over open wounds.

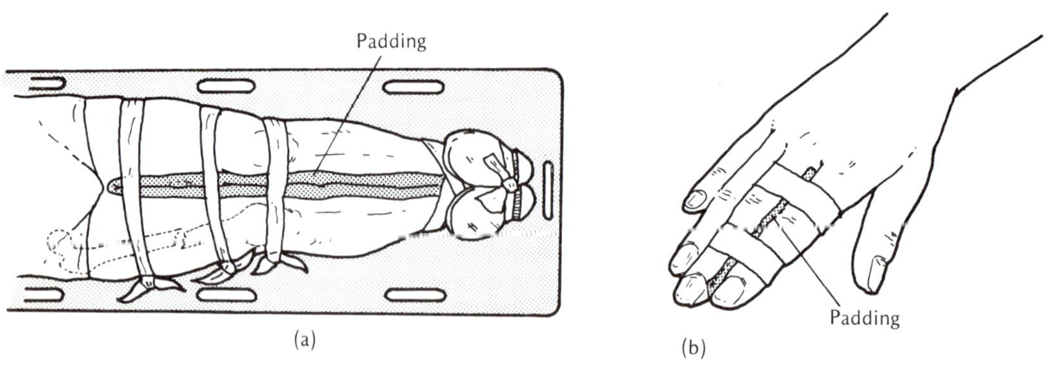


**Figure 20-71.** (a) Limb-to-limb splinting of the lower extremity and (b) the fingers.

2. Place a dressing over open fractures before application to avoid puncture.

3. Remove all sharp objects from the patient's clothing before application. Remove boots or shoes if application is to the lower leg or foot.

4. Inflate the splints periodically to test air capacity during storage periods.

5. Avoid temperature extremes, especially cold. These splints are extremely difficult to use when cold. The splints should be stored at temperatures between fifty and one-hundred degrees Fahrenheit if possible.

6. After use, the splint should be washed with soap and water or cold sterilized.

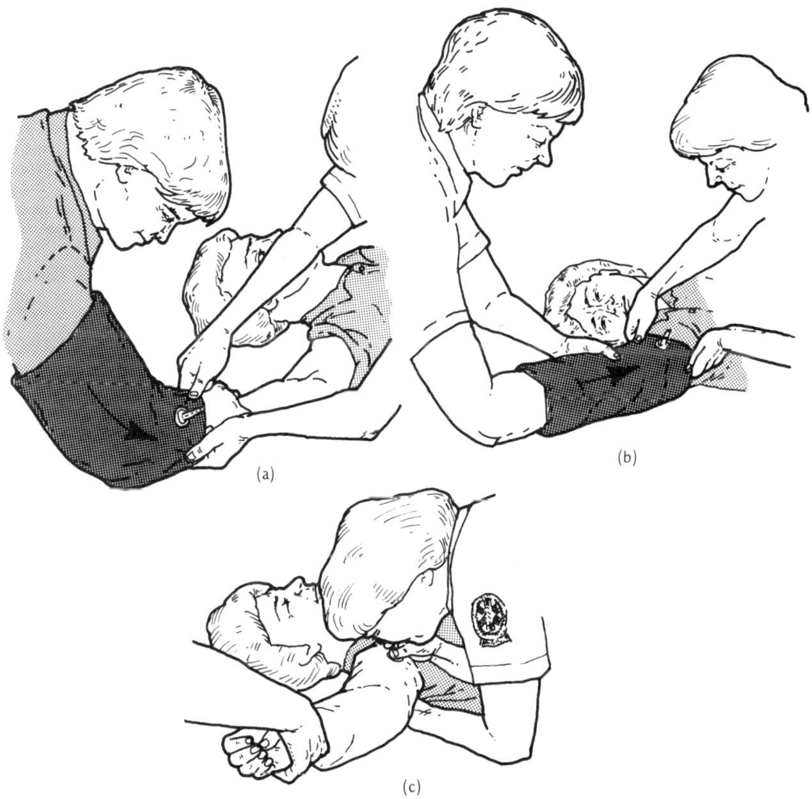

**Figure 20-72.** Procedure for applying a plastic air splint. (a) The injury is stabilized above and below the fracture site while traction is maintained. (b) The air splint is applied so that the zipper does not lie directly over an open wound or injury site. (c) The air splint is inflated until the injury is stabilized. Most patients will indicate relief of pain at point of stabilization.

7. These splints may be left on the patient for x-ray purposes.

8. Neurovascular assessment is impossible if they cover the hands and feet.

9. The EMT should always check the zipper of the splint for proper function before applying.

10. Plastic air splints are transparent, so the injured limb may be inspected regularly.

11. Plastic air splints should not be used for dislocations.

12. The circumferential pressure may aid in retarding hemorrhage.

Air splints should be inflated to a point where it feels good to the patient or you can easily indent the splint with your finger. Oral air splints are best used for simple nonangulated fractures. (See Fig. 20–72.)

### *Shock Trousers*

Shock trousers are used in shock management primarily to combat hypovolemia. However, their use in the stabilization and immobilization of pelvic and lower extremity fractures is well established. Since it is not uncommon for patients with pelvic and femoral fractures to lose 500 ccs of blood or more and develop shocky states, shock trousers are well suited for these injuries. Patients must be in a supine position for application of the trousers. If angulated compound fractures exist, the limb must be straightened and wounds dressed before trouser application. A traction splint may then be applied to the injured extremity over the trousers. All sharp objects should be removed from pants pockets before application. Inflating the trousers to 30–40 mm Hg will adequately immobilize the injury. The use of shock trousers will help reduce or stop hemorrhage and combat potential hypovolemia by redistributing lower extremity venous blood to the more vital organs (heart, brain, liver, and lungs). (See Fig. 20–73.)

## Traction Splints

Traction splints are designed to immobilize fractures by longitudinal pull, thereby aligning the distal bone fragment with the rest of the extremity. Commercially available traction splints include: (1) Thomas half-ring, (2) Sager, and (3) Hare.

The Thomas half-ring traction splint requires more manual preparation than the other types. This is because the leg cradles and ankle hitch are not premade for application.

The Hare traction splint is a telescoping one-piece device that has leg cradles and ankle hitch premade from Velcro webbing.

The Sager traction splint is a one-piece metal telescoping tube that is placed on the medial side of the lower extremity. It has leg straps for sup-

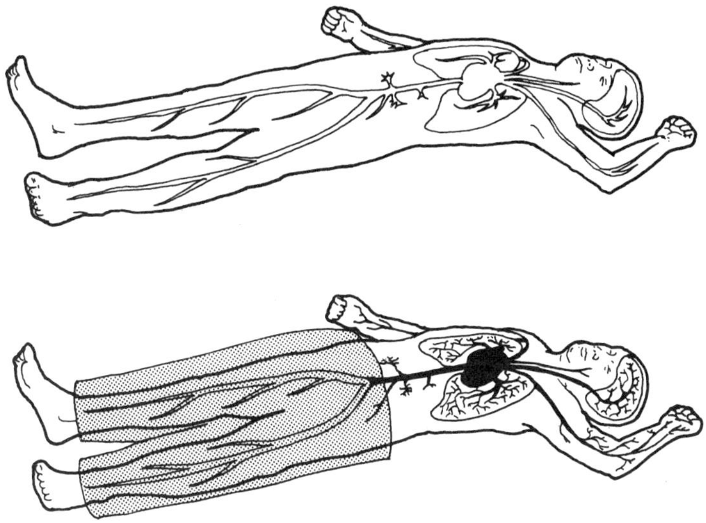

**Figure 20-73.** Shock trousers can be used to control bleeding and stabilize lower extremity fractures. Note the increased circulation to the more vital organs.

port, and a premade Velcro ankle hitch and weight calibrator for measuring the pounds of traction offered by its internal spring mechanism.

The EMT must remember when using these devices that when traction is applied at the ankle, countertraction is applied to the ischial tuberosity and perineum and this area must be well padded. The EMT should also be certain that ischial fractures do not exist. If there is doubt, rigid splints should be used. Two EMTs are required to apply any type of traction splint.

*Application of the Thomas Half-ring Traction Splint:* The EMT should always complete a primary survey of the patient and check the neurovascular status distal to the fractured area. The EMT may then proceed as follows (see Fig. 20-74):

1. Expose the injured area for inspection.

2. Explain the procedure to the patient and let him know that there may be pain while placing traction. Let him know that the pain should be considerably less after stabilization.

3. Have all necessary equipment prepared. This will include:

   a. three or four cravat cradles

   b. twist stick

   c. lock hitch attached to the end of the splint

   d. padding to be placed over the groin area

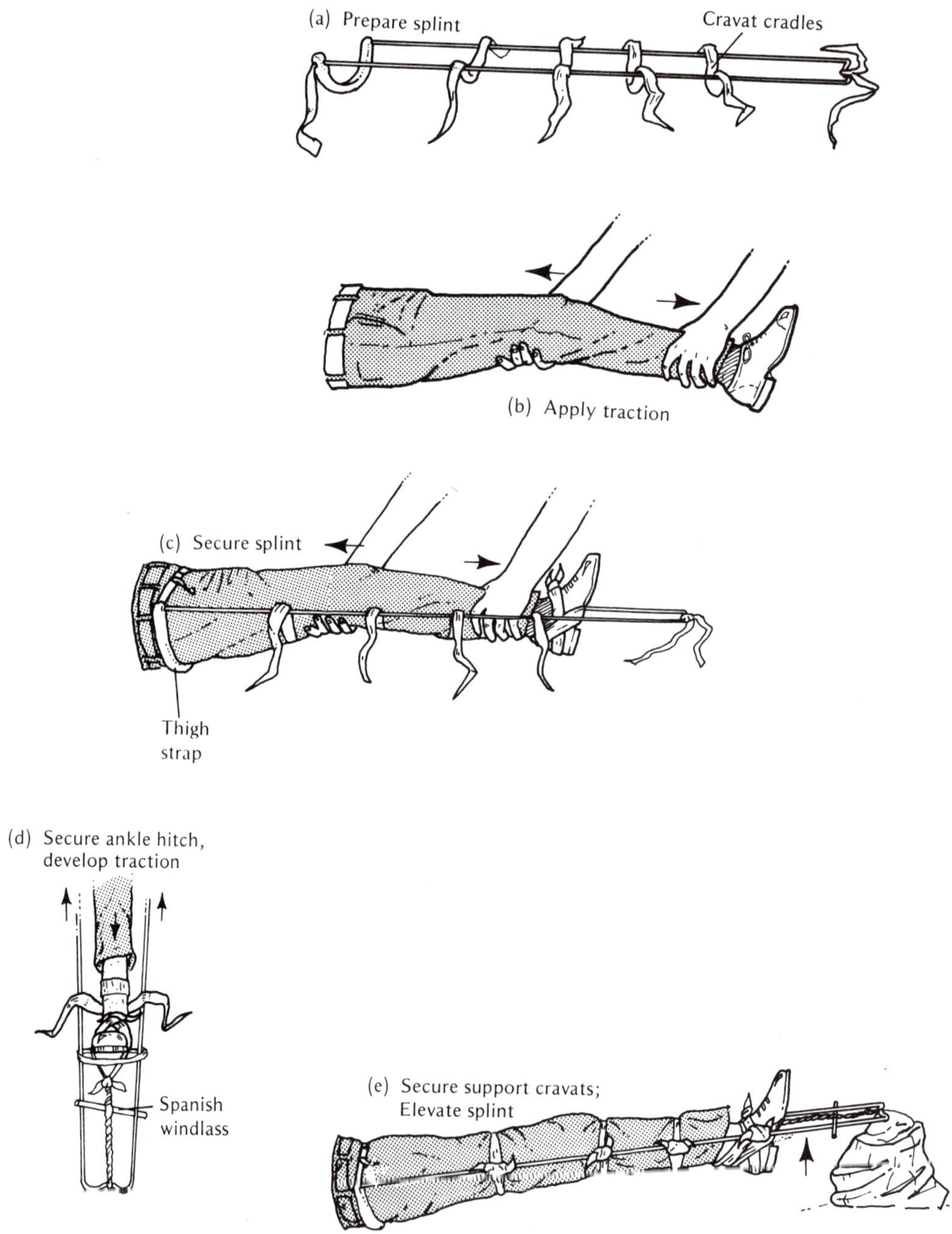


**Figure 20-74.** Procedure for applying the Thomas half-ring traction splint.

e. cravat or other material to tie off "Spanish windlass" (explained below)

f. splint placed next to injured limb

4. Patient should be in a supine position.

5. Apply ankle hitch, leaving the shoe or boot on. If ankle is not accessible, this step may be delayed until manual traction is applied.

6. While your partner stabilizes the area above and below the injured site, grasp the superior aspect of the patient's foot with one hand and posterior ankle with the other. With steady firm motion, straighten the extremity and maintain manual traction. The ankle should be elevated eight to twelve inches.

7. While maintaining manual traction, your partner now places the traction splint under the extremity, adjusting the padded half-ring against the perineum and ischial tuberosity. The perineum area should be padded.

8. The thigh strap is then secured.

9. The ankle hitch is then tied to the lock hitch.

10. The twist stick is then inserted through the tails of the lock hitch cravat and twisted until the traction is equal to your partner's manual traction. At this point, the twist stick is tied off and secured. (This type of traction with the twist stick is known as a "Spanish windlass.")(See Fig. 20–74.)

11. The leg cravats are then made taut, bringing the leg up between the splint. The ends of the leg cravats are then tied off at the side of the splint. They should not be tied off over the patient's leg.

12. The splint should be elevated eight to twelve inches.

13. The EMT should monitor distal neurovascular status en route to the hospital.

The patient's shoe or boot may be removed initially if there is doubt about injury. It is difficult to monitor neurovascular status with boots! If you place the traction splint on without footwear, be sure that the ankle and foot are padded to provide comfort and avert undue pressure, which may cause vascular compromise. It is also difficult to keep the foot and leg aligned properly with a bare foot. This is partly why it is recommended that footwear be left in place initially.

The use of this splint requires many hours of practice because of the manual preparation and team work involved. This is not an easy splint to apply if you have had little experience with it, but it works well if no other traction device is available.

*Application of the Hare Traction Splint:* The Hare traction splint utilizes attached Velcro straps on the splint that can slide under the patient's leg into the appropriate position. The splint also has a pre-prepared ankle hitch which contains a D ring that is attached to the S-ring on a ratchet traction system. The EMT may apply the splint in the following manner (See Fig. 20–75):

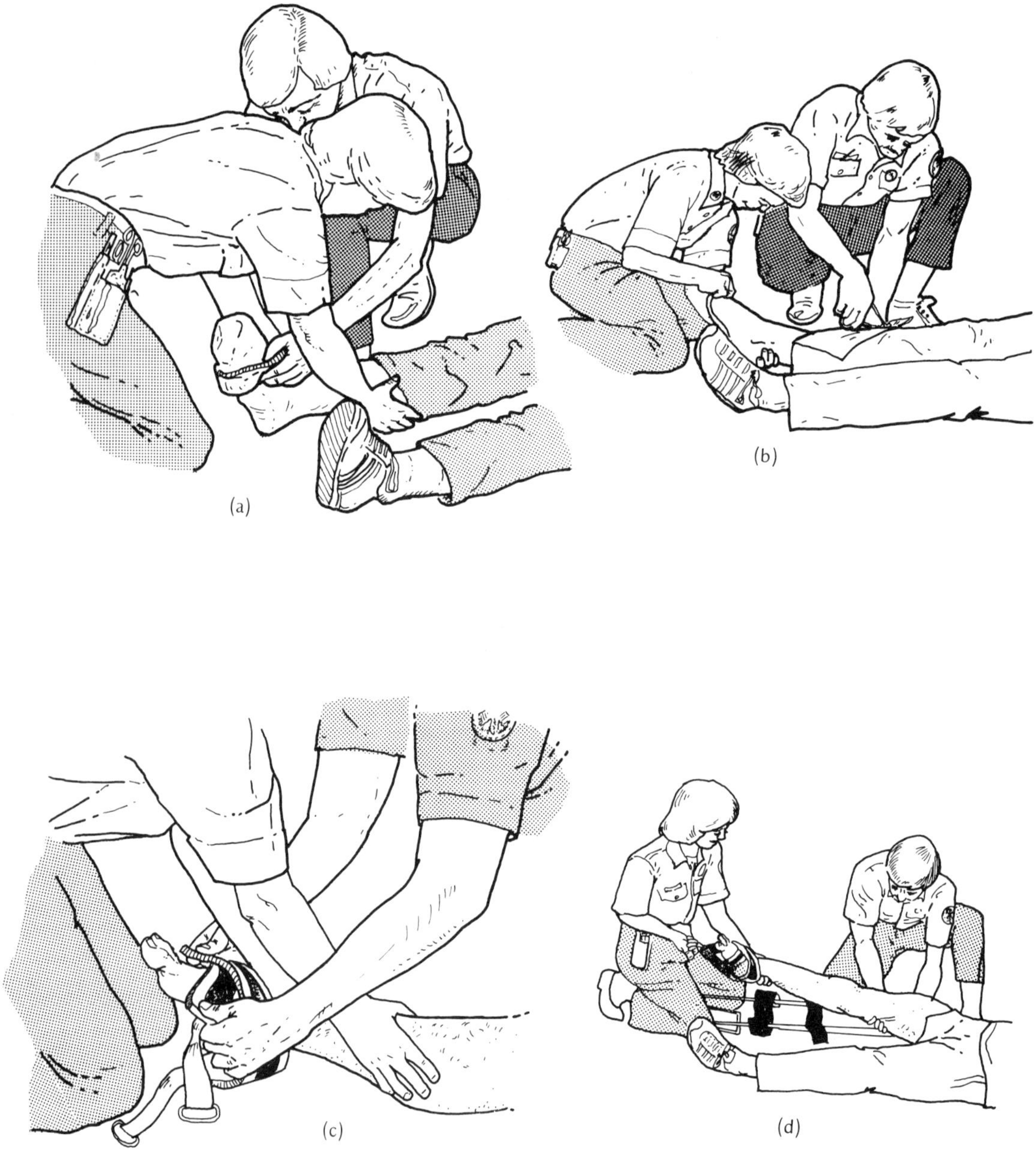

**Figure 20–75.** Procedure for applying the Hare traction splint. (a) EMT-A-1 removes the patient's shoe while the other EMT-A stabilizes the injured site. (b) EMT-A-1 exposes the injury site while EMT-A-2 supports the leg and palpates for the posterior tibial pulse. (c) EMT-A-2 applies manual traction to the injured limb while EMT-A-1 applies the ankle hitch. (d) EMT-A-1 positions the splint under the injured extremity while EMT-A-2 maintains

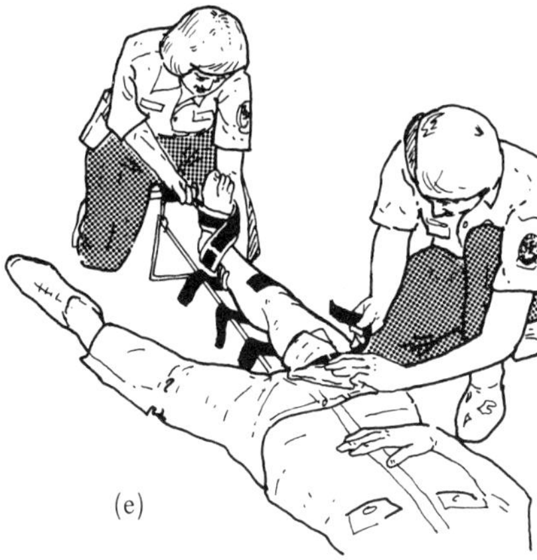

(e)

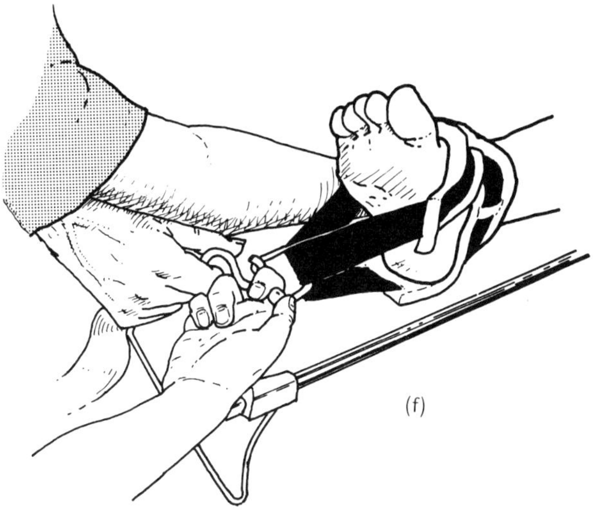

(f)

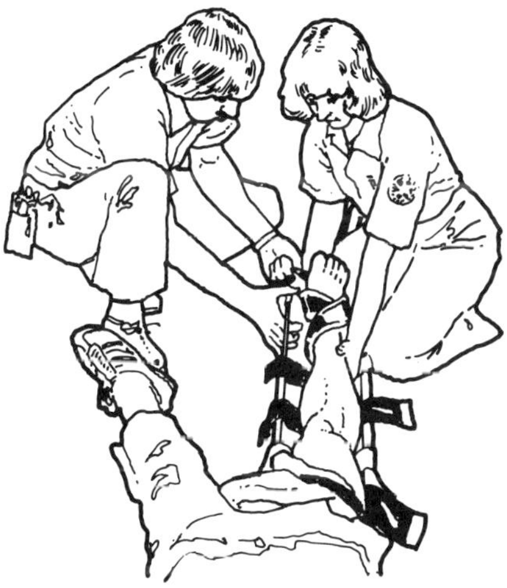

(g)

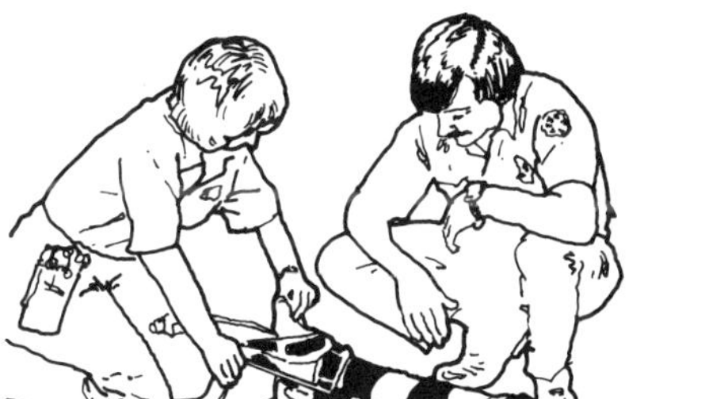

(h)

manual traction and elevates the injured leg. (e) EMT-A-1 places the splint snugly against the padded ischial tuberosity, applying the thigh strap in place. (f) EMT-A-1 places the S-ring through the D-ring of the ankle hitch. (g) EMT-A-1 applies traction by turning the ratchet until the mechanical traction equals the manual traction. (h) EMT-A-1 secures the Velcro leg support straps while EMT-A-2 positions the elevation stand of the traction splint.

1. Expose the injured area.
2. Explain procedure to the patient.
3. Place the prepared splint to the lateral side of the injured extremity.
4. Open and position the Velcro leg support straps so that the straps do not fit over the injury or knee.
5. Your partner stabilizes the injury above and below the fracture site while you apply the preprepared ankle hitch. The patient's shoe may be left on or taken off.
6. With steady movement the leg is straightened and manual traction is applied.
7. Your partner slides the splint under the injured extremity, placing it snugly against the ischial tuberosity. The groin should be padded.
8. He then secures the thigh strap in place.
9. At the ankle he places the S-ring through the D-rings and turns the ratchet until the mechanical traction is equal to manual traction.
10. After appropriate traction has been applied, the Velcro leg support straps are fixed in place.
11. The elevation stand attached to the splint is opened and the leg is elevated eight to twelve inches.
12. The EMT should then reassess neurovascular status.

*Application of the Sagar Emergency Traction Splint:* The splint is 30 inches long and weighs 2-3/4 pounds. It is constructed of two stainless steel tubes, one sliding within the other so that variable length may be obtained by telescoping the inner tube in and out. The outer shaft has a padded cross arm designed with compound curves to fit in the perineum (crotch) adjacent to the thigh. Velcro straps on the padded cross arm are provided to pull the pad snugly against the thigh in the lateral portion of the perineum. The distal end of the outer shaft has a locking device which permits extension and locking in position on the inner shaft; holes are drilled along the inner shaft to provide stops for the locking device. The inner shaft of the splint has a pulley shroud, pulley, and cable ring apparatus attached to an anchored internal spring, which permits application of force on the ankle when the splint is extended. The pulley is calibrated, permitting the operator to know the number of pounds of force applied. A general rule is to apply ten percent of the patient's body weight, up to a maximum of 25 pounds. There is an ankle harness with padding designed to fit around the ankle just above the medial and lateral maleoli. The harness is universal and fits around any size ankle or boot. The splint is applied as follows:

1. If possible, explain the procedure to the patient.
2. Expose the injured area.

3. Roughly measure the length of splint needed on the uninjured leg, extending the splint from the perineum to approximately 4 inches past the heel of the foot.

4. If the injured leg is angulated, straighten it and apply traction manually.

5. Place the padded end of the splint in the crotch, gently sweeping the genitalia of a male patient out of the way.

6. Pull the thigh strap securely around the upper thigh, drawing the crotch pad to the lateral side of the perineum.

7. Apply the ankle harness around the ankle above the medial and lateral maleoli.

8. Release the locking device and extend the splint until the desired amount of traction in pounds is obtained and noted on the calibrated pulley wheel.

9. Apply the longest 6-inch-wide elasticized strap over the splint and around the upper thigh.

10. Apply the second longest 6-inch-wide elasticized strap over the splint and around the lower thigh and knee.

11. Apply the shortest 6-inch-wide elasticized strap around the lower leg and splint.

12. Then apply the 1-inch-wide strap in a figure-eight over the ankles and feet.

13. Place the patient on a spine board and strap him to it in the usual manner. The patient is now ready for transport. (See Fig. 20–76.)

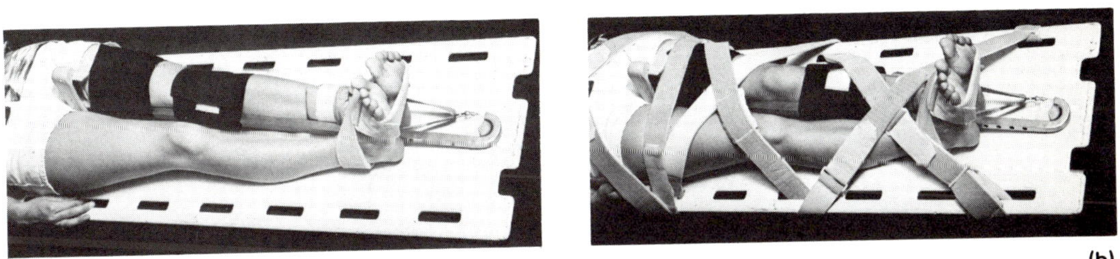

(a) (b)

**Figure 20–76.** (a) This patient has traction and splinting and is ready for strapping to the spine board. Note: Medial and lateral bone fragment movement and internal and external rotation of distal bone fragments are controlled with thigh straps and a figure-of-eight around the ankles and feet. (*Reprinted with permission of Anthony G. Borschneck, M. D., Minto Research & Development, Inc.*) (b) This patient is completely immobilized with thigh and leg straps, plus ankle and foot figure-of-eight strap. The patient is further immobilized on the spine board and is ready for transportation. (*Reprinted with permission of Anthony G. Borschneck, M. D., Minto Research & Development, Inc.*)

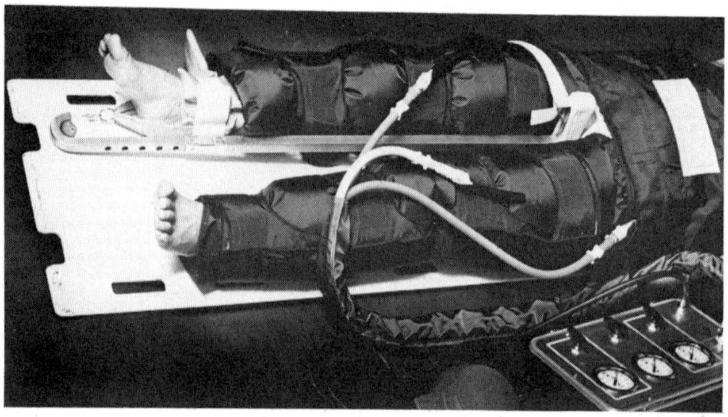

**Figure 20–77.** This patient has the Sagar emergency traction splint over antishock trousers. Fracture immobilization and traction is obtained by combined use of the splint and shock trousers. (*Reprinted with permission of Anthony G. Borschneck, M. D., Minto Research & Development, Inc.*)

If the patient is in shock and needs antishock trousers in addition to having fractures of the lower limb requiring traction, application of the Sagar Emergency Traction Splint is very quick and simple. Depending on the circumstances, the splint can be applied either before or after the application of the antishock trousers:

1. Fit the proper length of splint to the leg as above.
2. Apply the ankle harness.
3. Extend the inner shaft to the proper traction as noted in pounds on the calibrated pulley wheel.
4. Apply the thigh strap. (See Fig. 20–77.)

## SPECIAL CONSIDERATIONS

### Loading the Patient with a Traction Splint

The EMT should keep in mind that with a tall patient who has a traction splint on, the extended telescoping end may not allow clearance when shutting the rear door. Since most vehicles have a stretcher lock mechanism to keep the stretcher in place during transport, you cannot move the stretcher up to make clearance for the extended telescoping end of the splint. However, the patient can be placed feet first in the vehicle so that clearance is possible to close the door. If the EMT elects to transport the patient in this fashion, make certain that all necessary medical equipment is at hand at the opposite end of the vehicle, such as oxygen, bag-valve-mask, and airways. The transport of every patient is important, and the EMT should be cognizant of the potential hazards that exist when transporting the patient.

## Transporting

An important part of treatment related to musculoskeletal injury is the actual vehicle transport of the patient. The driver of the emergency vehicle has the potential of making a stabilized injury very unstable. The ride should be as smooth as possible, guarding against sudden stops and starts that jar the patient. We have all been witness to the effect of cresting a hill at a high rate of speed and being bounced into the air as we go over it. Not only can this restart bleeding and injure surrounding soft tissue, but it could convert a closed fracture into an open one! When driving, the EMT should pay particular attention in turning corners, going over railroad tracks, and driving on dirt roads with a "washboard" effect.

## Challenging Situations

Many situations will demand that the EMT move the patient from the position found to a more suitable one for total immobilization. This will often be the case in vehicle entrapment, and in those situations where fractures of the extremities exist and the patient is found in a prone position. If the patient is trapped in a vehicle, depending on what is injured and what is exposed for you to work on, you will probably have to wait for further definitive treatment until the patient is extracted. The EMT should take all possible advantages of stabilizing injuries while the extrication procedure is being done. Most of the time, at least, the upper spine can be immobilized. If the patient is found in a prone position, conscious and with a patent airway with musculoskeletal trauma, the EMT should capitalize on the position of the patient. Assess all possible injuries to the posterior head, neck, spine, back, and extremities. After this assessment, and with the help of at least two people, log-roll the patient into a supine position, stabilizing all possible fractures as you turn the patient, especially the cervical spine. If the patient is in a prone position and unconscious, the EMT must proceed in a systematic fashion, log-rolling the patient and protecting against all possible fractures. Determine the medical priorities and then immobilize fracture sites.

Gunshot wounds to the bones of the extremity must be immobilized quickly, especially if the victim has been shot in other body areas and is still conscious. These patients will go into a shock state (depending on the area shot), and as they do, their level of consciousness starts to deteriorate and they will get very restless and move about frantically. It is not uncommon, for example, that a patient who has had a femur shattered from a gunshot wound to flex his leg about. Centerfire weapons such as 357 and 44 magnums and 9mm handguns are notorious for this type of bone and body destruction, as well as shotgun blasts at point-blank range. These victims must be treated for shock on the scene and all bone fractures immobilized. Shock trousers are ideal for this type of patient.

## Basic Principles

Proper management of musculoskeletal injuries demands the understanding of patient approach, the injury itself, and complications that may occur during management. Important principles that the EMT should keep in mind with musculoskeletal injuries include the following:

1. Communicate with your patient. Let him know what you are doing and why.

2. Remove clothing from around the injury for inspection. Many injuries are missed by lack of careful assessment.

3. Always immobilize the joint above and below the injured site.

4. Always monitor the circulatory and nerve status distal to the injured site before and after splinting. In the upper extremity, check the brachial and radial pulse. In the lower extremity check the posterior tibial pulse and dorsalis pedis pulse. (The pedal pulse is often too difficult to palpate, especially in a moving vehicle.)

5. Active bleeding from fracture wounds may be controlled by direct pressure or application of an air splint.

6. Open wounds associated with fractures should be covered with a sterile dressing before splinting.

7. Never attempt to push exposed bone fragments back into an open wound. Traction may, however, draw bone fragments back into the wound—that is what traction is supposed to do.

8. Manipulation of the injured extremity should be kept at a minimum.

9. All splints should be padded to avoid excessive pressure, especially areas of the groin, axilla, and ankle.

10. Never attempt to straighten a fracture or dislocation involving joints unless directed by a physician.

11. Closed and open fractures not involving joints should be straightened when appropriate.

12. Never straighten a dislocation. (The only exception may be a posterior knee dislocation with arterial compromise.) In any case, the physician should be notified and he alone should give the order to straighten a dislocation.

13. Sprains and strains should be managed as if they were fractures.

14. Do not bind splints so tightly as to impair circulation.

15. Tourniquets are rarely needed to control bleeding.

16. If appropriate, traction splints can be used in conjunction with shock trousers.

17. When splinting or bandaging, always keep hands and feet exposed to monitor neurovascular status.

18. Never directly bind one extremity to the other unless padding exists between the areas.

19. Whenever you are in doubt about an injury, splint it.

20. Every good EMT should realize his own limitations when splinting fractures, and should request medical direction when in doubt.

## *References*

American Academy of Orthopedic Surgeons, Committee on Allied Health. *Emergency Care of the Sick and Injured,* 2nd ed. Chicago, IL: American Academy of Orthopedic Surgeons, 1977.

Anast, George T. "Physical Assessment of Long Bone Fractures," *Emergency Product News,* January/February 1977.

Barber, Janet M., and Budassi, S. A. *Manual of Emergency Care Practices and Procedures.* St. Louis, MO: The C. V. Mosby Company, 1979.

Borschneck, A. G., and Wayne, Marvin A. "Sagar Emergency Traction Splint: A New Splinting Device for Lower Limb Fractures," *The EMT Journal,* Vol. 4, No. 1, March 1980. St. Louis, MO: The C. V. Mosby Co.

Caroline, N. L. *Emergency Care in the Streets.* Boston, MA: Little, Brown & Company, 1979.

Erven, L. E. *Handbook of Emergency Care and Rescue.* Beverly Hills, CA: Glencor Press, 1976.

Frey, C. F. *Initial Management of the Trauma Patient.* Philadelphia, PA: Lea and Febiger, 1976.

Gardner, E.; Gray, D. J.; and O'Rahilly, R. *Anatomy: A Regional Study of Human Structure.* Philadelphia, PA: W. B. Saunders Company, 1975.

Gardner, A. W., and Roylance, P. J. *New Essential First Aid.* Boston, MA: Little, Brown & Company, 1971.

Gartland, J. T. *Fundamentals of Orthopedics.* Philadelphia, PA: W. B. Saunders Company, 1974.

Gazzaniga, Alan B.; Iseri, Lloyd T.; and Baren, Martin. *Emergency Care: Principles and Practices for the EMT-Paramedic.* Reston, VA: Reston Publishing Co., Inc., 1979.

Grant, H. D., and Murray, R. H., Jr. *Emergency Care,* 2nd ed. Bowie, MD: Robert J. Brady Company, 1978.

Hawken, Samuel M. "Injuries to Tendons and Ligaments," *Emergency Product News,* November 1977.

Henderson, J. *Emergency Medical Guide.* St. Louis, MO: McGraw-Hill Book Company, 1978.

Hoppenfield, Stanley. *Orthopedic Neurology: A Diagnostic Guide to Neurologic Levels.* Philadelphia, PA: J. B. Lippincott Co., 1977.

Looser, Kevin G., and Crombie, H. D. "Pelvic Fractures: An Anatomic Guide to Severity of Injury," *The American Journal of Surgery,* Vol. 132, November 1976.

O'Donnell, Thomas F; Brewster, David C.; Darling, Clement R.; Veen, Herman; Waltman, Arthur. "Arterial Injuries Associated with Fractures and/or Dislocations of the Knee," *The Journal of Trauma,* Vol. 17 No. 10, Oct. 1977.

Parcel, G. S. *First Aid in Emergency Care.* St. Louis, MO: The C. V. Mosby Company, 1977.

Stephenson, H. D. Jr. *Immediate Care of the Acutely Ill and Injured.* St. Louis, MO: The C. V. Mosby Company, 1978.

# Chapter 21

# Managing Emotional And Behavioral Problems

## NORMAL BEHAVIOR PROBLEMS OF VICTIMS AND BYSTANDERS

Sudden illness and injury produces stress in everyone involved: the victim, family, bystanders *and* the EMT. How you understand and manage that stress and the behavior problems that develop from it can make an important difference. Knowing what to do can make your job easier, and facilitate the recovery of the patient as well as the others associated with the trauma.

Once a patient believes he is critically ill, injured or in danger of death, a number of reactions are common. Professionals such as Dr. Elisabeth Kübler-Ross, who work with dying patients, have noted frequently occurring methods of coping with their terminal illness. Similar reactions have been found to be true for people who experience nonlethal trauma!

### *Emotional Shock and Confusion*

The shock of sudden illness or injury often elicits an initial reaction of disorientation, disorganization, and confusion. A disoriented person is one who has lost his bearings as to time, who or where he is. His behavior may become disorganized in so far as it is lacking order or any rational objective. Because of this, patients or bystanders will sometimes attempt a remedy which may seem irrational and ineffective. They may overreact—race from one thing to another, and only get in your way.

### *Anxiety and Fears*

Anxiety is an emotional experience resulting from a perceived threat to one's safety. A normal reaction to severe trauma includes anxiety symptoms such as sweating, shaking, weakness, nausea, and even vomiting.

Such tension can rise from a fear of the unknown as a result of the trauma. Fearful questions such as, "How much pain will I have? Will I be disabled? Will I die?" often occur in a patient's mind. A loss of control and sense of helplessness contribute to the anxiety. If the anxiety is severe enough, panic can set in. Good judgment disappears completely, and panic can be contagious.

*Denial*

Some people greatly minimize or ignore their problem. They may insist they're all right, when it's obviously not so or they may play down or dismiss their symptoms with words like "It hurts only a little" . . . "I can't believe this has happened," or behavior to that effect, e.g., trying to drive an obviously disabled automobile.

*Regression*

Under great pressure and stress, many of us temporarily regress to previously preferred, more primitive, and immature means of coping. An adult victim may behave like a child, e.g., throwing a temper tantrum, crying hysterically, sucking his thumb.

*Depression*

Whenever there is loss or threat of loss to our health or normal functioning, we usually experience some degree of depression. The depressed person may appear too quiet for the situation or he may become withdrawn and uncommunicative, partly in response to the shock.

*Anger*

When some people are frightened and helpless, they respond with anger. They may take it out on *you* by demanding unrealistic, immediate action, or questioning your competence: "Get him to a *real doctor* fast" . . . "Are you sure you know what you're doing?"

*Conversion Reaction*

In some patients, extreme anxiety can produce a conversion reaction, i.e., the individual unconsciously develops or "converts" the distress into a physical symptom such as blindness, deafness, or partial paralysis. Sometimes the person may demonstrate surprisingly little concern over the loss. The symptom usually serves some unconscious purpose, often symbolically to avoid painful emotions, e.g., the person who loses his sight after viewing a gruesome accident scene. Usually the symptom lasts only a short time and complete recovery of the lost function is achieved. Longer lasting reactions can be effectively treated with psychotherapy.

## Guidelines for Handling These Problems

As an emergency health professional you bring to the scene not only emergency medical skills, but also order and relief to a disordered, anxiety-ridden situation.

1. Serious physical illness and injury must be treated first, but do not ignore treatment of the psychological problems. Your manner of approach can significantly reduce the intensity of the early painful reactions to crisis.

2. To the shocked, confused, panicked, and despairing victim, you bring order, organization, calm, and hope. Identify yourself and take charge of the situation. An attitude of calm self-assurance needs to be communicated. Let your voice be firm and strong. Be sympathetic, yet businesslike. Especially for the confused, disorganized individuals, give clear, simple directions. Repeat them. The disoriented person needs to be reoriented with regard to time, place, person, and situation with calm, simple, concrete information.

3. Allow people to have and express their emotions. Telling them how they should or should not feel only adds to their confusion and guilt and may render them less cooperative. Give them permission to vent feelings. For example, "It's OK to cry—I know you're scared and hurt. We're doing everything possible." Even though a flood of emotions may seem to serve no immediate, rational purpose, it does serve to ultimately facilitate psychological recovery from the trauma.

4. As long as he is not harming himself or others, allow an upset, angry person to ventilate. He is deflecting his own sense of frustration and tension. *Don't take his attacks personally.* Recognizing his feelings without necessarily agreeing with him can de-escalate the rage considerably, e.g., "I know you're pretty angry and upset. We don't like what's happened either and we're doing everything possible."

5. Keep emotionally upset people and spectators away from patients. Interference by well-meaning bystanders is often caused by their observing a traumatic situation, identifying with the victim and feeling anxious and helpless enough to try something, even though it may be unproductive. Interference by the "helpers" can often be minimized by assigning them some simple, appropriate task. Should a bystander continue to interfere inappropriately, firmly confronting him with the unproductive effects of his behavior or removing him may be necessary.

6. If a patient's denial is interfering with emergency medical care, confrontation is necessary. An effective means of confronting includes the following elements:

a. Description of the behavior situation, e.g., "Mr. Thompson, your arm looks badly bruised and crushed."

b. An explanation of the consequences of continued denial, e.g., "Let me examine your arm. It could be broken and it won't heal properly unless treated."

7. Remember, even though a patient may be seriously injured, he is often sensitive and embarrassed by being examined. Damaged feelings can be as real as a damaged body. If possible, talk with the patient briefly before beginning your physical exam. Making some kind of human, caring, yet professional contact with the patient will reduce much anxiety and establish some trust. Be aware of an unclothed patient's embarrassment and make sure he is covered as much as possible to avoid curious stares by bystanders. Talking with a patient during your exam and medical procedure will help to reduce his anxiety and build some trust. Whenever possible, inform him of what you are doing and what will happen next. Minimize surprises.

8. The possibility of serious disability or death panics many patients to a degree that their anxiety may worsen their condition. If you are reasonably confident that their condition is not seriously disabling or life threatening, reassure them that this is the case. "You're not going to die." "You won't lose that leg." If their condition is not clear or is serious, you can tell them their condition is serious and that you are doing everything possible.

## SPECIAL BEHAVIOR PROBLEMS

### The Patient Who Refuses Transportation to the Hospital

Particularly perturbing is the patient who, in spite of a clear need for emergency medical treatment, refuses to cooperate. Your success in persuading him to accept help will depend upon your knowing his particular source of resistance. Ask him why he doesn't want help. He may or may not reveal his reasons directly. In all such cases, the patient should first be confronted with the reality of his physical condition and the serious, endangering consequences of his refusal to accept help. Other approaches depend upon the specific patient resistances.

### Domestic Disturbances

Domestic disturbance can sometimes be the most exasperating and high risk for the EMT. This is largely because you are entering a volatile situation where hostility may continue to pervade the atmosphere. Rage previously directed towards the original victim can sometimes be deflected toward you. Most violent acts, including murder, are inflicted by a family member or other close acquaintances. Often alcohol intoxication is involved and judgment and self-controls are poor. The assailant (a-sāl′ant) may even threaten the EMT if he assists the injured party. The

| Patient Resistance | Suggested Approach |
|---|---|
| 1. The patient has strong needs to demonstrate his toughness, manhood, etc. | 1. Reinforce and commend him for the strength and bravery he has already shown. If possible find some medical task he can do for himself, but emphasize the importance of obtaining additional help. |
| 2. Patient needs to demonstrate his independence. | 2. Increase his sense of choice. For example, *how* he goes to the hospital, *which* hospital he goes to. |
| 3. Patient fears legal charges or discovery of identity. | 3. Privately confront him with the consequences of endangering himself by refusing treatment. |
| 4. Fear of the unknown diagnostic or treatment procedures carried out at the hospital, questions of cost, etc. | 4. Explain in concrete step-by-step terms what most likely will happen to him once he arrives at the hospital. Emphasize the quality of the medical care that will be given when he arrives. Explain to him briefly any financial arrangements that can be made and emphasize the ultimate importance of his physical well being. |

In general, avoid arguing with the patient, since this will only tend to increase his resistance.

following guidelines have been found to be useful in managing such situations:

1. If there is suspicion of further violence, approach the scene slowly and calculate potential danger to yourself and others.

2. If risk of further violence seems likely, call or wait for law enforcement personnel to arrive.

3. When approaching the dwelling of a domestic disturbance scene, move to the side of the door frame, listen for cues of inside activities; knock on the door, announce your identity and your reason for being there. Proceed cautiously.

4. Avoid entering into the conflict itself. If possible, arrange to have the fighting parties separated with as much physical distance as possible before treating the injuries.

## Child Injury and Illness

Children are normally dependent people. They rely upon consistent routines and the availability of particular, familiar adults for reinforcement of their well-being and security. Sudden illness or injury greatly intensifies these needs. The changes accompanying pain, body injury, or unfamiliar emergency personnel and equipment tend to be more traumatizing for a child than an adult. For this reason, parents or other familiar caretakers should be allowed to maintain physically close, reassuring contact with the child as long as it does not interfere with treatment procedures. It is recommended that a parent accompany the child in the ambulance. Taking along a familiar toy, blanket, or other object can help reduce the child's distress and trauma.

The normally protective responses of parents are also magnified by such trauma. Occasionally, the severe distress of a child injury precipitates overreaction and overprotectiveness of the parent, which can ultimately interfere with the emergency treatment. An hysterical, crying mother may only worsen the child's distress. It will be necessary to help this person regain control before she can be helpful with the child. If this is not readily accomplished, some other familiar responsible adult should accompany the youngster.

Regardless of whether the parent was responsible for the child's trauma or not, he or she usually experiences considerable guilt and self-blame. Except in cases of obvious abuse or willfull neglect, criticism of the parent is usually unwarranted and counterproductive. A nonjudgmental, supportive attitude in addition to giving a parent some useful task is ultimately much more beneficial in allaying his distress as well as that of the child. In cases of suspected neglect or abuse, most state laws require an EMT to report the case to the proper authorities. Let the attending nurse or physician know about circumstances, if any, at the home or emergency scene that you think might aid or influence the future protection of the child.

## The Rape Victim

The victim of rape has just experienced a violent, degrading, often life-threatening trauma. She is apt to be in a state of stunned disbelief and may be agitated, incoherent, and emotionally upset. A strong sense of fear and having been violated predominates. The victim needs reassurance, warmth, and support. Give her permission to talk about the trauma and ventilate feelings if she wishes. If she is not ready to "open up," encourage her to talk and be with a responsible person whom she trusts as soon as possible. Primary medical concern is for treatment of injuries, prevention of venereal disease, and possible pregnancy. (Even though less than 5 percent of women who are raped become pregnant as a result, the fear of such a pregnancy can be devastating.)

The victim will also need assistance with the emotional impact of the trauma. It is common for her to experience considerable fear, rage, guilt, and depression for months after the assault. She will have difficulty telling and dealing with family and friends about it. There are a growing number of rape crisis teams, intervention centers, and trained professionals available to assist with the medical, legal, and emotional aspects of the crime. Be familiar with and encourage her to use these resources in your community.

## The Dying or Deceased Patient and His Significant Others

Issues of death are inescapable for the EMT in his daily work. As mentioned earlier in this chapter, Elisabeth Kübler-Ross in her work with dying patients has identified at least five phases experienced by most people when they are aware of their impending death: denial, anger, bargaining, depression, and acceptance. In spite of a rapidly growing interest in this area in the past number of years, death still tends to be an avoided subject in our culture. It is strongly recommended that the EMT directly consider his own attitudes about death, develop his own philosophy-belief system, and examine his own life and death issues. Some degree of personal resolution in this area will help him deal much more effectively with the death issues of others whom he encounters in his work.

### *Dying Patients*

In the case of patients who appear to be near death, the EMT is usually focusing most of his attention on life-maintenance procedures. If the patient is conscious or even partially conscious, it is usually helpful to communicate encouraging words to him to instill some hope and revitalize any life energy that remains. Experienced EMTs, paramedics, physicians, nurses, and other health professionals who work closely with dying patients have repeatedly been impressed with the impact that the patient's attitudes toward living and death have upon his ultimate recovery. Encouraging his will to live and life-supporting statements made to a critical patient even though he may appear unconscious may very well have a positive, nurturing effect. When all medical interventions have been completed and the patient knows he is dying, there may be a tendency for the EMT to avoid him. Don't. Dying patients often feel alone, are deeply lonely, and need close personal contact. Talk with him and, even more important, listen.

Despite all the best interventions, some patients will not respond to our efforts and will die. (Often the patient will be transported to the hospital before death is formally determined. There, it is recommended that the physician inform relatives of the death.) If the patient is clearly dead and you are still present at the scene, your attention may then need to be directed to nearby family and friends. You may not be a clergyman or want the role of the official proclaimer of bad news, but you are still a caring human being. Significant other people close to the dying patient experience coping mechanisms similar to those that he has used. Most frequently, but not always, their initial reaction to death is one of denial and numbness, followed by anger, grief, depression, and guilt and finally, much later, acceptance. Fortunately or unfortunately, all the bereaved do not experience the same coping mechanism at the same time. At any one moment each may be experiencing a different phase. For example, the wife may be dazed with shock and denial while a brother is screaming angrily and a daughter crying hysterically.

There is no one best way for the EMT to respond to them at this point. A simple response such as "We did everything possible," or a genuinely felt "I am sorry," may suffice. Should someone become hysterical, allow him to scream to vent his feelings as long as he does not harm himself or anyone else. It helps his grieving process. A genuinely felt caring touch on the shoulder may be all you need to communicate to that individual. You may wish to encourage physical support from some other significant acquaintance. Dr. Kübler-Ross recommends that as long as the dead patient is not badly mutilated, relatives be allowed to see the victim and if they wish, to have maximum emotional-physical contact with the deceased victim at this time, e.g., holding the body while allowing whatever words and strong feelings that naturally come forth to be expressed. Her studies have demonstrated that this process greatly enhances the reality of the death and consequently facilitates and shortens the mourning process.

## ABNORMAL BEHAVIOR PROBLEMS (PSYCHIATRIC EMERGENCIES)

A significant number of medical emergency calls are in response to the behavior of emotionally disturbed individuals, i.e., persons who are experiencing a psychiatric emergency. These are persons who are demonstrating a behavior, thinking, or mood disorder that is dangerous to himself or to someone else. The help of emergency health professionals is requested usually because the patient, family, or some other concerned person fears the patient has lost or is about to lose control.

### Causes and Precipitating Events

Psychiatric emergencies, "going crazy," having a "nervous breakdown," usually occur as a result of several factors. Disturbed individuals tend to have a history of coping poorly with stress. Often, they are currently or have been under the care of a mental health professional. In most cases there have been *recent* changes or events occurring in this person's life which present a *loss* or threat to him, e.g., divorce, death of someone close, health problems, job loss, etc. He may have just learned of the loss or he may have been struggling with it for some time with no success. He finally adapts a "crazy" or abnormal adjustment as an attempt to cope with the problem. *It is worth remembering that disturbed behavior may be the result of conditions other than mental illness.* Such behavior may have a physical basis, e.g., drug or alcohol intoxication, head injury, severe infections, chronic brain dysfunction, and hypoxia.

## General Approach and Assessment

In order to decide what to do with a disturbed individual, you must first assess the seriousness and roughly the nature of his disturbance. Here are some general guidelines:

1. You will need to take time to observe the patient and talk with him. You may first want to obtain information from family or bystanders. Ask them if he has a psychiatric history, what might be bothering him now, and the recent circumstances of his present emergency.

2. Make *personal* contact with him. Tell him who you are and what you are trying to do for him. Learn his name and use it frequently when talking with him.

3. Talk with him at *his* level, physically and personally. Don't tower over him or talk down to him. If possible get him to sit down with you.

4. Some things to look for as you talk with him:

a. *Physical Appearance*
—Is he dressed appropriately? Is he trembling or staggering?
—Does he show nervous mannerisms?
—Speech: Is it slowed or too fast?
—Does he seem drugged or intoxicated?

b. *Affect:*
—What is his mood? High? Depressed? Flat?
—Does his anger fit the situation?
—Can he control his feelings? Can he alter his behavior on request?
—Is he extremely frightened of some unknown or unreasonable thing?

c. *Orientation:*
—Does he know who and where he is? How he got there? Can he give the correct date? Can he explain what he's doing?
—Does he recognize you are an EMT?
—Can he answer questions or is he evasive and confused?
—Has he ever had psychiatric treatment or been in a mental hospital?

d. *Reality Testing:*
—Does he think people are plotting against him? Talking about him? Is he overly suspicious?
—Does he have grand ideas about himself?
—Is his thinking confused? Does he ramble or jump quickly from one topic to another with no clear connections between his thoughts?
—Does he talk to himself or hear voices?

—Does he see, smell, or taste, strange things?
—Does he have bodily ailments that are not possible?

e. *Dangerous Behavior:*
—Does he behave in a way dangerous to himself or others?
—Is he suicidal or despairing?
—Does he want to be hospitalized for his own safety or someone else's?

f. *Some information to get from others:*
—Have there been any major changes in behavior in the past few weeks or months?
—Are there any heavy stresses or pressures? Any recent deaths, divorce, or serious illnesses?
—Has he ever had psychiatric treatment?
—Has he talked of suicide or homicide? Does he have a fear of "going to pieces" or going "crazy"?
—Has he been withdrawn, explosive; changed his eating, drinking, recreational or work habits?

5. Be calm and listen to his story. You are not expected to provide in-depth psychotherapy, but let him know you care and are interested in *his* feelings, *his* view of things. Understand, but don't pity him. If he is relatively noncommunicative, comment on his behavior or apparent feelings and then ask open-ended questions such as, "You seem pretty upset. Tell me what happened," or, "It's pretty hard to talk about it. Let me try to understand what the pain is all about." Take your time. Silences are OK. Once he starts to open up, let him know you are listening and want to know more about him with encouraging statements such as "Uh huh . . . tell me more about that."

6. Supportive confrontation can be given to provide new information to the person about himself or his behavior and often implies a need for action or change on his part. "You seem pretty depressed and hurting right now. Seeing a doctor might help to relieve a lot of that pain," or, "You seem to be pretty much out of control right now and need to come with us where you can get some help getting it together again."

7. Stay nonjudgmental. Don't blame, threaten, or harshly criticize or you'll lose him.

8. Be honest. Let him know what you expect from him and what he can expect from you. Develop a plan of action and tell him what it is. "I think you're hurting a lot. The doctors can help you, and you need to go to the hospital." Lies, tricks, or surprises to get him to the hospital usually work against his recovery later and decrease critical trust in health professionals.

9. If you think a physical exam is necessary, gain the patient's trust first and keep talking with him during the exam.

10. Share your observations and information about the patient with

the mental health staff. By the time the patient sees them, he may regain control and minimize his problems. Your information can help them develop a more accurate assessment and treatment plan. In most cases, these patients require further evaluation and treatment by a mental health professional to determine whether hospitalization is necessary. If a patient is seriously disturbed, dangerous to himself or others, psychiatric (si″ke-at′rik) evaluation and hospitalization is needed. Legalities and procedures for transporting patients and hospital commitments vary from place to place. Generally, a person who is conscious and alert may be transported to the hospital only by his consent. If he refuses, law enforcement procedures are usually necessary, and appropriate officers must be summoned. Be familiar with the protocols and procedures in your community.

### Management of the Emotionally Disturbed

The common threat for most people who undergo a psychiatric emergency is their experience of loss of control. Their outside world seems to be out of control and, to an even greater degree, the sense of loss of being in charge of their inside world. Your job is generally to assist them with the initial stages of regaining as much control as possible, at least sufficient to transport them to where they can obtain further professional help.

## APPROACHES TO SPECIFIC EMOTIONAL AND BEHAVIORAL DISTURBANCES

### The Depressed Patient

Depression is currently considered to be the major mental health problem in the U.S. today. It is estimated that one in every ten adult Americans is depressed seriously enough to warrant professional attention. Depression is manifested by a sad, apathetic mood. Feelings of worthlessness, helplessness, and guilt are usually present. Increased social isolation is common. The depressed person's energy level is down, and he reports disturbances in his appetite, sleep, and sexual functioning. He may have thinking and concentration difficulties. Very little in life satisfies him. Preoccupation with physical health concerns are common. Physicians in general practice report that as much as one-third to one-half of the somatic symptoms presented by their patients are a manifestation of depression and stress. Many depressed people become sick and maintain an "I don't care" attitude about their illness. Such individuals need considerable warmth, caring, and can often benefit from professional help. Frequently they have suicidal thoughts and, if so, this should be explored further by the EMT. The depressed patient is most apt to come to an EMT's attention if suicidal behavior or threats have already taken place.

## The Suicidal Patient

Attempted suicide is the most frequent psychiatric emergency encountered by emergency health professionals. It is defined as behavior that is designed to end one's life or to give the appearance of such. Suicide is the ninth leading cause of death in the U.S.; the second among college age; and the third among fifteen to twenty-five-year olds. Women attempt suicide three times as often as men, but men succeed in killing themselves three times as often. (This is partly because men use more lethal means, such as guns and hanging.) Suicidal behavior is most apt to occur when a person suffers a significant personal loss such as in divorce, death of a loved one, loss of health or job. The suicidal person often feels very depressed, trapped, hopeless, and worthless. The suicidal behavior is often a communication of his hurt and rage to others—family, lover, or spouse. He is usually ambivalent about killing himself. *All* suicidal behavior should be taken seriously. Threats, even those that seen like manipulative gestures, are cries for help.

### *Suicidal Threat Management*

Most suicidal patients are ambivalent about killing themselves and 80 percent make last-minute attempts to communicate with someone. They often phone someone, which ultimately brings you to them. They should be kept on the line until you get there. When you arrive, look for methods and either discreetly remove them or talk the person into giving them up. "Look, we need to talk, but I can't talk to you with those pills (that knife, gun) in your hand." Encourage him to talk about his situation and listen hard.

As he talks, it is important for you to make some assessment of the suicide risk. Here are some questions that will help you evaluate that:

### *Risk Assessment*

a. If you can do it without being obvious, ask if he is planning to kill himself. If so, how much does he think about it? The more he does, the higher the risk. Do not be afraid to say "suicide." You won't be giving him any ideas.

b. Does he have a plan? The more detailed the plan the higher the risk. How available are the means? "Do you plan to shoot yourself?" "Do you have a gun?" "Do you have bullets?" "Do you know how to use them?" "*When* do you plan to kill yourself?"

c. *Previous attempts*—"Have you tried it before?" The more the prior attempts, the higher the risk. Eighty percent of successful suicides have tried it before.

d. Has anyone in your *family* tried it? It runs in families.

e. *Other factors*—The more alienated and lonely, the higher the risks.

*Alcohol*—Current use of alcohol in a depressed, suicidal person greatly increases the chances he will kill himself or try to.

Do not criticize or threaten him with punishment for his behavior. This tends to alienate him further, increase his feelings of guilt and rejection, and may even intensify his suicidal thoughts. Your caring, personal contact at this time may increase his openness for treatment later on. People may insist that they want to and have a right to die. Your attitude needs to be one of, "Today you may wish to die, tomorrow you may not. Let's give you a chance for reconsideration and outside help."

### *Trained Mental Health Professional*

As soon as possible, communicate your observations and risk assessment to emergency department and/or mental health personnel. Suicidal patients have been known to suddenly pull themselves together when they arrive in the emergency department. When interviewed by mental health professionals they may minimize their suicidality and can be erroneously released. It is not uncommon for such individuals upon returning home to make a more serious attempt only a few hours or days later.

High-risk people should not be left alone until they are in the hands of such a professional. Often they need to be hospitalized until the risk is considerably lowered.

### *Suicide Attempt*

If a patient has actually attempted suicide, his medical treatment receives top priority. Bleeding from self-inflicted wounds must be controlled. In drug overdoses, the patient may need treatment for respiratory depression or circulatory collapse. Collect pills and/or medication containers and bring them with you to the emergency department. If a patient is conscious, attempt to make *caring* personal contact with him, and, if he is able, encourage him to talk about his suicidal situation.

## The Hostile, Violent Patient

This patient is generally outraged and is usually ready to battle anyone. It is important to remember that in most cases, his rage is his response to some perceived threat and that beneath the surface there is considerable fear and a sense of hurt and helplessness. He may be responding to a personal loss or feeling unjustly treated. His anger may be displaced toward you.

### *Management*

1. Identify yourself and talk to him in low, calm, firm, and controlled tones. You must try to understand what he is angry about and convince him you care. For example, "You're pretty angry. . . . Tell me what it's about." You don't have to judge or agree with him, but don't challenge

his feelings. An attitude of, "I can understand why you might feel that way" can be helpful in defusing his rage.

2. Avoid arguments or escalation. The behavior of such a person can anger, disgust, repulse, or threaten you. Don't take his criticism or verbal abuse personally. Allow him to ventilate and save face. Shaming statements such as "You're acting like a child" will usually only increase his rage. Any threats directed toward him will escalate the hostility.

3. Avoid sudden movement or surprises. This increases the threat and the probability of violent acting out. Approaching him from the behind, the side, or head-on tends to increase his feelings of threat also. A gradual diagonal approach, that is, mid-way between the side and a face-to-face direction, has been found to be the least threatening.

4. If the patient appears near violent or is already out of control, don't attempt to take him to the hospital against his will without sufficient assistance. Three of you may not be enough to subdue him. If a patient is homicidal or has a weapon, and communication has been unsuccessful, let the police handle him.

5. Be sure to leave an escape route for yourself when approaching this patient. If possible, place yourself between him and a door whether in a building or in an emergency vehicle.

6. If your procedures allow for transporting a violent patient to the hospital, use padded restraints. A patient may be restrained by securing him to a stretcher, wrists and ankles first tied together with a cravat. His body may then be strapped to the stretcher itself. Explain to the patient that you must use restraints, that this is to protect himself and others from injury and that they won't be removed until he is safely transported.

## The Paranoid Patient

A paranoid patient is overly suspicious and distrustful. He is usually angry and uncooperative, believing most people are against him or out to persecute him. Delusions are often present, i.e., he has created a system of beliefs for himself that have little basis in reality. The delusion may be very complex, detailed, and organized. For example, one patient believed he was a victim of an FBI agreement with the Nazis following a World War II peace treaty. He insisted that the United States had agreed to permit the Nazis to continue drug experiments with certain *American* families, including his. Delusions of a complex plot or conspiracy designed to hurt him are common. He will question your motives, why you are here, or what you want. His anger camouflages deep feelings of fear, insecurity, and inferiority. He is often volatile and unpredictable.

There are different varieties of paranoid states. Some reactions occur in otherwise normally functioning persons who experience a severe stress or drug reaction temporarily. More often, the patient has already developed a psychotic condition such as schizophrenia (skiz″o-fre′ne-ah). A schizophrenic individual has poor contact with reality, his thinking is disorganized, and he tends to remain distant and alienated from people.

### *Management*

1. Look directly at him, but don't stare.

2. Maintain a friendly, concerned attitude but stay neutral regarding his anger. Be honest with him, but do not challenge or try to prove his beliefs false or ridiculous—"I know you're worried that the Martians are trying to kill you. But right now I see no danger. You seem to be under a lot of pressure and need to be in the hospital."

3. Before talking with anyone else nearby, ask his permission. Be honest about your plans—tell him what you will do next.

## The Hallucinating Patient

A patient is hallucinating when he experiences sensations and perceptions which have no basis in external reality. The experiences come from inside himself though *he* believes they are really out there. Hallucinations can stem from many sources, e.g., head trauma, electrolyte imbalance, brain tumor, drug or alcohol intoxication, or psychosis. In psychosis, hallucinations frequently are auditory. He may hear voices condemning him or telling him what to do. Drug- and alcohol-related hallucinations tend to be visual and tactile.

### *Management*

1. Identify yourself and your role.

2. Let the patient know that you believe his experience is real to him, but that you do not experience it. Ask him about his experience, e.g., "I don't hear them, but what do the voices tell you?" Trying to convince the patient his experience isn't real is futile.

3. Try to get the patient to focus on what is real—on concrete things like his surroundings, and his clothes: "It's cold here, isn't it?" "How did you rip your jacket?"

## The Disoriented, Disorganized Patient

The disoriented, disorganized patient may or may not know where he is or even who he is. His thinking often is disconnected, inconsistent, and aimless and his speech incoherent and rambling. He may be found wandering the street and muttering to himself. Often he is an older person. The description and management of this patient is similar to that presented for handling normal reactions to trauma.

*Management*

1. You need to give this patient what he doesn't have: structure, orientation, and organization. Firmly and clearly tell him who you are, where he is, and what the situation is. Keep your information simple and concrete.

2. Try to find out his name and where he lives. If he does not appear to be in need of emergency care, he might be returned to the care of a responsible person. If you feel he needs to go to the hospital to be seen by a doctor, tell him so. En route to the hospital you may need to repeat several times where he is and where he is going.

## The Overly Anxious and Phobic Patient

The extremely anxious patient, or one who may be having an anxiety attack, may demonstrate any number of symptoms: pacing, hand-wringing, tremors, tachycardia, vomiting, diarrhea, rapid speech, hyperventilation. He may believe he is having a heart attack or dying. Such individuals have usually reached this state as a result of excess stress. They tend to overcontrol or unconsciously deny strong, unacceptable feelings, e.g., rage towards a loved family member. Their feelings may be dammed-up to the point where the body's nervous system is overloaded and a sudden flood of anxiety is the escape valve. There is often an overwhelming sense of fear without knowing the source.

Whereas the anxiety reaction is more generalized, the phobic patient experiences a fearful response to a specific thing, creature, or situation. This may include high or enclosed places, elevators, crowds, and specific animals. His fear reaction objectively seems out of proportion to the actual threat. Specific phobias have been learned and can be unlearned. They are some of the more easily reversible disabilities.

*Management*

1. Separate him from other people who by this time may have become anxious themselves.

2. Tell him in a calm, slow voice who you are and what you're doing.

3. Ask him to describe his feelings and symptoms. Assure him this won't last forever, that he can be treated and his anxiety brought under control. Meaningless phrases as "Just relax, don't be nervous," "There's nothing to worry about," and "Pull yourself together," are usually not helpful. Explain in detail each step of his being transported to the hospital. If possible, minimize overstimulation—the less noise and glaring lights, the better.

## The Agitated, Manic Patient

The agitated manic patient is characterized by an excessive emotional excitement, rapid, disorganized thought process and excessive physical activity. He may be in a manic phase of a manic-depressive illness. Such an individual experiences cycles of extreme mood swings ranging from deep depression to periods of euphoric activity lasting days and even weeks. During this excited manic phase, he is apt to continue with little or no sleep and tends to exhibit many grandiose, overly confident ideas about himself. He is overly elated, talkative, and optimistic, although his thought processes tend to be disorganized. In acute episodes he may lose complete contact with reality.

### *Management*

Individuals in an acute state usually require hospitalization. Typically they harbour a strong desire for dominance and deeply resent any authoritative attempts to control their behavior. If cornered, restrained, or criticized too quickly or intensely, the agitated, manic individual's mood may quickly shift from one of extreme happiness to one of extreme anger and violence. Such an individual then needs to be managed in much the same way as a violent and/or paranoid patient.

## The Drug-Related Psychiatric Emergency

Narcotic withdrawal is one of the most frequent drug-related emergencies. This occurs when the person stops taking the narcotic upon which he has become physically dependent. Symptoms include restlessness, yawning, watery eyes and nose, sweating, dilated pupils, chills, nausea, and vomiting.

Serious lethal complications are more apt to occur when the drug has been "laced" with extraneous filler substances such as starch, quinine, or some less expensive drug. Such withdrawal is usually not dangerous, but symptoms can be relieved through a more gradual withdrawal in a hospital.

Amphetamine, barbiturate, and sedative withdrawal can be lethal if too sudden.

### *Management*

Be sure you can confirm whether the patient has been on "uppers" or "downers," since withdrawal signs may be similar.

The effects of hallucinogenic drugs, such as PCP, LSD, mescaline, and cocaine often include violence, disorientation, and paranoia and should be managed in a manner described earlier for these kinds of behavioral problems. If those behaviors are clearly drug related, the patient should additionally be reminded that his experience is not permanent and that the drug effects will wear off in a relatively short while (usually in a few hours and occasionally, in the case of PCP, in a few days). Many of the distressing effects of many drugs are worsened by the patient's refusal to accept what is going on inside of him. Often it is helpful to encourage him to not fight his experience and "flow with it" until it wears off.

*Summary*

Remember, every psychiatric emergency varies somewhat from the next and requires a different approach. Your personality is unique and you will develop your own strengths and style of intervention with psychiatric emergencies. What works for you may not work for your partner.

The guidelines presented here are based on considerable, tested experiences, but are *guidelines*, not rigid rules. Try them, and then refine them to fit your personality.

Remember, too, your observations will be valuable to mental health professionals who will do further diagnosis. Your early, on-the-scene intervention will greatly affect the recovery of the disturbed individual. Your attitude and manner, calmness and confidence, care and firmness will make a great difference in developing a favorable response in the patient—and will make your job easier.

## PERSONAL STRESS MANAGEMENT FOR THE EMT

As an EMT you have entered a "high-risk" profession, i.e., you have joined a number of other professions including police officers, air traffic controllers, and business executives, who experience an inordinate degree of on-the-job stress. You will be more susceptible to what is commonly referred to as "burn out." Because of this, it is important to be familiar with the symptoms and sources of burn out and to know what you can do to avoid or at least minimize its occurrence.

### Symptoms

What is "burn out" and what are the signs? A cetain degree of tension in every job is normal and necessary. We have to be aware of what needs to be done and feel at least some mild discomfort in order to be motivated to do our jobs. It is partly our experiencing at least some anxiety when we see a bleeding person that motivates us to intervene. This is *normal* stress. Sometimes, when the pressures become too intense or frequent, we experience considerable anxiety, lose a sense of control, and our performance suffers. This may occur when there are mass casualties and insufficient help. At this point, stress becomes *distress*. Because of the nature of the EMT's job, occasional periods of distress are to be expected. Sometimes these distress experiences become very intense or too close together with insufficient relief over a long period of time. This is when distress can lead to "burn out."

The symptoms of "burn out" or a prolonged distress syndrome will vary among individuals, but some of the more common signs include: physical and emotional exhaustion, irritability and argumentativeness, incessant complaining, dread of going to work, negative job attitude, loss of patience, or even a lack of concern for patients. Other signs include a generally negative, pessimistic and cynical attitude towards people and the rest of the world. Often a negative self-concept and loss of confidence develop. Partly as a result of work distress, the incidence of staff turnover, alcoholism, divorce, and job dissatisfaction is higher among EMTs than many other professions.

## Causes

The list of stress sources for the EMT is lengthy and variable. What may be distressing for one individual, another handles with ease. Because emergencies occur erratically, a part of you must be constantly on the alert to immediately respond to a call for your services. You risk life and limb every time you quickly maneuver through traffic. Upon arrival you don't know what awaits you. You're expected to quickly and accurately assess your patient and make an initial medical intervention. Your work often brings you in contact with people at their worst and on their own turf; they are inebriated, suicidal, on drugs, and so on. Especially if you work in a large inner-city area, your work may bring you in more frequent contact with minority groups—usually at their worst. Like police officers, you probably contact a disproportionately large portion of the problematic segment of these groups. Often an angry sense of cynicism and prejudice develops.

Upon arrival at the emergency department, physicians and nurses may criticize your treatment and rarely dole out praise. There is the additional distress of some of your patients dying. This is especially difficult when a patient is a child. Under this kind of pressure, co-workers are prone to take out their frustrations on each other. Team work is necessary, but can be a delicate operation dependent upon effective communication. Your partner may not like your style and vice versa. Supervisors can be hypercritical. Your salary may seem unfairly small when compared to other occupations requiring less skill and pressure.

There are often major discrepancies between your own image as an EMT and your perception of how others may see you, e.g., the public, police, and physicians. The public often has a glamorized, TV-influenced perception of your work as being colorful, exciting, dramatic, and heroic. Many people underestimate your skill and training, seeing you as just an "ambulance driver," or may become upset because you're not "a real doctor." There is often conflict with other emergency personnel as to the boundaries of responsibility for patients and who can legally or most effectively provide particular medical procedures. Generally, the greater the discrepancy between your own image and areas of responsibility versus that of the public and other professionals, the greater the stress.

Every EMT will need to shape and follow his own means of coping with stress that best fits his unique personality. The following general guidelines have been found to be particularly helpful for most people in high-risk professions.

## On-The-Job Stress Reduction

1. Be aware of your feelings and vent them. While you may need to temporarily control your anger and anxiety when in a tense working situation, it is important to express those feelings as soon as it is safely possible. Talk it over with your partner. Don't deny these emotions or withdraw from your peers.

2. Make optimal use of your break time. Do something absorbing that is as *un*related to your job as possible, e.g., playing chess, cards and other games, and light reading. If you still need to vent about that last bad run, do so—but don't dwell on it.

3. Accept your limitations. While it is important to notice what effect your treatment had on a patient, don't dwell on your mistakes. Above all, don't place yourself in the agonizing trap of "If I had only ________, the patient might have ________."

4. Avoid overinvestment in your patients; honest caring, but some detachment is necessary.

5. Cultivate cooperative relationships with coworkers. You need their support, and good working relationships produce greater job satisfaction. Playing the loner role precipitates greater alienation and rejection. Some interpersonal conflict is normal and expected among people who work closely together. Don't "gunny sack" those gripes, i.e., hide and store up your negative criticisms and annoyances. When problems with a fellow worker develop, try the following:

a. Clarify what's bugging you. Talk it over with a friend first if necessary, but don't let it stop there.
b. Find a time to talk about it with the person who is bugging you as soon as possible.
c. Describe the annoying behavior and your feelings about it, e.g., "John, I really like working with you, but when you cuss out all those suicides and other patients, I really get angry."
d. One or both of you "brainstorm" suggestions for changing the annoying behavior.
e. Be sure to demonstrate appreciation for any changes he makes in a positive direction. If it is an important issue, set a time for

getting together later to assess progress on the problem, e.g., "Let's try this for a week and talk abut it next Monday to see how it's working."

This method of negotiation for change with your partner may feel a bit awkward at first, but like any new skill, will become more comfortable and adapted to your personality. As a general rule of thumb, don't forget to give plenty of praise to your partner for the things he does especially well.

6. Keep breathing. Seriously. During tense moments we tend to unconsciusly hold our breath or breathe shallowly. This tends to increase stress and anxiety. During the tough times especially, breathe deeply to give yourself support and relieve the tension.

7. Laugh. People who maintain their sense of humor and perspective last longer. Take everything in your work too seriously, and it will take you. Those EMTs who can see the lighter side of their work go home happier.

## Off-The-Job Stress Reduction

No matter how effective you are with on-the-job coping, there will always be a residue of tension to bring home. Here are a few guidelines for dealing with the leftover pressure:

1. As much as possible, leave your work at work. Vent leftover job frustrations to your special person, but don't dwell on them.

2. Cultivate those significant other relationships. Whether this is a spouse or special friend(s), we all need someone with whom we can be more fully ourselves and feel safely supported.

3. Develop one or more recreational outlets, hobbies, or pastimes. Leisure time activities in which we can totally lose ourselves are musts for good mental health.

4. Keep physically fit. A balance of nutritious food and exercise is critical for good mental health. If you drink, do so in moderation. Excessive use of tension-relieving drugs or alcohol tends to produce more stress ultimately.

5. Cultivate your spiritual side. That deeper, less tangible part of you needs nourishment, whether it be church-related, yoga, or some other spiritually focused program.

6. If you've tried these guidelines for on- and off-the-job stress reduction and are still experiencing an excess of distress or "burn out" symptoms for an extended period of time, consult with someone who is trained to deal with personal problems, preferably a mental health professional. We all have blind spots in our personalities, and occasionally need an objective individual to help us deal with them. When something hurts emotionally for too long, a mental health check-up and possibly treatment is indicated.

*References*

Appelbaum, Steven. *Stress Management for Health Care Professionals.* Gaithersburg, MD: Aspen Publications, 1980.

Bach, George, and Goldberg H. Creative Aggression. New York: Doubleday & Co., 1974.

Burgess, Ann W., and Holstrom, L. L. *Rape: Victims of Crisis.* Englewood Cliffs, NJ: Prentice-Hall, Inc., 1974.

Girdano, Daniel, and Everly, G. *Controlling Stress and Tension.* Englewood Cliffs, NJ: Prentice-Hall, Inc., 1979.

Grollman, Earl. *Suicide: Prevention, Intervention and Postvention.* Boston, MA: Beacon, 1971.

Hatton, Corrine; Volente, M.; and Rink, A. *Suicide: Assessment and Intervention.* New York: Appleton Century Crofts, 1977.

Kübler-Ross, Elisabeth. "The Child Will Always Be There. Real Love Doesn't Die," *Psychology Today,* September 1976, pp. 48–52.

Kübler-Ross, Elisabeth. *Death and Dying.* New York: Macmillan, 1969.

Lipkin, Gladys, and Cohen, Robert. *Effective Approaches to Patient Behavior.* New York: Springer Pub. Co., 1973.

Pelletier, K. *Mind as Healer, Mind as Slayer.* New York: Dell Publishing Co. (Delta Press), 1977.

Selye, Hans. *Stress Without Distress.* New York: Signet, 1974.

# Chapter 22

# Acute Poisoning

The EMT is often confronted with a patient who has accidentally or intentionally ingested a poisonous substance. Young children, especially, come into contact with many items in the home which can cause an acute toxicological emergency. Among these are medicines, cleaning agents, aerosal sprays, cosmetics, and certain house plants. Some substances can cause serious illness and death when taken in sufficient quantities due to their adverse affects on the heart, lungs, kidneys, brain, and other vital organs. Others induce serious injury to the lips, mouth, esophagus, stomach, and intestines by their corrosive properties, for example, strong acids or alkalies. A few toxic items can be absorbed through the skin or inhaled, thus creating an acute poisoning. Since ingestions are the most common type of poisoning that the EMT is likely to encounter, these will be considered in detail.

## INGESTIONS

Preschool children aged two to five are constantly exploring their environment for new experiences, and may want to experiment with anything they find in the course of play. Since this age group is largely dependent upon the senses of taste and smell as a means of becoming acquainted with the world, eating and drinking strange substances is common. The cleaning supplies stored under a kitchen sink, the bathroom medicine cabinet, leaves and berries, house plants, and items in the basement or garage can become death-producing to a young child if ingested in sufficient quantities.

Many parents do not recognize that some items that are harmless when taken in normal amounts actually become poisonous if ingested in large quantities. For example, common substances such as table salt, alcoholic beverages, iron tablets, or aspirin can be potentially lethal for the individual who consumes unusually large quantities. It is therefore always important that an estimate be made regarding the quantity as well as the type of ingested substance.

Few adults are actually poisoned accidentally by ingestion, but rather intentionally consume an overdose of medicine or a toxic compound as a suicidal gesture. Occasionally, however, adults eat or drink substances that adversely interact with medicines they have been taking, and an acute poisoning emergency is accidentally created. For example, alcoholic beverages exaggerate the effects of certain agents such as sleeping pills, tranquilizers, or pain relief medications. Therefore, a careful history should be obtained when acute poisoning is suspected.

## SIGNS AND SYMPTOMS OF ACUTE POISONING

The EMT may learn from a history the exact nature of the poisoning including the agent, amount, and time of occurrence. However, in some instances, acute poisoning is suspected based upon signs and symptoms of a toxic crisis. Nausea; vomiting; excessive salivation (sal″ĭ-va-shun) or sweating; abdominal pain; dyspnea; burns of the face, mouth and throat; seizures; unconsciousness; dilation or constriction of pupils; and unexplained shock are among the more common manifestations exhibited by the poisoned patient.

The environment should be searched for clues such as open and empty medicine bottles, spilled liquids, open containers, or the odor of petroleum products or chemicals which might indicate that an accidental poisoning has occurred.

But, of course, immediate attention should be to the patient's basic life support, not to the exact nature of the suspected poisoning.

## PRINCIPLES OF INGESTED POISON MANAGEMENT

Poisons should be primarily managed by the principles of *preventing absorption* and *hastening the elimination of the substance.* Delaying the emptying of the stomach by giving milk, the induction of emesis, and lavage are examples of ways to delay or prevent absorption. Two to four hours are required for complete absorption of a poison. (Large doses of aspirin may take considerably longer.) Signs and symptoms become noticeable when enough of the substance has been absorbed to produce an undesired effect. The use of agents (antidotes [an′ti-dots]) to counteract the poison and render it harmless through an absorption process (e.g., activated charcoal) is an additional mode of reducing the possibility of poisoning. Elimination of the poison can be facilitated by administration of a cathartic (kah-thar′tik), by hemodialysis (he″mo-di-al′ĭ-sis) (using an artificial kidney) or forced diuresis (di″u-re′sis) (the elimination of urine). The use of these latter methods, of course, are only employed in specific types of severe poisoning that can be minimized by a more rapid removal from body tissues and fluids.

Each poisoning situation will be managed according to type of agent, the condition of the patient, the elapsed time since ingestion, and the preferences of the directing medical team.

## Immediate Assessments

The EMT should initially assess the basic elements of life support, airway, breathing, and circulation. Respiratory depression and cardiac arrest are not uncommon in severe instances of poisonings. Use mechanical airway and breathing adjuncts if necessary and provide supplemental oxygen if indicated. Use 100 percent oxygen for persons who have inhaled toxic fumes. (See Chapter 10.) The patient should be positioned in a semiprone, left side-lying position to minimize the risk of aspiration. Suctioning should be employed as necessary. It is advisable to auscultate the lungs frequently to ensure that there is a good air exchange and to detect noisy respirations characteristic of serious airway involvement. (See Chapter 17.) The mouth and throat should be inspected for evidence of redness, discoloration, or ulceration which could indicate contact with a corrosive substance. The EMT should also attempt to detect any peculiar breath odors which might provide clues to the ingested substance. Certain agents have classic associated odors. Gagging or choking may precede vomiting and accidental aspiration, so suctioning equipment should be immediately ready for use. Since some poisons affect the cardiac rate and rhythm, the apical pulse should be carefully monitored. The blood pressure is an important parameter of cardiovascular functioning and should be checked at least every five minutes because many poisons cause either a dangerous rise or a sharp fall. Shock states associated with acute poisonings should be managed as previously described. (See Chapter 11.)

Many toxic agents exert a stimulating or depressant effect on the brain and spinal cord. The EMT must be alert to changes in the level of consciousness, and expect confusion, drowsiness, coma, agitation, or excitement, dependent upon the properties of the ingested substance. Seizure activity is likely to occur in acute poisoning episodes and the EMT should exercise the usual precautions. The pupils should be checked frequently and dilation or pinpoint constriction should be noted since either phenomenon could provide a valuable clue in detecting an unknown substance.

If the patient vomits, the EMT should attempt to collect and save all emesis for later laboratory analysis at the hospital.

## Special Kinds of Poisonings

### *Iron Poisoning*

Iron poisoning is most common in toddlers who ingest a large amount of iron tablets. Vomiting or diarrhea colored with bright red blood may be noted within an hour or two post-ingestion since the substance is very irritating to the gastric and intestinal linings and thus induces hemorrhage. Upper abdominal pain is usually severe. Prompt emesis, lavage, and careful follow-up at the hospital is imperative.

### *Petroleum Products (Hydrocarbons)*

Kerosene, charcoal lighter fluid, mineral seal oil, furniture polish, turpentine, gasoline, lighter fluid, and insecticides in a petroleum-distillate base are the most common offenders, in rank order. An ounce or less of some of these agents can be lethal for the young child; three or four ounces are lethal for the adult.

An assessment should be made to determine the amount ingested. Sometimes an appropriate amount can be estimated by knowing how much substance was in a container before and after the ingestion. If the ingestion was witnessed, it is useful to know how many swallows were taken. (A small child ingests about 2 cc per swallow.) It is often difficult to assess from history how much was taken since gagging, choking, coughing, and spitting can affect the quantity actually ingested. If vomiting has occurred (it does in at least 50 percent of petroleum ingestions), check the airway very carefully since aspiration could have occurred at that time, as well as with the initial ingestion. *Collect and save all emesis* (em′ĕ-sis)!

The EMT should not spend precious time determining the exact type of hydrocarbon ingested or the amount. Attention should be given to airway maintenance and skin decontamination.

Look for redness, blisters, or irritation in the mouth and throat. Listen for breath sounds and note any dyspnea. Smell the breath for a volatile "fuel-like" odor which may be emitted. Most substances smell like they do in the container. An exception to the rule is turpentine, which gives off a violetlike fragrance. Violent coughing usually signifies that aspiration into the airways has occurred. The EMT should protect the airway by the semi-prone left side-lying position and administer supplemental oxygen at high flow for respiratory distress and cyanosis.

Do not induce vomiting with hydrocarbon ingestion unless specifically advised by supervising medical personnel.

### *Salicylates*

Aspirin, and occasionally oil of wintergreen, account for a large number of accidental poisonings, especially in younger children. "Baby aspirin" is pleasantly flavored and may be considered to be candy. Of course, oil of wintergreen is a pleasant fragrance that smells much like peppermint. Rapid, deep breathing, vomiting, sweating, thirst, and fever are among the common signs and symptoms. Some patients seize or have a change in the level of consciousness. A few may become comatose. If salicylate (sal′ĭ-sil″āt) poisoning is suspected, prompt emesis, lavage, and follow-up care at a hospital is crucial for the patient's survival.

Acetaminophen (as″et-am′ĭno-fen), a popular aspirin substitute for pain and fever, is also potentially lethal and requires prompt and definitive medical attention including the administration of the specific antidote. (See page 454.)

*Corrosive Acids and Alkalies*

Corrosive acids and alkalies include metal cleaners, bleach, disinfectants, household cleaners, paint removers, and automatic dishwasher compounds.

Severe burns of the lips, mouth and throat may be present and swelling of the throat may produce difficulty breathing. There may be blood-streaked vomiting and even shock.

In the event of the ingestion of corrosive acids or alkalies, the EMT should *not* induce vomiting, which would permit the caustic substance to injure the esophagus, throat, and mouth once again.

*Other Poisonings*

See Chapters 31 and 32 for a complete discussion of poisonous snakes, insects, plants, and marine life. See Chapter 23 for alcohol-related overdoses.

## Other On-the-Scene Activity

The EMT may be instructed to induce vomiting in the event of certain poisonings *before* transport to the hospital, particularly if a long transport (over thirty minutes) is anticipated.

The drug used in inducing vomiting is Syrup of Ipecac (ip′ĕ-kak). It produces emesis in ten to twenty minutes by its gastric-irritating properties and by its effect on a selected part of the brain that controls the reflex emptying of the stomach. Ipecac is given by mouth in doses of 15–30 cc (½ - 1 oz.) and followed by one or two glasses of water. It should never be given to an individual who is experiencing a deterioration in the level of consciousness, or if there has been an ingestion of a strong acid, alkali, or possibly petroleum products such as kerosene or gasoline. In these instances the vomiting would allow the substance once again to irritate the esophagus and mouth and threaten the airway.

The EMT must closely observe the patient who has been given ipecac to ensure that the vomiting does not threaten the airway. If feasible, the individual should be sitting up (or preferably walking) to hasten the emetic properties of the ipecac. *Save all emesis for later analysis by the receiving hospital.*

Lavage (lah-vahzh′) (washing out or "pumping" the stomach) may be necessary in cetain cases of poisonings, but the EMT would usually not be responsible for this procedure in the field. Lavage should take place in the hospital under careful management of physicians and nurses, since the airway can be compromised unless a rigid protocol is followed to minimize the risk of accidental aspiration.

### Other Prehospital Considerations

If a poisonous substance has been spilled on the skin, it should be removed by flooding the area with water. Tincture of green soap is useful to assist in removing pesticides, cyanides, hydrocarbons, and any oil-based agent which resists water alone. (Excess dry chemicals should be brushed away first, since the addition of water may result in a heat-producing chemical reaction.) Any clothing that has been soiled by toxic agents should be promptly removed.

The EMT should collect any containers or other environmental clues to an unknown poisoning agent and transport them to the hospital with the patient. Remember that many parents refill old bottles and cans with toxic substances and the label may not represent the actual contents. A soft-drink bottle may contain insect spray, or gasoline may be stored in a glass jug labeled "apple cider." It is possible for the hospital laboratory to identify a poison merely from examining residual material in an empty container, so such items should be retrieved from the home in all cases, since the treatment will be determined by the nature of the toxic agent.

## THE ROLE OF THE EMT IN POISON MANAGEMENT

The nature and scope of the role of the EMT in management of acute poisonings is dependent upon several factors including the type of poisoning, the condition of the patient upon arrival, the availability of direct medical supervision from a hospital or poison control center, the distance from the hospital, and others. The EMT may be directed to dilute the poison with milk or water, to induce vomiting, and, in rare cases to administer an antidote. Most often, the basic supportive care is provided and the patient is promptly transported to the hospital for definitive management and follow-up.

## POISON CONTROL CENTERS

Many communities are served by an areawide poison control center, which processes requests for direction in the management of poisonings. The receiver of the call at the poison control center obtains baseline information about the case and instructs the caller in a step-by-step manner about emergency management. (See Fig. 22-1.) In certain cases, such as unconsciousness or the ingestion of a known lethal substance, an ambulance would be dispatched immediately rather than risking private transportation to the hospital.

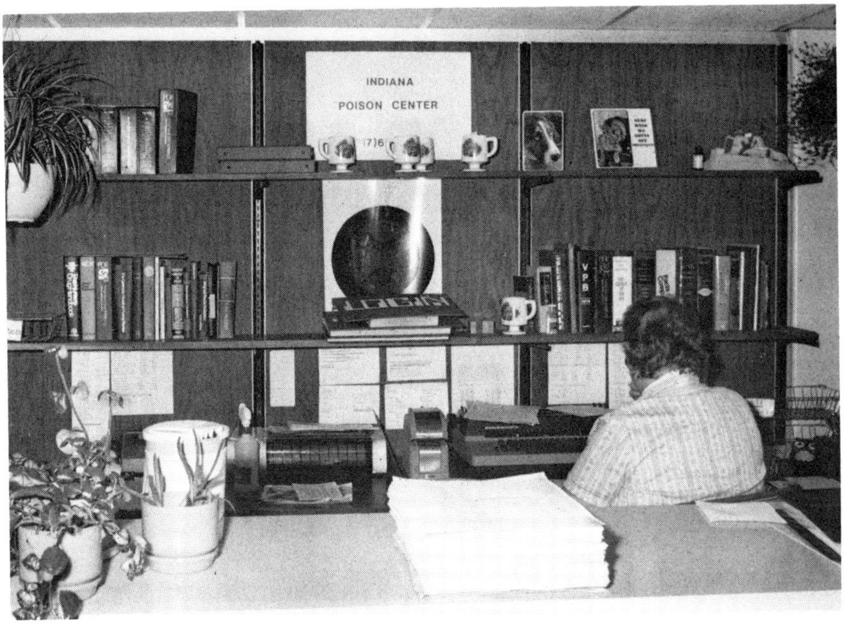


**Figure 22-1.** Poison control center. Full-time personnel with specialized training in poison management staff poison control centers. Protocols are accessed from microfiche, textbooks and other references, and cooperating commercial product and drug information networks in response to callers. *(Courtesy of Wishard Memorial Hospital, Indianapolis, IN)*

If the EMT receives a call from a frantic parent, friend, or the actual victim of an acute ingestion, of an overdose, or of a contact with a toxic agent, certain data should be systematically gathered for dispatching an emergency vehicle and for guiding emergency care which a poison control center might direct. Among this baseline information should be the name of the caller and the relationship to the patient; age and weight of the patient; type of ingestion or contact (name of poison, type, ingredients, amount); and the caller's evaluation of the severity of the problem. For example, is the patient alert, breathing, unconscious, coughing and choking, confused, etc? If skin or clothing have been contaminated, the caller should be instructed in techniques of surface decontamination including flushing the skin and removal of soiled clothing. Certain situations may indicate the need for producing immediate emesis by the use of ipecac or delaying the stomach's emptying, or diluting the toxin by the administration of milk. Of course, any oral intake of ipecac or milk is contraindicated in the presence of a depressed level of consciousness, seizures, or the loss of the gag reflex.

## SPECIFIC ANTIDOTES

Specific antidotes are not available for most poisons and the use of the "universal antidote" (still known to many from scouting or other first aid courses, consisting of tea, burnt toast, and milk of magnesia) is essentially ineffective and can be dangerous in certain instances. There are a few specific antidotes that directly counteract or block certain poisonings. These are reviewed in Table 22-1. Most EMTs will not be involved in the use of these in the field except for oxygen (specific for carbon monoxide) and pehaps naloxone (nal-oks'ōn) (Narcan) (specific for narcotics and a few other drugs).

TABLE 22-1. SPECIFIC ANTIDOTES

| *Poison or Agent* | *Antidote* |
|---|---|
| Carbon monoxide | Oxygen |
| Narcotics, dextropropoxyphene (Darvon), pentazocine lactate (Talwin), and diphenoxylate (Lomotil) | Naloxone (Narcan) |
| Mercury, arsenic, copper, lead, cobalt | British antilewisite (BAL) |
| Iron | Desferoxamine |
| Organophosphates insecticides (parathion, malathion) | Atropine, 2-PAM |
| Lead | Versene, penicillamine |
| Cyanide | Nitrite, thiosulfite |
| Methanol, ethylene glycol | Ethanol |
| Anticoagulants | Vitamin K |
| Acetaminophen | N-Acetylcysteine |
| Tricyclics, scopolamine, belladonna alkaloids, jimson weed, diphenhydramine (Benadryl) | Physostigmine |

## POISON PREVENTION

The EMT often has opportunities to instruct families in methods of prevention of accidental poisoning. For example, many homes have hazardous materials stored under the kitchen sink, in the bathroom, and in the garage or basement. Items such as drain cleaning crystals, automatic dishwashing detergents, pesticides, transmission fluid, antifreeze, paint thinners, and insect sprays are among the common and potentially lethal substances stored within easy access of the curious child. Parents should be warned of the danger in filling a soft-drink container with insecticides or a root beer jug with gasoline, since children may be expecting a treat rather than a poisonous agent. All containers of hazardous substances should be conspiciously labelled with the name of the contents and a classic poison label which may deter a child who has been carefully taught the dangers of poisons.

All medicines should have safety caps and be kept out of the casual reach of everyone since even vitamins and iron tablets pose a threat to life when ingested in excessive quantities. Even adults, on occasion, accidentally take someone else's drugs as a result of poor labeling, improper storage, or the mixing of several types of substances within one container. Careless practices such as keeping old or outdated medicine around for a future illness is a dangerous habit and self-medication of even over-the-counter drugs (such as aspirin, laxatives, or cold remedies) can be life threatening in certain combinations. Old and outdated drugs should be destroyed by flushing down the toilet. They should not be merely tossed into the waste basket in the kitchen or bathroom.

The EMT should recognize that certain families have several repeat instances of poisonings among children due to poor storage of hazardous substances in the home or lack of supervision of the youngsters by a responsible adult. Multiple or repeated instances of poisonings at the same home may be a form of child abuse and should be reported to the hospital physician and nurse staff for appropriate follow-up.

Many families have ipecac and poison control instructions in the home due to community action programs, public awareness campaigns, or the advice of the pediatrician. These practices, of course, should be strongly supported by the EMT, along with a program of proper storage of all potentially hazardous substances.

## *References*

Arena, J. M. *Poisoning: Toxicology, Symptoms Treatment.* Springfield, IL: Charles C. Thomas, Publisher, 1974.

Barber, J. M.; Stokes, L. G.; and Billings, D. M. *Adult and Child Care: A Client Approach to Nursing,* 2nd ed., St. Louis, MO: The C. V. Mosby Co., 1977.

Beamon, Richard F., *et. al.* "Hydro-carbon Ingestion in Children: A Six-Year Retrospective Study," *JACEP,* 5:771–775, October 1976.

Done, A. K., *et. al.* "Treatment of Salicylate Poisoning," *Modern Treatment* 8:528–551, 1971.

Hurwitz, Aryeh, and Klaassen, Curtis. "The Treatment of Poisoning," *Rational Drug Therapy,* Vol. 14, No. 3, March 1980.

Mahler, D. A. "Anticholinergic Poisoning from Jimson Weed," *JACEP* 5:440–442, 1976.

"Management of Acetaminiphen Overdose with N-Acetylcysteine," (Monograph) Fort Washington, PA: McNeil Consumer Products Company, January, 1979.

Pierce, A. W. "Salicylate Intoxication," *Postgraduate Medicine* 48:243–249, September, 1970.

Rumack, B. H. "Hydrocarbon Ingestion in Perspective," *JACEP,* 6:172–173, April, 1977.

Rumack, Barry H., and Bayes, Marc J. "Poisonings and Overdose," *Topics in Emergency Medicine,* Vol. 1, Number 3, October 1979.

# Chapter 23

# Alcohol-Related Emergencies

The EMT frequently is confronted with a patient who is ill or injured, and alcohol abuse is suspected, too. At other times, little or nothing is known about an individual who is "found down" and because of the environment, an assumption is made that the victim is drunk or has overdosed. Since there are several medical and surgical problems that are associated with signs and symptoms that could be easily mistaken for substance abuse, it is important that the EMT understand alcoholism-related phenomena and be able to differentiate it from other entities. Furthermore, alcoholism *by itself* can be associated with fatal complications due to metabolic phenomena. The purpose of this chapter is to provide the EMT with information about alcoholism and alcohol-related problems which is relevant to assessment and management in the field. Since management of the unconscious patient has been thoroughly discussed in Chapter 8, the emphasis here will be on the responding patient.

## RECOGNITION OF ALCOHOL—RELATED PROBLEMS

Alcohol intoxication and alcohol withdrawal can both be fatal in certain circumstances. These patients deserve to be treated as medical problems, not as social nuisances. It is tempting, at times, for health care personnel to be truly annoyed with the "drunks" who fall, hit their heads, get into fights, and use abusive language. It is imperative, however, that rough handling, punishment, or verbal reprimands be avoided. Such actions will not deter future use of alcohol and certainly are not helpful in managing the crisis at hand. A word of caution is in order, too, regarding our social biases about the appearance of the "drunk." A well-dressed and refined elderly lady can be acutely intoxicated, too. The EMT must be on guard and not make assumptions about the patient merely by his appearance or where he is found. A carefully taken history and a thorough physical assessment are vital to identification of serious alcohol-related problems.

There are certain alcohol-related emergencies which render the patient helpless in cooperating with a history and physical examination. However, family, friends or bystanders can often provide important information to you. It is valuable to know factors such as:

1. Time of most recent alcohol ingestion
2. Type of alcohol, e.g., beer, wine, whiskey, mixed drinks
3. Amount of intake

The amount of alcohol that is consumed is what is important, not just the type of beverage that determines the level of intoxication. Many alcoholics deny their real consumption of alcohol. It is common for an acutely intoxicated person to say, "But, I've just had two beers." Reassure the patient that you are there to help, and not to arrest him. Your only concern is for his health and safety. Your need for this information is to predict the nature of his problem, not to gather "evidence" of his substance abuse. Just the reassurance will often help in getting the patient to "open up" and be more realistic about his recent drinking history. Other information that is useful to elicit is in regard to previous problems of a similar nature. Specific questions which should be asked are:

1. What is the amount you usually drink?
2. Are you taking any medications?

Be careful to use the term *medications*, not *drugs*, since the latter word has a negative meaning to many patients, and they will say "no" emphatically, denying *illicit* drug use. It is sometimes helpful to say, "Are you on any medications prescribed by your doctor or are you taking any pills you bought at the drug store?" The purpose of this question relates to associated chronic or acute illnesses that might help your assessments or field management of the patient's problems.

3. How long has it been since you have eaten? (Alcohol is absorbed more quickly without associated food intake.)

4. Have you ever felt like this before or have you ever been in the hospital for this kind of problem? Another problem? When and for how long? Be sure to look for scars on the chest or abdomen which could provide clues to previous illness or injuries.

5. Are you under care by a clinic or private doctor for your drinking problem? (Patients who drink while taking Disulfiram (Antabuse) on an "alcohol-cure" program become quite ill if they consume alcohol.) (See page 462.)

A caring, kind approach during the history and assessment is important since many of these patients already feel that their lives are useless and that no one cares. Take this opportunity to convey that you are concerned for them.

## ALCOHOL INTOXICATION

Alcohol intoxication is a result of short-term drinking and the consumption of a large amount of alcohol. The inexperienced or occasional drinker, the person who drinks heavily and does not eat, or the drinker with a low body tolerance for alcohol may become intoxicated from considerably less than the one who has a long-term pattern of heavy consumption.

The type of beverage that one drinks is *not* the determinant of intoxication. Intoxication is related to the blood level of alcohol. Table 23-1 outlines the amount of alcohol found in the usual beverages, according to a typical serving. Note that the amount of alcohol in a typical serving does not differ appreciably. The differences in how quickly one becomes drunk is from the way he drinks. Gulping drinks such as distilled spirits (e.g., whiskey) is more common than "downing" several servings of wine in quick succession. Body weight is also an important factor, too. Larger individuals with normal organ systems can tolerate more alcohol than smaller persons, or even the elderly whose capacity for circulation and elimination is impaired by degenerative processes. Certain drugs also exagerate the depressant effects of alcohol. Sleeping medications, tranquilizers, antihypertensive agents, and mood-elevating drugs are among the examples.

The EMT should appreciate the meaning of blood alcohol levels, since these measurements are used to determine legal drunkenness. The amount of alcohol in a sample of venous blood is usually expressed in milligrams of alcohol per milliliter of body fluid or tissue. (Since mg/ml is a ratio of 1:1000, 1 per mille is equivalent to 0.1 percent.) In most states, an alcohol level of 0.15 percent is considered "under the influence" and 0.20 percent is "intoxicated." 0.10 percent is the common legal limit for operation of a motor vehicle. (i.e., two or three drinks.) A breath alcohol level may be useful in measuring a recent intake of alcohol, but it does not provide a reliable quantitative index as does blood levels.

Only serial blood levels can detect whether or not the patient has reached a peak of alcohol-related effects. Although it takes only a few minutes for alcohol to be absorbed into the blood stream, it is metabolized and excreted much more slowly. One drink of any type can be eliminated from the blood in one hour in a normal person. Any drinks beyond one per hour add to the blood level and thus to intoxication.

In order to perform the most meaningful assessments, the EMT should understand the effects of alcohol on the nervous system, responses, behavior, and performance of tasks.

## EFFECTS OF ALCOHOL

Changes in emotions and perceptions are primarily related to altered functions of the central nervous system. The changes begin and disappear on a continuum so it is difficult to compare a given emotion or perception

TABLE 23-1. ALCOHOL CONTENT OF SELECTED BEVERAGES

| *Type of Beverage* | *Typical Serving* | *Grams of Alcohol* |
|---|---|---|
| Distilled spirits (e.g. whiskey) | 1.5 oz. | 14–18 |
| Liqueur (cordials) | 1.5 oz. | 7–22 |
| Wine (table) | 2.5 oz. | 5–8 |
| Wine (dessert) | 2.5 oz. | 9–12 |
| Beer | 12 oz. | 9–18 |

TABLE 23-2. ALCOHOL INTAKE AND RELATED SYMPTOMS

| **Ingested Alcohol (Example: whiskey)* | *Blood Alcohol Level* | *Symptoms* |
|---|---|---|
| 2 ounces | 0.05% | Appears normal |
| 4 ounces | 0.10% | Emotions peak, exhilaration, boastfulness, belligerence, talkativeness, giddiness, remorse<br>Inhibitions are decreased<br>Slowed reaction time<br>Poor coordination |
| 6 ounces | 0.15% | Confusion; "under the influence"<br>Staggering gait<br>Slurred speech<br>Visual disturbances<br>Dizziness<br>Decreased pain response<br>Sweating<br>Tachycardia |
| 8 ounces (½ pint) | 0.20% | Decreased response to stimuli<br>Nausea and vomiting<br>Drowsiness, stupor<br>Acutely intoxicated<br>All symptoms listed for 0.15% blood alcohol level |
| | 0.30%–0.40% | Unconscious<br>Reflexes diminished or absent<br>Cool, pale skin<br>Low blood pressure<br>Tachycardia<br>Slow, labored respirations<br>Seizures |
| 24–32 ounces | 0.50% | Respiratory and cardiac arrest |

* Short time span intake; one to two hours.

to a sober state unless you know the patient well. (See Table 23-2.)

The EMT should appreciate that *heavy* doses of alcohol produce an amnesia, so an intoxicated person truly cannot remember a few minutes afterward about a given act or conversation. Behavior that would ordinarily be suppressed as taboo may surface. The individual may thus seem uninhibited and willing to do the unusual.

Mood changes occur and the intoxicated patient may appear hazy, withdrawn, or mellow. Depression is not uncommon for some; others become elated, talkative, and unusually social. The characteristics of the individual's personality and the environment seem to determine which extremes emerge. Self-confidence and self-esteem are generally quite high while the person is drinking. Speech, movement, facial expressions, and even handwriting change from normal patterns. Time intervals seem shorter to the average intoxicated person, too, so he cannot estimate the time required for a task, or realistically convey how much time has elapsed in a given situation. A rare intoxicated person, however, may feel that everything is happening too slowly.

Physiological reactions of nausea, vomiting, and dizziness occur in certain individuals. Others feel hot and flushed, and have reddening of the hands and face with the vasodilatory effect of alcohol.

Alcohol in high doses impairs the sensory functions, as well as the perceptual, mental, and motor ones. Awkwardness, visual disturbances, staggering, and slurred speech are among the more common manifestations.

The ability to change focus on problems is quite evident, undoubtedly contributing to the many accidents that involve an intoxicated person.

## MANAGEMENT OF THE INTOXICATED PATIENT

The main concern for the patient who is acutely intoxicated is airway management. Since vomiting and aspiration, as well as respiratory depression are quite common, the airway must be secured. Aspiration of emesis is a major cause of death, so the patient should be promptly placed in a left-lateral head-down position for transport. The respirations must be regularly assessed noting changes in the rate, depth, rhythm, and muscles involved in breathing (e.g., abdominal, intercostal, diaphragm). If there is an inadequate respiratory effort or if the air exchange seems poor, mechanical ventilatory assistance is in order.

The level of consciousness should be monitored. Peak blood alcohol levels are reached within thirty minutes to two or three hours after alcohol intake has ceased. If there is a decrease in the level of consciousness, the circumstances may be much more dire than originally perceived. Since seizures may occur during acute intoxication, seizure precautions are to be observed. (See pages 518–521.)

Vital signs should be monitored, especially if there is associated trauma to rule out acute hemorrhage and shock states.

Advanced EMTs may be instructed to draw venous blood samples, initiate an IV infusion, or place a nasogastric tube to decompress the stomach en route to a hospital.

## OTHER ALCOHOL–RELATED PROBLEMS

### Rum Fits (Drinking Seizures)

Seizures that occur while the individual is still drinking or during the first few days of abstinence may be induced by metabolic changes. A declining blood alcohol level, fluid and electrolyte imbalances, or a low blood sugar could be contributory. Since such seizures may lead to status epilepticus, the patient should be managed according to the protocol outlined in Chapter 27.

### Alcohol Withdrawal

Tremors, seizures, and hallucinations (hah-lu″sĭ-na′shunz) may occur as the blood alcohol level declines and the body adjusts its metabolic activity in response. These withdrawal problems may be mild or serious.

Mild alcohol withdrawal is often referred to as the "morning-after syndrome." Headache, tremors, irritability, nausea, and lethargy are typical characteristics. A simple plan of a high fluid intake, rest, aspirin, and time are usually the only management required.

There is also a very serious alcohol withdrawal phenomenon that occurs seven to twenty-four hours after cessation of alcohol intake. (Chronic drinkers may experience this while still drinking, if they have a blood alcohol level that is lower than their normal one.)

Signs and symptoms include insomnia (inability to sleep), nausea, vomiting, "the shakes," seizures, sweating, confusion, and auditory, as well as visual hallucinations (peaking at twenty-four hours post-withdrawal.) This aggregate of signs and symptoms must be carefully managed by the medical team or it can lead to *delirium* (de-lir′ĭ-um) tremens (DTs), which can be fatal. Signs and symptoms of DTs include: trembling, excitement, sweating, anxiety, gastrointestinal complaints, and precordial (pre-kor′de-al) pain. This so-called alcoholic psychosis involves visual and auditory sensations, usually of an unpleasant nature, such as seeing snakes, being chased, having rats climbing on the body, etc.

Delirium tremens begin at about seventy-two hours post-withdrawal and may continue for several days. The mortality rate for DTs is 10–20 percent. The EMT must be able to recognize alcohol withdrawal complexes promptly and understand their seriousness, so the patient can receive definitive care in time to ensure survival.

## Disulfiram (Antabuse) Reactions

Patients on an alcohol treatment program are frequently prescribed Disulfiram (di-sul′fi-ram) (or Antabuse), a drug that produces unpleasant effects when combined with alcohol. The purpose of the drug is to deter the person from alcohol ingestion. Alcohol in any form will produce the unpleasant effects. Certain cough syrups, fermented vinegar, food cooked in alcohol, and so forth, may produce an Antabuse reaction. Extrasensitive patients may even react to the use of rubbing alcohol or shaving lotion.

The effects of Antabuse (an′tah-būs″) remain for as long as two weeks, even if the individual has voluntarily withdrawn himself from the drug.

Signs and symptoms of an Antabuse reaction usually occur within five minutes to an hour after ingesting alcohol. There is a bright red flushing of the face, neck, and upper thorax. The person develops a throbbing headache and begins to perspire profusely. Hyperventilation, tachycardia, and hypotension follow soon, and there may be a decreased level of consciousness or even coma.

If the EMT encounters a patient with such symptoms, he should search for an Antabuse card or an identification bracelet that identifies him as an "Antabuse" recipient. Since metronidazole (Flagyl®) (a drug used to treat genital infections), and certain oral hypoglycemic (hi″po-gli-se′mik) agents can also produce such a symptom complex, they should also be considered as a precipitating factor.

The emergency management of an Antabuse reaction involves asking the patient to lie down and reassure him about what is going on. Use a semi-prone side-lying position, since vomiting is probable. (If possible, determine the amount of alcohol ingested. More than two or three drinks can produce shock and coma.)

Advanced EMTs may be instructed to initiate an IV and to place a nasogastric tube for decompression of the stomach.

En route to a treatment facility, the airway and vital signs should be judiciously monitored. Oxygen by nasal catheter may be useful for managing respiratory distress.

# DIFFERENTIATING ALCOHOLISM FROM OTHER CONDITIONS

The EMT must be on guard to differentiate alcoholism from adverse effects of drugs, diabetic reactions, and brain injuries. Any of these conditions can mimic alcohol-related phenomena, or can coexist with the ingestion of alcohol. It is vital to guard against labelling an individual with "acute intoxication," "alcohol withdrawal," or "under the influence" because it narrows your scope of assessment relating to other problems. A person who is drinking can have a head injury without obvious signs and symptoms, or a patient with a visible head injury can have an alcohol-related problem, for example. Approach each patient with an open mind to avoid the "tunnel vision" that can lead to faulty judgments that adversely interfere with prompt and definitive field management.

If the EMT cannot differentiate these problems, but can protect the airway and provide other basic life support measures, a valuable service will be rendered to any of these patients!

## *References*

Ansbaugh, P. "Emergency Management of Intoxicated Patients With Head Injuries," *JEN*, 3:9–12, 1977.

Greenblatt, D. J.: and Shader, R. I. "Treatment of the Alcohol Withdrawal Syndrome," in Shader, R. I., ed., *Manual of Psychiatric Therapeutics: Practical Psychopharmacology and Psychiatry*. Boston, MA: Little Brown and Company, 1975.

Gross, M. M.; Lewis, E.; and Hastey, J. "Acute Alcohol Withdrawal Syndrome," in *Biology of Alcoholism, Vol. 3, Clinical Pathology*. New York; Plenum Press, 1974.

Sachindra N. Pradhan, and Samarendra, N. Dutta, ed. *Drug Abuse: Clinical and Basic Aspects*, pp. 78–101, The C. V. Mosby Company, St. Louis, MO., 1977.

# Chapter 24

# Diabetic Emergencies

One out of every twenty people in this country either has diabetes mellitus (mĕ-li′tus) (sugar diabetes) or will develop it sometime during his lifetime. Half of the diabetics do not even know that they have diabetes until they develop a life-threatening complication. Diabetes is the third leading cause of death. Furthermore, it is a contributing factor in heart attacks and strokes, which are the two top-ranking producers of death. Diabetes affects all age groups and its incidence is increasing among older citizens. The EMT must be thoroughly familiar with the diabetic emergencies that are likely to present with an altered state of consciousness or coma. Immediate assessments and a careful history taking are vital for providing appropriate management of the patient.

## UNDERSTANDING DIABETES

Glucose, a type of sugar, is the primary fuel for body cells. The brain uses at least one-fourth of all available glucose to perform its vital functions. Since the brain cannot store glucose, it must be constantly supplied, just like oxygen. The amount of this sugar in the blood must remain fairly constant, between 60–120 mg/dl (mg per 100 ml) in order for the brain and other parts of the nervous system to be adequately energized. If the level of the "blood sugar" falls below 60 mg/dl, brain cells and their functioning may be seriously compromised.

*Insulin* (in′su-lin), a hormone secreted by the pancreas (pan′kre-as), regulates how fast the fuel (glucose) is consumed. Insulin works much like a carburetor, controlling the rate that fuel is supplied to cells for energy production. Muscle tissue, fat, and the liver cells each have a unique way of using glucose.

In individuals with a healthy pancreas, there is a constant monitoring of the blood sugar level and a secretion of necessary insulin in response. This organ, in effect, regulates carbohydrate metabolism. If the intake of carbohydrates is high and the blood sugar rises, the pancreas releases a correspondingly high quantity of insulin. If the blood sugar level falls below normal, the release of insulin is suppressed to keep the sugar in the blood. The cells must revert to an alternate mode of nourishing themselves when this happens. Like all "back-up" systems, there is a failure now and then, even in the most healthy individuals and emergency conditions ensue.

An individual with diabetes or with an inflamed pancreas is unable to produce insulin on a dependable basis. Muscle and fat tissue are unable to "take up" glucose from the blood although there may be more than an adequate circulating supply. In these cases, the liver senses the need for fuel and releases its sugar stores in the form of glycogen. The level of sugar in the blood rises even further, which can ultimately result in a hyperglycemic (high blood sugar) crisis. When the blood sugar level exceeds the kidney threshold for sugar, usually 180 to 200 mg/dl, the excess sugar spills over into the urine and the individual may lose sugar, salt, and water in large amounts. Essentially, the excess sugar in the blood acts like a diuretic (water pill) and dehydration will soon occur. At this point, the individual feels thirsty, and tends to drink a lot to correct the dehydration. Since the body is deprived of fuel, a diabetic feels tired and hungry. Excessive urinary output (polyuria [pol″e-u′re-ah]), extreme thirst (polydipsia [pol″e-dip′se-ah]), and increased appetite (polyphagia [pol″e-fa′je-ah]), are the classic symptoms of diabetes mellitus.

Ordinarily, the cells use glucose to produce energy, but when insulin is unavailable, proteins and fats (not carbohydrates) are metabolized. When proteins and fats are utilized, the metabolic by-products are acid, and they accumulate quickly. The high level of acids, coupled with a loss of base bicarbonates, induces acidosis (as″ĭ-do′sis). This acidosis, along with a water deficiency and electrolyte imbalances, adversely affects the brain and may produce coma, shock, and even death if insulin remains deficient. The administration of insulin, replacement of fluids, and correction of electrolyte imbalances will interrupt the protein and fat breakdown. Ultimately energy production will be resumed by the primary glucose mechanism.

Every day, diabetics must maintain a vital balance between diet, expenditure of energy, and availability of insulin. Some diabetics merely monitor their food intake and energy use to control their condition. Others take a drug by mouth to stimulate the pancreas to produce insulin. These drugs are called oral hypoglycemic agents. Other diabetics require insulin injections to meet daily needs. If outside factors affect the diabetic (e.g., they are unable to eat, do not take their medication, expend more than their usual amount of energy, or have an infection), the EMT may encounter this individual as a "diabetic emergency."

There are two major diabetic emergencies: (1) hypoglycemia (low blood sugar) or "insulin shock," and (2) hyperglycemia (high blood sugar), ketoacidosis (ke"to-ah"sĭ-do'sis), or "diabetic coma." Either condition can lead to unconsciousness.

## Hypoglycemia

Every diabetic who takes insulin or an oral hypoglycemic agent is subject to hypoglycemia if there is too much of the agent in the body for the amount of glucose present. In such instances, the blood is rapidly depleted of sugar and the brain does not have adequate access to glucose which is vital for its activity. This circumstance is induced when the individual takes too much insulin or an excessive dose of an oral hypoglycemic drug; the diet contains insufficient food to meet energy production needs; or there is an abnormal or excessive expenditure of energy that requires considerable glucose. In any of these situations, there is insufficient blood glucose to meet requirements. This hypoglycemia or "low blood sugar" triggers an emergency response of the sympathetic nervous system. Epinephrine (adrenalin), a hormone to assist in coping with stress, is released. Epinephrine facilitates an extra burst of energy to deal with the crisis.

When epinephrine is released into the blood stream, the diabetic may feel hunger pains or experience "butterflies in the stomach." This is nature's way of asking for food (glucose) to meet the need for energy. The pupils dilate and the individual experiences blurred vision. Sweating is also pronounced in response to epinephrine.

The brain of the individual with hypoglycemia, and deprived of glucose or oxygen, is irritable and restless. Changes in behavior (especially in children), weakness, and headache may occur. Eventually, seizures are likely to be induced as a result of energy starvation and chemical insults from electrolyte disturbances. At last, if intervention is not definitive, brain damage and death are possible.

## Hyperglycemia (Ketoacidosis)

Hyperglycemia is a life-threatening emergency caused by insulin depletion. Without insulin, the body cannot use glucose at the cellular level, so more and more sugar builds up in the blood stream. This can happen over several days or even hours. The following phenomena can cause ketoacidosis:

1. Failure of the diabetic to take insulin or an oral hypoglycemic agent as prescribed
2. Excessive food intake without compensation by more exercise

3. Coexistent illness, stress, pregnancy, infection, fever, menstruation, or surgery

4. Ingestion of drugs such as selected diuretics or corticosteroids (kor″tı-ko-ste′roidz), which increase blood glucose levels

Any of the four factors create a situation in which there is not enough insulin to convert glucose in the blood into energy production at the cellular level. Without energy, the patient becomes weaker and eventually is forced to use fat and protein to meet energy requirements. This process may take several days, but the consequences are certain.

The EMT who obtains information from the patient (who is still able to respond) may learn that he has not taken his insulin (or oral hypoglycemic drug) or that he has an unusual health problem or personal stress.

Dehydration is an early response to a high blood sugar level and the resultant excess volume of urine output. Of course, large amounts of sodium and potassium are lost during this phase of rapid water loss. Signs and symptoms of this hyperglycemic crisis include hot, dry skin that has lost its normal elasticity due to the water deficiency. Since dehydration is essentially *hypovolemia,* the pulse will rise and the blood pressure will fall as in other shock states. Electrolyte losses cause muscle cramping with abdominal pain and vomiting.

Acidosis develops over one or two days. As the body attempts to get rid of the excess acid, rapid, deep breathing ensues. These breaths of "air hunger" (Kussmauls' [koos′mowlz] respirations) are an attempt to reduce acid levels by "breathing off" the acid. If the EMT smells the patient's breath, it may resemble acetone (a sweet, overripe banana odor).

The brain begins to be dysfunctional as acid substances accumulate and their toxic effects are felt. There may be disturbed behavior or altered levels of consciousness, including coma.

## THE UNCONSCIOUS DIABETIC

The EMT should *not* assume that every diabetic patient encountered is suffering from a diabetic-related emergency. Diabetics may become unconscious from cardiac arrest, a heroin overdose, head injury, or excessive alcohol consumption, too! Of course, it is important for the EMT to have thorough details, if possible, about the diabetic patient's overall health status, since insulin shock or ketoacidosis are only two of many causes of unconscious states. The airway, breathing, and circulation are always the *highest* priorities, so the integrity of the airway must be assured at once. Remember that the patient will probably be confused or in an altered state of consciousness. Vomiting is probable, so great care should be taken to prevent aspiration.

The EMT must understand the relationship of insulin administration to the development of diabetic complications and also appreciate that oral

Table 24–1. Insulin Actions
(Onset, peak, and duration)

| *Type of Insulin* | *Onset of Action* | *Peak Action (in hours)* | *Duration* |
|---|---|---|---|
| Regular | ½–1 | 2–4 | 6–8 |
| Semi-Lente | ½–1 | 2–4 | 8–10 |
| Globin | 1–2 | 6–8 | 12–14 |
| NPH | 1–2 | 6–8 | 12–14 |
| Lente | 1–2 | 6–8 | 14–16 |
| PZI | 4–6 | 18± | 36–72 |
| Ultralente | 4–6 | 8–12 | 24–36 |

agents can lead to hypoglycemia, too. However, there may be subtle differences. On the scene analysis of data can be much improved if there is a clear understanding of when selected types of insulin "peak" (when their concentration is greatest and most likely to cause hypoglycemia.)(See Table 24–1.) Since some diabetics take more than one kind of insulin, this factor must be considered when anticipating reactions.

A chemically-sensitive sugar testing strip called Dextrostix may be used to rapidly determine an on the scene blood sugar level. (Since this requires a small blood sample, it may only be used by EMTs certified in invasive techniques.) This simple test is quite helpful in assessing the unconscious diabetic. Regardless, the EMT should arrange for prompt transportation of the patient to the hospital. Advanced EMT's may obtain blood samples, administer 50 percent Dextrose (sugar solution) by IV, administer naloxone (Narcan) and monitor the ECG to detect dysrhythmias induced by electrolyte imbalances. Intravenous fluids and oxygen are also components of the advanced EMT "diabetic" protocol in most communities. Formerly, EMTs were encouraged to give a sugar-enriched substance to a conscious diabetic. It is unlikely, though, that an ambulance would have been called if the patient were still alert enough for safe oral sugar intake. A gelatinlike concentrated sugar substance is commercially available for EMTs to place under the tongue or in the lining of the jaw. These sites are richly supplied with blood and promptly absorb sugar.

The EMT should suspect either hypoglycemia or hyperglycemia as a cause for coma in the diabetic patient. However, other causes should not be overlooked. Rather than trying to decide whether the blood sugar is too low or too high, it is safer to give glucose than to risk brain dysfunction and cellular damage due to *hypoglycemia*. Glucose may awaken the victim of low blood sugar and improve his condition almost miraculously within just a few minutes.

Transportation should not be delayed to permit time-consuming assessments to differentiate hypoglycemia and hyperglycemia. Assume that every diabetic patient who is unconscious needs sugar and administer it

TABLE 24-2. COMPARISON OF DIABETIC EMERGENCIES

| *Hypoglycemia* | *Hyperglycemia* |
|---|---|
| *Onset* | |
| Sudden (within minutes after insulin or oral hypoglycemic | May occur as gradual process over several days |
| *Causes* | |
| Too much insulin<br>Overdose of oral hypoglycemic agent.<br>Omission of meals<br>Excessive exercise before meals | Neglect of prescribed therapy<br>Intercurrent disease or infection; other drug therapy<br>Dietary indiscretion |
| *Signs* | |
| Pale skin; may be sweating<br>Shallow respirations | Reddened face<br>Kussmaul's "air hunger" respirations<br>Dry skin<br>Rapid pulse<br>Acetone "fruity" breath |
| *Symptoms* | |
| Hunger, nausea<br>Headache, dizziness<br>Fatigue, weakness<br>Blurred vision<br>Unusual skin sensations (e.g. burning, "crawling," tingling)<br>Diplopia (double vision) | Thirst<br>Headache<br>Nausea; vomiting<br>Abdominal pain<br>Poor (dim) vision<br>Dyspnea<br>Constipation |
| *Chemical tests* | |
| Urine tests negative for sugar and acetone<br>Dextrostix negative or very low for sugar | Urine tests positive for sugar and acetone.<br>Dextrostix positive; usually very high for sugar |
| *Response to treatment* | |
| Usually rapid when sugar is provided. | Very slow; requires insulin, hydration, correction of acid-base balance and electrolytes, and possibly ventilatory assistance and supplemental oxygen |

under the tongue, in the cheek lining, or by IV (for advanced EMTs). Assessment of vital signs and airway protection are, of course, essential EMT responsibilities enroute, since hypotension and vomiting are likely. Seizures should also be anticipated.

The EMT who understands diabetes and is skilled in its assessment and management may be instrumental in preventing brain damage and even death associated with diabetic complications.

*References*

Barber, Janet, M.; Stokes, Lillian S.; and Billings, Diane M. *Adult and Child Care: A Client Approach to Nursing,* 2nd ed., pp. 648–669, St. Louis; MO: The C. V. Mosby Company, 1977.

Barber, Janet M. "Diabetic Emergencies," *The EMT Journal,* 1:52–57, September 1977.

Barber, Janet M.; and Budassi, Susan A. *Mosby's Manual of Emergency Care, Practices and Procedures,* pp. 185–188. St. Louis, MO: The C. V. Mosby Company, 1979.

Gazzaniga, Alan B.; Iseri, Lloyd T.; and Baren, Martin. *Emergency Care: Principles and Practices for The EMT-Paramedic,* pp. 478–483. Reston, VA: Reston Publishing Co., Inc., 1979.

Guthrie, Diana W., and Guthrie, Richard A., eds. *Nursing Management of Diabetes Mellitus,* St. Louis, MO: The C. V. Mosby Co., 1977.

# Chapter 25

# Obstetrical Problems and Emergency Childbirth

An EMT is likely to be called upon at some time to manage an emergency delivery. This encounter can be extremely gratifying if the EMT is confident of the approach to imminent childbirth and understands exactly how to assist the mother and the newborn in the field. In this chapter, you will become familiar with the process of normal labor and delivery and will learn how to systematically assess and manage the mother and her baby during this time. Although the likelihood of complications in the delivery are small, the most important problems will be described along with recommendations for emergency care.

## FEMALE ANATOMY AND PHYSIOLOGY

The female anatomy of importance to pregnancy and childbirth consists of the ovaries, fallopian (fal-lo'pe-an) tubes, uterus (u'ter-us), and vagina (vah-ji'nah).

Each month, one ovary releases an ovum (egg); the ovum is transported to the uterus by the fallopian tube, which lies next to it within the pelvic cavity. If the ovum is not fertilized, it is discarded with the innermost lining of the uterus (endometrium [en-do-me'tre-um]) as part of the menstrual (men'stroo-al) flow. If the ovum is fertilized, it is implanted within the uterus, where it develops and grows. Two special "organs of pregnancy" protect and nourish the fetus during the pregnancy, the *amniotic fluid* and the *placenta.*

Early in pregnancy, a fluid-filled sac develops around the baby. This "bag of waters" is called *amniotic* (am"ne-on'ik) *fluid.* It cushions the baby, maintains an even temperature in the surroundings, and permits movement of the developing structures. The rupture of the amniotic fluid sac often denotes the onset of labor.

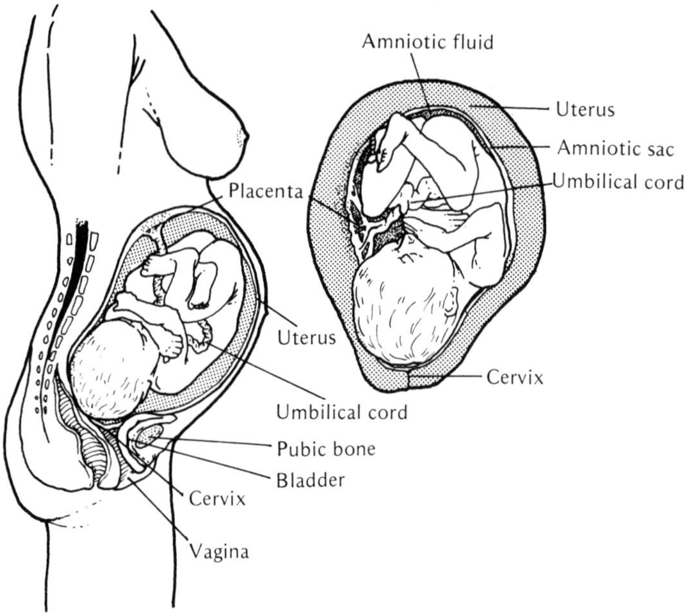


**Figure 25-1.** The female anatomy of pregnancy. Inset shows details of the amniotic fluid, placenta, and umbilical cord.

Another important structure called the *placenta* (plah-sen′tah) develops by the third month of pregnancy. The placenta has an important role in nourishing the baby, and functions much like a "root system" in connection with the maternal blood supply. The umbilical (um-bil′ĭ-kal) cord connects the baby to the placenta. One large vein and two arteries are contained in this rope-like structure, and transport a blood supply between the mother and the baby. The placenta is sometimes called an "afterbirth" by lay persons, since it is expelled after the baby is delivered.

The cervix (ser′viks) (the thickened structure at the base of the uterus) remains sealed with a mucus plug during pregnancy. Sometimes the expulsion of this blood-tinged mucus precedes other signs and symptoms of the onset of labor. When it is noted, it is referred to as "bloody show" or simply "show." The vagina has no special role in pregnancy until the onset of labor, when it is readied for its function as a "birth canal" for delivery of the infant. (See Fig. 25-1.)

## LABOR

Labor is the process by which the products of conception (the baby and the placenta) are expelled from the uterus. Ordinarily this event happens about forty weeks, or nine months after conception, but it may occur earlier if there are abnormal stresses affecting the baby's environment. For example, labor can be initiated early by an accident involving the mother, such as a fall or a blow to the abdomen. The EMT should be alert to this factor when assessing any woman of child-bearing age post-trauma. Infants of six months or more of age can survive outside the uterus if they receive prompt, definitive care. (See page 487.)

The onset of labor and its duration is highly individual, and although some "normals" can be outlined, the EMT should not be deterred from making careful assessments for the patient in question since the force of contractions, soft tissue resistance, the size and position of the infant, and even emotions affect the progress of labor. For example, labor normally is twice as long for the first baby than for later ones.

Labor is divided into three stages. These stages (1) prepare the cervix and birth canal for delivery, (2) expel the baby, and (3) expel the placenta and restore the uterus (u′ter-us) to its predelivery state within the pelvis.

The *first stage of labor* consists of a series of contractions, which become progressively stronger and occur more frequently until the cervix "thins out" and opens in response to the pressure exerted by the uterine muscles. The contractions characteristically begin subtly with cramplike pains that radiate from the lumbar region of the back to the lower abdomen. These "cramps" last from thirty to fifty seconds and occur every five to twenty minutes. Over several hours, in most women, the contractions become greater in intensity, lasting sixty to ninety seconds and the intervals between become shorter, only a minute or two. This first stage lasts about twelve hours for a primigravida (pri″mĭ-grav′ĭ-dah), (woman who is having her first pregnancy), and about six hours for the multipara (mul-tip′ah-rah) (woman who has delivered a child previously). The membranes, or "bag of water" that surrounds the infant, may rupture during this stage.

The *second stage* of labor is an extension of the first and ends with the delivery of the baby. The cervix is "thinned" and open and the head pushes down toward the perineum producing a reflex that causes in the woman a desire to "bear down" as if she were defecating. This urge cannot be controlled, and as the head progresses, the perineum bulges and the infant's scalp can be visualized during the height of each contraction. (This appearance of the scalp is called *crowning.*) Within a few moments, the head will be actually delivered, followed promptly by the shoulders and remainder of the infant. The second stage lasts about one hour in the primigravida and thirty minutes in the multipara.

The *third stage* of labor permits an additional "transfusion" of blood to the infant as postdelivery contractions force blood through the placenta and cord. The infant should be held at perineal level and the cord left unclamped until this vital reserve of blood is transferred to the infant. The process takes only three to five minutes and the placenta then separates from the uterine wall and is expelled. The delivery of the placenta is accompanied by a gush of blood.

Emergency delivery (or more appropriately, *unscheduled* or *un-*

*planned delivery*) provides the EMT an opportunity for a truly satisfying human experience.

The EMT's role in childbirth is essentially one of "standing by" while nature takes its course, and providing help and support to make the process safer for the woman and the infant. The process of birth must not be delayed, hurried, or interfered with by any individual in the field, since such injudicious tactics can harm both the woman and her infant.

The common reason for the EMT's getting involved in childbirth is that the woman is surprised by an unusually rapid progression of labor which does not permit a routine trip to the hospital for delivery. Such rapid labor courses are most prevalent in the multipara who has had several previous deliveries. As mentioned earlier, precipitating factors of accidents and abdominal injury or bleeding can also hasten the onset of labor and its progression. Classically, the EMT arrives just in time to permit a rapid assessment of the woman and either transport promptly or prepare for immediate delivery at the scene.

## ASSESSMENT

It is imperative for the EMT to gather on-the-scene information by both history taking and physical examination as time permits. The following data are essential for decision making:

1. *Reason for calling EMTs.* Did your membranes rupture? Are you bleeding? Remember that the membranes ordinarily rupture, signaling the onset of labor, or occur during the first stage. All women who have ruptured membranes or active bleeding should be transported. Bright red active bleeding is not normal and is indicative of an emergency requiring rapid response. (See page 481.) A small amount of "bloody show" (a brownish to reddish pink discharge) is normal and represents the displacement of the cervical mucus plug. The appearance of "show" accompanies the onset of true labor, but usually indicates that the delivery is several hours away—even for the multipara.

2. *Is active labor in progress, and if so, how far has it advanced?* Ask the woman about her "due date." Determination of whether or not this is a full-term pregnancy is important to anticipation of complications. (See page 481.) Is this her first baby or has she had several prior deliveries? Remember that labor often proceeds very rapidly in the multipara. What is the intensity of contractions and the interval between them? If the timing of contractions by palpation validate early labor, there is usually sufficient time for transport to a hospital. However, if the woman insists on bearing down or states that she feels like "moving her bowels," delivery is imminent, requiring your assistance. If time permits, examine the perineum for bulging during contractions or the appearance of the infant's scalp at the vaginal opening. Either of these phenomena do not permit time for transport, so prepare for the delivery.

Ideally, the delivery should be controlled and should take place under the best aseptic conditions possible. However, in the field, a bedroom, living room floor, or backseat of a car may not permit the luxury of sterility, good lighting, and proper equipment at hand. The EMT should be prepared to adapt skills and approaches accordingly, with utmost attention focused on the safety of the woman and her baby.

1. *Position the woman and reassure her.* The woman should lie down and bend her knees. Place a folded sheet or blanket under her buttocks to elevate the perineum off the surface. It is helpful to ask her to grasp her knees. The latter helps her to maintain her position and gives her a focus for "gripping" as labor pain becomes intense. As you prepare your equipment, explain your actions and reassure her as much as possible, that "everything is under control." If time permits (and it rarely does), record the patient's blood pressure, pulse, respiratory rate, and the fetal heart tones. (See Fig. 25–2.) Consider the possibility that the woman may vomit, and have a receptacle at hand and be prepared to manage the airway. (See Fig. 25–3.)

2. *Glove yourself and drape the woman.* One EMT should be at hand to assist and support the woman during the delivery and to care for the infant immediately after birth. The other EMT should put on sterile gloves and drape the woman, exposing only the perineum. (See Fig. 25–4.)

3. *Control the bleeding.* Encourage the woman to pant during each contraction to assist in controlling the urge to push. When the urge cannot be resisted and delivery is imminent, the EMT should place gentle pressure on the emerging head to avoid a precipitous "popping out" which can be harmful to both the woman (lacerations of the perineum) and the infant (intracranial hemorrhage). When the head is fully delivered, support it with your hands while nature rotates it to facilitate delivery of the shoulders. Make sure the cord is not around the infant's neck. If it is, remove it by slipping it over the head. Do not pull on it since tearing it could result in fatal hemorrhages for both the woman and the baby. If it is too tight for removal, clamp it in two places, and cut it between the clamps. If there are membranes covering the infant's face, snip them with sterile scissors, at the nape of the neck, and pull them from the nose and mouth. (See Fig. 25–5.)

4. *Assure the infant's airway.* As soon as the head is delivered, a bulb syringe should be used to suction the mouth and nose. Although infants are "nose breathers," the mouth and throat should be cleared first, with the head being held in an extended position. Oral and pharyngeal aspiration should always precede nasal aspiration, because the latter often causes reflex inhalation which could result in secretions being drawn into respiratory passages. (See Fig. 25–6.)

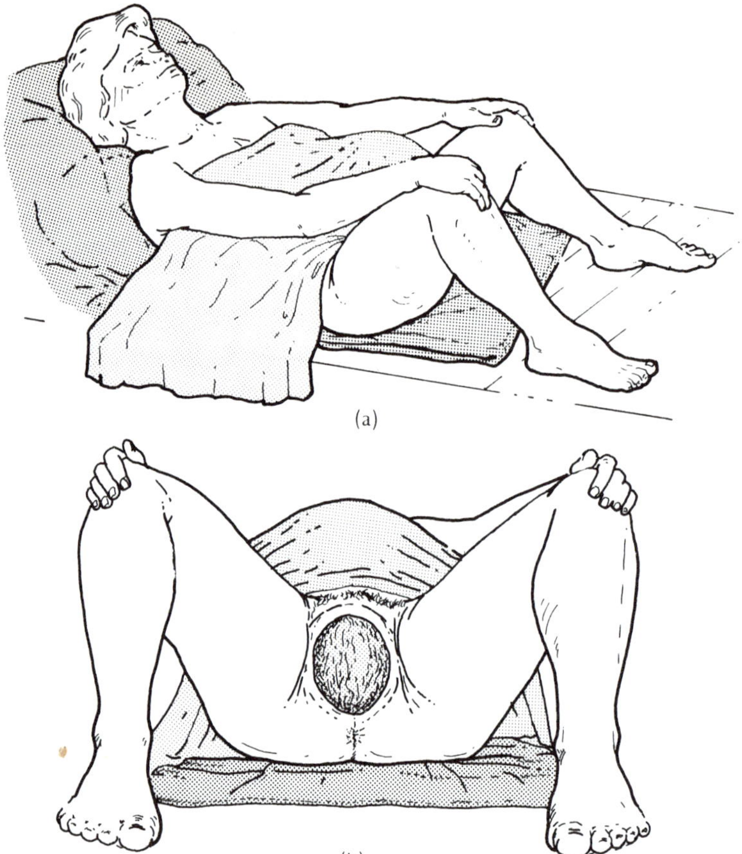

(a)

(b)

**Figure 25-2.** Position of mother for delivery. (Note that the hips are elevated on a folded sheet and that the feet are apart and flat on the bed or other surface. Having the mother grasp her knees aids in maintaining the position. (b) Appearance of the perineum during "crowning" of the infant's head.

5. *Complete the delivery and note the time. Resuscitate as necessary.* Delivery of the shoulders may be facilitated by guiding the head downward to deliver the anterior shoulder and then upward for the posterior shoulder. The delivery of the remaining parts will follow promptly. Note the time and inform the woman about the sex and condition of the baby. Hold the infant's body at the level of the perineum, on its side, in a head-down position and suction the airways once again. Spontaneous breathing should be initiated by the first cry. If not, dry the infant vigorously to stimulate respirations. When airway and breathing are assured and the heart rate is above one-hundred beats per minute, the cord can be clamped and the infant dried and warmed for transport. If respirations do not occur, begin CPR. (See page 485 and Chapter 10.)

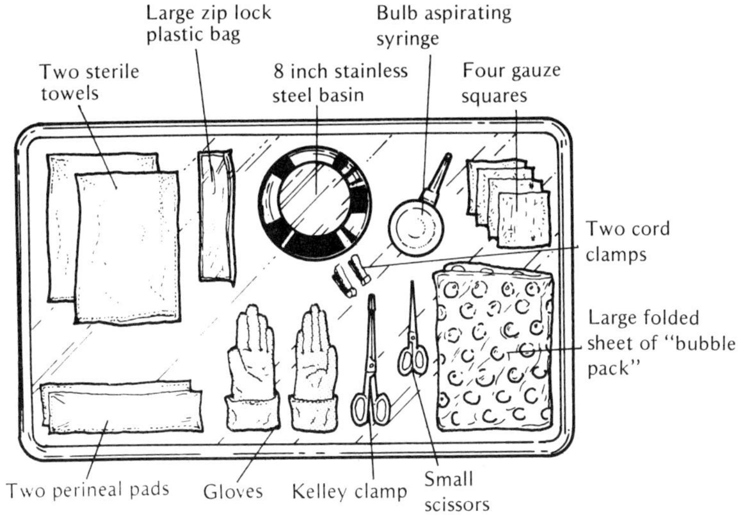


**Figure 25-3.** Suggested contents of an emergency delivery kit for field use.

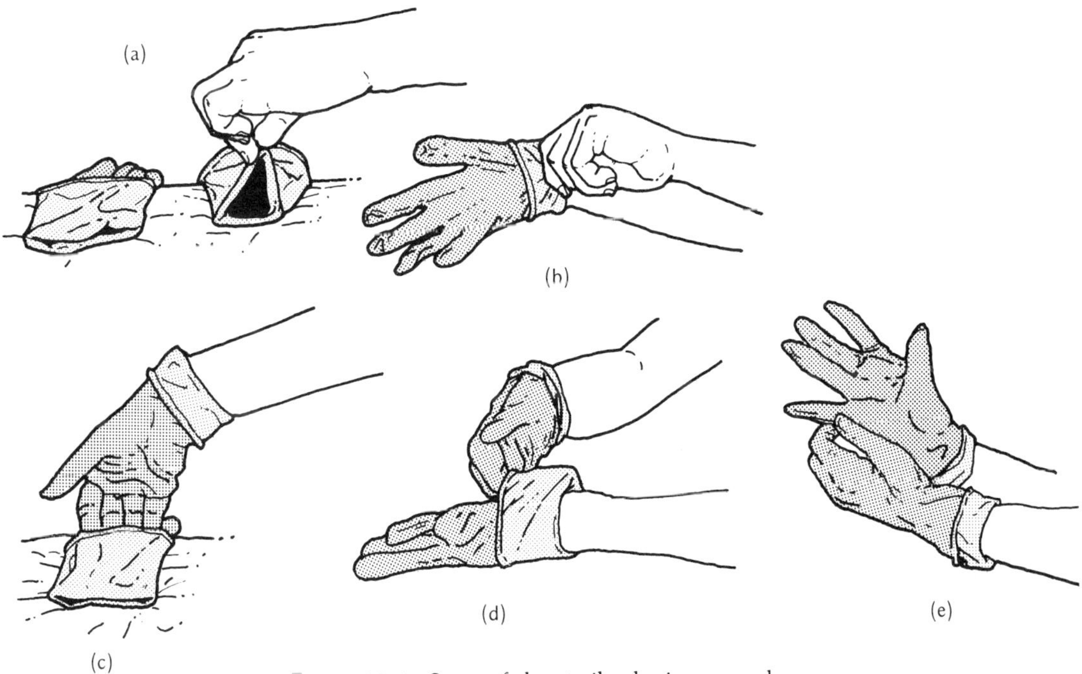


**Figure 25-4.** Steps of the sterile gloving procedure.

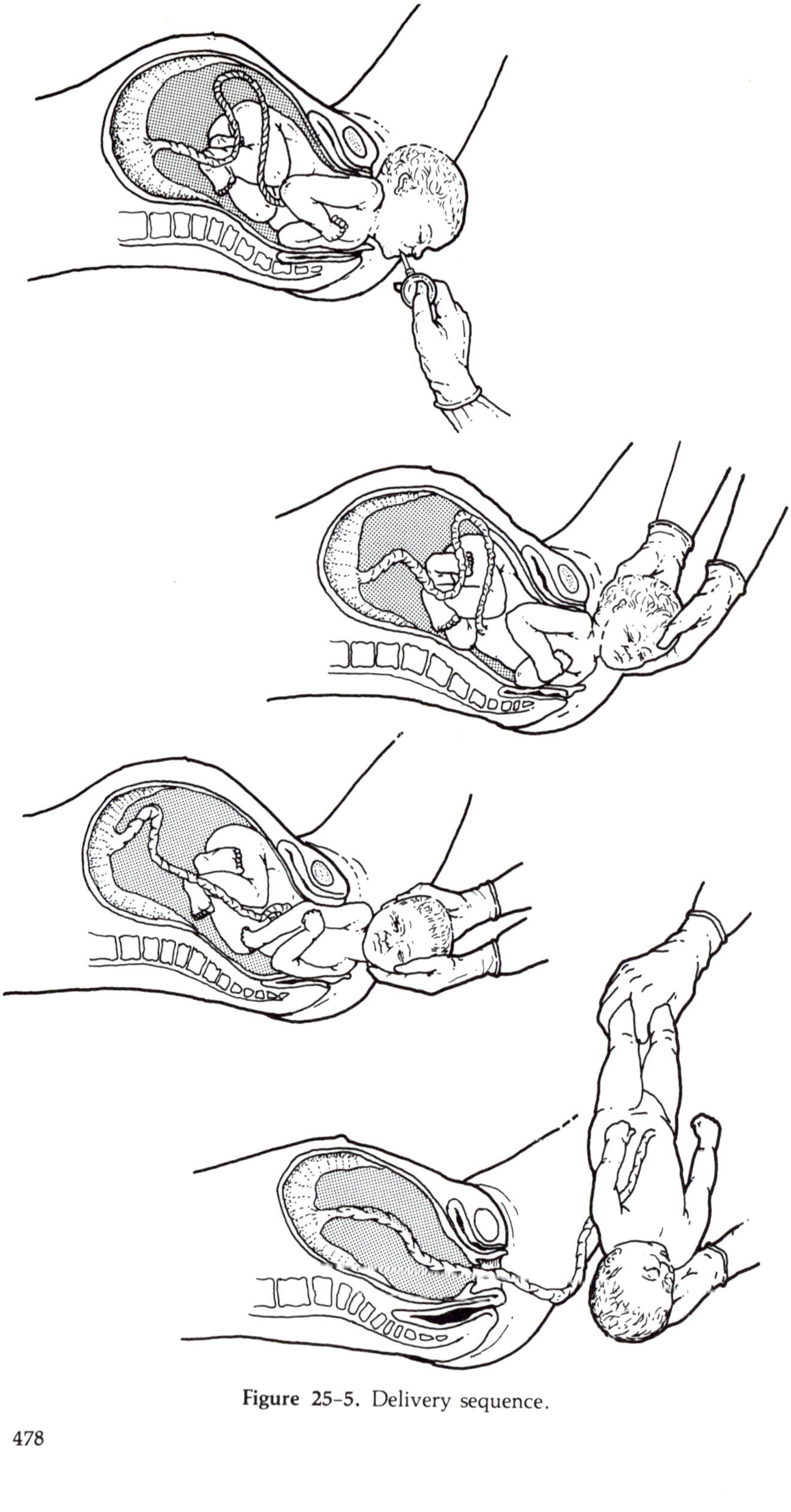

**Figure 25-5.** Delivery sequence.

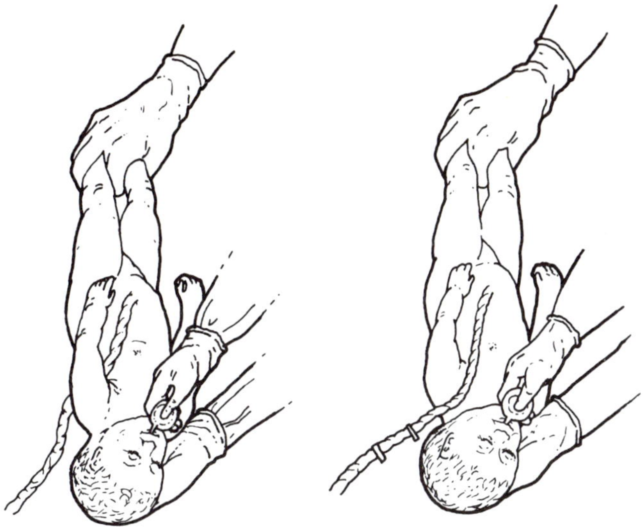

**Figure 25-6.** Suctioning airway with bulb syringe. Note that head is held in an extended position.

6. *Clamp the Cord.* After the cord stops pulsating, three to five minutes) clamp it in two places. (See Fig. 25-7.) If you do not have sterile supplies, do not clamp or cut the cord. Merely keep it wrapped with the baby after its delivery, keeping it at the level of the baby until all pulsations cease. The first clamp should be placed six to eight inches from the infant and the other clamp about two inches distally (close to the placenta). Cut the cord between the two clamps with sterile scissors. Apply another umbilical clamp on the cord three to four inches from the baby. Position the infant on his side with a slight head-down position. The head should be extended but *do not hyperextend* the neck since this latter maneuver tends to

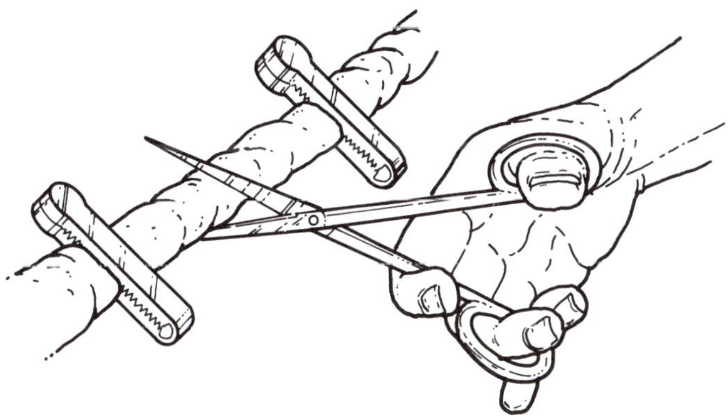

**Figure 25-7.** Cord clamping and cutting procedure.

kink and obstruct the tiny airway. (See page 176.) If feasible, the head should be slightly lower than the feet in order to pool secretions in the cheek for easy removal by the bulb syringe. Furthermore, this position causes the tongue to fall to the side, making the airway more secure. Dry thoroughly and cover snugly with a warm blanket, aluminum wrap, plastic or bubble pack. *Keep the infant warm!* Heat loss in a newborn results in rapid utilization of oxygen and sugar stores leaving him vulnerable to hypoxia and hypoglycemia. (See pages 487–488.) If possible, place the infant close to the mother to conserve the tiny infant's body heat.

7. *After Care of Placenta.* During the final stage of labor, the placenta will be delivered along with a gush of blood. The EMT will note that the cord advances farther out of the vagina and that the uterus becomes round and rises noticeably upward in the abdomen. The woman may then bear down to expel the placenta. (Occasionally, it will not separate without physician manipulation. The EMT should never attempt to force the expulsion of the placenta since it could result in a fatal hemorrhage for the mother if it is torn. If there is heavy bleeding post-delivery, promptly transport the mother and baby. (See Fig. 25–8.) The placenta should be contained in a basin or bag for transport to the hospital along with the woman and her infant. The physician will carefully examine the placenta to ensure that it is normal and is intact since even a small fragment remaining in the uterus can result in hemorrhage and infection.

8. *Prepare Woman for Transport.* Place the woman on clean linens and place a sanitary napkin over the perineum. If there are large lacerations of the perineum, active bleeding can be controlled with pressure, using sterile 4 × 4s. Lower the legs gently and provide a blanket for additional warmth and comfort. One EMT should carefully massage the uterus to keep it contracted to prevent further bleeding. (See Fig. 25–9.) Vital signs should be monitored as time permits. If the women does not object, the baby may be put to the breast since the sucking will assist in contracting

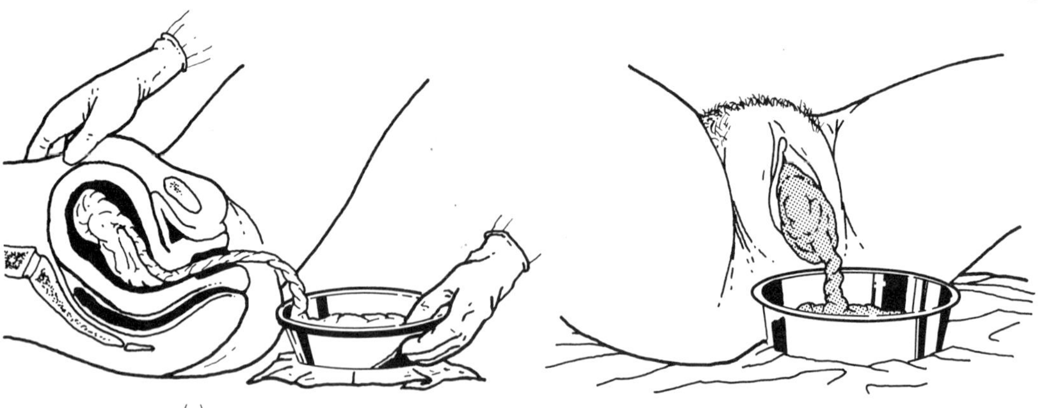

(a) (b)

**Figure 25–8.** Delivery of placenta: (a) lateral view; (b) perineal view.

the uterus and arresting the hemorrhage. If there is a lengthy transport (over thirty minutes), antishock trousers may be applied to control the hemorrhage. (See page 215.) Oxygen should be administered and the shock position employed. Advanced EMTs or Paramedics may be advised to initiate IV fluid therapy.

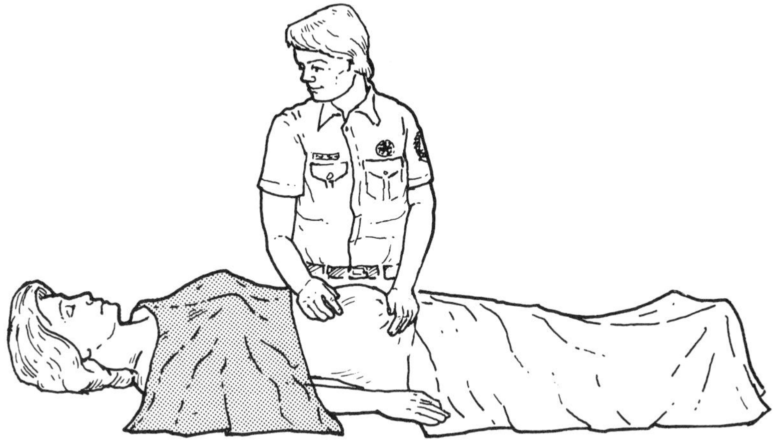

**Figure 25–9.** Technique of uterine massage to control bleeding after delivery. One hand is placed above the pubic bone to prevent downward displacement. The opposite hand is cupped around the uterus and gently rotated until the organ is firm. Do not overmassage the sensitive uterus!

## Multiple Births

If multiple births are expected or if the abdomen is large post-delivery, an additional delivery may be at hand. Labor usually begins within ten to fifteen minutes after the first birth, with delivery accomplished in thirty to forty-five minutes. (If the second baby is attached to the same placenta as the first baby, the placenta delivery will be delayed, of course, until the second birth has occurred.) Essentially, multiple births are managed in the same manner as single ones. Since twins may be smaller or even born prematurely, they require the special handling of a "high risk" neonate. (See page 487.)

# COMPLICATIONS OF PREGNANCY AND DELIVERY

## Excessive Bleeding

Hemorrhage can occur prior to delivery from early separation of the placenta. This complication can occur anytime within the last three months of pregnancy. There will be profuse bright, red bleeding, pain and signs of

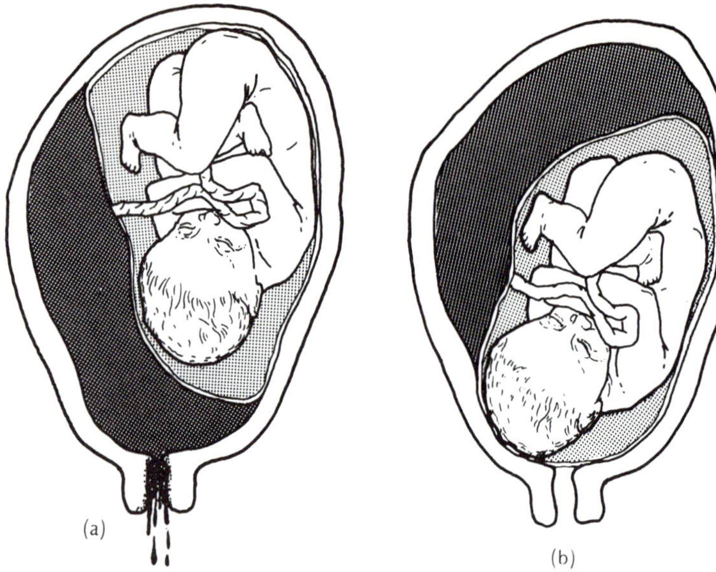

**Figure 25–10.** Placenta-related complications resulting in (a) visible bleeding and (b) concealed bleeding.

shock. There may be an absence of fetal heart tones if more than half of the placenta has separated, thus depriving the fetus of circulation. If EMTs encounter profuse bleeding in a pregnant woman, they should manage the shock state using the usual measures (see Fig. 25–10) and transport at once to the hospital for surgical intervention.

Another cause of excessive bleeding prior to delivery is the result of the placenta being misplaced in the uterus. If, for example, it covers the opening to the cervix, it may spontaneously induce bleeding, especially in the seventh or eighth month of pregnancy when continued mechanical pressure of the developing fetus is exerted on the cervix. The hemorrhage is painless, as opposed to the one discussed in relation to the early placental separation.

The woman should be managed for the shock state and transported promptly to a hospital.

## Prolapsed Cord

Occasionally the baby's cord will push down through the cervix and vagina ahead of the baby, and will be visible at the vaginal opening. The baby's heart rate will be indicative of fetal distress (see page **481**). The cervix will clamp off the cord during contractions preventing circulatory exchange between the mother and infant. In the event of a prolapsed (pro′lapst) cord, place the woman on her left side and elevate her hips.

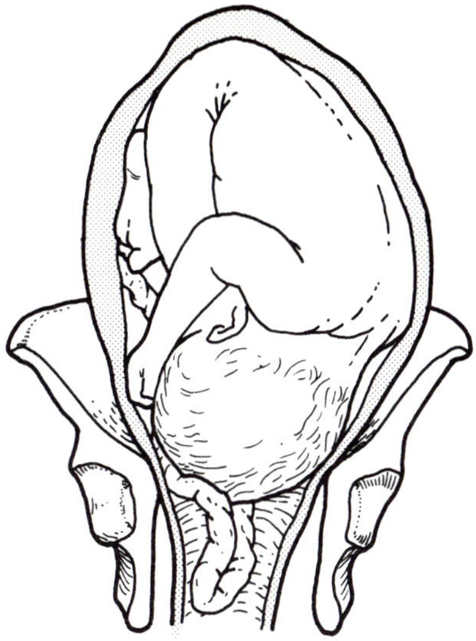

**Figure 25-11.** Prolapsed cord. Note that the infant's head is compressing the cord and interrupting blood supply.

Give high flow supplemental oxygen (8*l* by nasal cannula) and transport at once to the hospital for surgical intervention. Do not attempt to manipulate the cord, but do continue to monitor it for pulsations to estimate the amount of fetal distress to be anticipated upon delivery. (See Fig. 25-11.)

## MECHANICAL PROBLEMS IN DELIVERY

In addition to complications which have already been discussed, there are emergencies during labor due to (1) the fetus' being too large to pass through the pelvis or (2) its being in an abnormal position for delivery.

There is little that the EMT can do in the field if the fetus is too large to be delivered vaginally. Prolonged labor with strong, frequent contractions and no signs of impending birth should cause the EMT to suspect this problem. Often a diabetic mother produces an unusually large baby and this problem should be anticipated if diabetes is a factor in the maternal history. Certain congenital anomalies such as hydrocephalus, which distends the head, will also cause delivery difficulties. Prompt transport to the hospital for cesarean (se-sa′re-an) section is the appropriate mode of management.

### Abnormal Positions or Presentations for Delivery

There are many possible variations in the position of the baby for delivery, but fortunately, those that interfere with labor and those which complicate or prevent vaginal delivery rarely occur. (See Fig. 25-12.)

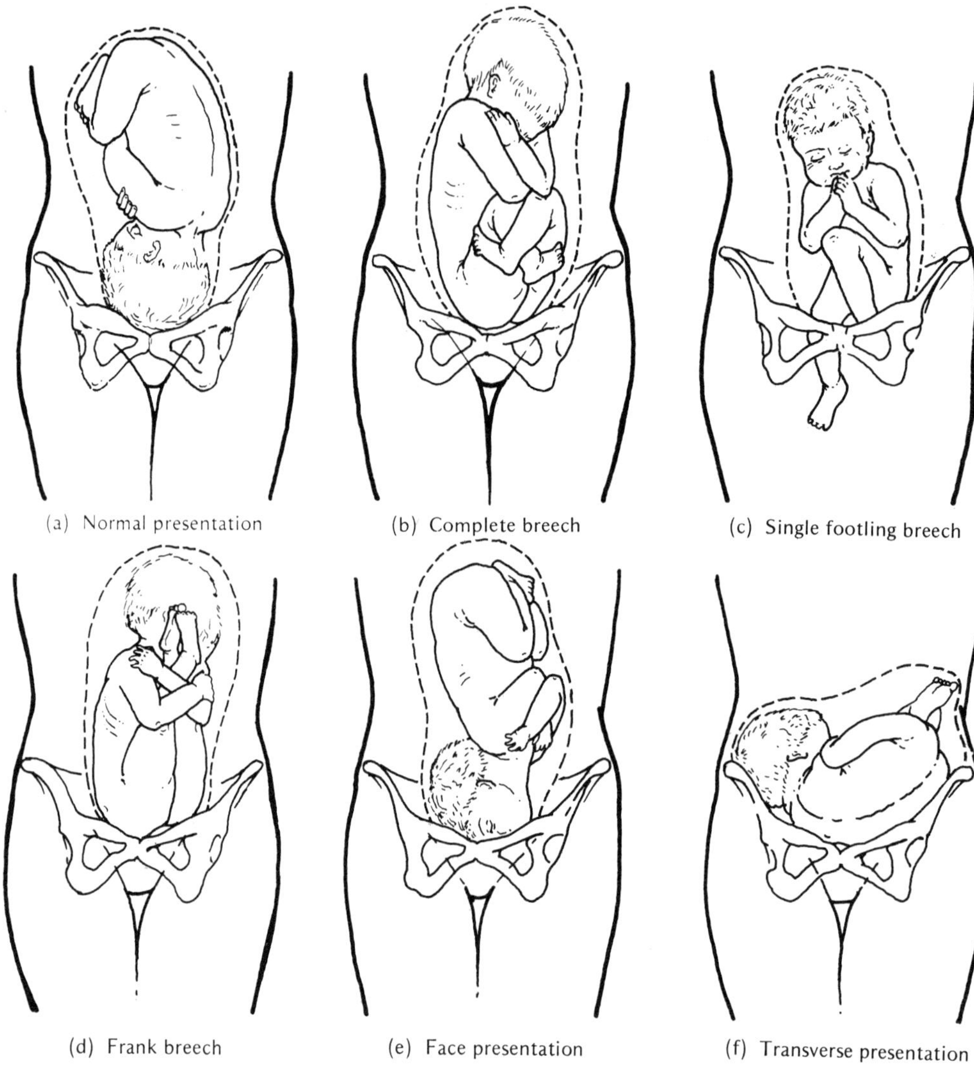


**Figure 25-12.** Variations of obstetrical presentations: (a) normal position for delivery; (b) complete breech; (c) single footling breech; (d) Frank breech; (e) face presentation; (f) transverse presentation.

However, the EMT should be prepared to recognize and manage certain abnormal positions. Table 25-1 outlines the characteristics of selected variations of position, the attendant dangers, and suggested field strategy appropriate for the EMT.

TABLE 25-1. FIELD MANAGEMENT OF ABNORMAL PRESENTATIONS

| *Abnormal Presentation and Its Characteristics* | *Dangers of the Presentation* | *Field Management* |
|---|---|---|
| *Breech.* The baby presents by the buttocks or feet, rather than the head first. | Fetal distress from *cord compression* against the vaginal wall by the head. Threat of hypoxia and meconium aspiration. (See page 486.) Intracranial injury can occur from the head's rapid descent (rather than gradual) through the pelvis. | *Buttocks Presentation* (See Fig. 25-12.)<br>1. Instruct woman to push with contractions to deliver buttocks. Legs will follow. *Do not pull—allow contractions to propel infant.* Support baby as arms are delivered.<br>2. Deliver the head by placing a finger in the mouth to flex head as it appears over the perineum. Suction mouth and nose. Place traction on the shoulders. Have second EMT apply pressure over pubic bone to complete delivery.<br>*Feet Presentation*<br>If both feet present, the delivery can be accomplished. If a single arm or single foot presents, a complex delivery problem requiring expert medical intervention is at hand. The EMT should prepare the patient for prompt transfer to a hospital. |
| *Face.* The face looks up rather than down toward the perineum as it presents. Scalp may be seen but labor does not progress. | Head cannot proceed through pelvis in some instances. Delivery is not accomplished despite strong regular contractions and the woman pushing. | Prompt transfer to hospital for forceps assistance. |

## Neonatal Distress

### *Resuscitation of the Newborn*

The normal neonate breathes a few seconds after delivery. Respirations are rapid (thirty-five to sixty per minute) and are irregular in rhythm due to the immature respiratory center. Infants are "nose-breathers" and tolerate mouth-breathing rather poorly. To compensate for the inefficiency of his respiratory pattern, the neonate has excessive hemoglobin (red blood cells that carry oxygen) and an unusual ability to take in a heavy load of oxygen from the lungs during inhalation.

The neonate who has an arrest is usually *not* the victim of a heart-related problem. The arrest state in neonates usually is due to prolonged hypoxia prior to delivery. Some causes are a prolapsed cord, placental abnormalities, breech presentations, and similar complications that interfere with cord blood flow and the oxygenation of the fetus.

The severely distressed baby who is not getting enough oxygen from its placental lifeline may initiate a desperation respiratory effort in the uterus and, consequently, aspirate amniotic fluid contaminated with waste products such as meconium (me-ko′ne-um)(fetal stool). Obviously in the event of this aspiration, the infant is at risk.

## Meconium Aspiration

Meconium is the fetal stool or waste products eliminated by the bowel during intrauterine development, which contains mucus, fine hair, and other by-products of growth. It is a greenish black, tarry substance. Ordinarily, this stool is not passed from the baby's rectum until after birth, but if there is a low oxygen supply for any reason, there is a tendency for the bowel to become hyperactive and for the anal sphincter to relax, permitting the passage of the stool into amniotic fluid. At the same time the oxygen-starved infant struggles to breathe and aspirates some of the intrauterine fluid and the meconium.

Amniotic fluid is normally colorless. The EMT should be alert to dark-stained amniotic fluid in which the green-black infant stool may be visible as flecks or even large particles. Stained amniotic fluid signals a dire emergency for the infant since any aspiration of this substance often leads to death from respiratory complications. Occasionally meconium may be seen on the infant's scalp as the "crowning" occurs. (See Fig. 25–2.)

If stained amniotic fluid is detected, the EMT must be prepared to deeply suction the airway with a DeLee suction catheter (Fig. 25–13.) as

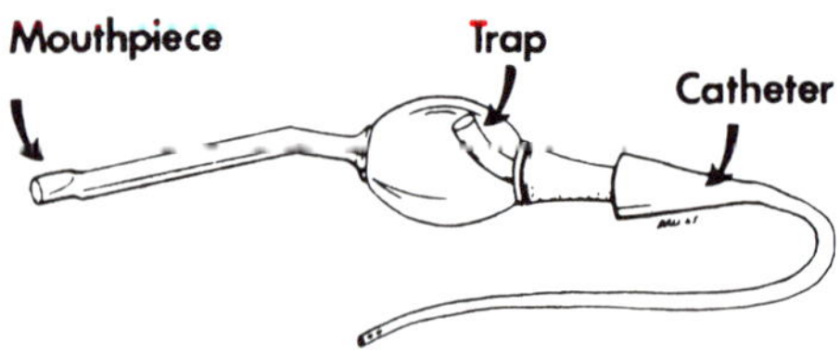


**Figure 25–13.** A DeLee suction device for use in neonatal airway management.

soon as the head is delivered and before shoulder delivery. If the majority of the meconium-containing fluid is suctioned from the upper air passages prior to the first breath, the infant's chances for survival are much greater.

## Cyanosis

Cyanosis is a bluish discoloration of the skin and mucous membranes due to poorly oxygenated blood in capillaries close to the skin's surface. In neonatal assessment it is essential to differentiate between central and peripheral cyanosis. *Central* cyanosis affects the mucous membranes, tongue, and skin and results from poor oxygenation of arterial blood. This condition is abnormal after the first few minutes of life. *Peripheral* cyanosis is bluishness of the extremities *only*, especially when the infant is cold. This condition may last for several weeks. The EMT should observe for central cyanosis. If the chest, abdomen, and membranes in and around the mouth do not "pink up" after several minutes of ventilatory effort, a severe cardiac or respiratory problem exists and transportation to a hospital should be promptly facilitated.

## Care of the High-Risk Infant

The EMT may deliver a premature infant, or encounter one of low birth weight (less than five and one-half pounds). These infants appear small, have little fatty tissue on the arms, legs and buttocks, and have heads that seem unusually large. Since the infant has not fully developed within the uterus before birth, he demands special attention of the EMT to facilitate survival.

*Oxygenation* is of utmost importance since the cardiovascular system is immature. With the head in a "sniffing position," oxygen should be provided at 10–12 *l*/min. and respirations assisted by a neonatal bag-valve-mask. (Note that oxygen accumulator tubing is directed at the face.) Watch for chest expansion. Do not compress the nose in an attempt to seal the mask well. Infants are nose-breathers.

*Keep the infant warm!* The premature or low birth weight infant has little fat to insulate his tiny body and requires considerable attention to ensure that he is kept warm. Warmth prevents the unnecessary utilization of oxygen and sugar which is burned by the body to produce heat. Warmed blankets, chemically activated hot water packs wrapped in towels, and the mother's body may be used to provide external sources of heat. An aluminum or plastic bubble blanket may be employed to insulate and protect the tiny infant.

## Vaginal Bleeding

The EMT may be called to assist a woman with vaginal hemorrhage. She may be in shock or impending shock from the blood loss. Vaginal bleeding may be caused by a complication of pregnancy or be related to other pathology of the uterus. The field management consists of placing the woman in shock position and transporting, carefully monitoring vital signs en route.

*References*


Barber, Janet M. and Budassi, Susan A. *Mosby's Manual of Emergency Care: Practices and Procedures.* St. Louis, MO: The C. V. Mosby Company, 1979.

Barber, Janet M. "Neonatal Resuscitation," *EMT Journal,* 2:79–83, Dec. 1978.

Gazzaniga, Alan B.; Iseri, Lloyd T.; and Baren, Martin. *Emergency Care: Principles and Practices for The EMT-Paramedic.* Reston, VA: Reston Publishing Company, Inc., 1979.

Jensen, Margaret Duncan; Benson, Ralph C.; and Bobak, Irene M. *Maternity Care: The Nurse and the Family.* St. Louis, MO: The C. V. Mosby Company, 1977.

Chapter 26

# Pediatric Emergencies

Children who are ill or injured deserve special consideration of the EMT. They are not only unique in their size, but in their communication skills, behavioral responses to pain and discomfort, and physiological reactions to illness or trauma. It is useful to know how to initially approach the child of various ages who is sick or hurt.

## THE SICK CHILD

Recognition of a sick child is usually the role of a parent, caretaker, or school teacher who notices a change in appearance or behavior that could indicate illness. For example, a child who does not want to play or to eat, or who whines, cries, or fusses may be ill or at least experiencing discomfort. A preschooler may be able to tell you where it "hurts" or can perhaps point to a spot on his body that is painful to move or to touch. Older children can often provide vivid descriptions of what is wrong. This information, when combined with objective assessments such as vital signs and a head-to-toe survey may reveal a specific problem which requires EMT management.

EMTs should also be prepared to estimate the weight of a child. The hospital management team will require this information to select the proper size equipment in their preparation to receive the patient and to plan the type and amount of fluid therapy as medications. Table 26–1 provides a general guideline for weight estimation.

Do not hesitate to ask the parents (or even the child himself). Often they are able to supply a near accurate weight readily.

### Respiratory Assessment

Abnormal breathing phenomena may be the initial clue to childhood illness. Recognition of unusual patterns requires that the EMT know the normal patterns of infant and childhood respirations. Both visual (looking) and auditory (listening) assessments must be made.

TABLE 26-1. TABLE OF ESTIMATED WEIGHTS

| *Age* | *Kilograms* | *Pounds* |
|---|---|---|
| Newborn | 3–5 | 6–11 |
| 1 Year | 10 | 22 |
| 3 " | 15 | 33 |
| 5 " | 20 | 44 |
| 8 " | 25 | 55 |
| 10 " | 30 | 66 |
| 15 " | 50 | 110 |

From *Mosby's Manual of Emergency Care.* (Used with permission of author)

### *Looking*

The respiratory rate should be counted by observing abdominal excursions in infants and thoracic (chest) excursions in the older child. Respirations should be counted for a full minute since variations are likely over shorter time intervals. Note whether or not there is a struggle in breathing or if the respirations seem to be an exhausting process. The appearance of restlessness, cyanosis, retractions, and/or nasal flaring indicate respiratory compromise. (See pages 306–307.)

Healthy newborns are "nose-breathers" and do not tolerate mouth breathing well. The usual rate is rapid (thirty-five to sixty breaths per minute) and excursions are shallow. Considerable motion of the diaphragm is noted. It is not unusual for newborns to exhibit irregular rhythms or patterns of breathing due to the immaturity and instability of their respiratory mechanisms.

As an infant proceeds through the first year of life, the chest wall muscles develop and grow stronger. Thus, their role in the respiratory process is greater, and the diaphragm plays a less significant (at least less visible) part in air exchange.

Pre-schoolers (two to five year olds) and school-aged youngsters breathe at a rate of twenty to twenty-five breaths per minute. The rate does not change appreciably until adolescence when it stabilizes at twelve to twenty breaths per minute, the rate characteristic of the average adult.

### *Listening*

Breath sounds should be assessed by use of the stethoscope to determine if both lungs are involved in air exchange and to detect any sounds of obstruction. Grunting, stridor, wheezing, rales, and rhonchi may be noted. While listening for breath sounds, the apical pulse should be counted since an elevated pulse rate is often linked to interferences with oxygenation. Review pages 307–310.

Other factors which affect respirations should also be considered in the initial assessment such as obesity, fever, exercise, drugs, and stress. (See Chapter 17.)

## Cardiovascular Assessment

The examination of the heart and circulatory status is a vital part of the initial approach to the ill child, and includes determining the pulse rate and blood pressure. It is imperative that the EMT know the normal values for the pulse and blood pressure in order to recognize any significant alterations which might indicate that there is something "immediately wrong" with the child. The pulse rate will rise in conjunction with fever, anemia, blood loss, certain heart diseases, and during periods of excitement. In addition to counting the rate, the characteristics of the pulse should be noted. For example, a strong pulse beat that is followed by a weak beat (pulsus alternans) suggests that the heart is in a weakened state. Although there are a variety of names for unusual pulse patterns, it is sufficient for the EMT to detect irregularity and to describe its characteristics. If time permits, the apical pulse should be counted simultaneously with a radial, or brachial, or femoral pulse.

The apical area in a school-aged child is at the fifth intercostal space in the midclavicular line. In younger children it is higher and more medial.

Blood pressure is a significant factor in cardiovascular assessment, both in illness or acute injury of the child. It is important that an appropriate cuff size be used. The width of the cuff should encase approximately one-half to two-thirds of the upper arm. (See page 152.) The child's arm is supported at the level of the heart during the actual recording. The systolic pressure is the initial sound heard and the diastolic pressure is the muffling or disappearance of sound. (See page 152.) Most authorities indicate that for children, the diastolic reading is most accurate if the muffling point is used, not the complete disappearance of any sound. This is an important distinction in blood pressure measurement of a child from that of the adult. If a pediatric cuff is unavailable, an adult cuff may be used on the thigh. In a child less than one year old, the systolic pressure in a thigh is approximately equal to the arm's reading. In older children, it may yield a 10–40 mm Hg higher reading. Diastolic pressures usually do not vary.

Children younger than one year usually have inaudible blood pressures unless a special electronic stethoscope is used which amplifies the sounds considerably. Pulsating neck vessels, cyanosis, pallor, and edema are other signs related to certain disorders of the heart, circulation, or the respiratory system. The presence of these should be noted and conveyed to the medical team at the hospital. Table 26–2 outlines normal pediatric vital signs.

## Temperature

Small children (especially infants) have a poor temperature-regulating system, and the temperature reading readily reflects changes in the body's functioning or the environment. An infant or older child who has an ab-

TABLE 26-2. PEDIATRIC VITAL SIGNS

| | *Pulse* | *Respirations* | *Blood Pressure* |
|---|---|---|---|
| Newborn | 120–160 | 60 | 69–90/20–60 |
| 1 Year | 80–140 | 25 | 65–95/25–65 |
| 3 " | 80–120 | 20 | 70–100/30–70 |
| 5 " | 70–115 | 20 | 70–100/30–70 |
| 7 " | 70–115 | 25 | 70–100/30–70 |
| 10 " | 70–115 | 30–35 | 90–120/50–80 |
| 15 " | 70–90 | 18 | 102–140/50–70 |

normally high or low body temperature is seriously ill. Furthermore, the mere presence of either extreme will cause the body to expend considerable energy in trying to resume a normal temperature status.

Fever is the most common problem in children up to one year of age. A *fever* is an elevation above 99.4°F. (37.4°C.). *Hyperpyrexia* is an elevation above 106°F. (40.6°C.). Ordinarily, until a temperature reaches the stage of *hyperpyrexia,* it is not of serious concern except to signal that "something is wrong." However, at the hyperpyrexic level, the central nervous system may be adversely affected, resulting in delirium or seizures. This is especially true in the preschool-aged child.

A *febrile* (feb′ril) child (one with a fever) may be initially detected by noting a flushed face, sweating, restlessness, and tachycardia.

Infections, dehydration, drug reactions, central nervous system disease, and heat stroke are among the possible causes for fever.

The EMT should *not* sponge the child with cool water or alcohol in the field, since such an effort may actually aggravate the condition by driving heat from the skin surface to the inner parts of the body where it can cause serious harm to vital organs. Sponging may also induce shivering, which is actually a *heat-generating* reaction; this, of course, only makes the situation worse.

Children should be lightly covered during transport to prevent exposure to drafts or other stimuli, which could initiate shivering. If seizures occur, they should be managed according to the usual procedure. (See pages 518–521.)

Fever accompanied by vomiting, diarrhea, or rashes can suggest a serious problem requiring prompt intervention.

## Vomiting and Diarrhea

The presence of vomiting and diarrhea in the infant or young child usually represents a significant illness. The rapid loss of fluids and electrolytes (e.g., sodium and potassium) from the body can be fatal in a few hours after onset, especially in an infant or the very young child. Losses are more devastating in the child than the adult, primarily because of the immaturity of certain fluid-regulating systems such as hormones and the kidneys.

An infant or young child who has vomiting and diarrhea for an hour or two will become weak and perhaps unresponsive. Fontanels may be sunken (see page 501), and the skin will take on a grayish color or appear to have lost its elasticity (turgor).

When vital signs are assessed, fluid loss will be evident by a weak, rapid pulse and a declining blood pressure. Cardiac output may be reduced enough to be reflected in cyanosis of the skin surface.

Since vomiting and diarrhea result in water loss (water is a natural mode of heat transfer outside the body), fever may result merely from this dehydration of tissues. Of course, fever that occurs in connection with vomiting and diarrhea could indicate a serious infection. The EMT who encounters this combination should consider the child infectious and exercise great care in handwashing and equipment clean-up post-transport to prevent the transfer of disease-producing micro-organisms.

## Rashes

A skin rash may be indicative of superficial irritation of the skin (e.g., diaper rash) or a sign of systemic disease. Certain rashes are characteristic of allergic reactions or of a childhood illness such as measles or scarlet fever. Each of these rashes have unique characteristics and distribution on the body surfaces. Since the EMT will not be familiar with all variations, a description of any skin lesions should include the following points:

*Location or Distribution*—Face? Arms? Mouth and throat? Trunk? Chest? Back? All over?
*Color*—Red? Brown? Black? Purple?
*Presence of Blisters*—Do the lesions appear to contain fluid or pus?
*Other Characteristics*—Are lesions flat or raised? Moist or dry and crusty? Are there open ulcers (sores) or breaks in the skin?

One particular rash, *petechiae* (pe-te′ke-e), should always be promptly recognized by the EMT. *Petechiae* are tiny, red or purple lesions that are sharply outlined. They accompany serious infectious diseases such as meningitis (men″in-ji′tis) or a bleeding disorder and must be reported immediately as a significant finding.

## Other Skin Assessments

The skin is an important reflection of a child's general state of health. Normally, it should be warm, dry, well colored, and free of any lesions or discoloration. Poor nutrition, inadequate circulation, metabolic disease, and blood disorders may be detected by abnormalities in the skin.

*Jaundice* (jawn′dis) is a yellowish discoloration of the skin and mucous membranes that accompanies some liver diseases such as infectious hepatitis or obstructions in the bile ducts around the liver and gallbladder.

Jaundice, of course, is indicative of a severe problem and should be noted and reported.

Early yellowish skin discoloration can be readily detected in the scleral (white) portion of the eyes, usually before it becomes apparent elsewhere. Itching is common with jaundice, so evidence of "scratching" should be viewed with suspicion and noted.

There are certain skin manifestations which are common in child abuse. The EMT must be alert to classic types of skin "clues" that suggest either willful abuse or neglect. (See pages 496–497.)

### Chest and Abdominal Pain

Most children cannot identify or specifically complain of chest pain until they are four or five years old. The EMT, therefore, must be alert to any clues which indicate chest-related problems. (See Chapters 17 and 18.) Oxygen should be administered if there is evidence of dyspnea or cyanosis.

Abdominal pain evokes characteristic responses, even in very young children. Infants, for example, often will cry or draw up their legs onto the abdomen if they have discomfort. An older child may exhibit rigidity of the abdominal wall and tend to "guard" it from being touched or examined. Acute abdominal problems in the young child may be accompanied by vomiting, diarrhea, constipation, or abdominal distention. These signs and symptoms of distress deserve specific medical study, since they may be indicative of a serious underlying problem.

## SPECIFIC MEDICAL PROBLEMS OF THE CHILD

### Respiratory Distress Due to Airway Obstruction

All airway obstructions deserve prompt management, particularly those which totally obstruct the airway. A young child may aspirate coins, parts from toys, buttons, and certain small, hard food items. Peanuts are commonly aspirated by the small child, resulting in airway obstruction. Signs and symptoms of obstruction will be dependent upon where the item lodges and whether or not any air is passing the obstruction.

Anatomical obstructions should always be suspected, such as the tongue falling back, enlarged tonsils, or thick secretions. Since infants are nose-breathers, the EMT should suction the nares to ensure their patency. If the tongue is seemingly creating an obstruction, it can be displaced forward and an airway placed if necessary.

A complete obstruction of the upper airway is marked by profound air hunger and the absence of breath sounds. Cyanosis will be quickly apparent.

A partial obstruction of airways may be detected by choking, coughing, stridor, noisy breathing, and respiratory struggle.

The EMT should not make attempts to remove a foreign object unless there is serious compromise of ventilation. Attempts at removal or changing the child's position may result in the migration of the object into lower airways or may in some instances convert a partial obstruction to a complete obstruction.

Oxygen administration is useful to compensate for poor ventilation, but care should be taken not to change the child's position. Back blows or the Heimlich maneuver may be tried. However, none of these field actions should preclude rapid transportation to a hospital. (See Chapter 10.)

Advanced EMTs or EMT-paramedics may try to remove a foreign body using a laryngoscope (lah-ring′go-skōp) or in certain cases, to perform a surgical airway opening called a *cricothyrotomy* (kri″ko-thi″rot′o-me).

## Inflammation of the Respiratory Passages

Medical conditions that produce inflammation and swelling of certain respiratory structures can contribute to an obstructed airway. Epiglottitis (ep″ĭ-glo-ti′tis), bronchiolitis (brong″ke-o-li′tis), and asthma are examples.

*Epiglottitis* is a potentially fatal respiratory tract infection that involves the *epiglottis,* (the tissue that overlies and protects the larynx and trachea during swallowing). The epiglottis becomes inflammed, swollen, and blocks air flow.

Epiglottitis usually occurs in children who are two to seven years old, but may occasionally occur in infancy. The onset is sudden with a high fever and hoarseness. The child will have what is called the 3 Ds—*drooling, dysphagia* (dis-fa′je-ah) (difficulty swallowing), and respiratory *distress.* The airway may be so obstructed that pallor or cyanosis is evident. Classically, the patient with epiglottitis will lean forward with the head extended like a turtle in an effort to breathe. The drooling of saliva occurs because swallowing is too difficult or painful. Inspiratory stridor (stri′dor), a "brassy" cough, irritability, and restlessness are not uncommon.

If the 3 Ds (or other evidence suggesting epiglottitis) are noted, the EMT *should not attempt to examine the child.* A simple maneuver such as looking at the throat could induce a spasm of the larynx and thus totally block the airway and induce respiratory arrest.

The child should be permitted to remain close to the parent(s) for *immediate* transport to a hospital. Separating the child from his parents could evoke struggling or crying, which might create even additional complications to an already critical situation.

The hospital should be informed by telephone or radio about the critical problem en route, so that the appropriate medical team members can be summoned to manage the child at once upon arrival.

Infectious laryngotracheobronchitis (lah-ring″go-tra″ke-o-brong-ki′tis) (croup) may be confused easily with epiglottitis, although its risks for airway obstruction are less than epiglottitis. The EMT should suspect the worst and err if need be on the conservative side, and manage either of the conditions as a life-threatening crisis.

*Bronchiolitis* is an infection of the bronchioles caused by a virus. Ordinarily it affects children less than two years old. Dyspnea and wheezing are the usual manifestations of this problem and it is easily confused with asthma.

Field management of bronchiolitis is similar to that of asthma. (See page 310.)

The child should be promptly transported to a hospital in an upright position to facilitate breathing. Supplemental oxygen, by nasal cannula, is usually advised to relieve hypoxia. Advanced EMTs or EMT-Paramedics may be instructed to initiate an IV since hydration and a route for medication administration is essential.

## Sudden Infant Death

The EMT may respond to a call in which an infant is "dead upon arrival." Grief-stricken and panicked parents may summon emergency assistance merely because they do not recognize an alternative, or cannot permit themselves to accept that the child is dead. This grief response is typical in situations of the "sudden infant death syndrome (SIDS) or "crib death."

SIDS is a phenomenon that accounts for one out of ten deaths in the first year of life. The infant, usually between one and six months of age, dies in his sleep with no apparent contributing illness. Parents often respond with guilt and wonder if they failed to recognize that the child was sick, or perhaps wonder that the child might have been in distress and that they did not hear him because they were entertaining, watching TV, or asleep.

The EMT should reassure parents that such deaths are not predictable or preventable. They are not due to suffocation. Care should be taken in summoning police or the coroner, since many parents may perceive that you suspect child abuse or neglect.

Certain local protocols may dictate that the EMTs perform CPR, even on an infant who apparently has been dead for several hours, so that the parents will feel that "everything possible" has been done.

## Child Abuse

EMTs are often confronted with circumstances that suggest that a child has been neglected or willfully harmed by caretakers. Any act that involves physical abuse, emotional torment, sexual assault, or parental neglect of a dependent child is termed *child abuse.* Child abuse is not confined to families of a particular social class, economic status, ethnic or

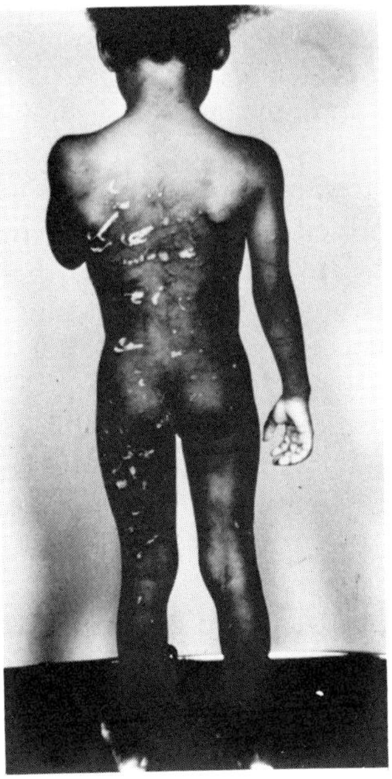

(a)

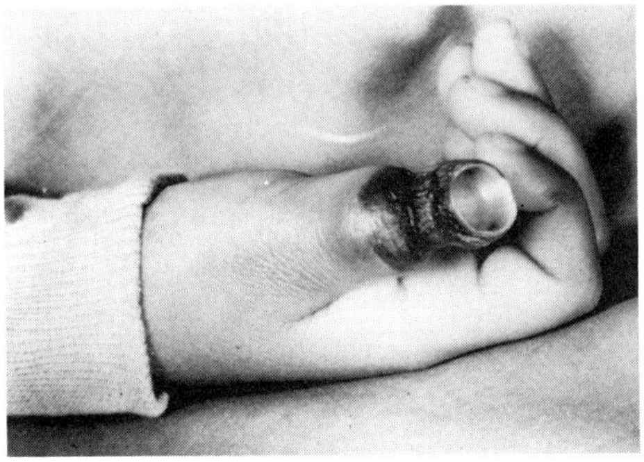

(b)

**Figure 26–1.** Examples of injuries of child abuse. (a) Multiple beatings using different objects. (b) Gangrenous thumb. Parents used rubber band around thumb to prevent thumb-sucking. *(Courtesy of Pediatrics Dept., Wishard Memorial Hospital, Indianapolis, Indiana)*

cultural background. It is recognized as a major source of pediatric trauma and accounts for many deaths each year. It is essential that the EMT promptly identify the classical findings of child abuse and take appropriate steps to facilitate the child's protection.

Common indications of child abuse include: cigarette burns, rope marks, human bites, bruises on the trunk (chest and abdomen), malnutrition, rope or "switch" marks, and fractures that are atypical for the history of injury.

Parents of abused children offer explanations of the "accident" that are contradictory and tend to be evasive in answering questions. They may seem to be angry about the injury and show little or no concern for the child's feelings.

The EMT should report suspected child abuse to the appropriate community agency, according to protocol established for such reporting. A victim of suspected child abuse should always be transported to a hospital for protective care until the proper authorities have investigated the findings that suggest maltreatment. (See Fig. 26–1.)

## THE INJURED CHILD

One out of every three deaths in children up to fourteen years of age is a result of trauma. In addition to this fatality rate, thousands more are injured and have lifelong handicaps. Recreation, vehicular crashes, and falls are the most frequent causes of serious pediatric trauma. Recently, however, crimes of violence have become a growing cause. Stabbings, gunshot wounds, and child abuse account for many injuries that have devastating consequences.

The initial approach to the injured child is an important factor in the successful management. An injured child is upset and is fearful of anyone who is trying to help. Since very young children cannot express themselves in specific verbal terms, they may respond with loud, protesting behavior such as screaming, biting, and kicking. The EMT should recognize that such actions are the child's feeble attempts to control what is happening. An unresponsive child postinjury should be viewed with caution since a lack of activity may signal shock or other serious consequences.

The child's reaction to injury is greatly influenced by others. Children quickly "tune in" to the responses of those around them so they should be protected, if possible, from panic-stricken or hysterical adults in the environment.

If there are no immediate needs for life-saving intervention, the child should be approached gradually and gently in an attempt to gain his confidence. When examining the injuries, the known sources of pain should be manipulated last to avoid setting up an early, generalized state of discomfort. It is useful to tell the child that you are about to touch or handle an injured part and that it will hurt. Honesty assists in gaining the child's trust in you.

Be friendly and human with your relating. Ask the child his name and tell him yours. Reveal what your are doing and why. Use eye contact as a mechanism of communication, and speak in short, simple sentences. When it is necessary to give instructions, state them as a command. Say, "Lie very still while I am examining your leg." Avoid saying "Don't move now." "Don't" rules are threatening and intimidating to the youngster.

Occasionally an EMT may encounter a child whose overactive and combative behavior may make examination of injuries and their management quite difficult, and it is sometimes tempting to overwhelm the child with power and size. Such actions should not be used, since they convey hostility and exaggerate the impact of trauma. A gentle, firm approach that communicates warmth and understanding is much preferred.

Always be as honest as possible. If an action will be painful, tell the child. For example say, "I am going to move your leg and it will hurt. It's OK if you cry." An honest and accepting relationship will do much to build confidence so vital to both the parents and their child.

There are times when a crying or struggling youngster may require physical restraint to facilitate examination or treatment. Since fears of pain, body mutilation, and death may be foremost in the youngster's mind, the EMT must make an effort to explain everything that is being done and why. Having all equipment at hand and well organized is desirable since any delays usually exaggerate anxiety.

Children should not be given a chance to choose when choosing is not practical. For instance, it is not wise to say, "May I put this splint on your leg?" Instead, indicate what you are doing and ask for his cooperation. Be sure to tell the child how he can help you. Involving him in your activity will lessen feelings of being "victimized."

Even very young children have a need for privacy and their modesty should be respected. Avoid removing underclothing or exposing the child's body. Shield areas being examined or exposed with a towel, blanket, or an article of clothing.

Parents or loved ones on the scene may make the situation more difficult for the EMT. It is usually not advisable to ask them to leave. Rather, their aid should be enlisted to reduce their feelings of helplessness. Involve them in decision making when feasible and permit at least one individual to accompany the child to the hospital in the ambulance. Such simple considerations may assist in gaining the cooperation and respect of parents as opposed to alienating them to a state of helplessness and uninvolvement. Parents may fear separation from the child even more than the child fears separation from the parents!

### Obtaining a History and the Basic Examination

Preschool children may be unable to provide a reliable account of an accident, but the older child may be an excellent historian. The EMT should merely say, "Tell me about your accident." Do not suggest certain sequences of events or probe with specific questions. Either of these latter approaches tend to place the child on the defensive and may tend to foster dishonest responses. If bystanders are present, it is useful to get their story, too. Pay particular attention to observations about the child's behavior immediately prior to and following the accident. Facts such as seizures or unusual actions *prior* to the accident, or unconsciousness *following* the accident, may help to determine the cause or potential consequences of the incident.

Encourage the child to tell you what is "hurt" and to touch or point to it. Equally important are the behavioral responses. Remember that fear of punishment for a wrongdoing or forbidden act that resulted in injury is likely to make the child minimize the seriousness of it. Essentially the child feels that he deserves to hurt. By-standers or friends may assist with other meaningful data such as a history of a bleeding disorder, diabetes, or epilepsy, which could considerably influence the management of injuries.

## INITIAL CONSIDERATIONS POST–TRAUMA

### Airway, Breathing, and Circulation

The airway should be cleared if necessary and oxygen therapy initiated if there is shock (see Chapter 10), cyanosis, or respiratory distress. Breath sounds should be noted since there may be serious internal chest injuries even though the ribs may not be fractured.

Vital signs must be taken and compared to the normal for the age group. Since on-the-scene excitement may influence these, continue to assess them every five to ten minutes to determine if there is stabilization or deterioration of the child's condition. Weight, of course, should be estimated to assist in initial management with equipment, fluid, and drugs. (See Appendix 1.) Signs and symptoms of shock should be noted.

## Shock

A child's response to trauma often includes rapidly developing shock. Even losses of relatively small amounts of blood can lead to shock in the young patient. The EMT should assume that all children are potentially "shocky."

Shock becomes apparent in the small child when the fluid volume (water or blood) is reduced by 15–20 percent. The heart rate will accelerate and the blood pressure may fall. The pulse may become weaker, but more rapid. Since a child's heart rate varies from 70–160 and can exceed 200 if crying, tachycardia *alone* is not a good indicator of a shock state. Other signs and symptoms of developing shock include: shallow respiration, pale, cool cyanotic extremities, a weak cry, lethargy, or even unresponsiveness in severe cases. Infants who have been in shock for an extended period and whose body temperatures are low may develop *sclerema neonatorum* (skle'rah ne"o-na-tor'um), a yellowing and tallowlike hardening of the subcutaneous fat.

In addition to careful management of the airway and institution of measures to combat shock (positioning, fluid therapy, and the application of antishock trousers) (see page 215), it is imperative that the child be kept warm, since heat loss can increase demands for oxygen, thus aggravating the shock state.

## Head to Toe Assessment

When performing an examination of the injured child, begin with a visual inspection of the body. Obvious injured parts should be moved or touched later in the examination when the EMT has gained the child's confidence. Be sure to avoid focusing on the apparent injuries that are easily seen, such as burns or open fractures. Internal injuries of the head, chest, and abdomen are less obvious, but surely more life threatening.

Pediatric injuries are influenced by anatomical variations of the growing child. Several of these directly affect the vulnerability and response of organs to injury. Following is a brief review of the most significant ones that require consideration during the head-to-toe assessment.

### *Head and Neck*

The infant and very young child's head is expandable due to the fontanels (fon"tah-nelz) (the "soft spot" in the skull of an infant before bones completely fuse and harden), and suture (su'chur) lines (the point where

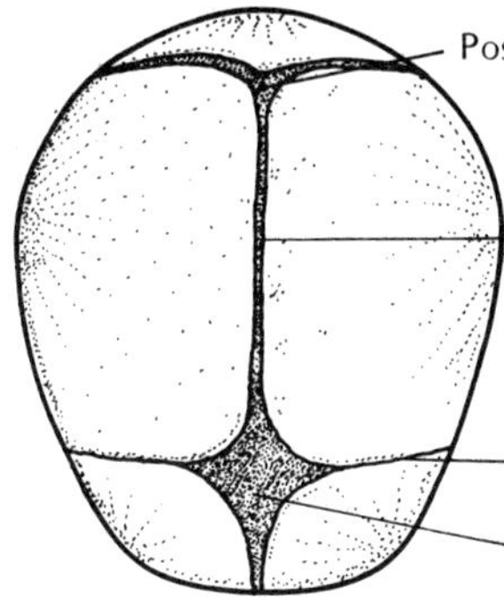


**Figure 26–2.** Fontanels and suture lines of an infant's skull.

two bones meet and are not yet fused). Consequently, the head can adjust to additional intracranial volume from bleeding or edema formation. (See Fig. 26–2.) Sometimes the direct evidence of increased intracranial pressure can be obtained by observing the fontanels with the infant at rest.

The head and neck of the infant are vulnerable due to their poor muscular protections and their high vascularity (because the bones are growing). Serious injury to these structures may result from bleeding and mechanical compression of the cord.

The EMT should always suspect cervical spine injuries even though they are rare. Backboards, sandbags, and logrolling are indicated as in the adult. (See Chapter 15.) A careful assessment should include a search for *subcutaneous emphysema.* This condition is due to air in tissues and can be noted by the crackling feel of the tissue, similar to compressing course styrofoam. Subcutaneous emphysema of the neck would probably indicate a break in a major airway (bronchus, trachea, etc.) which allows air to escape to surrounding tissue. The discovery of this phenomenon indicates the need for speedy transport of the child to a hospital.

The movement and strength of all extremities should be assessed. Abnormal posturing must be noted, particularly decorticate and decerebrate posturing. (See Fig. 15–3a, b.)

Head injuries are common in the child since their head is pliable, thin, and soft. Furthermore, since the head comprises a larger percentage of total body weight in the very young, it is proportionately larger than in the older child or adult and, therefore, tends to make the child "top-heavy."

The level of consciousness is a crucial component of the assessment since it reflects the dynamic consequences of injury. Lethargy or general unresponsiveness may mean serious brain damage or may be indicative of shock. A high-pitched cry, irritability, seizures, or agitation should be viewed with alarm.

Pupillary assessments should also be made.

The skull should be palpated for swelling, lacerations, or deformity. Rhinorrhea (discharge of cerebrospinal fluid through the nose) and otorrhea (discharge of cerebrospinal fluid through the ears) should be noted since they indicate leaking cerebrospinal fluid. Bleeding from the nose and ears also suggest a serious skull fracture. Facial bones should be palpated, too, and any structural deviations noted.

Children with head injuries should be placed in a semi-Fowler's position and supplied supplemental oxygen by mask. Poor oxygenation is detrimental to the child since it contributes to cerebral edema. (See page 276.)

Shock does not occur as a result of intracranial bleeding, except perhaps in an infant or tiny child. Consequently, shock should be attributed to some injury other than head injury, such as fractures of long bones, chest injuries, or intra-abdominal bleeding.

### *Chest and Abdomen*

The child's chest organs are encased by a rather soft, flexible rib cage, and the abdomen has a poorly developed thin, muscular wall overlying the highly vascular organs such as liver and spleen. In addition, the child's liver is proportionately larger than the adult's and it tends to protrude slightly from the lower margin of the rib cage, making it an excellent target for injury. Both the liver and the spleen bleed profusely when damaged, and can create life-threatening hemorrhage within minutes post-trauma.

The child's abdominal wall is not thick and strong like the adults, and any direct impact will permit the stomach, small bowel, and pancreas to strike the anterior projections of the vertebral column. Blunt trauma can cause rupture of the stomach and bowel, especially if they are distended with contents.

The chest of an injured child should be inspected for abrasions, edema, discoloration, and any other apparent signs of injury. The flexible chest of a small child "gives" considerably, and may damage underlying organs by impact without any rib fractures. Any signs or symptoms of trauma to external tissue of the chest should cause the EMT to suspect soft tissue injury to the lungs, heart, and large blood vessels. Since the lower portion of the rib cage partially covers the liver and spleen, any evidence of impact here should raise suspicion of internal bleeding.

The rib cage should be palpated for fractures, and subcutaneous emphysema and abnormal movements such as paradoxical chest movement or paradoxical respirations (See Chapter 17.) The lungs should be auscultated to ensure the presence of breath sounds on both sides over the entire lung field.

The abdomen should be scrutinized for distention, bruises, or abrasions. Any tenseness, rigidity, or tenderness during palpation could indicate rupture of abdominal organs or internal bleeding. Bulging or tenderness of the flank can point to kidney injury. If the time permits, the EMT should measure the abdominal girth (see page 341) to assist in evaluating the extent of distention since ruptured organs or internal bleeding can produce a rapidly expanding abdomen. This abdominal girth measurement is even more valuable if the EMT has a prolonged transport time with the child.

Children have backs as well as fronts! Always include a thorough assessment of the posterior chest wall, the spine, and the outline of the pelvis. Discoloration or bruising at the lumbar spine level ("small of the back") should be viewed with suspicion and carefully communicated to the hospital personnel, since it usually means serious internal injury and bleeding, especially related to the renal system. Fractures of the pelvis or vertebral column are common with such injuries.

### *Urinary System*

A child's kidneys are poorly protected due to poor surrounding support tissue and because they lie mainly within the abdomen. The kidneys of both adults and children are highly vascular and extremely fragile, thus they bruise and bleed with even a seemingly minor impact.

A child's bladder can be nicked or torn, especially with pelvic fractures. It can be ruptured readily if it is full at the time of severe impact to the anterior abdominal wall. Watch for a hematoma formation (see above) at the level of the lumbar spine, since this is a common indicator of retroperitoneal bleeding that accompanies renal injury.

Children who have high impact injuries to the pelvis and perineum (especially boys) run a risk of cutting the urethra (the tube that transports urine from the bladder during voiding). With such an injury, the child may sense an unusual urgency to void, particularly if the bladder is full. This voiding should be discouraged until the child reaches the hospital, if at all possible, since the act of emptying the bladder can allow urine to drain into the pelvis, producing an even more serious complication of trauma. (See page 337.) The EMT should note any drops of blood on the underclothing or on the child's penis or perineum, which classically accompany certain injuries to the urinary tract system. If the child *does* void, the EMT should collect the urine and transport it with the child. Blood in this urine sample can be detected by the hospital laboratory and can assist greatly in the evaluation of injury to the urinary tract.

### *Skeletal System*

Children's bones are growing rapidly and thus are soft, flexible, and richly supplied with blood. Many fractures are incomplete due to their flexibility, resulting in torus (to′rus) (buckle) or the classic "greenstick" fracture. (See page 364.)

All suspected fractures and dislocations should be identified and carefully splinted according to the usual procedure.

Careful examination of the arterial blood supply to extremities should be made by palpating the peripheral pulses. This is extremely important in possible fractures of the humerus or femur, since vascular damage frequently is associated with these injuries.

Color or temperature changes are likely to accompany circulatory insufficiency. Of course, observing for signs and symptoms of shock should also be a high priority, particularly if there are fractures of long bones which bleed profusely or if multiple traumatic injuries are present.

## Transportation of the Injured Child

The child should be transported promptly with attention to monitoring both vital signs and the general condition. The airway must be guarded with utmost vigilance, since vomiting tends to follow the psychic trauma of a serious accident. An advanced EMT or EMT-Paramedic may be instructed to insert a nasogastric tube to relieve gastric distention and thus prevent vomiting. This is especially valuable in the event of assisted ventilation, since forced air delivery can contribute to gastric distention.

Children have relatively small airways for the size of their tongue. Any lacerations of the tongue should be closely watched since the bleeding or associated edema could rapidly lead to an obstructed airway.

The child who is injured should be comforted by gentle contact and conversation—even if there appears to be unresponsiveness. Touching the child and offering statements of comfort and encouragement are quite significant in reassuring the frightened, young patient!

*References*

Barber, Janet and Budassi, Susan. *Mosby's Manual of Emergency Care.* St. Louis, MO: The C. V. Mosby Company, 1979.

Barber, Janet M. "Tips on Assessment and Management of Pediatric Trauma," *EMT Journal,* 4:66–71, March 1980.

Boles, R. "The Immature Airway," *Emergency Medicine,* 10:56–57, February, 1978.

Dube, S. K. and Pierog, S. H. *Immediate Care of the Sick and Injured Child.* St. Louis, MO: The C. V. Mosby Co., 1978.

Gazzaniga, Alan V.; Iseri, Lloyd T.; and Baren, Martin. *Emergency Care: Principles and Practices for the EMT-Paramedic.* Reston, VA: Reston Publishing Co., 1979.

Gratz, Rene, Resnick. "Accidental Injury in Childhood: A Literature Review on Pediatric Trauma," *J. Trauma,* 19:551–555.

Melker, R. "Resuscitation of the Newborn, Infant and Child," *Critical Care Quarterly,* 1:49–63, May 1978.

Pascoe, Delmar J. and Grossman, Moses. *Quick Reference to Pediatric Emergencies,* 2nd ed. Philadelphia, PA: J. B. Lippincott, Company, 1978.

Reece, Robert M., and Chamberlain, John W. *Manual of Emergency Pediatrics.* Philadelphia, PA: W. B. Saunders Company 1974.

Surgical Staff, The Hospital for Sick Children, Toronto, Canada. *Care for the Injured Child.* Baltimore, MD: The Williams and Wilkins Company, 1975.

Touloukian, Robert J. ed. *Pediatric Trauma.* p. 646. New York: John Wiley and Sons, 1978.

# Chapter 27

# Patients with Special Problems

The EMT may be confronted with patients who are challenges since they present a dysfunction in communication or because their age and/or physical handicaps pose on-the-scene dilemmas. In this chapter, each of the "special" patient groups will be discussed along with tips for EMT assessment and management in the field.

## THE BLIND PATIENT

The blind patient may not always be with a guide dog, a white cane, and other hallmarks of the visually handicapped. Your first clue to blindness may be the patient's being confused when you approach or begin to perform an initial assessment. Be alert to the presence of dark glasses, eye prosthesis, a Medic Alert Identification tag, or other items which could suggest blindness. Of course, if the patient is conscious, you can politely inquire if you suspect blindness by saying something like, "Sir, can you see me?" Blind persons will respond promptly to communicate their unsightedness.

The individual who has a view of his world often is dazed and disoriented from an accident or injury. This feeling of "Where am I? What happened?" is exaggerated in the blind. They cannot see where they are, who is helping them, or determine what has happened by merely looking at the surroundings. The EMT can do much to acquaint the blind patient with what is going on.

First, tell the patient who you are and why you are with him. For example, say, "You were crossing the street and a child on a bike ran into you. I am Dave, an Emergency Medical Technician who is here to help you." Reassure the individual exactly where he is and who is at the scene. Physical contacts such as a handshake are helpful, since they provide information about your size, strength, and personality. If you use any equipment or supplies or perform a procedure, explain exactly what you are doing and why. At each step, relate your activity. Also include *when* you are doing something, since you do not want to frighten the patient with a surprise. Be as exact as possible, and advise the individual if there are delays or changes. For instance, "You have a small cut here on your arm. I'm going to wash it off with some water I have in this bottle now." "I am going to help you onto this stretcher in a minute." "I'm waiting for Jim, my partner, who will be helping me lift you." If you find it necessary to leave the patient for a moment, let him know, since otherwise he will assume you are still there. When you return, re-establish your presence by stating, "I'm back now. I had to get my box of supplies from the ambulance."

A blind person is like anyone else, except that you must "paint a picture" for him about his surroundings. Be explicit in communications. We tend to abbreviate much of our speech and expect the receiver to "see" what we mean through visualization of our activities, our facial expressions, and the environment.

If the blind individual is not seriously ill or injured, and can walk, the EMT should bend his arm and permit the individual to grasp it just above the elbow. This will permit him to feel the direction of your movements. Never grab the blind person's arm to lead him. Of course, warn the patient of anything in the path which could frighten or injure him, such as a curb or a revolving door.

A guide dog should be permitted to remain with the patient, even in the ambulance, unless he interferes with treatment. If conditions require that the dog be separated from his master, advise the patient and inquire who should be contacted to temporarily assume responsibility for the animal. Most guide dogs have a harness plate with specific emergency information.

If an individual other than the master must handle the dog, use the leash, not the harness, which is reserved for guide purposes only. The dog is accustomed to walking to the left of the master and usually is more comfortable if permitted to assume this position with an alternate handler.

The blind patient will be comforted by an EMT who seems self-assured and at ease with him. When in doubt about what to do, or how you can help him, merely ask rather than attempt a trial and error approach that will frustrate both of you!

## THE DEAF PATIENT

The deaf, like the blind, may find themselves in a real predicament in an emergency situation, since they cannot respond to verbal questions or benefit from sounds from the environment which ordinarily provide clues to what is going on. The deaf may point to the ear, or to the ear and mouth, with an index finger, to tell you that they are deaf. Some shake their head in a "I don't understand" message. Occasionally they may gesture indicating that they want to write a message. If they attempt speech, it may be of unusual voice quality, lacking normal tone and inflection. Others may use sign language to communicate their dilemma. When EMTs identify the deaf patient, there are some specific approaches that will facilitate communication.

Not all deaf individuals have always been hearing impaired. Some, however, were deaf at birth. The age and type of circumstances that resulted in the hearing loss may affect how the individual communicates. Certain patients use sign language or lip reading; others use writing to convey messages. The EMT should be prepared with a paper and pen for the latter. Remember that the patient's inability to hear does not mean that he is not intelligent or that he fails to understand what is happening.

If time permits, an interpreter may be obtained, but this service is limited to certain communities. Consequently, an EMT should be prepared to use alternate modes of "talking" with the individual who is deaf.

It should be understood that shouting will not facilitate communication with the deaf. If someone is "hard-of-hearing," particularly the elderly, greater volume may help, but a distinct voice and slow speech is more valuable in conveying your message. If lip-reading is used, look at the person as you speak. Good lighting is essential for facilitating lip-reading, too.

Some individuals may have hearing aids. This should alert the EMT to the fact that the individual has some hearing ability and thus he should speak distinctly, slowly, and in a natural tone. Shouting not only distorts sounds, but can be interpreted as hostility.

Avoid gestures without speech, and use facial expression and physical contact to convey warmth and understanding that is normally expressed verbally to patients. If the individual has glasses, he should be encouraged to wear them in order that he can make full use of visual cues, thus compensating for his hearing impairment.

A patient who relies on sign language may be thwarted in communication when IV's, restraints, or other equipment prevent free use of the hands for gesturing or writing messages. If feasible, the dominant hand should remain free for facilitating signs or using a pen. See Appendix 6 for sign language.

## THE OBESE PATIENT

Every practicing EMT seemingly will eventually be required to deal with a patient whose weight exceeds 350 pounds. There are multiple problems in assessment, treatment and use of equipment with extremely obese patients which deserve discussion.

### Assessment

It is almost impossible to do a thorough examination of the extremely obese patient in the field with a team of just two or three EMTs. Common tasks such as listening for breath sounds, recording vital signs, palpating the abdomen, and searching for swelling or signs of surface trauma become complex when the patient is overweight. For example, listening and palpating is complicated by heavy layers of fat. The pulse may be hard to find, the abdomen virtually impossible to evaluate, and the observable breath patterns may be obscure due to excess fat which envelops the chest and abdomen. Although a large thigh cuff may be used to assess the blood pressure in an arm, readings may be difficult to obtain, since sounds are poorly transmitted through several inches of fat. Furthermore, the normal landmarks used in assessment reflect the relative position of bone structures. In the obese patient, these landmarks may be hidden deeply under fatty tissue.

### Treatment

Controlling bleeding or starting an IV are real challenges for the EMT who is treating an obese patient since vessels are deeply imbedded in fat. For example, bleeding can be controlled by pressing an artery against a bone. In the obese individual, the fatty tissue acts like a cushion and prevents contact of the artery and bone.

Defibrillation and other aspects of cardio-pulmonary resuscitation are complicated by obesity, and adjustments in procedures must be made. (See Chapter 10.)

### Equipment

Antishock trousers, cervical collars, traction splints, blood pressure cuffs, and even stretchers are made for the normal-sized patient. Stretchers, particularly the hinged models, may collapse under weights exceeding 400 pounds. The safety belts may be too short for use without extension parts. A scoop stretcher may be helpful or the use of a blanket to scoot the patient from place to place or the floor may be necessary in extreme cases.

The EMT should take great care to avoid hurting himself while lifting or moving a heavy patient. Several strong individuals, even up to eight or ten, may be required. (See Chapter 5.)

It is imperative that the EMT remain composed when dealing with the obese patient. Occasionally jokes and humor, or remarks are exchanged due to the tension and frustration which is present. Care must be taken to avoid this pitfall. Remember, most obese individuals have a serious or chronic illness, and demand careful field assessment and a respectful acceptance by the EMT.

## THE MENTALLY RETARDED OR BRAIN–DAMAGED PATIENT

The EMT may be involved in an emergency care response for a patient who is mentally retarded or is brain damaged. This patient can be a child or an adult. In many instances you can identify this individual with special needs at once, due to the initial appearance or behavior. Often there are accompanying physical handicaps, too.

## Mental Retardation

Mental retardation is a form of brain dysfunction characterized by impaired or incomplete mental development. The individual has a limited ability to learn and to implement learning. The degree of retardation varies from mild to severe. It is thought to occur from genetic defects, complications of pregnancy or childbirth, and a wide variety of illness and injury-related circumstances.

The EMT should be aware that not all mentally retarded patients have obvious physical abnormalities and that their appearance and behavior may not initially provide a clue to their needs. Most importantly, this individual will require the use of communication techniques that are designed to build confidence and trust and convey a sense of caring. (See Chapter 21.)

## Brain Damage

Additionally, all patients who are brain-damaged do not have problems in comprehending. For example, about one-fourth of the individuals with cerebral palsy have normal mental capabilities despite their inability, in some cases, to coordinate extremity movements, walk, talk, or write in a normal manner. One out of three persons with cerebral palsy have hearing difficulties, however, and this factor must be taken into consideration as you talk with your patient. Airway management may be complicated because of excessive salivation and difficulty in swallowing. They may have uncontrollable movements of limbs, especially when attempting a purposeful act and may become very excited when confronted with an unfamiliar problem such as an accident or injury. Of course, they are involved in numbers of accidents due to their lack of coordination, frequent seizure activity, and in some instances, poor judgment due to mental deficiencies or perceptual problems of vision or hearing.

Caring for a patient with brain damage is often a real challenge and requires considerable patience and understanding. Assessment of injuries may be complicated by the supports, braces, or slings the individual routinely wears to aid his ability to sit, stand, or walk. The EMT must understand that the individual's inability to "hold his arm or leg still" for example, is a product of brain damage, *not* an unwillingness to cooperate. Often spasticity, rigidity and other dysfunctional movements become exaggerated when the brain-damaged person is ill, injured, or consciously trying to complete a purposeful act. *Patience* is a must for the EMT in such cases since the patient may view impatience as nonacceptance or anger.

In dealing with a mentally retarded or brain-damaged patient, family members, teachers, friends, or neighbors may be valuable sources of information about the past history of illness, current problems, medications, and so forth. They may also be able to offer hints about how you can communicate more effectively with the individual and in some cases, may actually be able to serve as a "go-between" interpreter.

Slow, gentle, kind, and accepting behaviors described earlier are in order for this group of special patients.

## THE ELDERLY PATIENT

With the growing number of elderly in our society, an EMT needs to be aware of some of their special needs. They are victims of increasing illnesses as they become older and not uncommonly, are involved in accidents due to their failing eyesight, hearing, or neuro-muscular coordination. Many live alone and with limited income. This factor sometimes contributes to poor health, since they tend to eat poorly and may not get to the clinic or physician's office for a needed prescription on time. When you inquire why they haven't been "eating right" or taking their prescribed medication, they may tell you that they are waiting for their Social Security check or pension check. Every EMT who regularly practices will also become acquainted with the problems that loneliness causes for the elderly. They may call an emergency service just so they have someone to visit them and talk to them. Others enjoy the special attention of riding to the hospital in an ambulance!

The inferior, often crowded housing for the elderly also contributes to frequent bouts of illness, especially in winter months when they can't afford to buy enough fuel to keep their rooms warm or to make repairs on doors and windows to keep out the cold. Insects, poor plumbing, and architectural defects may add to the elderly's housing problems, too.

Of course, the picture is not so bleak for all of the elderly, but the EMT must understand that, in general, many are living in marginal circumstances where neither human or physical needs are met.

The elderly who has diminished sensory input may be confused. There may be impairments in vision, hearing, and memory for recent events, which result in the patient's inability to connect the series of circumstances that have led him to his current surroundings. The EMT should continually reinforce the patient's orientation of where he is, to whom he is talking, and what is happening to him. Elderly individuals who are blind, deaf, or paralyzed may rely heavily on the sense of touch to know that someone is present to help. Touching expresses warmth and reinforces a sense of security and trust.

The EMT should realize that all older people do not have circulatory disorders, arthritis, or poor mental functioning. However, these are some classic physical changes. Others involve the declining adaptation of the central nervous system. Hypothermia is common, for example, due to inefficiency of regulatory mechanisms, and a reduction in well-nourished muscle tissue with a rich blood supply. Bones and joints stiffen and muscles weaken with inactivity. Breathing problems often are noted when the rib cage stiffens and does not permit good chest expansion. Digestive processes are not as efficient in the elderly, and constipation and other abdominal complaints are common. Their lack of teeth or ill-fitting dentures, coupled with a low budget, a preference for soft foods and sweets, and little desire for fluids may contribute further to poor diet habits.

The EMT should not address the patient by names such as "Grandma," "Grandpa," or "Old-Timer." These are depersonalizing and demeaning and indicate loss of his individuality and identity. Use his proper name throughout your interactions with him.

Be patient with the elderly. They need extra time to think, to make decisions, and to act. In aging, the brain undergoes changes which make organization of thoughts a more lengthy process. If the brain receives too many messages at once, they must wait to be handled in turn, when circuits are free (much like calls to an overloaded switchboard).

Talk to the elderly in short, simple sentences. When messages are too complex, their response may be one of confusion. Instructions or information should be given in small units, and simple tasks. Do not expect the coordination of many details. If feasible, demonstrate what you want them to do. This seems to aid in their comprehension. Speak slowly, listen attentively, and exhibit an interest in what is being said by your patient. If the EMT follows these guidelines, communication will be considerably more meaningful and mutually satisfying.

When transportation to a hospital is required, be patient as the elderly attends to household details as they leave. Take care in lifting and moving since they have stiff muscles and joints. Their skin is also very thin and fragile and can be easily torn if subjected to friction such as sliding them over on a sheet to the stretcher. Gentle lifting is always in order for the elderly—not only because it protects their skin, but because it conveys your caring and understanding of their special needs.

## THE PATIENT WITH A CARDIAC PACEMAKER

The EMT may initially notice a cardiac pacemaker device on a small box implanted in the chest. (See Fig. 27–1.) The box may be clearly outlined and can be palpated under the surgical incision in the chest wall. Some patients have an external battery-pack which is fixed to the outside of the chest, but these are usually present in hospitalized individuals for emergency support. (Few individuals would be sent home with the external device.)

A cardiac pacemaker provides an electrical stimulus to the heart and replaces or supplements the heart's conduction impulses. Certain heart conditions disrupt the electrical stimulus for normal conduction, and outside mechanical assistance is required to stimulate the heart to beat with regularity. Pacemakers may be required on a temporary or a permanent basis, depending upon the kind of damage of the myocardial cells.

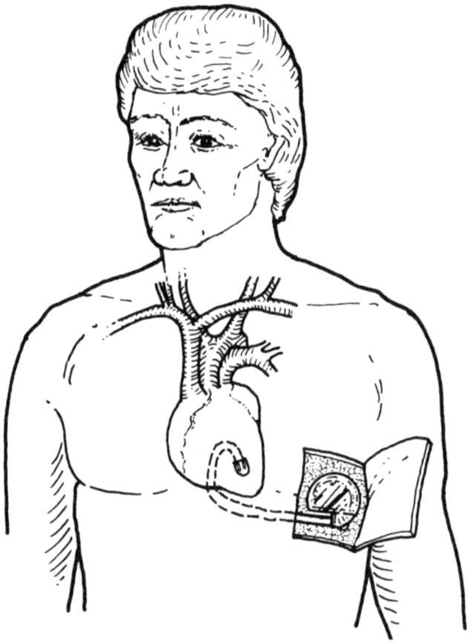

**Figure 27–1.** Patient with implanted pacemaker

An EMT who identifies a pacemaker should note its presence and consider pacemaker malfunction as a possibility for medical problems experienced, such as chest pain, dizziness, or fainting. These signs and symptoms might point to abnormalities in heart rate or rhythm due to a dysfunctional or malfunctioning pacemaker.

## THE PATIENT WITH A COLOSTOMY OR URINARY TRACT DIVERSION

A *colostomy* (ko-los′to-me) is a surgically-created opening in the abdominal wall to permit the elimination of fecal material. The need for this operation may be due to cancer, bowel obstructions from other causes, or ulcerative disease. A colostomy may be temporary for a few months until the bowel heals, or may be permanent in some instances. There are several terms for variations of this opening, depending upon its type and location. For example, if it is done at the ileum of the bowel, it is called an *ileostomy* (ĭl″e-os′to-me), at the jejunum, a *jejunostomy* (je″joo-nos′to-me), at the cecum, a *cecostomy* (se-kos′to-me). Drainage from the opening will be either liquid stool or formed stool, depending upon the location of the stoma. Stomas in the upper bowel or small intestine usually have liquid drainage, while in the colon or large intestine, the stool is usually well formed. Of course, diet, certain medications, and illness can affect the character and amount of drainage, too.

The EMT will readily note this abnormal opening because ordinarily it is covered by a plastic-bag pouch to collect the fecal material. If there are abdominal complaints such as constipation, obstipation (no stool passage or gas expulsion), or abdominal distention with pain, the EMT should arrange for transportation to the hospital. Occasionally patients with cancer or ulcerative disease of the gastrointestinal tract will bleed through the stoma. Of course, gastrointestinal bleeding can lead to shock, and prompt intervention is in order.

A surgical opening into the abdominal wall can also be created when a disease of the kidneys, bladder, ureters, or urethra exists which requires a bypassing procedure. Like a colostomy, it may be a temporary or permanent opening to permit urinary elimination. If the bladder has been removed, the ureters may be implanted into the bowel to allow the urine to be eliminated along with feces, or they may be brought out onto the abdominal wall. Other surgical procedures require the patient to wear a receptacle for urine collection on the abdomen or more commonly on the leg. (See Fig. 27–2).

A Foley catheter may be in place to control urinary incontinence. A tube is anchored in the bladder by a small balloon, and urine is permitted to drain into a plastic bag or semirigid plastic container. (See Chapter 36.) On occasion, these catheters become dislodged or obstructed, resulting in bladder distention and discomfort for the patient. Unless the EMT is skilled in the procedure for catheterization, the patient should be transported to a hospital for further care.

Bleeding, infections, or obstruction to the outflow of urine are the most common problems for these patients. The EMT will need to arrange for prompt transportation to a hospital in such instances.

If questions or problems arise regarding any of the bowel or bladder diversions and their management, the patient and the family can usually provide meaningful assistance for on-the-scene management.

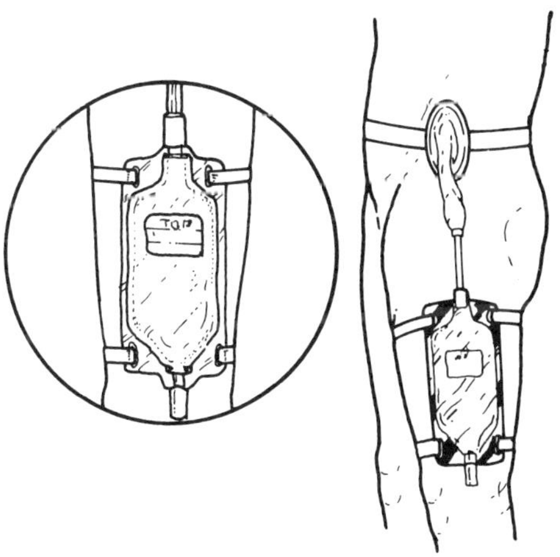

**Figure 27–2.** One type of external collecting device for patients with urinary or bowel diversion.

## THE PATIENT WITH A TRACHEOSTOMY OR LARYNGECTOMY

A *tracheostomy* (tra″ke-os′to-me) is the creation of an artificial opening into the trachea to permit breathing. The patient's anterior neck may have a metal or plastic plate over the opening (stoma) or it may be merely a hole (stoma) permitting air passage. The latter stoma is typically created after removal of the larynx (voice box) for cancer control.

A tracheostomy is characterized by the presence of a tube that is passed into the trachea between tracheal cartilage rings. (See Fig. 27-3.) A laryngectomy (lar″in-jek′to-me) opening is large and round and the tracheal lining can be noted at the skin line. (See Fig. 27-4.)

Persons who have undergone surgery for either a tracheostomy or laryngectomy require special adjuncts for speech production, so the EMT may experience difficulty in obtaining information from this patient.

Ventilation problems with these patients require prompt and skilled attention. Air cannot get to the lungs via the nose and mouth, and the patient depends on his stoma (sto′mah) entirely.

*Suctioning.* Fluid or mucus can block the stoma and create respiratory distress. The EMT should promptly suction the patient if evidence of suffocation is apparent. Before suctioning the tracheostomy, the catheter should be moistened with sterile water or saline, since the tracheal-bronchial tissue is delicate, and unnecessary friction must be avoided to prevent irritation. In emergencies, deep suctioning as demonstrated in Fig. 27-5 may be required. To suction the left bronchus,

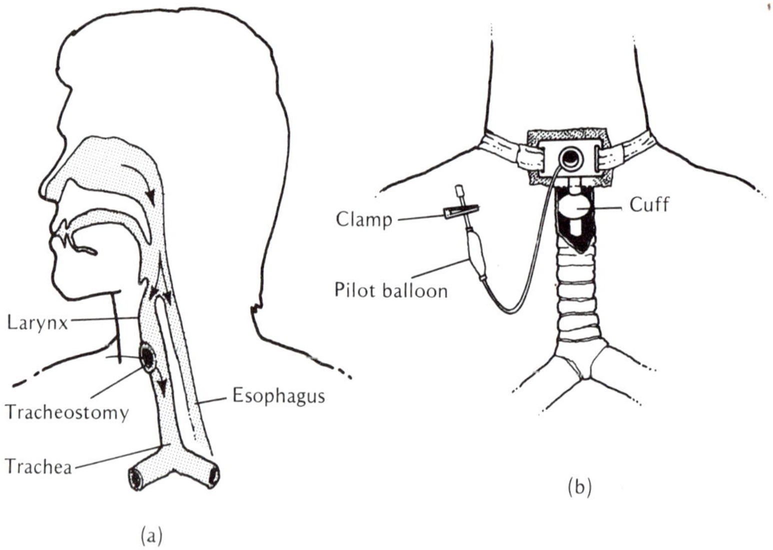


**Figure 27-3.** Tracheostomy: (a) airway structural relationships; (b) external appearance of tracheostomy tube. Inset shows details of tube placement.

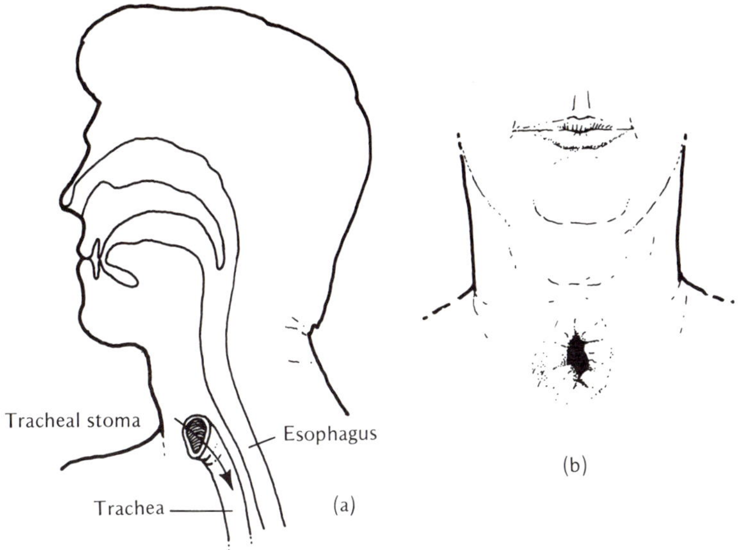


**Figure 27-4.** Laryngectomy: (a) airflow pattern through stoma; (b) external appearance of laryngectomy stoma.

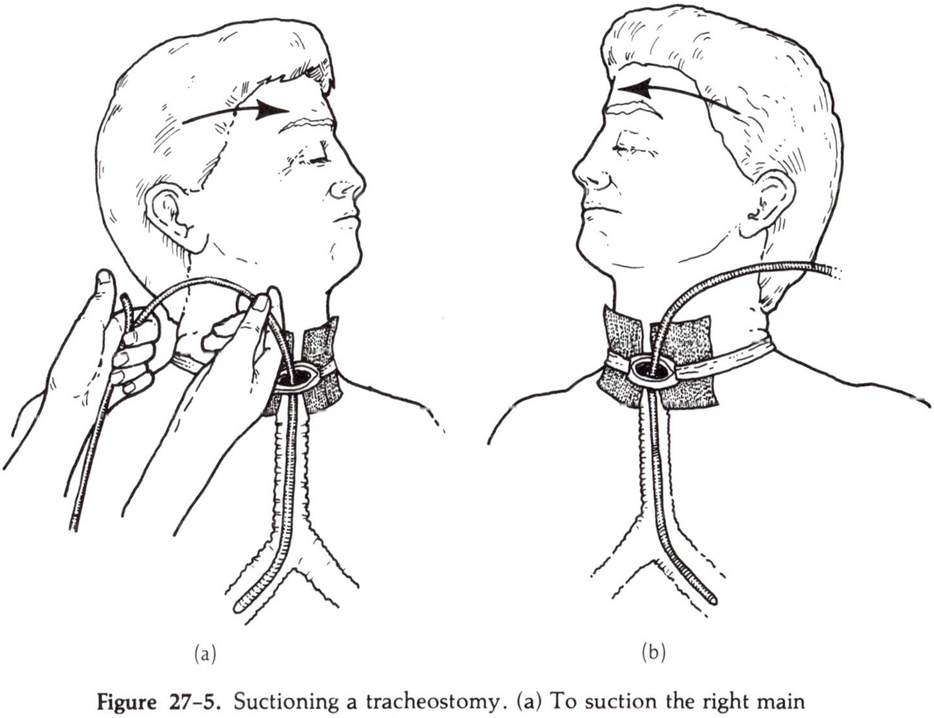


**Figure 27-5.** Suctioning a tracheostomy. (a) To suction the right main bronchus, the chest is turned slightly to the right and the head is turned to the left. (b) To suction the left bronchus, the chest is turned slightly to the left and the head is turned to the right.

the patient should be positioned on the left side (or the chest turned to the left) and the head turned to the far right. To suction the right bronchus, the opposite directions should be employed. As the catheter is passed downward, suction should not be used. (The vent should be open.) When the catheter is at the desired depth, the vent hole should be closed off with the finger or thumb, creating the suctioning force. As the catheter is withdrawn, it should be rotated between the thumb and forefinger for improved results and to lessen mucosal lining trauma. Suctioning usually stimulates coughing which helps to "bring up" secretions. The catheter should be removed during hard coughing to prevent the buildup of undue pressure in the airways.

When the suctioning is complete, the catheter should be cleansed by drawing water or saline through it. If the nose, mouth and throat also require suctioning, another catheter should be used to prevent cross-contamination.

A tracheostomy tube may become accidentally dislodged from violent coughing or a struggle to breathe. If this occurs, the EMT should promptly spread the trachea vertically with a hemostat or tracheal dilator to establish a ventilation channel until the tube can be reinserted. (See Fig. 27–6.)

If artificial ventilation is required for resuscitation, mouth to stoma assistance is required. Place your mouth directly over the stoma and deliver breaths in the usual manner. It is not necessary to close off the mouth and nose of the patient, to remove dentures, or concern yourself with the position of the tongue. The head should be kept in straight alignment and the shoulders must be slightly elevated to maximize the patency of the opening.

Many EMT units have a tracheostomy tube adapter for the bag-valve mask unit to ventilate patients with tracheostomy tubes. The adapter is not to be used in the stoma, however, unless a tracheostomy tube is in place, since it can be easily lost into the trachea by accidental disengagement from

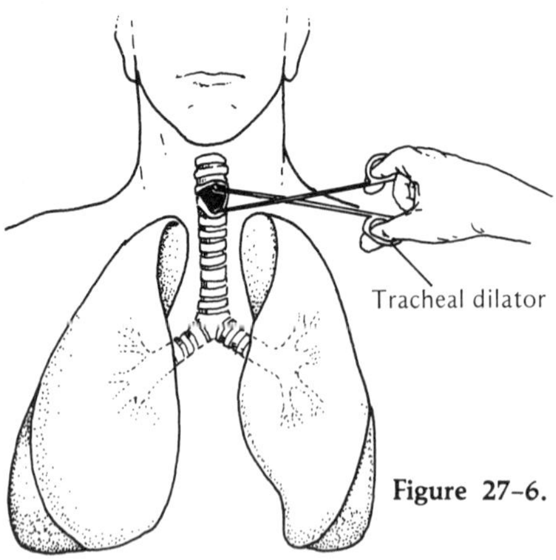


**Figure 27–6.** Procedure for conserving the airway if a tracheostomy tube is accidentally dislodged.

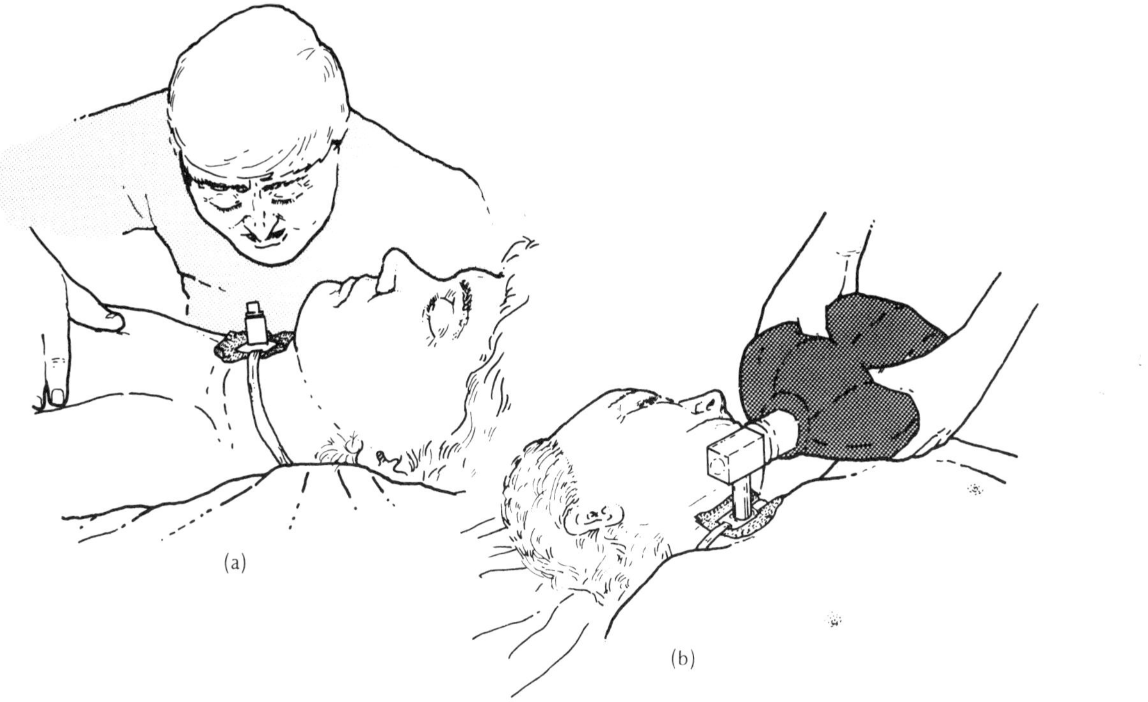


**Figure 27-7.** Emergency ventilation of patient with tracheostomy. (a) Mouth-to-tracheostomy tube using adapter. (b) Bag valve-mask technique.

the bag and a satisfactory seal cannot be attained. (See Fig. 27-7.) For additional principles and techniques of resuscitation, see Chapter 10.

## DIALYSIS-RELATED EMERGENCIES

The EMT may encounter a patient who is having routine renal dialysis and has an external shunt to access circulation. Most shunts are located in the forearm, ankle, or groin. The shunt permits the attachment of the "artificial kidney machine" time and again without surgical procedures being required each time. (See Fig. 27-8.) Between dialysis treatments, the shunt's arterial and venous lines are connected, wrapped, and protected with a dressing to prevent dislodging. Occasionally, these

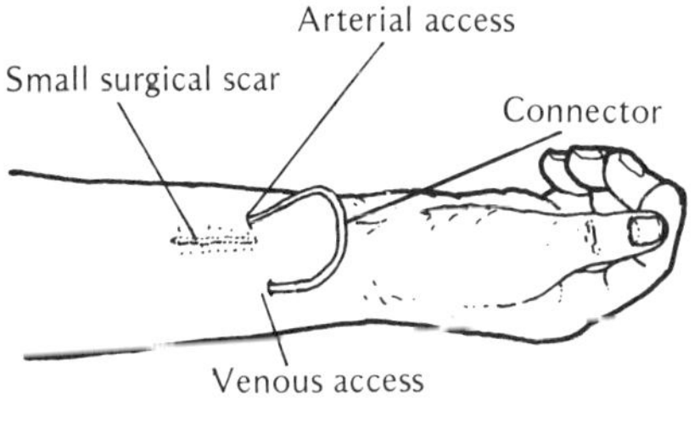


**Figure 27-8.** Schematic representation of external dialysis shunt.

shunts "clot off" or bleed, and the patient will summon medical help. There is little that the EMT can do in the field except to control bleeding. Definitive emergency care at a hospital is indeed indicated.

## THE SEIZURE PATIENT

Seizure disorders represent a dysfunction of the brain, usually overactivity of certain cells. A *seizure* is a sudden change in sensation, behavior, muscle activity, or level of consciousness. There are many types of seizures and a variety of suspected causes including infection, alcoholism, fever, trauma, metabolic disturbances, and interferences with the brain's blood supply. The EMT must appreciate that a seizure is not a disease, but a symptom, of an underlying problem within the central nervous system.

*Epilepsy* (ep′ĭ-lep″se) is a condition in which the patient has recurrent episodes of seizure, but in which there is no defined or known causative problem. Epilepsy ordinarily has its onset between early childhood and young adulthood. It involves seizures of several types but does not affect any physical or mental processes, and the individual can continue a normal lifestyle in most instances if he complies with the regimen of anti-convulsant medications. The regular use of these agents controls seizures by raising the threshold for their onset. Among the most common drugs are: Phenobarbital, phenytoin sodium (Dilantin®), primidone (Mysoline®) and diazepam (Valium®). EMTs should suspect seizures as one cause of unconsciousness if a patient is found to have such drugs in a pocket or handbag, or among a medicine supply within the home. Since many seizure patients carry wallet cards or wear a Medic-Alert tag, the EMT should always check for these.

Although patients take their medications regularly, it is possible for seizures to occur as a result of unusual stress upon the body. Fatigue, fever, infections, pregnancy, constipation, and menstrual periods may be factors that contribute to a lowering of the threshold for seizures. A careful history from the patient, the family, or friends may be useful in identifying these underlying causes of stress.

### Types of Seizures

#### *Neonatal Seizures*

The newborn may have seizures that are easily missed since they are unique in their signs. The only clues that the tiny infant is seizing may be unusual posturing, rigidity, or apnea. Tremors, loss of muscle tone, spasmodic crying, facial twitching, chewing movements, or shivering movements may also be indicators of neonatal seizures. If such patterns are recognized, the EMT's major responsibility is airway support and prompt transport to a hospital.

### *Febrile Seizures*

Young children, six months to about six years, may have a seizure in response to fever due to the brain's inability to adapt to a sudden increase in temperature. These seizures typically accompany upper respiratory tract infections. Treatment is aimed at the underlying cause of the fever. (See page 156.)

### *Petit Mal Seizures*

Certain patients have petit mal seizures, which are essentially momentary lapses of consciousness. A blank stare or a transient "unawareness" or "dropping out" may be the only evidence of seizure activity. Petit mal seizures are seldom involved in an emergency medical response.

### *Jacksonian Seizures*

This type of seizure is marked by hyperactivity of certain muscle groups. There may be involvement of an arm or a leg, usually progressing to adjacent areas on the same side of the body. There is no loss of consciousness.

### *Psychomotor Seizures*

Psychic phenomena are experienced without recall. Motor behavior may involve purposeless activity such as hand wringing or picking at clothes. Emotions that occur at the same time may reflect anger, fear, rage, or frustration. Speech may be nonsensical or rambling.

### *Grand Mal*

The grand mal seizure or *convulsion* is the type of seizure that concerns EMTs most often. There is a sudden loss of consciousness due to brain hypoxia and alternating tonic (contractions) and clonic (successive contractions and relaxations) movement of arms and legs. Since the diaphragm is temporarily paralyzed, respirations cease and cyanosis is evident. Head and face muscles jerk and there may be dyspnea and "frothing at the mouth." Some patients are incontinent during the attack, especially with regard to bladder control.

If grand mal seizures occur successively without an interim period of consciousness, a condition called *status epilepticus* exists. Status epilepticus is a grave disorder due to brain hypoxia incurred during repeated seizures. Respiratory arrest, hypertension, fever, and elevated intracranial pressure accompany these repeated seizures.

*Status epilepticus is a dire emergency* requiring intensive care. Airway maintenance and supplemental oxygen are key factors in patient protection. These successive seizures may recur until anticonvulsant drugs are administered in large doses and the airway is well stabilized. During status epilepticus, vital signs should be carefully monitored and supplemental oxygen administered. The EMT who encounters a patient having repeated seizures should arrange for prompt transfer to a hospital, protecting the airway and breathing en route.

## Emergency Management

Some people who have repeated seizures or frequent bouts of seizures are warned a few minutes ahead by an *aura.* An aura is a highly individualized sensory experience including "seeing," "hearing," "tasting," or "smelling" something. Most are unique to the seizure victim, who usually experiences the same sensation before each seizure. For example, one may see green lights, hear an imaginary train, taste bananas, or smell cloves immediately prior to losing consciousness. The experienced seizure patient will have enough warning to lie on the floor, call for help, and take some measures for self-protection. Auras do not precede seizures far enough in advance for the attack to be thwarted, but do permit some opportunity to prevent injury.

When an EMT is responding to a "seizing patient" call, it is likely the attack will be over upon arrival at the scene, since most seizures last only a minute or two. However, some individuals have one seizure after another without regaining consciousness between. These seizures are called *status epilepticus* and can be life-threatening, since they result in severe brain hypoxia.

There is little that an EMT can do during the seizure except to protect the patient from physical harm during the violent "jerking" of arms and legs. Do not restrain the individual, since soft tissue injuries and even fractures could result. Do, however, take precautions such as moving furniture and padding hard surfaces to prevent extremities from striking objects that could result in injury.

Airway protection is the most crucial part of caring for the patient with seizures. Loosen clothing at the neck and encourage an adequate airway by positioning the head and neck. Protect the tongue from being bitten by placing a plastic "bite stick" or oropharyngeal airway in place at the onset of the seizure. Do not try to force any object into the mouth *during* the seizure. Prying the mouth open could injure the jaw muscles, which usually contract violently. Never put your fingers into the mouth of a seizing patient because a serious bite injury could result—perhaps even loss of fingers!

Many patients who seize "turn blue" or become cyanotic during the attack. Lay people often think that this is due to the tongue falling back into the throat, thus obstructing the airway. Rather, the cyanosis results from a momentary paralysis of the diaphragm and chest muscles, which interrupts ventilatory efforts. Since the brain is dependent upon oxygen for its functioning—even to induce seizure activity—the hypoxic interval actually is thought to serve as a factor in limiting or interrupting the seizure. The EMT should reassure the family that, despite this cyanotic episode, no one's life is endangered by this brief period of respiratory arrest. Repeated seizures with cumulative hypoxia insults to the brain, however, are dangerous and life-threatening.

Immediately after a seizure the airway may require suctioning, since secretions build rapidly. Some patients appear to be "frothing at the mouth" during an attack, due to the copious secretion of saliva. Use of a bag-valve-mask with supplemental oxygen helps to raise the threshold or resistance to additional seizures by improving the brain cell environment. The patient's head should be positioned to encourage good air flow, too. It is also advisable to keep an oropharyngeal airway in place in the event of a second seizure.

The EMTs on the scene should take care not to stimulate the patient after a seizure. Most will lie unconscious for awhile or desire to sleep. (This period following a seizure is called the *postictal state.)* Avoid talking, moving, or any other activity that would perhaps provoke an additional attack. If the patient has had more than a single seizure, advanced EMTs may be instructed to initiate IV fluids or to administer anticonvulsant drugs.

It is advisable to transport all patients experiencing seizure to a hospital for follow-up, since many factors could be operant in inciting the attack. A developing infection, trauma, or coexistent disease process could be contributory.

During transport, primary attention should be given to airway protection and ventilatory support. Use the left-lateral semi-prone position and adjuncts to ventilation as indicated. (See Chapter 10.) Monitor vital signs and reassure the patient as he wakes up from the attack.

The EMT's record should include the following factors. If an aura was present, it should be described. Note whether movements were generalized over the body or limited to certain limbs or one side of the body. Any unusual respiratory complications or injuries that occurred should be documented as well. Since many individuals having *grand mal* seizures become incontinent during the attack, this information should also be noted in the record. Pertinent observations on the scene and a complete report is helpful to the physician in evaluating the seizure episode and planning treatment.

## THE PATIENT WITH A COMMUNICABLE DISEASE OR INFECTION

Communicable diseases and infections of many types can pose a risk to an EMT during field management. It is important to understand the hazards of commonly encountered infections and how to ensure self protection and guard against transmission of disease to others. In this section, selected communicable processes will be discussed as they relate to field management by the EMT.

## Local Infections

Although the skin provides protection for most body tissue, microorganisms readily enter if it is broken or unhealthy. Lacerations, burns, bruises, poor circulation, and malnutrition are examples of factors that can contribute to an invitation for infection. Inflammation is the response of tissue to infection, and readies the tissue for repair.

Signs and symptoms of inflammation are redness, swelling, warmth, pain, and possible loss of motion if joints are involved. Redness, swelling, and warmth result from increased vascular activity in the affected area as the body sends additional blood cells to fight the invading organisms. When arterial vessels dilate (get larger), the walls permit circulating fluid to flow into the surrounding spaces. The purpose of this outpouring is to plug space between cells, which tends to block off the injured or infected tissue. Congestion is created with the increased circulation, and the "walling off" process often results in a throbbing sensation or even pain. Certain blood cells engulf and destroy the microorganisms over a period of hours or days, depending upon the nature of the infection and the resistance of the individual. When these "destroyer" cells are heavily concentrated, an abscess may form. Finally, there is complete resolution of the inflammatory process as the tissue repairs are completed. Scars or other permanent alterations of the tissue may occur in response to certain kinds of infections.

If the body is unable to successfully localize and destroy the invading microorganisms, a systemic infection may result. Fever is one sign of the onset of such a process. Others may be quite general. The patient may feel tired and weak, and may lack the usual amount of energy before becoming frankly ill from the infection.

Certain infections are termed "communicable" or easily transferrable from one person to another. These are of special concern to the EMT. Any patient known or suspected of having a communicable disease requires added precautions during field management and transport to protect the EMTs and their subsequent patients.

## Tuberculosis

Tuberculosis affects primarily the lungs, but can affect almost any organ of the body. Respiratory tuberculosis is transmitted from one person to another by moist air containing the causative organism. Close contact with a tuberculosis patient can result in acquisition of the disease, particularly if resistance is low as a result of a cold, sore throat, or other illness. Poor nutrition and fatigue also predisposes one to acquiring an infection.

Tuberculosis is transmitted easily via expired air and secretions from the nose or mouth. The EMT should avoid direct exposure to the patient's expired air as he talks, sneezes, or coughs. (Some local units may suggest the wearing of a mask by either the patient or the EMT to prevent transmissions.) Oxygen masks, emesis basins, tissues, or linens deserve special handling after use with the patient with tuberculosis. Local units usually have specific guidelines for aftercare of equipment used in conjunction with a patient who has a communicable disease.

Careful handwashing is the EMT's best protection against tuberculosis and most other communicable diseases, but masks may be employed for respiratory infections and gloves for wound or skin infections.

## Hepatitis

Infectious hepatitis is a viral infection of the liver. (Other noninfectious forms of hepatitis may also occur as the result of toxins, usually drugs or chemicals.) *Jaundice,* a yellow discoloration of the skin, is a characteristic late symptom of the disease when the liver is unable to excrete bilirubin, the pigment of hemoglobin detoxification. When the pigment is absorbed by the blood, it colors the skin and sclera of the eyes, giving them a decidedly yellow cast. Laypersons sometimes refer to hepatitis as "yellow jaundice." There are two distinct types of viral hepatitis, infectious and serum, each posing different hazards for the EMT.

Infectious hepatitis is transmitted by fecal contaminants. Occasionally, some authorities have indicated that it may be spread by the respiratory route or blood. Unless the EMT comes in contact with the patient's stool (or underwear which could be contaminated), he is in little danger of contacting this type of viral hepatitis.

Serum hepatitis, however, poses a special threat to EMTs who do invasive procedures such as starting an IV or drawing blood. In serum hepatitis, the offending organism is carried in the blood. If the EMT is accidentally stuck by a needle that has been used with this patient, prompt medical attention is essential to prevent contracting the disease. Serum hepatitis is common among drug addicts who inject themselves with contaminated needles used earlier by someone else with the virus.

EMTs exposed to viral hepatitis may be advised to take immune serum globulin (gamma globulin) to reduce chances of acquiring the disease.

Linens, needles, airways, or other equipment that could be contaminated with virus deserve isolation and special handling according to unit operational guidelines. Handwashing is perhaps the best defense for the EMT against contracting viral hepatitis, too.

## Infected Wounds or Skin Lesions

Certain patients may have infected wounds or skin lesions that harbor infectious organisms. Most can be readily recognized by their foul appearance and odor. Purulent drainage (pus) may or may not be evident.

Foul drainage, warts, ulcerations, and irritated skin around genitalia may be the result of venereal disease processes. Although venereal disease is transmitted primarily by sexual intercourse or contact of any two moist mucous membrane surfaces (mouth, eyes, vagina, penis, or rectum), they are possibly communicable through cuts, sores, or broken skin surfaces such as even a hangnail. Again, the EMT should use careful handwashing techniques after contact with these patients. If accidental needle punctures are incurred, these should be reported and should be medically managed in certain instances. Linen and other equipment or supplies that are contaminated require special handling too.

Infected wounds or skin lesions may need to be touched in the process of field assessment or care. If so, sterile gloves should be available for the EMT's protection, and to aid in preventing the introduction of additional contaminants into the affected skin. Any wounds that have foam-like drainage or are surrounded by subcutaneous emphysema require prompt medical attention, since they reflect invasion of especially dangerous gas-forming organisms. Gas-forming organisms rapidly destroy tissue and result in gangrene, and are highly contagious!

## Other Communicable Diseases

Many types of communicable diseases are prevalent in certain areas of the country or are seasonal. Some migrate in epidemics (for example, influenza), and thus are hazardous from time to time. Others, such as measles, mumps, or chickenpox, are seldom of concern since most adults have had the disease as a "childhood disease." However, vulnerable adults (those not previously exposed, pregnant, or debilitated by acute or chronic illness), must exercise special precautions when caring for patients with a communicable disease.

*References*

Barber, Janet M.; Stokes, Lillian G.; and Billings, Diane M. *Adult and Child Care: A Client Approach to Nursing,* 2nd ed. St. Louis, MO: The C. V. Mosby Co., 1977.

Barber, Janet M., and Budassi, Susan A. *Mosby's Manual of Emergency Care: Practices and Procedures.* St. Louis, MO: The C. V. Mosby Co., 1979.

Chitwood, Donna, "The Deaf Person in an Emergency," pp. 66–69, *Emergency Product News,* October 1977.

DeDominicis, Carla "Pleasantly Plump," pp. 55–58, *Emergency Product News,* October 1977.

Magilvy, Joan K., and Magilvy, Douglas B., "Your Patient Is Deaf: Comments on Working with the Deaf Person in an Emergency," *The EMT Journal,* 1;50–51, September 1977.

Saltzman, Joel "What To Do When Treating a Blind Person," *Emergency Product News,* pp. 31–33, October 1977.

Teichmann, Peter, "Emergency Care of the Aging," *Emergency Product News,* pp. 75–76, October 1977.

# Chapter 28

# Burns and Lightning Injuries

EMTs are frequently faced with patients who have burns over a major portion of the body. When such injuries occur, there is extensive trauma to the body's largest organ, the skin. In adults, almost 20 pounds of skin covers the entire external surface of the body. Skin is also called the *integument* (in-teg′u-ment).

Functions of the skin are vital to life. In addition to its cosmetic characteristics, it is a first line of defense against microorganisms, trauma, and temperature extremes of heat and cold. Skin also is watertight and prevents the escape of body fluids that nourish and support tissue or organs. Regulatory processes related to the maintenance of body temperature are largely dependent upon the skin's role as a sensory organ that perceives heat, cold, pressure, position changes, and pain.

The skin is composed of two distinct layers, the *epidermis* (ep″ĭ-der′mis) and the *dermis* (der′mis). The *epidermis* is the outer layer of the skin and is made up of a protein substance called *keratin* (ker′ah-tin). The epidermis varies in thickness over the several body surfaces, and is heavier in areas of exposure where more protection is needed, such as over the hands and feet. Cells in the epidermis are shed continuously and are replaced by cells that migrate upward from the second layer of skin called the *dermis.*

The *dermis* is the living tissue of the skin and contains blood vessels, nerves, oil glands, and sweat glands, as well as hair follicles and nail beds. Each of the components of the dermis is designed to adapt to changing body conditions and to respond to environmental stimuli. Since the dermis depends upon the epidermis for protection, it is severely endangered and functionally impaired when the dermis is injured or destroyed as a result of burns.

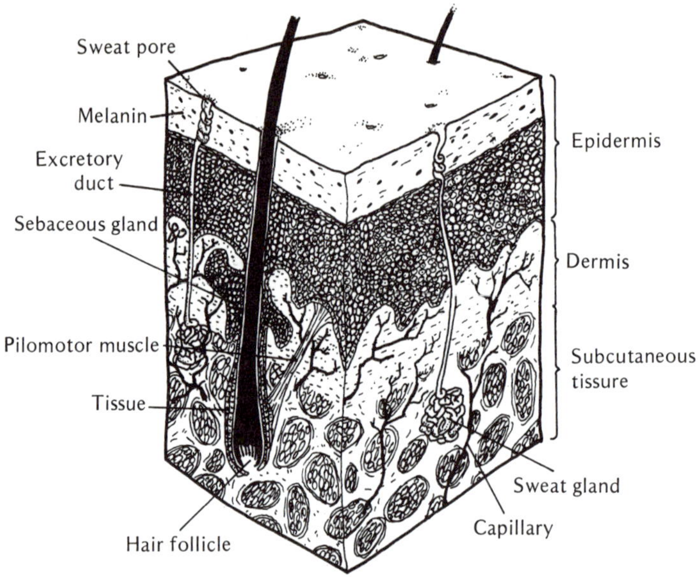


**Figure 28–1.** Layers of the skin and its derivatives.

## BURNS

Burns are tissue injuries caused primarily by heat, electrical or radiation energy, chemicals, or friction. The severity of a burn is determined largely by the amount of body surface involved, and the depth of tissue damage. Other factors, such as anatomical location of the burn, related chronic disease, or concurrent injury all affect the patient's chance for survival. The EMT should be prepared to assess a burn injury in the field, since initial management is largely affected by this data.

The *body surface area (BSA)* involved in the burn is estimated according to precalculated percentages representing body parts or skin surface. Two examples of models are the Rule of Nines (see Fig. 28–2) and the Lund and Browder Chart (see Fig. 28–3). The latter is preferred by many burn centers, since it makes appropriate adaptations for children of various ages.

*Burn depth* refers to the type and extent of damage to various tissue layers. Historically, these "depths" have been described as "degrees" of burn. Three different degrees are described in Fig. 28–4. Recently, many clinicians merely refer to "partial thickness" or "full thickness" burns to denote the involved skin. "Full-thickness" burns are those in which the entire dermis is affected. The EMT must appreciate that in the field, particularly if the patient has other injuries, there may not be clear data to estimate burn depth. Even in the hospital, after the wound has been cleaned and all dead tissue removed (debridement [da-brēd' ment]), the extent of real damage may not be apparent until three or four days later.

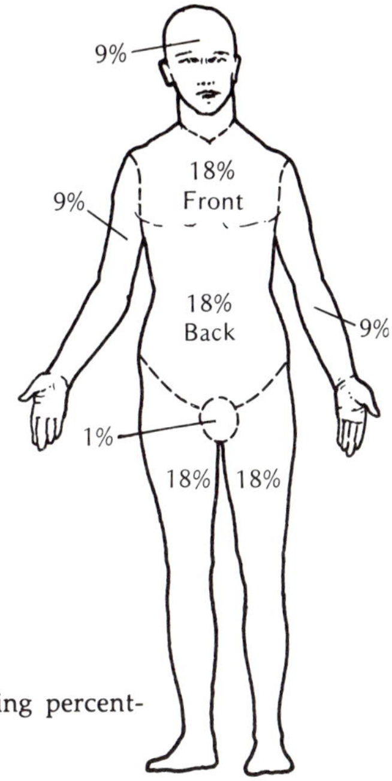


**Figure 28–2.** "Rule of Nines" for calculating percentage of body burned.

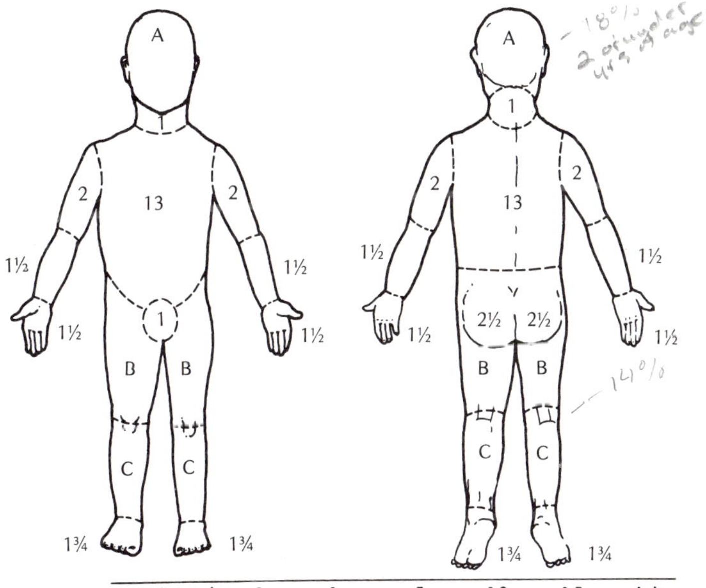


| AGE (years) | 0 | 1 | 5 | 10 | 15 | adult |
|---|---|---|---|---|---|---|
| A - ½ of head | 9½ | 8½ | 6½ | 5½ | 4½ | 3½ |
| B - ½ of one thigh | 2¾ | 3¼ | 4 | 4¼ | 4½ | 4¾ |
| C - ½ of one leg | 2½ | 2½ | 2¾ | 3 | 3¼ | 3½ |

Total % burned ——————— 2° + ——————— 3° = ———————

**Figure 28–3.** Lund and Browder method for assessing the extent of burn injury; this method takes into account changing body surface areas due to growth.

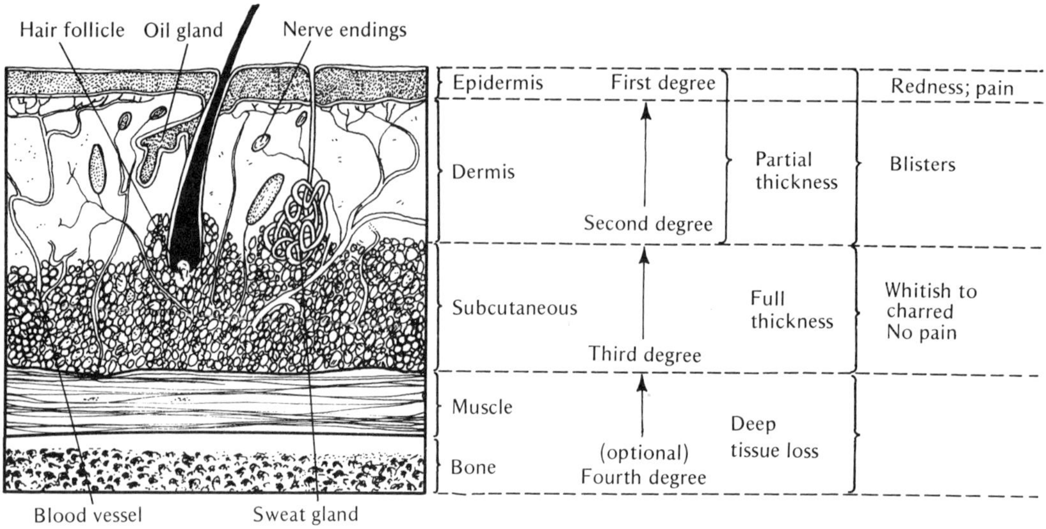


**Figure 28-4.** Classification of burns according to type and degree.

Other factors important to determining the severity of the burn is to note which anatomical surfaces are involved. Burns that affect the hands, head, feet, or genitalia always tend to be more difficult to treat. Burns that are circumferential (ser″kum-fer-en′shal) (completely encircle a limb, for example), are also prone to complications, primarily as the result of interference to blood flow, as the swelling (edema) becomes marked. Patients who have such injuries should be transported to the hospital, even though the percentage of the burn seems relatively small. A burn at the wrist, although only 1 percent of the BSA, could result in the loss of a hand from circulatory interferences induced by postburn edema. All electrical burns, too, should be transported to a hospital for follow-up.

Burns that occur in the very young and the elderly, in conjunction with other trauma (fractures, dislocations, internal injuries), or to an individual with chronic or acute illness (diabetes, heart disease, kidney problems, pneumonia), have a more precarious outcome than those affecting a healthy young adult. The EMT should be cognizant of these variables when gathering and conveying an initial burn history and status report to a treatment center.

## On the Scene Management

The EMT is frequently the first medically trained individual who encounters the burned patient. The care that is provided initially will often influence the final outcome for the victim, so it is imperative that attention be given to all aspects of care in a systematic manner. Airway problems, of course, are assessed and managed as the first priority and followed by other facets of basic life support as required.

The EMT, like other members of the health care team, are often engrossed with the burn wound and fail to consider other possible injuries. Spinal cord trauma, fractures, and internal bleeding must always be suspected if there has been an auto accident, explosion, or fall associated with the burn. Of course, the usual measures should be taken for these related problems, i.e., controlling hemorrhage and shock, splinting of fractures, and careful assessment of the level of consciousness.

## Chemical Burns

Chemical burns should be managed by flushing the skin with large amounts of water. If a dry chemical is involved, the skin should be carefully brushed to remove as much of the substance as possible *before* flushing with water, since adding water to certain dry chemicals results in a heat-generating process that could add to the burning.

The EMT should take care not to become "contaminated" with the hazardous chemicals. If accidental contact with personal clothing or the skin occurs, remove the affected garments and flush the skin as soon as possible to avoid burns.

If a chemical has gotten into the eyes, the eyes should be flooded with large amounts of water (for at least 5 minutes for acid burns and 20 minutes for alkali burns), followed by covering them with a dry, sterile dressing. If the individual is wearing contact lenses, they should be removed initially to ensure that the entire eye is flooded. A flask of intravenous normal saline with tubing attached makes an ideal irrigation apparatus for field use. (See Fig. 16-2, page 292.) All chemical burns to the eyes should be transported to a treatment facility for further evaluation and care by an ophthalmologist.

## Electrical Burns

All electrical burn injuries should receive careful attention, since a seemingly small wound can be accompanied by hidden damage to muscle, nerves, and blood vessels over a large area.

Electrical injury produces intense heat that travels along nerve tissue routes and destroys them. The heart and lungs may be affected, too, and the EMT should be prepared to deal with resultant cardiopulmonary arrest. *All* electrical burns should be transported for evaluation and care.

## The Burn Wound

The burn wound should be evaluated as the last factor in the multiple trauma examination using one of several methods such as the Rule of Nines or the Lund and Browder formula, the latter formula being preferred for children. It is helpful also to calculate the percentage of unburned surface to minimize the usual tendency to overestimate the percentage of BSA involved.

Any smoldering or damp clothing should be removed, but garments adhering to the skin should not be torn away. Do not break any blisters or apply anything to the wound! Although ice and cooled compresses have been used to alleviate the pain of small-area partial-thickness burns, they are not recommended for extensive burns since they unnecessarily lower body temperature.

The wound may be rinsed with saline solution, however, to remove surface debris. A dry (preferably sterile) sheet is ideal for covering the wound during transport to the hospital. Since edema formation can occur early after the burn has occurred, it is important that EMTs elevate involved extremities and remove any constricting jewelry (rings, bracelets, or watches) that could subsequently interfere with circulation.

### Other Prehospital Care

Vital signs should be obtained for baseline values and monitored closely. A blood pressure cuff or monitoring leads can be safely placed over burned areas if necessary.

The distal pulses in burned extremities should be checked frequently throughout the transfer. The use of antishock trousers in prolonged transports should be avoided if there are lower extremity burns since they may compound problems of edema and circulatory deficit.

EMT-Ps may initiate an IV infusion of Ringer's lactate on persons with major burns using a large-bore device.(Some authorities do not advocate prehospital fluid infusion for burned patients unless there is shock already present or if the hospital is more than thirty minutes away.) Of course, extremities with circumferential burns should not be selected for IV fluid administration, since developing edema could impede the flow. Surgical entry into a vein (venesection) [ven″e-sek′shun] may be necessary in selected instances. The flow rate should be monitored cautiously.

The EMT should reassure and comfort the victim as much as possible. Procedures and their rationale should be explained. The patient should be told what events will take place at the hospital upon his arrival.

Highflow oxygen, suctioning, and supportive ventilation should be provided as needed, especially for inhalation injuries.

## UNDERSTANDING INHALATION HAZARDS

EMTs are likely to encounter accidents on the highway, in industry, or in the home that pose environmental hazards to the rescuer. It is imperative that sources of poisonous fumes be well known and that the EMT be familiar with ways to minimize their harmful or even lethal effect during prehospital care.

A few respiratory injuries are related to direct causes of pulmonary insult such as inhalation of steam, superheated gas, or toxic fumes. Unfortunately, when a victim has inhaled hot gases, edema rapidly obstructs the upper airways and prehospital care teams can do little to aid this individual unless they are skilled in creating surgical airways. (See Chapter 10.) The most commonly encountered respiratory problems are due to smoke inhalation.

Smoke consists of particulate matter suspended in a gas. It characteristically contains large carbon particles coated with chemical by-products of the burning process that irritate the airways on contact causing constriction, edema, and even hemorrhage.

## Carbon Monoxide

Carbon monoxide (CO) is the most classic of inhalation injuries that occurs in relation to burns. Carbon monoxide is a colorless, odorless, tasteless gas produced by incomplete combustion of burning materials. It is present in relation to most fires or associated with combustion devices, but is usually undetectable since it is nonirritating. Common causes are exhaust fumes from automobiles; charcoal grills used in a poorly ventilated space such as tents, campers, or inside the house; and furnaces with poor ventilation.

Carbon monoxide passes unchanged through the lungs and combines with hemoglobin (producing carboxyhemoglobin [kar-bok″se-he″mo-glo′bin]) and displaces oxygen since its affinity for hemoglobin is about 200 times greater than oxygen. It also interferes with the release of oxygen from its carrier in the blood. Its harmful effects, of course, are related to tissue hypoxia.

Signs and symptoms of low concentration (about 20 percent carboxyhemoglobin) may be limited to a throbbing headache. As levels of carboxyhemoglobin reach 50 percent there may be confusion, dizziness, dilated pupils, visual disturbances, a full bounding pulse, nausea, dyspnea, and even syncope (fainting) on exertion. When levels approach 70 to 80 percent, coma, seizures, respiratory failure, and death may occur. EMTs should appreciate the fact that if carbon monoxide is inhaled quickly in high concentrations, there may be no early warning signs such as the throbbing headache or dizziness. Victims of carbon monoxide poisonings may not be cyanotic although they are suffering from hypoxia. Instead, they may appear flushed due to the blood's cherry-red color induced by the high levels of carboxyhemoglobin. Furthermore, victims of smoke inhalation can have significant hypoxemia without any signs or symptoms.

The major initial treatment for carbon monoxide inhalation is humidified oxygen. Of course, the airway should be cleared and ventilations supported as necessary. It is essential to remember that many noxious gases create a central nervous system depression that reduces tidal volume (the volume of air exchanged during breathing), although the respiratory rate remains within normal limits. Bag-mask assistance may be necessary to facilitate adequate oxygenation.

## Other Noxious Gases

The majority of noxious gases that can pose threats at the scene of an accident are the result of burning synthetics, particularly plastics. When one considers the number of everyday applications of these materials in cars, homes, aircraft interiors, and personal products, it is evident that they pose many potential inhalation-related injuries. Electrical wiring, insulation, mattresses, car seats, synthetic fiber carpeting, and items of clothing that contain plastics are commonly found smoldering nearby as an EMT extricates and cares for a burn victim. Merely breaking a window may be a valuable technique to improve the ventilation space by allowing fumes to escape and, of course, reduce the risk of carbon monoxide build-up.

The earliest signs of noxious gas inhalation are shortness of breath; wheezing, coughing, and burning of the nose and throat; lightheadedness; irregular pulse; chest pain; nausea; fainting; and irritation of the eyes. A victim who exhibits respiratory distress or who is unconscious when recovered from a burning environment should be assessed for these signs and symptoms of toxic inhalation. Look for singed nasal hairs, a rasping cough, hoarseness, soot or blood in the sputum, and any difficulty in breathing. The characteristics of the ventilatory effort are far more important than the rate of respirations. Since noxious inhaled substances depress vital centers, be ready to assist breathing using a bag-valve-mask unit. Care should also be taken to survey the scene to identify sources of toxic fumes. This information may alert the hospital team to potential dangers and offer insight regarding later developing manifestations of inhalation injuries.

Since persons tend to breathe more deeply on exertion, it is recommended that the victim be encouraged to avoid any exercise so that ventilation can be maintained at a minimal rate and depth. If cooperation can be elicited, instructions should be provided to prolong the duration of expiration to reduce the time that pulmonary irritants are in touch with the lower airways. Breath holding or shallow breathing may also be advised to confine particles and irritants to conducting airways.

On occasion, EMTs encounter individuals who have been exposed to heavy smoke but are not experiencing acute distress. However, they should be evaluated at a hospital (often admitted for twenty-four-hour observation) to ensure that hidden airway damage will be detected promptly and managed definitively.

# COMMUNICATING WITH THE HOSPITAL ABOUT BURNS

If the EMT can establish radio communication with the hospital, the following information should be relayed regarding the burn patient:

1. Name and age of patient
2. Description of burn and history of incident, if known
   a. Percentage and areas involved
   b. Depth of burn (as estimated by initial appearance)
   c. Type of burn (chemical, steam, flame, scald, etc.)
3. Condition of airway and vital signs
4. Description of any known medical complications or associated injuries
5. Current status of treatment
   a. Airway management including oxygen administration
   b. Fluid therapy
   c. Wound care
   d. Other

## LIGHTNING INJURIES

Injuries due to the effects of lightning are not a common occurrence. It has been estimated that between 150 to 300 persons die each year in the United States from direct or indirect contact from lightning.

Lightning is a natural phenomenon that occurs from the collision of ice particles in the clouds, being carried upward by warm air and downward by cooler air. Because of a large buildup of negative electrical charges in the bottom of the cloud and the positive charge of the earth, an attraction of negative and positive charges occur resulting in a bolt of lightning. It has been estimated that the current from such a bolt of lightning contains between 12,000 and 200,000 amperes, and takes between 1/100 and 1/1000 of a second to strike the ground.

Patients with lightning injuries who are not responsive and in cardiac arrest should have CPR started immediately. Resuscitation efforts should continue for an extended period of time. There have been many cardiac arrest victims from lightning injuries who have successfully been resuscitated without sequelae. This is because the 4–6 minute rule for brain cell death does not apparently apply.

It is thought that cell degeneration is halted for an indeterminate period of time because when the electrical force passes through the body, all cell metabolism stops, therefore, requiring a longer period of time for the body's cells to begin degeneration.

The EMT should check for entrance and exit wounds caused by the electrical force. The patient should have shoes and socks removed to facilitate observation of exit wounds which are commonly found on the feet.

The EMT should provide the following treatment and care with lightning injured patients:

1. Provide a patent airway and give oxygen 4–6 *l*/m by mask. Begin CPR if required.

2. The heart should be monitored if possible. These patients usually have dysrhythmias.

3. An IV of Ringers Lactate solution should be administered if available by advanced EMTs or Paramedics.

4. Continuous monitoring of the blood pressure, pulse and respiration are necessary.

5. The resultant burn should be treated as any other type of electrical burn.

6. The patient should be transported in a semi-Fowler's position if conscious, and a supine position with head turned to one side if unconscious.

7. The EMT should alert the emergency department as to the condition of the patient, the treatment given en route and the estimated time of arrival.

## Prevention

Lightning is a natural occurrence and should be taken as a warning to one's health and safety. Tips on how to avoid injury by lightning during a thunderstorm include the following:

1. Stay out or get out of the water during a thunderstorm (this includes the bath tub.)

2. Stay clear of any single tall object. They are prime targets for lightning.

3. Stay off the telephone (unless it's an emergency,) because lightning may travel through the wires to the caller.

4. If in a car during a lightning storm, stay in it. It is well-grounded because of the tires.

5. Discard all sporting equipment, such as golf clubs, fishing rods, aluminum ball bats, etc.; they are good targets for lightning.

6. If afield with no apparent protection, head for dense small trees, ravines, or valleys.

7. Do not run during a storm.

8. If indoors, do not stand between an open door and open windows, as lightning may strike in a linear fashion, between the door and window along a current of hot or moist air.

9. Do not ride motorcycles, golf carts, bicycles, tractors, etc. If riding, park and stay clear until the storm passes.

10. Groups of persons such as campers and hikers should spread out, staying several yards apart, so that if lightning strikes, the smallest number will be affected.

## *References*

Apfelberg, O. B.; Masters, F. W.; and Robinson, D. W. "Pathophysiology and Treatment of Lightning Injuries," *The Journal of Trauma*, Vol. 14 No. 6, 1974.

Caroline, Nancy L. *Emergency Care in the Streets.* Boston, MA: Little, Brown and Company, 1979.

Coleman, T. H. "Deaths of Lightning," *Penn. Med.*, 72:56–58, 1969.

Cooper, Mary A. "Lightning Injuries: Prognostic Signs for Death," *Annals of Emergency Medicine*, 9:3, March 1980, pp. 134–138.

Edlich, R. F., *et al.* "Emergency Department Treatment, Triage and Transfer Protocols for the Burn Patient," *JACEP* 7:152–158, 1978.

*Emergency Product News*, 9 (4), June 1977.

Fabbi, Don. "Field Treatment and Management of Electrical Burns," *Emergency Product News*, June 1977, pp. 77–79.

Fisher, J. C. "Immediate Care of the Burn Victim," *Emerg. Prod. News* 9(4):58–59, 1977.

Gursel, E., and Tintinalli, J. E. "Emergency Burn Management," *JACEP*, 7:209–212, 1978.

Harding, J., and Walraven, G. "Prehospital Management of Burn Injuries: A Case Study," *Emerg. Prod. News*, 9(4):34–37, 1977.

Lankford, T. Randall. *Integrated Science for Health Students.* Reston, VA: Reston Publishing Company, Inc., 1979.

Simmons, R. "Emergency Management of Electrical Burns," *JEN*, 3:14, 1977.

Weigel, Edwin P. "Lightning: The Underrated Killer," *NOAA Magazine*, April, 1976, p. 9.

Wikin, Jonus H., and Taussig, Helen B. "Delayed Reactions to Celestial Flashes," *Emergency Medicine*, May 15, 1979, pp. 63–64.

# Chapter 29

# Heat-Related Illnesses

The human body maintains a constant internal (core) temperature within ±1°F every day of our lives unless a heat-related illness develops. This constant internal body heat is generated as an end product from cellular metabolism.

The surface (skin) temperature of the body varies according to the surrounding environment rising or falling, depending on the surrounding ambient [am'be-ent] temperature.

When referring to the patient's temperature, one refers to the internal or core body temperature. The average normal body temperature is considered to be 98.6°F or 37°C. Body temperature above this value is called a *fever.*

When referring to the body's ability to lose heat to the environment, one refers to the surface or skin temperature. An area in the brain called the *hypothalamus* regulates the amount of heat loss in the body. It does so by responding to temperature changes in cerebral blood flow and thermoreceptors located in the skin. When internal body temperature rises, so does the rate of cellular metabolism, thereby generating more heat. The more heat generated the higher the metabolic rate, and so on, creating a heat production cycle. This heat-producing cycle is normally broken or kept constant by the body's ability to peripherally dilate blood vessels which allow heat to escape from the skin surface by radiation and conduction. When air currents pass across the skin, additional heat is lost by convection. As body temperature increases sweat glands are stimulated and sweat travels to the skin surface. Once this salt and water mixture is exposed to dry passing air currents, it is evaporated, which cools the body. Heat loss by evaporation is the major cooling system of the body. However, when very humid and hot surrounding air temperature approaches that of the body temperature with little air movement, the body temperature may continue to rise even though sweat continues to pour from the body. This is because the high humidity of the surrounding air is already maximally saturated with water vapor and will not take on any additional moisture.

In any environment where surrounding temperatures approach that of body temperature and the atmosphere is humid, chances of heat-related illnesses are greatly increased. Illnesses related to heat are heat cramps, heat exhaustion, and heat stroke.

## HEAT CRAMPS

Heat cramps are painful muscle spasms, usually in the arms, legs, and abdomen or those muscles which perform most of the work for the body. Heat cramps may develop in anyone in a setting of vigorous exercise or work, hot humid environments, or industrial or steel mill occupations. Hot weather and prolonged sun exposure, therefore, are not necessary components for heat illness to occur. When the patient sweats and loses water, he also loses electrolytes, sodium, and chloride. Water loss in the body causes the patient to be thirsty. He may drink water, but he does not replace the much-needed sodium chloride or salt. Since normal muscular activity is based on a strict balance of salt and water on a cellular level, depletion of water and sodium chloride causes the muscles to cramp.

### Treatment

The EMT should perform a rapid primary survey to rule out possible injuries. Remember that peripheral vasodilation causes heat to be lost to the environment, but may also cause fainting (heat syncope) because of venous pooling of blood.

The patient should be moved to a cool place or shaded area. Muscle spasms may range from minor to severe. The EMT should massage affected areas. The patient with heat cramps needs sodium chloride replacement. The EMT should give the conscious patient a salt water mixture to drink. One teaspoon of salt in one quart of water or electrolyte/glucose drink, such as Gatorade®, Body Punch®, or Sportade® should be administered. Heat cramps are easily reversed once the patient's salt intake is accomplished. This heat-related illness is usually self-limited and requires little or no additional medical direction.

Generally, persons who are prone to heat cramps need a higher salt intake than others when working or exercising in hot, humid environments. Patients should be informed to take proper amounts of salt by tablet form or by commercially available electrolyte/glucose drinks.

Vital signs should be closely monitored and if a low or decreasing blood pressure exists, a more serious developing heat illness such as heat exhaustion or heat stroke may be ensuing.

## HEAT EXHAUSTION

Heat exhaustion (heat prostration, heat collapse) is the most common of the heat-related illnesses and occurs to persons who work or exercise in a hot, humid environment. Heat exhaustion occurs due to severe water depletion in the body from sweating without adding more fluid to the system. Because victims essentially become dehydrated and because peripheral blood vessels are dilated to reduce body heat, venous blood is pooled, decreasing peripheral and cerebral perfusion and causing a mild

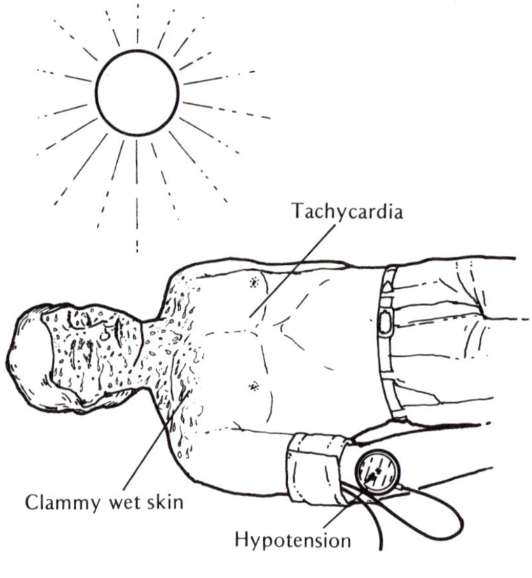


**Figure 29–1.** Heat exhaustion produces hypotension and hypovolemia through loss of water and salt.

state of shock. Heat exhaustion is a step further into the heat syndromes. Because of decreased cerebral and peripheral perfusion, weakness, faintness, giddiness, nausea, and headache are common. The skin is clammy and moist and may be pale or flushed. The patient is usually sweating profusely. A loss of one liter of water per hour is commonly lost. Because some salt is lost in sweating, both salt and water combined cause electrolyte (e-lek′tro-līt) imbalance causing muscle cramps, although not always present in heat exhaustion.

Heat exhaustion usually produces a temperature between 39° and 40°C. This may help distinguish it from the more severe heat stroke. The patient's blood pressure may be slightly decreased because of vasodilation. Tachycardia (tak″e-kar′de-ah) and thready pulse may be detected. (See Fig. 29–1.)

## Treatment

The patient should be moved to a cool or shaded area and placed in a shock position with the extremities elevated eight to twelve inches. Oxygenation is important. Administer 100 percent oxygen.

If the patient is conscious give a salt solution (one teaspoon of salt in one quart of water or an electrolyte/glucose drink). Clothing should be removed appropriately and the EMT should fan the patient to cool him, but not to the point of shivering, since this will only increase heat production. The patient should promptly return to a normal state with rest and fluid replacement. However, if the vital signs are not stable, the patient should be transported to a medical facility.

Muscle cramps may be massaged to reduce pain. Some patients may not drink because of unconsciusness, nausea, etc. These patients must be taken to the hospital immediately for treatment. Intravenous therapy must be instituted to replace fluids.

## HEAT STROKE

Just as in heat cramps and heat exhaustion, heat stroke (sunstroke, hyperpyrexia [hi"per-pi-rek'se-ah], hyperthermia) occurs to those persons who are exposed to hot, humid environments while working or exercising. Heat stroke is caused by the accumulation of body heat because of the failure or inadequacy of heat regulatory mechanisms. Because the body cannot lose heat by normal regulating mechanisms (primarily sweating), the internal body temperature rises. Increased body temperature, above 105°F, causes irreversible damage to the nervous system and body organs on a cellular level. The important point here is that of increased body temperature! The patient may still be sweating (although uncommon) and still be having a heat stroke. It is the internal body temperature that is the culprit in cellular destruction, possibly causing hypoxia; electrolyte imbalance of water, sodium, and chloride; and severe acidosis, leading to death. (See Fig. 29–2.)

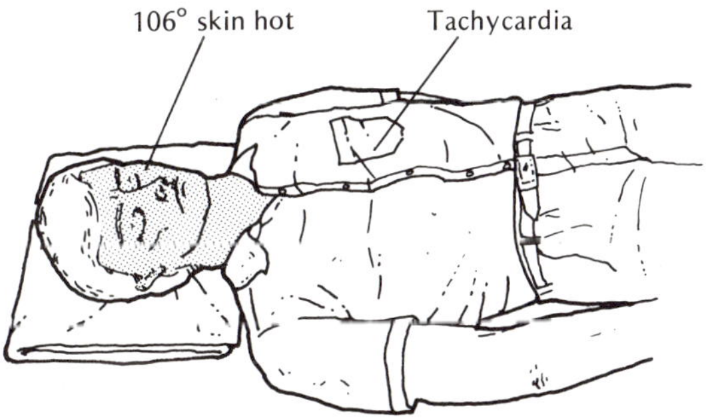


**Figure 29–2.** Heat stroke results from failure of the brain's heat regulatory center, causing an increase in body temperature.

### Factors

#### *Exercise*

Individuals who exercise strenuously, even well-conditioned athletes, are susceptible. Many sports training programs are notorious for contributing to an unreasonable share of heat stroke deaths. In fact, heat illness, as a consequence of football activities, is second only to head injuries as a cause of death in American football. The sport of jogging is another activity that generates large numbers of heat illnesses.

*Age*

The aged are more prone to heat illness than younger individuals because their mechanisms for thirst are depressed, thereby decreasing proper fluid intake.

*Heart Disease*

Heart disease predisposes victims to heat illness because the individual cannot appropriately adapt to changes in environmental or physical stress.

*Obesity*

Obesity is considered a risk factor because of the lack of physical conditioning.

*Drugs*

Drugs that affect the body to decrease sweating mechanisms, to peripherally dilate blood vessels, to increase the metabolic activity or affect the heat regulation center of the body predispose the individual to heat-related illnesses.

Drugs that decrease sweating include:

Atropine
Scopolamine

Drugs that affect the central heat regulation activity centers include:

*Phenothiazines*—(antipsychotic or psychosedative drugs)
- Thorazine
- Sparine
- Vesprin
- Serentil
- Mellaril
- Compazine
- Stelazine
- Trilafon
- Dartal
- Prolixin
- Permitel

*Tricyclic antidepressants*
- Tofranil
- Elavil
- Pertofrone
- Norpramin
- Aventyl
- Vivactil
- Sinequan
- Adapin

Drugs that peripherally vasodilate and increase metabolic activity include:

| | | |
|---|---|---|
| Amphetamine | Nitrous oxide | Ethylene |
| LSD | Halothane | Ethyl chloride |

### *Alcohol*

Alcohol not only predisposes a person to heat-related illnesses, but to hypothermia as well.

## Signs and Symptoms

### *Central Nervous System*

One of the first factors to be noted because of increased temperature and decreased cerebral perfusion is an onset of confusion. Irrational behavior, change or loss of consciousness, and convulsions are not uncommon. (See Table 29–1.)

### *Circulatory System*

The patient in early stages of heat stroke maintains a normal blood pressure. However, because of peripheral vasodilitation and therefore venous pooling, the blood pressure will decrease as time goes on. Hypovolemia also occurs because of the water and sodium chloride loss. Heart disturbances in the elderly are common, leading to heart failure and pulmonary edema. Myocardial infarction and death from heart failure or dysrhythmia may also occur with heat stroke.

TABLE 29–1. SIGNS AND SYMPTOMS OF HEAT RELATED ILLNESSES

| | *Heat Cramps* | *Heat Exhaustion* | *Heat Stroke* |
|---|---|---|---|
| Temperature | Normal | Usually normal, but may be slightly elevated or subnormal | Increases rapidly; may reach 43°C (109°F) |
| Blood Pressure | Normal or slightly depressed | Slightly decreased | First elevated, but later decreased |
| Respirations | Normal | Rapid | Slow and deep: later Cheyne-Stokes |
| Pulse | Fast | Rapid and weak | Rapid and full: later thin and weak |
| Skin | Pale, moist, cool | Pale, cool, moist | Hot and dry |
| Diaphoresis | Profuse | Profuse | Usually absent |
| Level of Consciousness | Normal | Stuporous | Early loss of consciousness |
| Nausea and Vomiting | Mild nausea, rarely vomiting | Both present, may be prolonged | Usually not present |
| Muscle Cramps | Severe and painful spasms | Occur in most cases; mild | Seizures and severe cramps may occur |

*Renal System*

Because of hypovolemia and hypoperfusion, the kidneys fail to work normally. The kidneys cannot concentrate the urine enough (a mechanism that helps keep water in the body) and, therefore, urine has been described as looking like "machine oil." Renal dialysis may be necessary for the heat stroke patient.

## Treatment

Heat stroke is a true emergency. Recognition is paramount and time is crucial in this heat-related illness to reduce body heat. The patient should be removed to a cool place or shaded area. Since respiratory (pulmonary edema) and cardiac problems are commonly involved, oxygen should be administered (100 percent) by mask. The EMT should remove the patient's clothing where appropriate and begin immediate cooling by placing cold wet sheets on the patient. The patient should then be fanned to promote cooling. Chemical cold packs, if available, should be placed about the neck, armpits, and chest to further reduce body heat. The patient's temperature must be lowered to at least 39°C and stopped at that point to avoid hypothermia. If the patient develops seizure activity, the EMT should protect the patient from harming himself. Place a bite stick in the mouth to prevent tongue biting and guard the airway. These patients may die even if treated. Patients who do survive often have central nervous system damage.

Vital signs should be monitored and temperature reduction continued enroute to the hospital. If possible, radio or call the emergency department so that they may prepare for your arrival.

## Prevention

Heat-related illness can be avoided or reduced in severity by understanding and recognizing the illness. The EMT should relay preventative information to the patient, should he decide not to go to the hospital. Important points to cover are:

1. *Acclimitization* (ah-kli″mah-ti-za′shun). Persons not used to hot, humid environments should gradually become accustomed to heat exposure. This causes the body to increase blood and fluid volume, reducing salt concentration in the sweat, thereby reducing its loss. The person should gradually expose himself thirty minutes a day for at least a week and then build on extended exposure time. Although being in good physical condition does not prevent heat-illness, it does improve heat tolerance. Obesity contributes to heat susceptibility, so reduction in weight should take place if the person is to be exposed to a hot and humid environment for any length of time.

2. *Alcohol Avoidance.* - Alcohol should be avoided while one is exposed to hot, humid environments because alcohol suppresses the antidiuretic hormone production leading to excessive loss of water.

3. *Clothing.* - When exposed to long periods of sunlight in hot weather, a light-colored hat should be worn to shield the rays of sunlight. The head is very vascular and heat radiates greatly from it. On the other hand, if ambient temperatures approach body temperature, the head can take on heat radiated by the sun. Be sure to take the hat off when in a cool or shaded area for effective cooling. Remember that light-colored clothing reduces heat input from direct sunlight. However, all clothing reduces evaporation. In direct sunlight or air temperatures above 95°F, the wearing of light-weight clothing increases comfort.

4. *Fluid Intake.* - Water loss by sweating must be replaced if heat related illnesses are to be avoided. Drink whenever you are thirsty. Persons who are not used to hot and humid environments tend to drink less than what their bodies actually need. Salt should be sprinkled on food during break periods or throughout the days or weeks of environmental exposure. Electrolyte/glucose drinks are excellent for salt and fluid replenishment. Salt tablets are fine to use, but may cause gastric disturbance in some people.

5. *Pace.* - People tolerate heat to different degrees. Each person should pace himself and realize his limitations. If the heat seems to be intolerable, stop and rest in a cool or shaded area.

## *References*

American Academy of Orthopedic Surgeons, Committee on Allied Health. *Emergency Care of the Sick and Injured,* 2nd ed. Chicago, IL: American Academy of Orthopedic Surgeons, 1977.

Guyton, A. C. *Textbook of Medical Physiology,* pp. 831–843. Philadelphia, PA: W. B. Saunders Co., 1971.

McElroy, C. "Update on Heat Illness," *Topics in Emergency Medicine,* Vol. 2, No. 3, Oct. 1980, pp. 1–18.

Murphy, R. J. "Heat Illness," *J. Sports Medicine,* 1(4):26–29, 1973.

Myerson, G. "Heat Stress," *Wilderness Adventure,* August 1977. pp. 30–32.

Shibolet, S; Lancaster, M. D.; and Dono, Y. "Heat Stroke: A Review," *Aviation, Space, and Environmental Medicine,* 47(3):280–301, March 1976.

Sturzenberger, A. J. "Differentiating Among Heat Syndromes," *JEN,* July-August 25–28, 1978.

# Chapter 30

# Injuries Due To Cold Exposure

In the chapter on heat-related illnesses, we discussed how the body tries to dissipate heat to maintain the body's internal (core) temperature. We discussed how surface (skin) temperature varies according to the surrounding air temperature and that if the body does not conserve water and certain electrolytes, heat illness ensues.

Cold or freezing injuries may occur when the body cannot generate enough heat, especially to the periphery (hands and feet). Let's discuss how the body conserves heat in response to cooling and how the body loses heat to the surrounding environment when exposed.

## BODY RESPONSE TO COLD

Body temperature must be maintained within ± 1°F of 98.6°F to insure proper metabolic functioning. When the hypothalmic area of the brain is cooled below approximately 37°C (98.6°F), internal body mechanisms are activated to increase or conserve body heat. (See Fig. 30–1.)

### Heat Conservation

The body automatically responds to decreased internal core temperature in two major ways:

1. *Peripheral vasoconstriction* The arterioles close to the skin surface constrict so that warmed blood from the internal organs (heart, brain, liver, lungs, etc.) is kept from losing heat at the skin surface. Remember that peripheral vasodilation takes place to dissipate heat. Peripheral vasoconstriction is one of the first compensatory mechanisms of the body to occur to prevent heat loss. Because the ability of vasoconstriction is important as a first line of defense against the effects of cold, it makes sense that persons with vascular disease or agents that affect proper vasoconstriction are more susceptible to cold injury. These persons include diabetics, alcoholics, the elderly, and persons on certain medications.

2. *Cessastion of Sweating* The ability to perspire stops when the body temperature drops below 37°C (98.6°F). Evaporative cooling of the body, therefore, is not possible. This mechanism further keeps the internal body temperature in check.

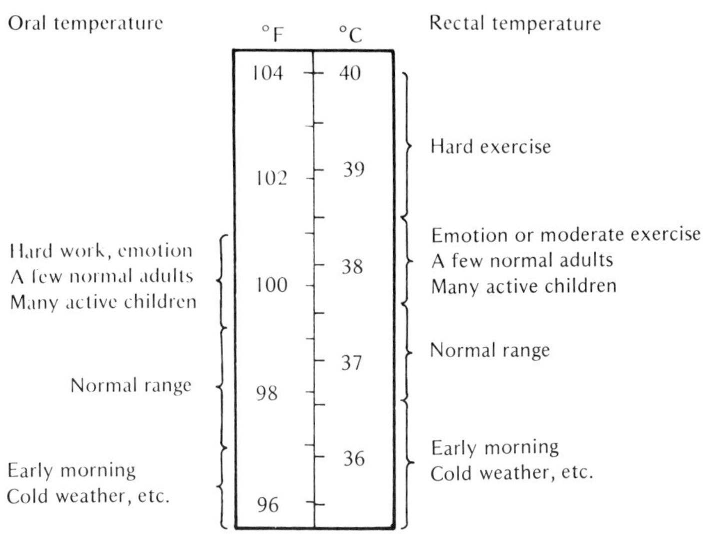


**Figure 30–1.** Internal body temperature fluctuates with normal daily activity.

*Body Insulation*

Another way in which heat is conserved is by our skin and subcutaneous tissues, especially subcutaneous fat. Fat can be an important determinant in length of survival in the cold because it conducts heat only one-fourth as rapidly as do other tissues. On the other hand, this may help explain, in part, why obese individuals may have trouble dissipating heat to the environment. Women generally have better body insulation than men because of the thicker layer of subcutaneous fat. This surface insulation helps keep heat-generating organ tissues warm when external temperatures drop.

Premature infants and low birth weight infants are particularly vulnerable to body cooling because they do not have sufficient subcutaneous fat to help keep them warm.

*Pilo—Erection:*

Heat can also be conserved by a body mechanism called pilo-erection. However, this mechanism in humans is not effective because our hair is sparse. When the body shivers to generate heat, the hair on the body surface stands on end. This is called pilo-erection and is caused by pilo-erector muscles around each hair shaft that contract, forcing the hair to stand on end. Because humans do not have enough hair, the only effect from this mechanism is the characteristic "goosebumps" or "gooseflesh." This natural mechanism is effective only in animals. The effectiveness of conserving heat by animals in this fashion occurs as follows. When the hair stands on end, a layer of air is trapped over the skin, serving as an insulator against heat transfer from the body to the environment.

## Increased Production of Heat

The body also responds to a decreased core temperature by increasing heat production. There are three major ways the body increases heat production in response to a falling core temperature: shivering, increasing metabolic rate, and releasing thyroid hormones.

### *Shivering*

Located near the heat-regulating center of the body (*hypothalamus*) are thermoreceptors that respond to nerve signals from the skin when body temperature begins to drop. The stimulation of the thermoreceptors cause skeletal muscles to increase their tone, thereby increasing muscle metabolism, which generates more body heat. As much as 50 percent increase in heat production can occur after shivering begins.

### *Increased Metabolism*

When body temperature starts to drop, the sympathetic nervous system is stimulated. Chemicals in the body called epinephrine (ep′ĭ-nef′rin) and norepinephrine are released in the blood from this stimulation, and increase the rate of cellular metabolism. Therefore, food eaten is broken down faster than usual, producing heat.

### *Thyroid Hormone Release*

When body cooling occurs, a hormone called thyroxin is released in the body which also increases cellular metabolism. This hormone is not im-

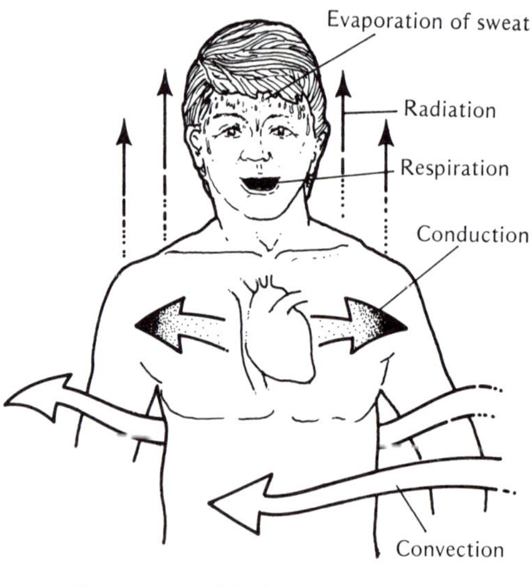


**Figure 30–2.** Mechanism of heat loss.

mediately released in response to the cold, but takes several weeks for the thyroid gland to be stimulated and increase in size to prepare for the release of thyroxin. Military personnel exposed to cold harsh climates for several weeks experience a 20 to 40 percent increase in the size of their thyroid glands. Their metabolic rate is also increased 16–20 percent above normal. Eskimos have even a higher rate of metabolism from living in cold environments. The body's ability to conserve and generate heat is inherent and responds to a drop in core temperature at approximately 37°C (98.6°F). We think little about these protective properties because they automatically take place.

Let's talk now in more detail how the body loses heat in response to environmental conditions or natural physical phenomena.

## HEAT LOSS

The body may lose heat in five major ways: radiation, conduction, convection, evaporation, and respiration. (See Fig. 30–2.)

### Radiation

Body heat is lost by radiation in the form of infrared heat rays being emitted from the body to the surroundings. Heat loss from the body varies directly with the temperature difference between the temperature of skin and average temperature of the surrounding environment. If the body surface temperature is greater than the environment in which the body is located, heat is radiated to the environment. Because the head and neck are so vascular, heat radiates from these areas more rapidly than other body areas.

The body surface absorbs infrared heat rays very effectively. White or black skin absorbs radiant heat in the same proportions. However, light rays from the sun are reflected more effectively by white skin. Black-skinned individuals reflect sunlight only in small amounts. Therefore, dark skin absorbs more heat than white skin in sunlight. Remember, every object that is not at absolute zero temperature radiates heat. Therefore, the walls of buildings, floors, and other objects radiate heat to our bodies, especially when the temperature is higher than our body temperature.

### Conduction

Heat loss from conduction occurs when body heat is directly transferred to another object. Heat loss from this mechanism is very minute. As one sits in a chair, the body's heat is conducted to the chair until the chair warms to a temperature to that of the surface body temperature. After this point, the chair acts as an insulator to prevent further heat loss. Conduction of body heat to the environment represents a larger percentage of heat loss.

## Convection

The movement of air is known as convection and the removal of heat from the body by convection air currents is commonly called *heat loss by convection.* In actuality the heat must first be conducted to the air and then carried away by convection currents. Factors important in cold injury development are temperature of the air and velocity of the wind.

### *Windchill*

When the wind increases, air that lies close to the skin surface is being constantly replaced by cold air, therefore increasing heat loss of the body by convection currents. The wind combined with low temperatures may rapidly cause injury depending on the above factors. The body can usually stand longer periods of cold exposure when there is no wind because no new air layers are being added to the skin, thereby decreasing body heat loss by convection. When the wind is added to the already low temperature, the skin picks up the difference and relates the cold as being colder than it actually is. The term *windchill factor* and associated charts have been developed to estimate what the temperature would be if there were no wind. Table 30–1 shows the combined effect of wind and temperature and the chilling effect it has on the body. Remember that the skin can be injured by the windchill factor by freezing underlying tissues once the surface heat has been lost. The windchill factor can only affect flesh, not inanimate objects such as car engines and wood. Temperatures to

TABLE 30–1. A WIND-CHILL CHART.

*Cooling Power of Wind on Exposed Flesh Expressed as an Equivalent Temperature (under calm conditions)*

| Estimated wind speed (in mph) | Actual Thermometer Reading (°F.) | | | | | | | | | | | |
|---|---|---|---|---|---|---|---|---|---|---|---|---|
| | 50 | 40 | 30 | 20 | 10 | 0 | −10 | −20 | −30 | −40 | −50 | −60 |
| | EQUIVALENT CHILL TEMPERATURE (°F) | | | | | | | | | | | |
| calm | 50 | 40 | 30 | 20 | 10 | 0 | −10 | −20 | −30 | −40 | −50 | −60 |
| 5 | 48 | 37 | 27 | 16 | 6 | −5 | −15 | −26 | −36 | −47 | −57 | −68 |
| 10 | 40 | 28 | 16 | 4 | −9 | −24 | −33 | −46 | −58 | −70 | −83 | −95 |
| 15 | 36 | 22 | 9 | −5 | −18 | −32 | −45 | −58 | −72 | −85 | −99 | −112 |
| 20 | 32 | 18 | 4 | −10 | −25 | −39 | −53 | −67 | 82 | 96 | −110 | −124 |
| 25 | 30 | 16 | 0 | −15 | −29 | −44 | −59 | −74 | −88 | −104 | −118 | −133 |
| 30 | 28 | 13 | −2 | −18 | −33 | −48 | −63 | −79 | −94 | −109 | −125 | −140 |
| 35 | 27 | 11 | −4 | −21 | −35 | −51 | −67 | −82 | −98 | −113 | −129 | −145 |
| 40 | 26 | 10 | −6 | −21 | −37 | −53 | −69 | −85 | −100 | −116 | −132 | −148 |
| (wind speeds greater than 40 mph have little additional effect.) | LITTLE DANGER<br>In < 5 hr with dry skin<br>Maximum danger of false sense of security | | | | Increasing Danger<br>Danger from freezing of exposed flesh within one minute | | | GREAT DANGER<br>Flesh may freeze within 30 seconds | | | | |
| | Trenchfoot and immersion foot may occur at any point on this chart. | | | | | | | | | | | |

INSTRUCTIONS

MEASURE local temperature and wind speed if possible, if not, ESTIMATE. Enter table at closest 5°F interval along the top and with appropriate wind speed along left side. Intersection goves approximate equivalent chill temperature. That is, the temperature that would cause the same rate of cooling under calm conditions., Note that regardless of cooling rate, you do not cool below the actual air temperature unless wet.

these objects are absolute. The cooling effect of wind can be seen in the example when the outside temperature is 5°F, coupled with a ten-mph wind, makes the skin interpret the coldness as 15°F below zero. Every person who may be exposed to environmental extremes for any length of time, for whatever reason, should be cognizant of the cooling effect of the windchill factor and how to interpret its effect by the use of the chart.

### *Water Chill*

Heat transfer in water is about 25 times faster than in air of the same temperature. Water chill therefore, becomes extremely important when a patient has accidentally been immersed in cold water. The EMT should remember, too, that injured patients lying on a cold wet floor, ground, or roadway lose heat rapidly because of the wetness in cold environments. Perspiration-soaked clothing in cold weather is also a dangerous situation because of the rapid heat conduction from the body to the environment.

Table 30-2 shows life expectancy when the body has been submerged in cold water wearing normal clothing.

## Evaporation

When one perspires and the sweat reaches the skin surface, the water vaporizes and evaporates as the wind sweeps across the body. This evaporation further reduces the body temperature. As previously mentioned, perspiration-soaked clothing is a chilling factor in cold environments and should be replaced if possible.

## Respiration

Air that is inhaled in a cold environment is warmed as it enters the lungs. Constant cold air that is being inhaled warmed and exhaled adds to an overall heat loss in cold weather. Fortunately, heat loss from respiration is minimal.

Table 30-2. Water Chill Table (Adapted from *Emergency Medical Services*, July-Aug. 1977, "Immersion Hypothermia," by Alan M. Steinman and Lou Parris)

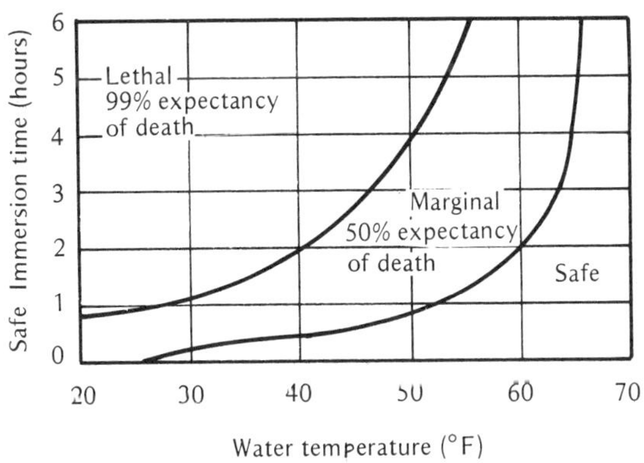

If body heat is allowed to escape from the core, or if the surface (skin) temperature is subjected to the extreme cold for a protracted period of time, general body cooling or local tissue injury may occur. Injury to the body may occur in two general ways when environmental temperatures overcome tissue temperatures:

1. Local tissue injury (frostbite)
   a. Frostnip (incipient frostbite)
   b. Superficial frostbite
   c. Deep frostbite
   d. Trenchfoot
   e. Chilblains
2. General body cooling (hypothermia)
   a. Accidental
   b. Immersion

It is important that the EMT know how frostbite injury ensues so that proper identification and treatment may occur.

## PATHOPHYSIOLOGY OF FROSTBITE

Frozen flesh, the actual damage of frostbite, occurs at the arteriole, capillary, and venule level of the body's circulatory system. Remember that cells of the body are nourished by oxygen in the blood in arterioles given up to the capillaries, then travel through the capillary wall and feed the cells. Carbon dioxide and other waste products are taken back into the capillaries, delivered to the venules and returned to the right side of the heart where the blood is pumped to the lungs for reoxygenation. When the body is chilled, the arterioles constrict to conserve body heat. If the chilling is brief the bloodflow to the capillaries is slowed down or directed to other nearby arterioles and capillaries not yet affected by this chilling response. However, if the chilling is intense, the vasoconstriction in the arterioles in the cold tissues can totally occlude the passage of blood. If this occurs for only a short period of time, no damage occurs because muscle tissue of the body can go for awhile without oxygenation. If the occlusion of blood to the tissue lasts for longer periods of time, the chance of injury to the arteriole itself, and to the surrounding tissue, can be great.

When a capillary bed is chilled to the point of inactivity, the arterial blood bypasses the capillary entirely and travels directly from the arteriole to the venule, a compensatory mechanism of the body called *capillary shunting.* (See Fig. 30–3) This mechanism is the body's last chance effort to keep the chilled area of the body warm and continue the otherwise blocked circulation. Because adjacent areas of tissue are frozen, chilled blood is taken back toward the heart causing an overall general cooling of the core.

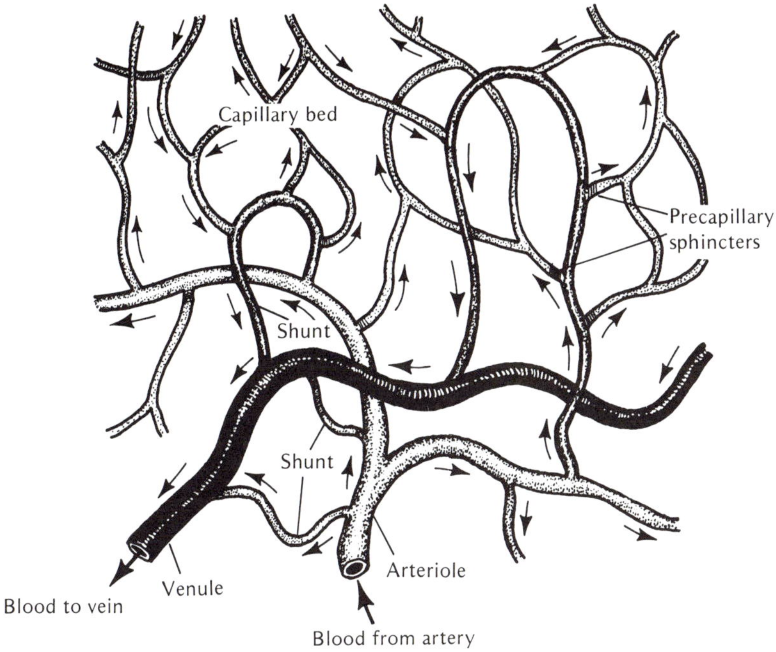


**Figure 30-3.** A capillary bed. Note how blood is shunted from arteriole to venule.

If temperatures are below freezing, tissues will begin to freeze immediately after circulation has been stopped. Ice crystals start to form and grow between the cells (extracellularly). If the source of cold is not removed, these extracellular crystals continue to grow, deriving the water for their growth from the contents of adjacent cells. When this occurs, intracellular dehydration may take place and disrupt normal cell function. Tissues that are highly susceptible to frostbite include muscles, nerves, and blood vessels. Tendons, ligaments, and bone are resistant. It is not necessary for injury to tissue to occur with temperatures below freezing. If conditions are such that coldness exists and stays cold long enough to result in vasoconstriction and prolonged blockage or even a major slowdown of capillary circulation, injury may occur to any exposed area of flesh.

## Local Tissue Injury - Frostbite

### *Incipient Frostbite (Frostnip)*

Frostnip occurs in cold weather and affects those areas of the body usually exposed the most, or peripheral body areas that are farthest from the trunk. They include the nose, ears, cheeks, chin, hands, and feet.

The area affected by frostnip usually turns white (blanches) and has a tingling or burning sensation which gives way to numbness. Frostnip comes on slowly in persons who are active in the outdoors, so that the person may or may not be aware of its occurrence. Because the EMT works in an environment that is less than desirable and under extreme weather conditions when treating patients, it is best to employ the buddy system of frostnip detection when patient evacuation is lengthy in cold weather. With this system, each partner alerts the other as to areas of the body which are starting to turn white from the cold. Frostnip is usually self-limited and the person usually warms himself by blowing warm air into his cupped hands or placing his warm hand over his cheeks or ears. Frostnip can and should be treated, in the field or on the trail, by warming the affected area.

### *Superficial Frostbite*

Frostnip rapidly gives way to superficial frostbite if not noticed and treated. With superficial frostbite the skin and superficial tissue layers beneath the skin become solid from freezing. If you depress the skin gently, though, the deeper tissues will be soft and resilient. The skin will have a white or waxy appearance and will be numb.

After warming, the frostbitten area will first be numb and turn mottled or purple in color. Then the area becomes edematous with a stinging and burning sensation. Blisters may occur and slowly dry up and become hard and black in one and one-half to two weeks. Swelling will usually subside with bedrest, but will persist longer if the affected area is not rested. Throbbing and burning of the affected area may last for weeks depending on the severity of the exposure. After the swelling finally disappears, the skin will peel and remain red and tender, be extremely sensitive to the cold, and perspire abnormally for a long time.

### *Deep Frostbite*

Deep frostbite is the last in the continuum of local cold injury. Damage to the tissues includes the skin, subcutaneous tissue, muscle, and blood vessels. The affected area will be hard and solid and cannot be depressed when touched. The skin color turns pale or gray. After rewarming, tremendous swelling takes place that may last for weeks. Blisters appear in about three days. During this period there will be decreased mobility of the injured part, and a blue violet or grey discoloration of the skin takes place. Sharp throbbing pain may be experienced after the first couple of days and lasts from two weeks to two months. Blistering will finally dry up, turn black and slough off, leaving a very sensitive red layer of new skin which may or may not return to normal. Itching and perspiration may persist for more than six months after the injury, and the frostbitten area will suffer lengthy or permanent sensitivity to cold. In extreme cases of deep frostbite, which have not been rewarmed rapidly, permanent loss of some tissue almost invariably occurs. Gangrene of the tissue usually occurs and the affected part may have to be amputated.

## Incipient Frostbite

Only frostnip may be treated in the field or on the trail. Frostnip can be safely and effectively treated by applying warmth to the affected body part. This may be placing the hands in the armpits or blowing warmed air into them. Parts of the face can be warmed by your hands or your partner's. The only effective way to treat frostnip of the toes or feet is to take off your footgear and rewarm them on the spot. After rewarming, put on dry socks. Remember not to lace back your shoes or footgear tightly. Circulation, as we know, is a determinant in frostbite. The affected area should never be rubbed, as this may cause further damage.

## Superficial and Deep Frostbite

There is absolutely no way to estimate how severe frostbite actually is in the field until after rewarming the injured part. (See Fig. 30-4.) Active rewarming is necessary for superficial and deep frostbite.

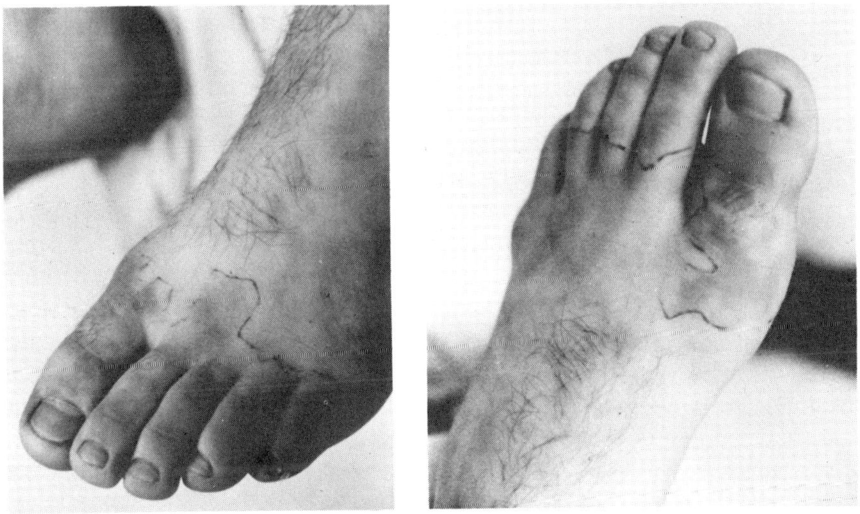

**Figure 30-4.** The EMT-A cannot estimate how severe frostbite injury is in the field. This patient sustained superficial frostbite to both feet; recovery was uneventful. Note the color difference between the toes and rest of the foot. (Courtesy of Gareth Gilkey, M.D., Medicine Dept., Wishard Memorial Hospital)

*When Transportation To a Medical Facility is Imminent*

1. Perform a primary assessment and rule out possible spinal injury. Resuscitate if necessary.

2. Remove the patient from the cold, windy, or wet environment by stretcher or Stokes Basket.

3. Perform a secondary assessment. The coldness of the patient may distract your attention from other illness or injury.

4. Record and monitor vital signs. Take a rectal temperature with a low reading thermometer. The patient may be hypothermic.

5. Remove wet clothing including hats, boots, socks, and replace with warm blankets.

6. Do not rub the affected body parts.

7. Apply oxygen by face mask at 4–6 *l*/min.

8. Transport patient in a fashion that is comfortable to him.

9. Remember that the frostbitten parts have no feeling. Place them in a comfortable position without putting any pressure on the area.

10. Alert the designated medical facility as to the nature of your patient's illness or injury.

*When Transportation to a Medical Facility is Not Possible*

If afield, keep the patient walking as long as possible. Even if the body part is frozen, walking will not injure it any more than it already is. Once you can get to shelter or a home, active rewarming must be instituted. The affected frostbite areas must be immersed in a warm water bath for thawing. Remove wet clothing and replace it with dry articles or cover the patient with warm blankets.

With a thermometer, warm a container of water to 100°F–105°F (37.7°C–40.5°C). The water should be heated separately by fire or stove and then added to the container. Place the affected parts (usually the extremities) in the warmed water. Do not let him touch the sides of the container. The water should completely surround the frozen parts. Once the frozen parts enter the water it will reduce the temperature. Warm water will have to be added periodically to keep the temperature between 100°–105°F. When replacing warm water, remove the extremities and stir the added water to maintain constant temperature throughout the container. Because the patient has no pain perception, it is always best to remove the frozen parts while adding warm water. Rewarming takes about thirty to sixty minutes. As the affected area begins to thaw (approximately ten minutes) there will be no pain, but toward the end of thawing, the part will start to throb, burn and ache. Since this will be quite uncomfortable, analgesics may be necessary.

After thawing, the part should be covered lightly with sterile dressings after patting the skin dry. Cotton or gauze should be placed between the fingers or toes to keep adjacent skin areas from contacting each other.



If transport can be instituted to a medical facility, carry the victim to the emergency unit, elevate the injured area and keep the patient warm.

## General Treatment

1. If the frostbitten part is warmed or thawed on the trail or in the field, the victim at that point becomes a stretcher case and must be carried. If he is allowed to walk, serious loss of tissue will be almost certain to occur.

2. If the patient is conscious and has a good airway, have him drink warm fluids.

3. Do not let the patient drink alcohol or smoke.

4. Never rub or massage a frostbitten part.

5. Never rub the area with snow or try to thaw the area in cold water.

6. When rewarming the affected area, never add water warmer than 105°F.

7. Do not let the patient test the warm water with the frozen part. Always test it with a thermometer.

8. Do not try and rewarm the affected area by exercising it. This may increase tissue damage.

9. If blister formation occurs, do not rupture or pick them.

10. Use a nonalcoholic-base antiseptic solution when cleansing the rewarmed part.

11. Never cut off any tissue, even if it looks dead.

## Prevention of Frostbite

Being in sound physical condition, utilizing proper clothing, and using common sense are the best assurances against frostbite. Chances of frostbite are increased with injury, illness, hunger, hypoxia, and exhaustion. Following these suggested tips will reduce the chance of frostbite in the field:

1. Dress according to weather conditions to maintain general body heat. In cold winds and wet environments, protect the head, neck, inguinal and axillary regions or those areas from which considerable body heat may be lost. Unprotected body parts in environmental extremes promote rapid heat loss through radiation. The amount of heat loss from an unprotected head for example, in ratio to the total body heat loss, has been estimated to be the following:

| *Temperature* | *Heat Loss* |
|---|---|
| at 60°F (15.5°C) | 33% |
| at 40°F (4.4°C) | 50% |
| at 5°F (−15°C) | 75% |

2. Avoid clothing that binds or is so tight that circulation is impaired, especially on the hands and feet.

3. Follow the layer principle of wearing clothes. Dress by wearing several shirts, vest, and coat. If perspiration occurs, remove a layer of clothing. Keep feet and hands dry.

4. Never touch metal objects with bare skin in extreme or moderate cold temperatures when the hands are moist or wet. Caution should be used when loading cameras or handling fuels. The freezing point of gasoline is near −70°F and its rapid rate of evaporation as well as its extreme chill makes it dangerous.

5. Do not smoke or use alcohol in cold environments.

6. Eat plenty of the right kinds of food to maximize output of body heat. At low altitudes in cold weather, fats and carbohydrates should be ingested. Proteins are least important as a high energy food for heat. At altitudes above 10,000 feet, carbohydrates are most important. Digestion takes place differently in people at higher altitudes.

7. Toenails and fingernails should be kept trimmed to a reasonable length.

8. Blisters should never be ruptured.

9. Gloves or mittens made of horsehide should not be worn since they tend to dry out very stiff after being wet.

10. If you become frostbitten afield, try to keep calm. The increased anxiety will cause you to perspire causing further chilling.

11. If you have been the victim of frostbite before, take great care to protect the area from further damage.

12. Always have your tetanus toxoid vaccination up to date.

## OTHER COLD-RELATED INJURIES

### Chilblains

Chilblains are lesions that occur to bare skin surfaces when exposed to temperatures of 60°F (15.5°C) or cooler for prolonged periods of time. The injury to those affected areas, usually the hands or feet, take form as red, swollen, tender, and hot areas that itch. Thses signs are due to injury of the skin layers and peripheral capillary circulation impairment. Chilblains are chronic and recur in the same body areas during cold weather.

Women and children are most often affected because of the constant unprotected exposure of bare areas such as the legs. Once the skin and capillary damage has been established, there is no treatment other than to protect the affected areas when exposed to the cold and prevent reoccurrence.

## Trenchfoot - Immersion Foot

Trenchfoot is an injury that develops in the lower extremities when exposed for long periods of time (hours to days) to water or mud at temperatures between 32°F and 50°F (0°C–10°C).

The primary damage occurs at the capillary circulation level, which is impaired, causing injury to the skin, subcutaneous tissue, nerves, and muscles. Tissue necrosis and gangrene may be the aftermath of extended exposure.

The affected area will be waxy white, mottled, cold and swollen with numbness. Clothing and footgear should be removed and replaced with dry, warm clothes or blankets. The injured area should be gently rewarmed and cleaned with a nonalcoholic solution, after which it should be covered with a sterile dressing. After rewarming, the extremity will become red and swollen and blisters may form. Because of the possible skin, nerve, and muscle damage, the affected area may be impaired for months or years after exposure causing disability.

## Systemic Hypothermia

Systemic hypothermia or general body cooling results when the body's core temperature falls below 95°F (35°C.)

As previously discussed, the body may lose heat in a number of ways when unprotected or as a natural physical phenomenon. As a review, they include radiation, conduction, convection, evaporation, and respiration. When the body cannot compensate for these heat loses, both the shell (skin) and core (internal organs) body temperature drops, resulting in a hypothermic state. In frostbite only the shell temperature drops, creating local tissue damage but the core temperature is maintained.

## Predisposing Factors

Hypothermia is generally discussed in two types of settings, hypothermia by accident and by water immersion. Besides the natural physical phenomena of heat loss, other factors come into play that may predispose the patient to hypothermia.

### *Accidental*

Accidental hypothermia occurs when there is a drop in core temperature where the body is exposed to a cold, windy, or wet environment. Accompanied with the above setting, the patient very often has an acute medical problem but his heat-regulating center is not affected. This is often seen in the elderly, neonates, alcoholics, the unconscious, drugged, or immobile, and the patient who becomes exhausted while exposed to a cold environment.

*Elderly*

The elderly are more susceptible to accidental hypothermia for several reasons. The aged lose important compensatory mechanisms that increase heat production when going from a warm to a cold environment. Their peripheral vessels do not constrict adequately to contain body heat; therefore, they have frequent feelings of coldness. Because of age, they may be less mobile causing a decrease in muscle activity and, therefore, not generate much heat.

*Neonate*

The neonate has similar problems when exposed to a cold environment because developmental changes to generate sufficient heat have not occurred. They have less body insulation in the form of subcutaneous fat; they have an inadequate ability to shiver; and they have a larger surface-to-body-mass ratio making heat loss occur more rapidly. This is one of the reasons why newborns should be warmly wrapped in the field after delivery. The development of accidental hypothermia is even a greater risk in premature or low-birth-weight infants.

*Alcoholic*

Hypothermia is seen more often in the alcoholic than any other type of patient in the United States. The main reason for this is that after alcohol ingestion, the patient has a euphoric warm feeling when out in a cold environment. Alcohol gives this warm feeling because it dilates peripheral vessels and therefore heat is dissipated quickly. As the patient passes out or falls asleep in the alleyway or a snowbank, or off the roadside in a car, he may die of hypothermia. Alcohol depresses the central nervous system and acts as an anesthetic to decrease sensation and motor function. It is not surprising that so many intoxicated and alcoholic patients are treated for and die from cold exposure.

*Drugs*

Some drugs interfere with the body's ability to either generate or conserve heat. (See Table 30–3.) Patients who have been prescribed these medications should take necessary precautions in cold weather.

*Illness/Injury*

All victims of illness or injury found down in the field, exposed to a cold environment for a protracted period of time, should always be suspected for hypothermia. Automobile accident victims are often subject to prolonged stays in extreme weather conditions, awaiting the arrival of

TABLE 30-3. DRUGS THAT MAY LOWER BODY TEMPERATURE

| | |
|---|---|
| **A. *Antidepressants*** | |
| Adapin | Nardil |
| Amtryl | Norpramin |
| Aventyl | Pamelor |
| Deprol | Parnate |
| Elavil | Pertofrane |
| Endep | Presamine |
| Etrafan | Sinequan |
| Imavate | Tofranil |
| Limbitrol | Triavil |
| Marplan | Vivactil |
| **B. *Barbiturates*** | |
| Alurate | Kinesed |
| Belap | Levsin |
| Butabarbital | Levsinex |
| Buticaps | Mebaral |
| Butisol | Nembutal |
| Carbrital | Oxoids |
| Donnatal | Plexonal |
| Donphen | Repan |
| **C. *Psycho-Sedatives*** | |
| 1. *Meprobamates* | |
| Equagesic | Miltown |
| Equanil | Miltrate |
| Meprobamate | PMB |
| Meprospan | Pathibamate |
| Milpath | SK-Bamate |
| Milprem | |
| 2. *Phenothiazines* | |
| Chlorpromazine | Prolixin |
| Compazine | Stelazine |
| Mellaril | Temaril |
| Phenergan | Thorazine |
| Pro-Banthine | Vesprin |
| **D. *Tranquilizers*** | |
| Ativan | Valium |
| Serax | Verstran |
| Tranxene | |

(Adapted from *Cold-Related Injuries.* John Goll, Wishard Memorial Ambulance Service)

aid. These patients should be protected against the cold, windy, and wet conditions as rapidly as possible.

### *Emotionally Disturbed*

The emotionally disturbed patient is also a great risk to cold exposure. This is because the patient may have an altered sense of the existing environment, and he is probably on some type of medication that will lower his body temperature.

The EMT must remember that a cold environment is not a requirement for hypothermia to develop. Factors such as wind velocity, moisture, clothing, duration of exposure, poor physical condition, illness, and injury comprise important roles in hypothermia. Most victims are stricken in temperatures between 30°F to 50°F (−1°C–10°C).

*Immersion*

Depending on weather conditions, physical condition, body size, clothing and water temperature, a person may develop hypothermia after being submerged in cold water.

Generally, all patients should be considered hypothermic when involuntarily submerged in cold water. At temperatures of 50°F (10°C) or lower, a person may develop hypothermia in a very few minutes. Immersion hypothermia, unlike accidental hypothermia, is rapid depending on weather and temperature conditions. Cold water that surrounds the body causes heat loss about twenty-five times faster than heat loss by air. Accidental and immersion hypothermia are treated in the same manner.

## SIGNS AND SYMPTOMS OF HYPOTHERMIA

As the body temperature begins to drop below 95°F (35°C), the patient will start to exhibit different signs and symptoms. These changes can be broken down into several stages of developmental hypothermia.

| *Stage* | *Core Temperature* | *Signs/Symptoms* |
|---|---|---|
| Mild | 98.6–95°F (37–35°C) | Initially B/P, pulse and respiration increase. Fatigue, sensation of coldness. Shivering (may be delayed or absent). |
| Moderate | 95°–90°F (35–32°C) | B/P, pulse and respirations start to decrease. Difficult speech, loss of hand control. Memory lapse, mood changes, combative; may have violent shivering. |
| Marked<br>Harsh movement of the patient at this stage may cause ventricular fibrillation | 90–82°F(32–28°C) | B/P and pulse may be imperceptible, respirations hard to detect, pupils dilated, amnesia, shivering decreased to constant muscle tension or rigidity. Heart irregularities; tachycardia, or bradycradia may exist. Acetone odor to breath. The characteristic "J" or Osborne Wave of hypothermia starts to appear on the ECG. (See Fig. 30-5.) |
| Severe | 82–77°F (28–25°C) | Irrationality proceeding to unconsciousness. Muscle rigidity similar to *rigor mortis*. Skin may be edematous and cyanotic, loss of reflexes. Pulmonary edema may develop. The "J" or Osborne Wave becomes more prominent. Bradycardia leading to ventricular fibrillation likely. |
| Profound | 77°F or below (25°C) | Cardiopulmonary arrest. Death. |

The primary goals in the treatment of the hypothermic patient are to increase the core temperature to normal values and to protect the patient from further chilling. It is important to realize that the hypothermic patient has lost the ability to generate his own heat and that the EMT must provide the necessary heat for him. There are two major ways in which heat may be added to the victim: by *external* means and *internally*. External methods of rewarming include warm water baths, hot water bottle, electric blanket, camp fires, and any other means by which external heat can be radiated to the victim.

Internal rewarming is usually performed in those medical facilities that have experience with hypothermic care and can provide more extensive therapy, such as peritoneal dialysis, warm water enemas, warm gastric lavage (lah-vahzh'), cardiopulmonary bypass (in cardiac arrest), warm IV fluids, warmed humidified oxygen, intrathoracic irrigation with a warmed solution, and drinking warm fluids.

Most of the time the EMT will be able to transport the patient to a medical facility without much delay. In those situations in which evacuation is imminent and there will be no delay to the hospital, perform a rapid primary assessment before moving the patient. Check the ABCs and rule out spinal injury. With care, place the patient on a stretcher and carry him to the emergency transport unit, for completion of the secondary survey. The patient compartment should be as warm as possible. Remove all wet clothing from the patient very gently. It is better to cut the clothing; avoiding jerky movement created by tugging and pulling of his clothes. (Remember that at temperatures between 82°–90° the heart becomes very irritable and that mechanical stimulation may cause the heart to fibrillate.) A warm blanket should be placed on the stretcher so that the patient has an insulated layer on which to lie. Remove wet clothing and cover the patient with warm dry blankets. The EMT should attempt to get all baseline vital signs including a rectal temperature. (All emergency units should carry a low reading thermometer which registers below 92°F ((33.3°C). If the patient is unconscious, place him in a left-lateral position. If he is conscious, a semi-Fowler's position is fine. In any state, oxygenation is important (4–6 *l*/per min. by face mask should be administered). Airway suctioning may be necessary because decreased body temperature decreases the cough reflex and increases respiratory secretions. If the hypothermic patient has shallow breathing, it does not necessarily mean that respiratory difficulty exists. Because of the cold state of the body, metabolism is decreased; therefore, the body needs less oxygen. Unnecessary use of mechanical airways including endotracheal intubation may cause ventricular fibrillation or a more depressed respiratory rate. Warm oxygen may help to raise the core temperature while enroute to the medical facility. Oxygen from a standard source run through a warm water bath of 47°C will make the delivery temperature of oxygen to the patient at about 40°C. (There is a commercially available device that can be connected to standard oxygen in ambulances and helicopters.)

If the patient is conscious, do not let him perform any work; have him lie quietly. If warm drinks are available and his airway is clear, have him drink, as this will help increase his core temperature. The patient should be checked for frostbite, as it often accompanies hypothermia. Other possible injuries should be looked for as well. The coldness of the patient often distracts the EMT from identifying other problems. Vital signs should be monitored every five to ten minutes and irregularities noted on the patient's report form.

Patients with core temperatures below 90°F (32°C) are often mistaken for a DOA because of dilated pupils, muscle rigidity, no audible heart beat, decreased respiratory rate, and a very slow pulse. If you start CPR on a hypothermic patient who is not in cardiac arrest, the mechanical stimulation of chest compressions may cause the patient to develop ventricular fibrillation. If possible, monitor the heart rate by taking an ECG. This may be the only sure way of detecting a heart beat. Arrhythmias are common such as atrial fibrillation, atrial flutter, tachycardias, or bradycardias. The characteristic "J" or Osborne wave may be noted following the QRS wave on the ECG. (See Fig. 30–5.) If the patient is in cardiopulmonary arrest, start CPR and continue until arrival at the hospital. Efforts to cardiovert the cold patient will probably be unsuccessful because the heart has to be rewarmed before successful cardioversion.

If the hypothermic patient is in cardiac arrest, continue resuscitation measures no matter how bad the patient may seem. These patients have survived after twelve to fifteen hours of CPR without deleterious effects.

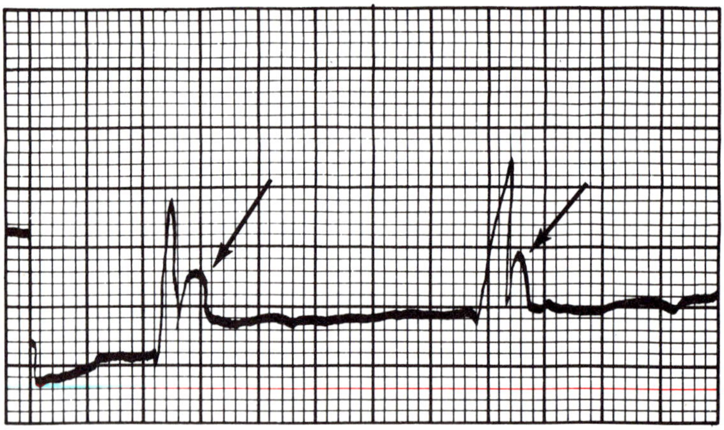

**Figure 30–5.** The characteristic "J" or Osborne wave of hypothermia.

Remember their chances are better than the normothermic patient because they require minimal oxygen. The EMT should remember that no hypothermic patient is a dead patient until *warm and dead*!

During transport the driver should avoid bumps and turns as much as possible; sudden starts and stops should be kept to a minimum. The heart is irritable and may develop ventricular fibrillation. You should always alert the designated hospital regarding the patient you will be bringing them.

When evacuation by helicopter is going to be instituted, make certain that the immersed hypothermic patient is well protected. Remember that wind causes a tremendous increase in the rate of evaporation and heat loss. A one-hundred mph wind can be generated from the rotor wash of a helicopter. If an immersion victim is to be transported by helicopter, windproof the patient as best as possible, especially around the head and neck.

If the patient cannot be evacuated to a medical facility within a reasonable period of time, start rewarming procedures as soon as possible. In back country, make camp as soon as possible. Remove the patient from the cold, windy, or wet environment. Replace wet clothing with dry clothes, preferably those with insulating properties, such as wool, fiberfill, or down. If the patient is conscious, have him drink warm fluids and eat easily digestible, high carbohydrate foods. If a fire can be started, have the victim absorb as much of the radiant heat as possible by placing a heat reflector behind him. Another way of providing heat to the patient in adverse field conditions is to sandwich the victim against one or two normothermic persons and wrapping them in a sleeping bag or blankets. If hot stones or other warm substitutes are available, place them on the blanket-covered body where there is least insulation, namely the inguinal area, lateral chest area, and around the neck. Cover the patient once again to keep the heat in.

If the patient cannot get to a medical facility, but can get to a shelter such as a cabin, home, or place where water can be heated, start rewarming as follows. Replace wet clothing with dry, insulated ones. If the patient is conscious, have him drink warm drinks and eat easily digestible, high-carbohydrate foods. Heat from hot water bottles, or electric blankets will help. Immersing the victim in a warm bath may help raise the core temperature rapidly. (See Fig. 30-6.) However, rewarming a patient too fast can be hazardous. This is termed *rewarming shock.* As the core is warmed rapidly, the blood moves to the peripheral circulation where it is still cold and where the tissues are acidic from anaerobic metabolism. As the blood moves back to the heart, it is cooled again and further chills the patient. Likewise, the acidic cold blood is pumped through the heart, making the heart susceptible to ventricular fibrillation. The patient's chance of survival depends on rewarming. If warm water immersion is to be used, heat the water to 105°–110°F, not any hotter. Keep the victim's arms and legs out of the container for the first thirty minutes, and continue adding warm water, making sure it is between 105–110°F.

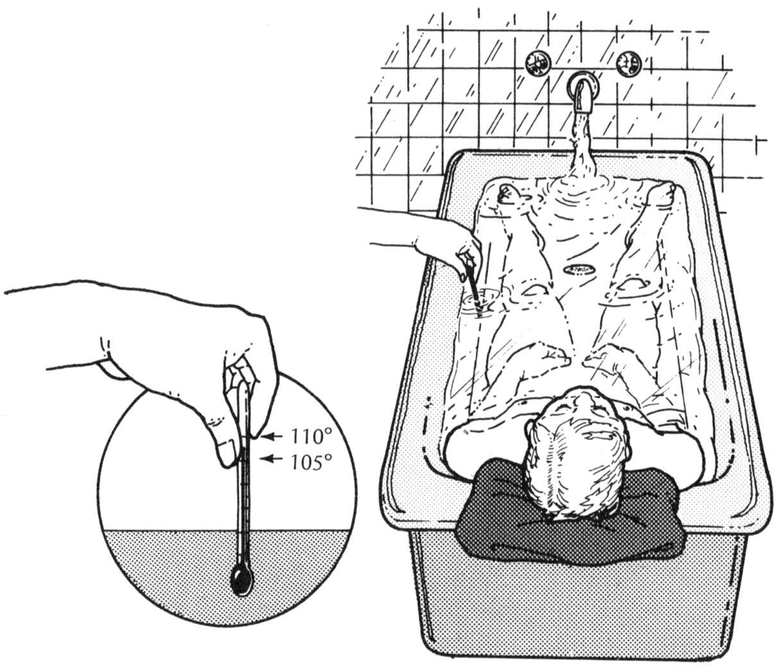


**Figure 30-6.** Warm water immersion of the hypothermia patient must be done slowly to avoid rewarming shock. The EMT-A should maintain water temperature between 105°–110°F.

*References*

American Academy of Orthopedic Surgeons, Committee on Allied Health. *Emergency Care of the Sick and Injured,* 2nd ed., pp. 309–316. Chicago, IL: American Academy of Orthopedic Surgeons, 1977.

Avery, W. M. and Fairall, L. A. "Hypothermia: The Silent Killer," *Emerg. Med. Services* 26–29, Jan/Feb 1979.

Bangs, C. C., "Dos and Don'ts of Immediate Treatment," *RN,* pp. 42–44, Nov. 1979.

Bangs, C. "Early Recognition and Treatment of Cold Injuries." Proceedings of Mountain Medical Symposium, Yosemite Institute, 1975.

"Chilled to the Core," pp. 173–175. *Emergency Medicine,* Jan. 15, 1979.

Day, R. L.; Caliguiri, L.; Kamenski, C.; Ehlich, F. "Body Temperature and Survival of Premature Infants," *Pediatrics* 34:171–181, 1964.

Freinkel, N.; Singer, D. L.; Arky, R. A.; Bleicher, S. T.; Anderson, J. B.; Silbert, C. K. "Alcohol Hypoglycemia in Carbohydrate Metabolism of Patients With Clinical Alcohol Hypoglycemia and the Experimental Reproduction of the Syndrome With Pure Ethanol," *J. Clin. Invest* 42: 1112–1133, 1963.

Goll, J. "Drugs That Affect Body Temperature." Indianapolis IN: Wishard Memorial Hospital, August 1980.

Grant, H. D. and Murray, R. H., Jr. *Emergency Care,* 2nd ed., pp. 378–385. Bowie, MD: Robert J. Brady Co., 1978.

Guyton, A. C. *Textbook of Medical Physiology*, 4th ed., pp. 831–843. Philadelphia, PA: W. B. Saunders Company, 1971.

McSwain, N. E. "Thermal Control Due to Environmental Extremes," *The EMT Journal*, pp. 63–67, December 1978.

Motil, K. J., and Blackburn, M. G. "Temperature Regulation in the Neonate," *Clinical Pediatrics*, 12:634–639, Philadelphia, PA: 1973.

Reuler, J. B. "Hypothermia: Pathophysiology, Clinical Settings and Management," *Annals of Int. Med.*, 891:519–527, 1978.

Steinman, A. M. "Immersion Hypothermia," *Emergency Med. Services*, pp. 22–25, July/August 1977.

Stine, R. J. "Accidental Hypothermia," *JACEP* 6:9, pp. 413–516, Sept. 1977.

Volker, C., and Bunce, G. "Hypothermia—The Cold Weather Killer," *Emergency Med. Serv.*, pp. 46–49, Feb. 1978.

Washburn, B. "Frostbite: What It Is, How to Prevent It—Emergency Treatment," pp. 4–22, A publication of the Museum of Science, Boston, 1975.

Weyman, A. E.; Greenbaum, D. M.; Grace W. J. "Accidental Hypothermia In an Alcoholic Population," *Am. J. Med.*, 56:13–21, 1974.

# Chapter 31

# Bites, Stings, and Irritations From Arthropods

There is no place in North America where human beings are totally free from the toxic or irritating effects of arthropods (invertebrate animals such as insects, spiders, and crustaceans). Although rare, some arthropods (ar′thro-podz) pose a serious threat to life mainly due to the allergic response to their venom or saliva. Other arthropods have irritating or annoying effects to people and do not present a great medical concern. (See Table 31–1.)

The EMT should not only be able to treat the patient with local or systemic effects induced by a venomous or irritating arthropod, but be able to possibly identify it. Just as identification of pills or liquids are important in ingestion poisonings, so is the identification of the arthropod who has injected his potential poison. On occasion, the EMT will be in the environmental setting where the bite, sting, or irritating injury has taken place. If possible, the EMT should bring the offender to the hospital along with the patient for positive identification. One should not go out of the way, however, to capture the offending arthropod and thus lose sight of properly attending to the patient!

The EMT will observe some of the worst living conditions. These living conditions harbor many kinds of disease-transmitting arthropods that affect people (especially if cats, dogs and other animals abound), such as lice, fleas, ticks, bed bugs, spiders, and other arthropods that thrive in trash-strewn surroundings. The EMT should be alert to the presence of the arthropods and report their possible effects on the patient to the attending nurse or physician at the medical facility.

Most arthropods are active from May through October and therefore, more calls for first aid will be through these months. However, some arthropods are active the year around. As a general rule, most venomous and irritating arthropods are prevalent in the southern half of the United States. This is because of the more mild environmental conditions and benign winters. Arthropods that harm or irritate man do so either by biting, stinging, or both. Generally, a bite is an offensive maneuver used to obtain food. The bite is intended to kill or anesthetize a victim for the purpose of nourishment. A sting is used by certain arthropods as a defensive maneuver and is not intended to kill its victim. Therefore, the lethal mixture of venom in certain snakes and spiders contribute to the more severe medical problems encountered with their inflictions. Whereas the stings from bees, wasps, hornets, etc. are less potent in venom, their medical consideration comes from within our bodies to the potential allergic reaction we have to the protein fraction of the venom of the arthropod. Signs, symptoms, and treatment of arthropod injuries are found in Table 31–2.

## STINGS FROM ARTHROPODS

### The Hymenoptera—Bees, Wasps, Yellow Jackets, Hornets, and Ants

This insect order is of medical importance to us because the stings from Hymenoptera (hi″men-op′ter-ah) cause twice as many deaths as from the bites of rattlesnakes. This is due primarily to the allergic response the victim has to the injected venom. These insects sting their victims as a defensive maneuver. A sting is caused by the anatomical injection of a device known as a stinger into the flesh of a victim. For the most part, the stinger is a defense weapon used as a vehicle for venom, and differs in form and location from one insect species to another. Bees, wasps, yellow jackets, hornets, and fire ants have a stinger, which connects with a venom gland, located in the terminal portion of their abdomen. Stings can only be incurred by the female species, since the stinger is a modification of her egg-depositing organ.

About 50 percent of the deaths that occur from this group of insects are attributed to the honey bee. (See Fig. 31–1a.) Most of these deaths occur within the first hour after the sting. The honey bee's stinger, unlike other stinging insects in this group, is barbed (see Fig. 31–1b), so, once injected into the flesh of its victim, it becomes anchored. Therefore, when an attempt is made by the insect to fly or crawl away or when it is brushed off, it loses a portion of the posterior abdominal contents, including the venom sac that connects it to the stinger. Because of this trauma, the bee subsequently dies. If the EMT arrives at the scene and the patient has a honey bee stinger still attached, he should scrape the stinger off the victim. This can be done by using the fingernail, a knife, or some other sharp-edged object. (If a knife is used, caution should be used to avoid cutting the patient!) If the stinger is pulled off the victim, the squeezing grip on the venom sac will force more venom into the wound of the patient. The remaining group of insects (wasps, yellow jackets, hornets, and ants) (see Fig. 31–2) do not have barbed stingers and, therefore, have the ability to

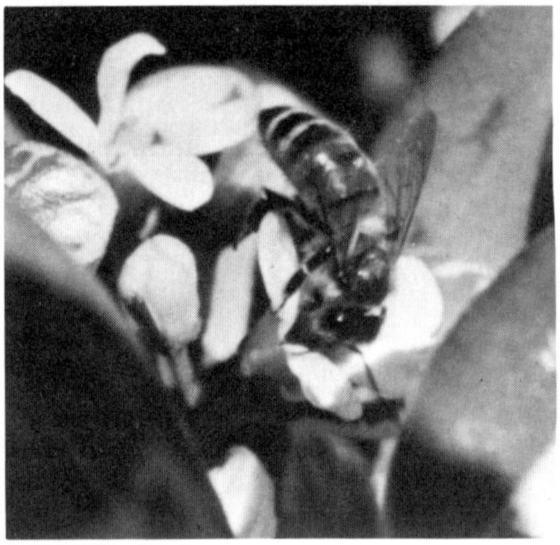

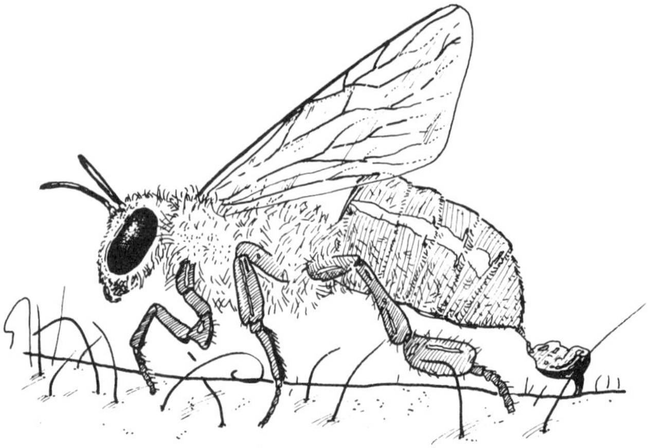

(a) (b)

**Figure 31-1.** (a) The honeybee. (b) Because the stinger of the honeybee is barbed, it becomes anchored in the skin.

sting their victims repeatedly, injecting more venom into the wound. This group of insects tend to swarm their victim, especially when their nesting quarters are disturbed, some species being more aggressive than others (yellow jackets and velvet ants).

*Venom*

Each species has its own distinct toxin, although there are some similarities. The venom of Hymenoptera contains a complex mixture of enzymes and nonemzymatic proteins which interact with human body tissues, causing local to severe reactions. Certain body chemicals

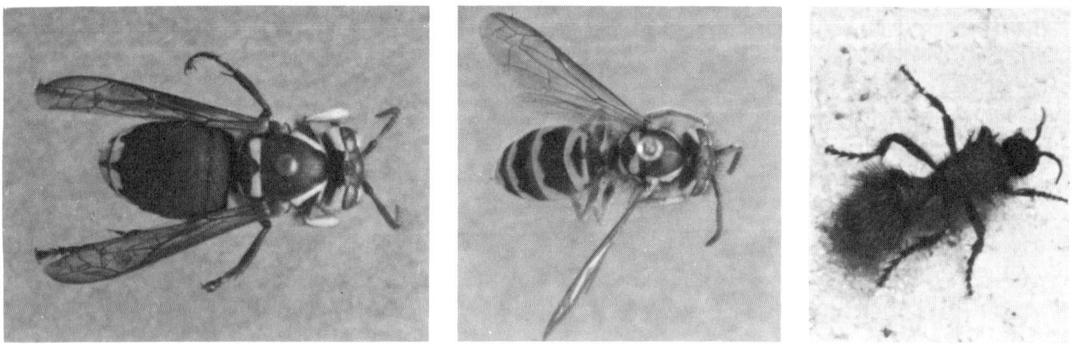

(a) (b) (c)

**Figure 31-2.** (a) Bald-faced hornet; (b) yellow jacket; (c) velvet ant. (Courtesy of Terry L. Biery, Captain, USAFR, BSC, Rickenbacker AFB, Ohio) (histamine, kinin, etc.) are released in response to the foreign protein in venom and if the victim is hypersensitive to the venom, he may develop an anaphylactic (an″ah-fı-lak′tik) shock reaction within minutes.

## Ants

Female ants have a stinger at the posterior tip of the abdomen. Species that can be quite dangerous in the U.S. include the fire ants (Solenopsis) and harvester ants (Pogonomyrmex). Both species can be easily identified by the mounds they build. The fire ant builds his mound high (three to thirty-six inches), leaving vegetation undisturbed around the home. (See Fig. 31–3a.) Harvester ants build a rather flat or slightly elevated mound and usually destroy all vegetation around their home (two to ten feet in diameter). (See Fig. 31–3b.) Harvester ants are also two to three times larger than fire ants. These ants are predominately found in the southern half of the U.S. They will attack in mass when their mounds are disturbed, the worker ants taking up the defense. These insects can sting repeatedly and can bite as well. Thousands of these ants can attack within minutes. It is no wonder why some deaths have been reported, due to envenomation of these ants. Intoxicated individuals have been known to pass out near ant mounds or "sleep it off" on the mound because of the softness of the mound, only to awaken with hundreds of stings! Anaphylactic shock is the greatest medical concern with envenomation.

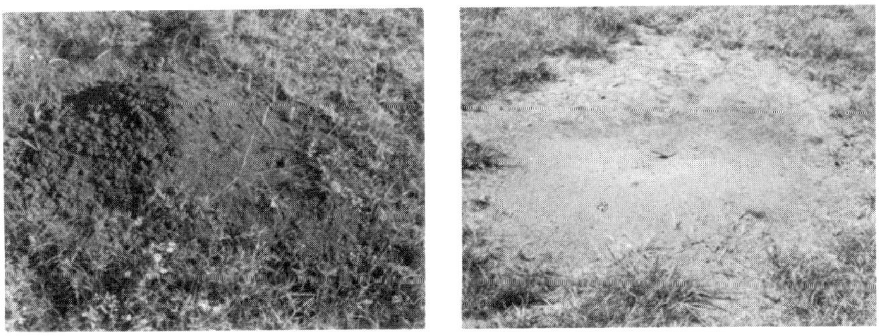

(a) (b)

**Figure 31–3.** (a) Fire ant mound; (b) Harvester ant mound. (Courtesy of Terry L. Biery, Captain, USAFR, BSC, Rickenbacker AFB, Ohio)

## Scorpion Stings

Scorpions are relatives of spiders and all are poisonous, some species more so than others. There are approximately forty species of scorpions in the U.S. Of these, only one is known to possess lethal venom, the sculptured scorpion (Centruroides sculpturatus). This deadly species is localized to Arizona and its neighboring states. Stings from scorpions are a

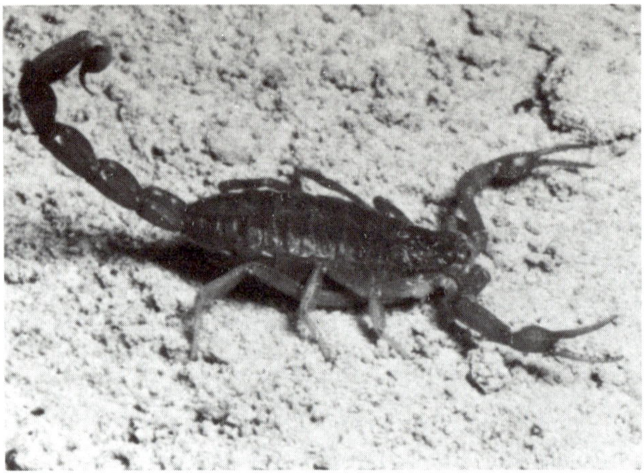

**Figure 31-4.** Scorpions are most prevalent in warmer climates. This poisonous species is found in Arizona. (Courtesy of Terry L. Biery, Captain, USAFR, BSC, Rickenbacker AFB, Ohio)

problem of considerable medical importance in Arizona, since scorpions kill more people than do poisonous snakes. Scorpions have their stinger or telson located at the terminal portion of their tails. (See Fig. 31-4.) They are nocturnal creatures and hide by day under rocks, leaves, lumber, and other similar places when outdoors. Favorite haunts when indoors include closets, shoes, stored newspapers, and cluttered areas. Children are stung more often than adults, which probably accounts for the high mortality rate. Most stings occur to the hands or feet of the victim.

The venom of the sculptured scorpion is principally neurotoxic. This accounts for the minimal local tissue reaction when stung. Death may occur due to respiratory and circulatory collapse.

## BITES FROM ARTHROPODS

A bite from an arthropod is caused by vicelike jaws (Chelicera) or a beak that pierces the flesh of a victim. The bite from different species of arthropods affects each person differently and the signs and symptoms from their toxin or saliva will vary considerably. The variations are based on these factors:

1. Location of the bite
2. Allergic reaction
3. Toxic chemical composition in the injected saliva
4. Bacterial infection of the wound

5. Immunity development

6. Retention of the bits and pieces of the animals' mouth parts in the wound

Arthropods in this category that bite or pierce the skin of their victims include: ticks, spiders, centipedes, true bugs, mites, and flies.

## Ticks

These eight-legged creatures are relatives to the spider and first cousins of insects. They can be found almost anywhere on earth, primarily along pathways in the woods and on uncleared land. They feed entirely on blood, usually of animals, but sometimes of humans. Once on the body they attach (usually the head, neck, and groin) by burrowing their heads into the skin of the victim (host) to feed on their blood. With their barbed piercing organs, they take a firm grip on the skin and suck blood for anywhere from fifteen minutes to several days, until they are full.

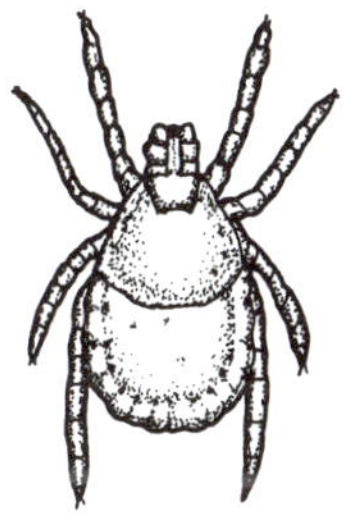

**Figure 31–5.** The wood tick.

The body of this spider relative is very flat, when not engorged with blood, and is difficult to feel when it crawls over the skin and hard to locate once embedded in hairy areas of the body. (See Fig. 31–5.) While most tick bites are not painful, and the victim may not even be aware he is being fed upon, the wounds caused by the bites of some species are severe. The wood tick (*Dermacentor andersoni*) is responsible for tick paralysis. Tick paralysis is due to the neurotoxin introduced in the victim while the tick is feeding. The victim of tick paralysis becomes very irritable, does not eat, and generally feels sick. Intermittent bouts of pain begin in the lower extremities, followed by ascending flaccid paralysis. If the paralysis reaches the respiratory system, the patient will die from respiratory failure. If the offending tick is found and removed, the symptoms will disappear.

Ticks also carry spotted fever, tularemia, relapsing fever, and a number of other diseases. In areas infested with ticks, it is unwise to sleep or sit on the ground. Clothing should be examined carefully at least once a day and ticks destroyed. When children play outdoors in wooded places, they should be inspected twice a day, and any ticks that have attached themselves should be removed carefully.

*Removal*

If the tick is swollen from feeding, special care should be taken not to crush it, so the skin is smeared. A slow, steady pull with tweezers will usually make the tick release his grip. Because the tick has breathing holes on both sides of his body, a dab of petroleum jelly or fingernail polish will cause him to withdraw his mouth parts in a few minutes, so he can be removed more easily. The EMT should wait a full ten minutes before removal procedures are initiated. In this way, one can be almost certain that resistance will be minimal and all of the tick will be removed.

*Treatment*

After the tick is removed, the EMT should place the offender in a container and bring it along with the patient. The wound should be wiped with an antiseptic solution. The EMT should make certain that he washes his hands and tweezers (if used) with soap and water or rinses them with alcohol.

In areas where ticks are a problem, the EMT should check each patient for infestation and remove them.

## Spiders

Almost all spiders are poisonous, but most are too small to harm man. Spiders have fangs connected to their jaws associated with a venom gland. Like most biting arthropods, spiders use their fangs to inject venom into their prey to anesthetize (ah-nes′the-tiz) it, then feed upon their body fluid for nourishment.

In the U.S. only two species of spiders are of considerable medical importance:

1. the black widow (Lactrodectus mactans)
2. the brown recluse (Loxosceles reclusa)

These spiders are venomous and can cause medical grief when not identified by the victim or EMT as the cause or injury of illness.

*Black Widow Spiders*

These spiders are found in every state except Alaska. They are more prevalent, however, in the southeastern portion of the United States. Like most venomous arthropods, the female species of the black widow spider creates the greatest medical concern. Although the male species has lethal venom, he is one-fifth to one-third her size and his bite cannot penetrate the thickness of skin. This shiny black spider is approximately one-half inch long and has a characteristic reddish orange hour glass on the underside of her round abdomen. This characteristic marking does have some variations. There could be only a red button or two red dots. (See Fig. 31–6.) The black widow spins her irregularly shaped web near the ground as a general rule. Other web sites, however, can be found in wood piles, loose

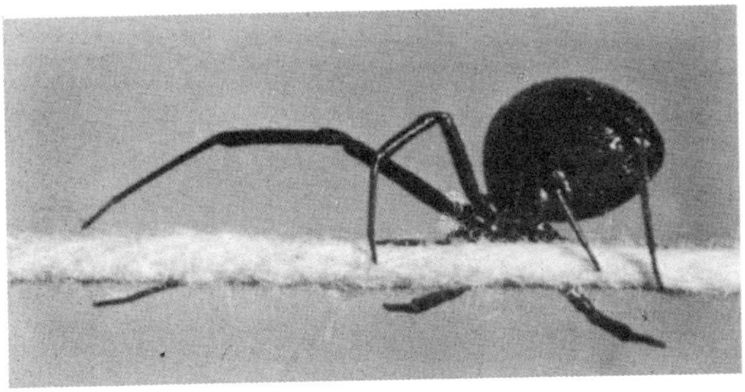

**Figure 31–6.** The female black widow spider. A reddish-orange hourglass-shaped marking on the underside of the abdomen helps to identify her. (Courtesy of Terry L. Biery, Captain, USAFR, BSC, Rickenbacker AFB, Ohio)

bark, seldom used storage areas, barns, water faucets, and outhouses. It would be a good practice to clear webs with a stick or with gloved hands, especially seats of outhouses before sitting! The black widow can live as long as two years.

Humans are often bitten and envenomized when the web is disturbed (as sitting) or when the spider is trapped against a body part. The venom of the black widow is neurotoxic; therefore, local tissue reaction will be minimal. If untreated, envenomation will produce muscle spasms, increased blood pressure, nervousness, and possibly cardiopulmonary arrest.

Healthy adults usually survive envenomation from the black widow without serious medical complications. However, bites from this spider incurred to children pose a great medical concern, because of their size in relation to the amount of injected venom. Elderly patients, and patients with underlying cardiac or respiratory illnesses also pose a serious medical concern if bitten. The EMT should, as in all stings or bites from unknown arthropods, try to establish the offender's identity or *modus operandi.* (See Table 31–3.) The patient's past medical history is also pertinent information to ascertain, especially if the patient has heart, respiratory, or high blood pressure problems. Fortunately, there is a specific antivenin for the black widow spider bite.

### *Brown Recluse Spider (Brown Spider, Violin Spider)*

The brown recluse is most commonly found in Arkansas, Kansas, Missouri, and Oklahoma. Its range, however, extends into several states including: Alabama, Georgia, Illinois, Indiana, Iowa, Kentucky, Louisiana, Ohio, Mississippi, Tennessee, and Texas. Several localized populations of the brown recluse, probably imported from the south central states, have been reported from Arizona, California, Wyoming, Pennsylvania, Washington D.C., New Jersey, North Carolina, and Florida.

The brown recluse is about one inch long, including leg span. Its color

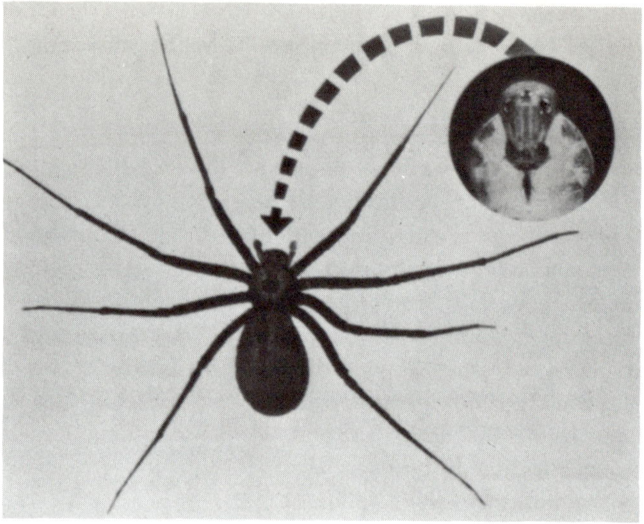

**Figure 31–7.** The brown recluse or brown spider. Note the violin-shaped marking behind the eyes. (Courtesy of Terry L. Biery, Captain, USAFR, BSC, Rickenbacker AFB, Ohio)

varies from yellow-tan to dark brown. Characteristics that make this spider identifiable include three pairs of eyes (most spiders have eight eyes) and a violin-shaped marking, extending from the area of the eyes to the abdomen. (See Fig. 31–7.) Both the male and female are dangerous. This spider is mostly nocturnal and seeks its prey in darkness. It can be found indoors where it rests by day in closets, boxes, littered areas, and other undisturbed places where it is dry. Outdoors, it can be found under rocks, loose bark, and other undisturbed protected areas (hence the name recluse). This harmless looking spider is nonaggressive and will seek shelter when distrubed. The victim is usually bitten in several ways: putting on clothing in which the spider is hiding; stepping on the wandering spider at night; rolling over in bed onto the spider; or cleaning closets or other storage areas where the spider has its web.

The venom of the brown recluse is cytotoxic (kills tissue cells) and in some patients, hemotoxic (destroys red blood cells). The term given to red blood cell destruction is *hemolysis* (he-mol′ĭ-sis). This serious complication of envenomation is indicated by the appearance of bloody or dark colored urine.

Although the bite from a brown recluse spider is rare, it can produce large areas of tissue scarring and possibly death. Unfortunately, there is no specific antivenin for the brown recluse spider bite.

## Centipedes

Centipedes are multisegmented arthropods, ranging in size from one to ten inches or more. There is one pair of legs on each segment and according to species, they vary from fifteen to one-hundred pairs of legs or more.

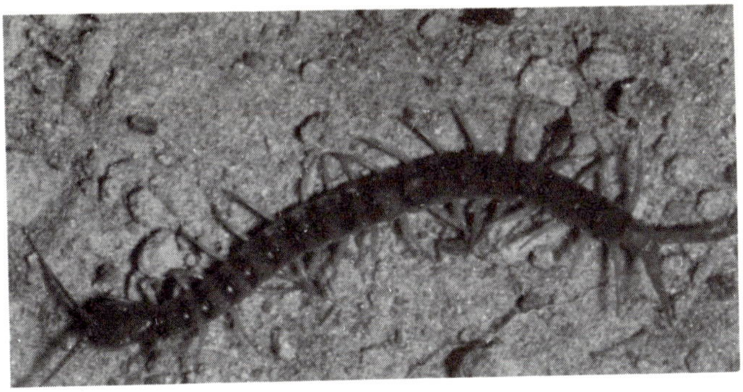

**Figure 31-8.** The centipede is nocturnal and most are found in the southern half of the U.S. (Courtesy of Terry L. Biery, Captain, USAFR, BSC, Rickenbacker AFB, Ohio)

(See Fig. 31-8.) Although centipedes are located throughout the U.S., they are most numerous in the southern states. All centipedes are poisonous, but most are too small to harm man. However, if even the smallest centipede succeeds in breaking the skin, it can cause intense pain. Centipedes inject their venom through two powerful jaws, located behind their head. A centipede very common in Arizona, Scolopendra heros, is very large and can inflict an extremely painful bite.

Most centipedes are nocturnal and hunt for prey which consists of insects or other small arthropods. In the daytime, centipedes hide under rocks, loose bark, stones, leaves, cracks, crevices, and other moist, protected places. Centipedes cannot inject venom through their segmented legs. Most bites occur when they are picked up, stepped on, rolled over on, or otherwise trapped against the body.

## True Bugs

Almost anything that crawls or flies is considered a bug in the eyes of most people. As a general rule, insects have six legs, three body segments, a head, thorax and abdomen, and one pair of compound eyes. In contrast, spiders and their relatives have eight legs, eight simple eyes, a cephalothorax (combined head and thorax), and abdomen. Bugs are insects. Ones that concern us include: the Conenose bug (Triatoma sanguisuga) and wheel bug (Arilus cristatus). Both insects can produce local tissue reactions or anaphylactic responses in their bitten victims.

### *Conenose Bug (Kissing Bug)*

This insect is generally located in the southern half of the U.S. Its size ranges from one-half inch to one and one-half inches, and it has orange and black color markings noticeably on its abdominal periphery.

This family of insects (Reduvudae) has a characteristic cone-shaped head which helps to identify it, hence, the name "conenose bugs." (See Fig. 31-9.) This insect has a very flat back which allows it to hide in small

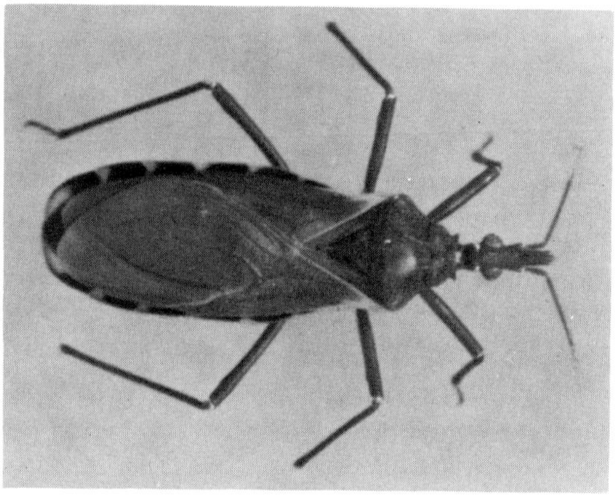

**Figure 31-9.** The conenose or kissing bug. (Courtesy of Terry L. Biery, Captain, USAFR, BSC, Rickenbacker AFB, Ohio)

cracks and crevices. It is a nocturnal insect that feeds on blood when seeking its prey at night. Although usually feeding on small animals, it will readily feed on humans in their absence. It is commonly referred to as a "kissing bug" because it occasionally takes a blood meal from around the lip area of humans. Other common sites of attack include the hands, arms, feet, head, and trunk. It is not known to bite through clothing.

### *Wheel Bug*

The wheel bug occurs in the southern two-thirds of the U.S. This light-grey insect is about one to two inches in length and has a head similar to that of the conenose bug. The identifying characteristic of this insect is a cogwheel-like crest located on its thorax, hence, the name "wheel bug." (See Fig. 31-10.)

Wheel bugs feed by day on soft-bodied insects that are found on vegetation and debris. Victims are usually bitten when they either pick up the insect or make accidental contact when working around vegetation. The insect penetrates the skin by using its long beak, or proboscis, and injects its salivary fluid normally used in killing its prey.

Its bite can be avoided by positive identification and keeping a distant neutrality from it. The wearing of gloves when handling vegetation and debris can also reduce the risk of being bitten by this unusual insect.

## Biting Flies

There isn't a true outdoorsman who does not know the effects of biting flies. The two groups that affect man most in producing extremely irritating bites include the black fly (Simulium venustum) and the sand fly (Psychodidae).

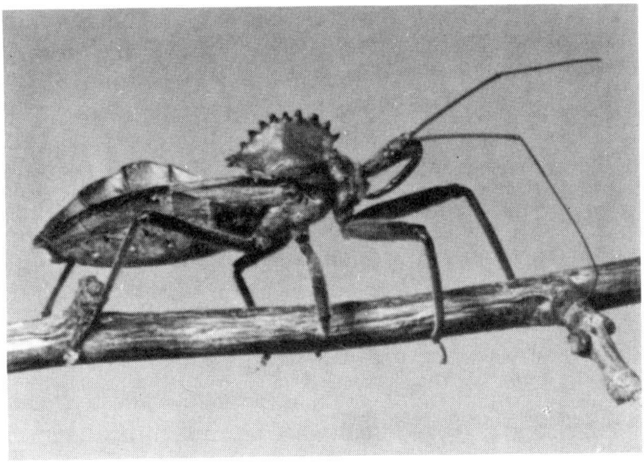

**Figure 31-10.** The wheel bug. (Courtesy of Terry L. Biery, Captain, USAFR, BSC, Rickenbacker AFB, Ohio)

*Black Flies*

Of approximately eighty or more different species known to occur in the United States, black flies that inhabit the northern United States, Canada, and Alaska are far more famous because of their numbers. The term *black fly* is somewhat misleading, since color patterns of this insect are gray to tannish-yellow. Generally, the females are the blood suckers. The males have piercing mouth parts to suck blood, but they are usually too small to penetrate the skin. Black flies are small ranging in size from one to five mm. They have a characteristic humped back with a tiny head that droops. (See Fig. 31-11.)

Black flies are outdoor daytime biters and tend to settle down about dusk. They are rarely found indoors. What makes black flies extremely an-

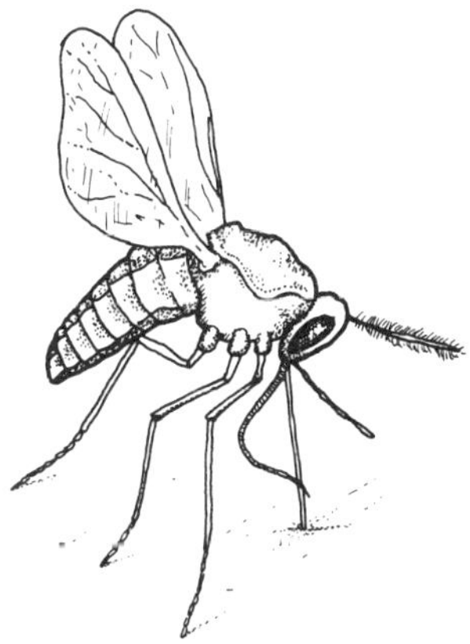

**Figure 31-11.** The black fly. Note the characteristic humped back and drooping head.

noying and unbearable is that they occur in enormous swarms. These creatures have ruined many a well-planned trip!

For breeding and development, they are found in areas where there is swift flowing, well-aerated water. Some species breed continually from early spring to late autumn. Because of the vast number of rivers in Canada, the country is notorious for black fly seasons!

In season, the black fly is just about inescapable. Their size enables them to maneuver through tent netting and loose clothing. Persons planning trips where the black fly exists should take head netting that is tightly woven and wear insect repellent on all exposed skin surfaces.

### *Sand Flies*

The sand fly is particularly a nuisance in southwestern United States. As with the black fly, it is the female that is the blood sucker. Unlike black flies, the sand fly usually bites only at night and is active only when there is little or no wind. During the day, they hide in dark cracks and crevices of buildings, in vegetation, hollows of trees, etc. Characteristically, they fly at slow, weak, noiseless hops that one can follow. Although most species feed on cold-blooded animals, some will take a blood meal from man. Unlike black flies, they are not aquatic, and breed in places where there is darkness, humidity, and organic matter, which serves as food for the larvae (lar′ve). The sand fly is a carrier of disease and can cause medical concern when it occurs in overwhelming numbers. Its bite is extremely painful. Prevention rests with proper protection in dress and application of insect repellent on exposed skin surfaces.

Similar biting flies that cause painful bites include: the buffalo gnat, and biting midges (popularly called "Punkies" and "no-see-ums"). Protection against these small insects is the same for black and sand flies. See treatment on page 585.

## Lice

Lice are not generally thought of as a medical concern because most people have never had association with them.

As an EMT treating different people in all sorts of environments and situations, the likelihood of being exposed to lice will be increased. It is important that the EMT recognize these creatures as being lice and take precautions against their spread by informing the triage nurse once at the hospital, and taking proper care in cleaning the emergency vehicle once the transport is completed. There are three species of lice that one may encounter when examining a patient. They include:

1. Crab louse (Pthirus pubis)
2. Head louse (Pediculus humanus capitis)
3. Body louse (Pediculus humanus humanus)

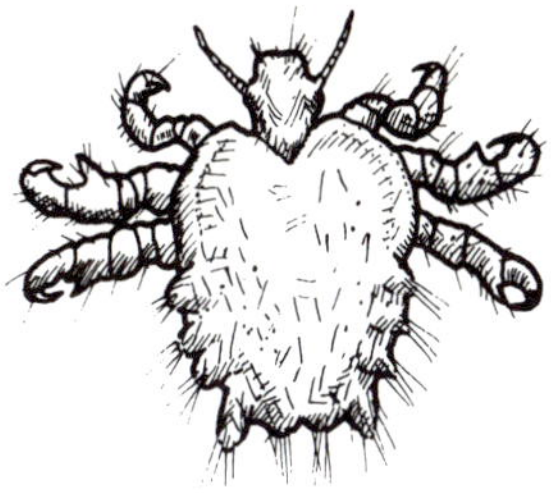


**Figure 31-12.** The pubic louse.

*Pediculosis* (pe-dik″u-lo′sis) is the medical term used when there is lice present on any part of the body. All three species of lice suck blood and cannot exist away from their host for very long periods of time.

### *Crab Louse*

This louse is also called the pubic louse, and to have them is popularly known as having the "crabs." This creature gets its name from its appearance—it looks like a crab. (See Fig. 31-12.) Crab lice are very stationary in habit and stay attached at a point on the skin for days. They particularly infest the pubic region of adults, but may also infest armpits, eyelashes, beards, and mustaches. Crab lice are often transmitted by sexual contact and can be considered, in a sense, a venereal disease. The lice may also be transmitted by contacting clothing used by the infested person. Crab lice generally infest human adults and not prepuberty individuals. The bites of crab lice cause extreme itching and the human skin usually discolors with long infestation. The louse attaches its eggs on the coarse hair of the body.

### *Head Louse*

This type of louse is about two to three mm in length and occurs especially on the head. These lice are easily transmitted by physical contact. The louse attaches its eggs onto the hair of the body.

### *Body Louse*

This louse can be found any where on the body, but tends to be common where clothing comes in contact with the body for continual periods of time, such as the underwear, waistline, and armpit. This louse usually stays on clothing, where it lays its eggs. It usually moves to the skin only when feeding. These lice may be transmitted by physical contact, or by contacting objects (usually clothing) used by the infested person. (See Fig. 31-13.)

All lice irritate the skin and cause extreme itching. Their saliva causes small red pimple formations after a bite. Scratching the area, which is

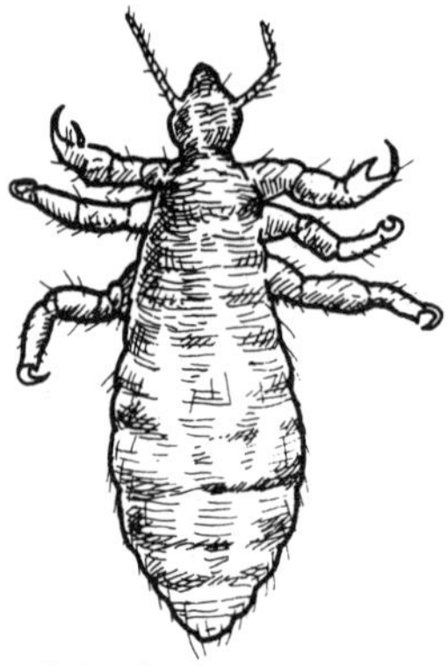

Pidiculus humanus

**Figure 31-13.** The body louse.

always a necessity, sometimes leads to infection of the bitten area. Severe infestation can lead to general tiredness, irritability, depression, and body rash. Persons who are continually infested with lice, such as "winos," bums, and indigents, develop pigmented and hardened skin, a condition known as *"vagabond's disease."*

All lice are generally treated in the same fashion. Persons who have been infested should steam clean, burn, or fumigate clothing. A lotion such as Kwell® may be used to clean the body. EMTs who have come in contact with a person with lice will usually automatically start itching, even if contact has not been made!

Clothing should be changed and washed in hot water or steam, and a Kwell® or a similar shampoo should be used. The vehicle, if contaminated, should be taken out of service and fumigated, especially all linen.

## Vesicating and Urticating Arthopods

Arthropods that cause vesication (ves″ĭ-ka′shun) (blistering) include the blister beetles. Arthropods causing urtication (ur″tĭ-ka′shun) (burning and itching) include certain species of caterpillars.

### *Blister Beetle*

This soft-bodied beetle ranges in size from one-half inch to one inch in length and has considerable color patterns of irridescent black, purple, and brown. Blister beetles are found, generally, in the western half of the U.S. (See Fig. 31-14.)

These insects feed on other insects and are generally found on vegetation. They are readily attracted to bright light and many human exposures occur when the insect lands on the person in this fashion. A clear amber colored fluid called cantharidin is contained in adult blister beetles. When the beetle lands on the skin and is brushed away, the pressure of touching the insect causes the fluid to be released from its leg joints and other segmented areas of the body. It is this fluid that causes blistering. The bee-

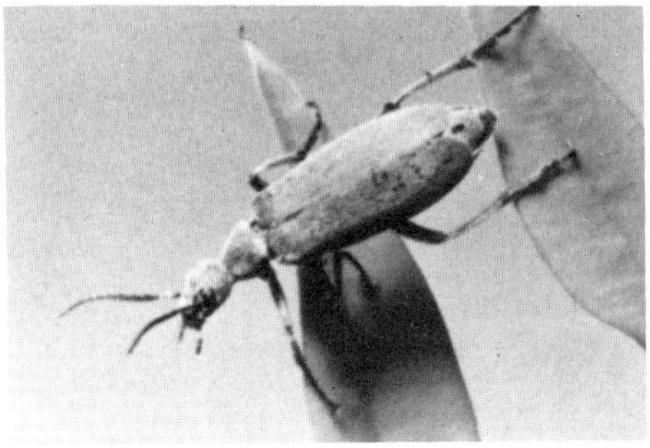

**Figure 31-14.** The blister beetle exudes the chemical Cantharidin from its joints when disturbed. (Courtesy of Terry L. Biery, Captain, USAFR, BSC, Rickenbacker AFB, Ohio)

tle is most active during the months of summer; therefore, most cases of exposure occur in July, August, and September.

Prevention lies with identifying, but not handling the insect. If the insect lands on the skin, it should be blown off, rather than brushed or picked off, since this will result in the release of the insect's vesicating fluid.

*Caterpillars*

Caterpillars are larvae of moths and butterflies. Certain species contain protective hairs that connect with a poison gland and when they are disturbed, the hairs break off or become attached to the intruder, allowing venom to enter the skin. These nettling hairs cause an intense burning and itching sensation when contact is made with the skin. This is especially true if the nettling hairs enter the eye. There are several species of caterpillars that can cause irritating effects to man. Three very common caterpillars that are reported more so than others as causing irritation include (see Fig. 31-15):

1. Io Moth Caterpillar (Automeris io)
2. Puss caterpillar (Megalopyge opercularis)
3. Saddleback caterpillar (Sibine stimulea)

These caterpillars are found in the central and southeastern portion of the United States. Prevention of exposure rests with identifying, but not touching the caterpillar.

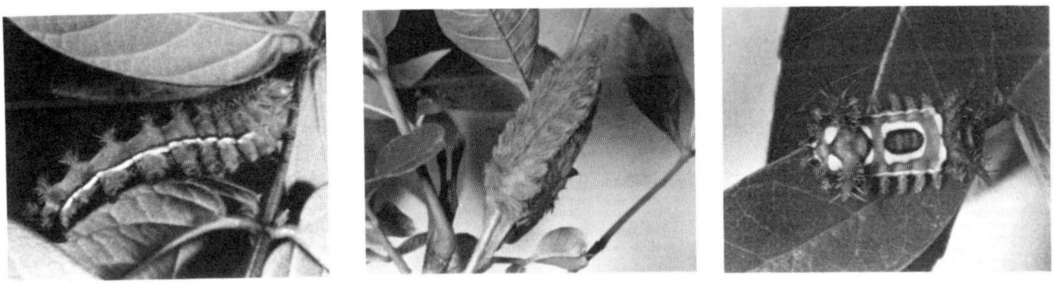

(a) (b) (c)

**Figure 31-15.** (a) The Io moth caterpillar; (b) the puss caterpillar; (c) the saddleback caterpillar. (Courtesy of Terry L. Biery, Captain, USAFR, BSC, Rickenbacker AFB, Ohio)

TABLE 31-1. CLASS AND ORDER OF ARTHROPODS OF MEDICAL CONCERN

| *Class—Insecta* | | | |
|---|---|---|---|
| *Order—Hymenoptera* | *Order—Lepidoptera* | *Order—Diptera* | *Order—Hemiptera* |
| Stinging Insects | Nettling/Irritating Caterpillars | Biting Insects | Biting Insects |
| Honeybee | Puss caterpillar | Black fly | Wheel bug |
| Bumblebee | Saddle back caterpillar | Sand fly | Conenose bug |
| Wasps | Io moth caterpillar | Deer fly | |
| Hornets | White moth caterpillar | | |
| Yellow jackets | Buck moth caterpillar | | |
| Ants | Tussock moth caterpillar | | |
| | Brown-tailed moth caterpillar | | |
| | Range caterpillar | | |

| *Class—Arachnida* | | |
|---|---|---|
| *Order—Araneida* | *Order—Scorpionada* | *Order—Acarina* |
| Biting spiders | Stinging arthropod | Sucking arthropod |
| Black widow | Scorpion | Ticks |
| Brown recluse | | Lice |

| *Class—Chilopoda* |
|---|
| *Order—Scolopendromorphia* |
| Biting arthropod |
| Centipedes |

Table 31-2. Signs, Symptoms and Treatment of Arthropod Injury

| *Mechanism of Injury* | *Arthropod* | *Signs/Symptoms* | *Treatment* | *Complications* |
|---|---|---|---|---|
| Stings | Honeybee<br>Bumblebee<br>Wasps<br>Hornets<br>Yellow jackets<br>Ants | *Local reaction*<br>Pain at sting site,<br>Redness, swelling, itching | Stinger of honeybee should be scraped away. DO NOT PULL OFF. | The more rapid the onset of symptoms, the more severe the reaction is likely to be. |
| | | *General reaction*<br>Hives, abdominal pain, nausea, vomiting, anxiety. | Apply antiseptic solution to sting site. Apply coolant (ice bag or chemical cold pack) to sting site. | Stings of the head, face, and neck tend to cause more serious effects. |
| | | Constriction feeling in chest, wheezing. | Elevate part.<br>Keep patient warm. | Anaphylaxis.<br>Secondary infection |
| | | *Shock Reaction*<br>Any of the above, plus cyanosis; hypotension; incontinence; asthma; bloody, frothy sputum: glottal or laryngeal edema; unconsciousness | Put patient in shock position if necessary. | |
| Stings | Scorpions | Initial pain at sting site, followed by numbness.<br>Muscle spasms, nausea, vomiting, incontinence, hypersalivation.<br>Respiratory and circulatory depression<br><br>Scorpion stings produce little or no swelling or discoloration of local tissue. | Apply lymphatic/venous tourniquet above the sting site.<br>Apply local coolant.<br>Keep patient warm.<br>Put patient in shock position if necessary.<br>*A specific antivenin exists for scorpion envenomation.* | Secondary infection |

TABLE 31-2. SIGNS, SYMPTOMS AND TREATMENT OF ARTHROPOD INJURY

| *Mechanism of Injury* | *Arthropod* | *Signs/Symptoms* | *Treatment* | *Complications* |
|---|---|---|---|---|
| Bite | Black widow spider | Pinprick feeling at bite site, followed by numbing.<br>Pain within fifteen munutes.<br>A bite on the lower extremity can produce severe abdominal muscle cramping becoming rigid and tender.<br>A bite on the hand or arm produces intense back, chest and shoulder pain, and pain on inspiration.<br>Systemic symptoms may include:<br>hypersalivation, nausea, vomiting, weakness, increased blood pressure. | Apply antiseptic solution to bite area.<br>Apply ice locally<br>*A specific antivenin exists for the black widow.* | Death may occur in children and elderly patients.<br>Secondary infection. |
| Bite | Brown recluse spider | Bite may or may not be felt.<br><br>*1–3 hours*: Bitten area becomes painful and swollen. Blisters form around bite site.<br><br>*18–24 hours*: Bite site turns cyanotic and purple.<br><br>*2–7 days*: Tissue cells die and skin area turns black.<br><br>*2–4 weeks*: Blackened dead cells fall off leaving an ulcerated pit in the skin.<br>Ulcerated pit fills with scar tissue. | Apply antiseptic solution to bite area. DO NOT USE ICE on bite area since the cold will constrict the already compromised blood vessels and increase the tissue necrosis.<br>The spider should be salvaged for positive identification.<br>Ulceration may be avoided by surgical tissue.<br><br>Excision at the hospital if done within four hours after bite. | Nonhealing wound.<br>Secondary infection. |
| Bite | Centipede | Intense pain at bite site.<br>Two red puncture wounds from bite.<br>Redness, some swelling<br>Burning ache for four to five hours. | Wash area with soap and and water or antiseptic solution.<br>Apply ammonia in 10 percent solution.<br>Apply cool wet dressing for pain. | Secondary infection.<br>Allergic response to toxin. |

| | | | | |
|---|---|---|---|---|
| Biting/ sucking | Conenose bug | Mild to no pain at bite sites.<br>There are several reactions, depending on sensitivity:<br>1. Papule with a central redspot.<br>2. Small vesicles grouped around bite site with swelling and little redness.<br>3. Urticaric lesions with central redspots and edema.<br>4. Hemorrhagic nodules to blistering lesions on hands and feet. | Wash area with soap and water or antiseptic solution. | Anaphylatic shock.<br>Secondary infection. |
| Biting/ sucking | Wheel bug | Intense pain at bite site, subsides within three to six hours. | Wash area with soap and water or antiseptic solution. | Anaphylactic shock.<br>Secondary infection. |
| Biting/ sucking | Black flies<br>Sand flies<br>Deer flies<br>Buffalo gnats<br>Biting midges | Except for the black fly, there is intense pain at the bite site. It is thought that the black fly uses an anesthetic during the bite.<br>Since it is not felt, the first thing noticed is a drop of blood on the skin.<br>Within one hour, intense pain, itching and local swelling. | Wash area with soap and water or antiseptic solution.<br>Oral antihistamines may be indicated.<br>*The use of active insect repellent such as "Deet" (Diethyl-toluamide) keeps the insects at a distance.* | Death has been reported from anaphylaxis.<br>Secondary infection. |
| Blistering | Blister beetle | Pain at site where insect released clear amber fluid (Cantharidin).<br>Blistering of skin. | Wash area with soap and water or antiseptic. Do not rupture blisters. Self-limiting. | Secondary infection. |
| Nettling | *Caterpillars*<br>puss<br>Saddle back<br>Io | Burning pain at nettling site, may be followed by numbing sensation.<br>A double row of spine tracks may be seen with the saddle back or Io.<br>Systemic reaction may include: nausea, vomiting, fever, and headache. | With cellophane or adhesive tape, strip away the spines on the skin surface.<br>Keep affected limb away from the eyes. Apply ice packs to the area. | Anaphylaxis has been reported.<br>Irritation of the eyes from spines. |

TABLE 31–3. HABITS AND EFFECTS OF VARIOUS ARTHROPODS

| *Insect* | *Average Length in MM (10 mm=3/8 in.)* | *Usual Location* | *Method of Attack* | | *Time of Activity* | | | | *Local Reaction* | | | | | *Distribution of Lesions* | | | *Residua* |
|---|---|---|---|---|---|---|---|---|---|---|---|---|---|---|---|---|---|
| | | | | | | | | | *Onset* | | *Duration* | | | | | | |
| | | | *Bite* | *Sting* | *Day* | *Night* | *Dusk* | *Dawn* | *Immediate* | *Delayed* | *Hours* | *Days* | *Weeks* | *Single* | *Scattered* | *Grouped* | |
| Bumblebee | 20–25 | Flowers | | X | X | | | | X | X | X | X | | X | | | None |
| Honeybee | 10–15 | Flowers | | X | X | | | | X | X | X | X | | X | | | None |
| Mud-Dauber Wasp | 20–25 | Orchards Garbage Pails | | X | X | | | | X | | | X | | X | | | None |
| Yellow Jackets | 10–15 | Orchards Garbage Pails | | X | X | | | | X | | X | | | X | | | None |
| Hornet | 20–30 | Wood Flowers | | X | X | | | | X | | X | | | X | | | None |
| Harvester Ant | 7–9 | Vegetation Kitchen | | X | X | | | | | | | X | | X | | | None |
| Fire Ant | 6–7 | Fields | | X | X | | | | X | | | X | | | | X | Pigmented Macules Occasionally Nodules |
| Stable Fly | 6–7 | Barns | X | | X | | | | X | | X | | | X | | | None |
| Horse Fly | 10–20 | Barns | X | | X | | | | X | | X | | | X | | | None |

| | | | | | | | | | | | | | | | | | |
|---|---|---|---|---|---|---|---|---|---|---|---|---|---|---|---|---|---|
| Deer Fly | 7–9 | Cattle | X | | X | | | | X | | X | | | X | X | | None |
| Black Fly | 1–5 | Woodlands Running Water | X | | X | | | X | | X | | | X | | X | | Nodules Scars |
| Sand Fly | 1–4 | Woodlands | X | | | X | | | X | | | X | | | X | | Bluish Spots |
| Biting Midges | 0.6–5 | Marshlands | X | | | | X | | X | | X | | | | X | | None |
| Chigger Mite | 0.2–1 | Vegetation | X | | X | | | | | X | | X | | | | X | Hyperpig-mentation |
| Ticks | 5–15 | Vegetation | X | | | | | | | | X | X | | X | X | | Granulomas |
| Brown Recluse Spider | 10–15 | Closets Attics | X | | | | | | X | | X | X | | X | | | Scar |
| Black Widow Spider | 10 | Basements Out Houses | X | | | | | | X | | X | X | | X | | | None |
| Tarantulas | 15–20 | Vegetation | X | | | | | | | | | | | X | | | None |
| Scorpions | 15–200 | Stones and Sand | | X | | X | | | X | | X | | | X | | | None |
| Wheel Bug | 20+ | Vegetation | X | | X | | | | X | | X | | | X | | | None |
| Kissing Bug | 20+ | Bedroom | X | | | X | | | | X | | X | | | | X | None |

Table 31–4. Signs, Symptoms and Treatment of Injuries from Venemous Marine Animals

| *Mechanism of Injury* | *Type of Marine Animal* | *Signs/Symptoms* | *Management* | *Complications* |
|---|---|---|---|---|
| Traumatic lacerations | Shark<br>Alligator gar<br>Great barracuda | Tremendous soft tissue loss.<br>Possible amputations. | Control bleeding.<br>Support airway.<br>Guard against shock. | Shark attack has a 85 percent mortality rate!<br>Shock<br>Secondary infection |
| Stings | Jellyfish<br>Hydras<br>Corals<br>Sea anemones | Intense pain where stinging cells (nematocysts) have touched the skin.<br>Joint and muscle pain.<br>Respiratory difficulty.<br>Severe red rash.<br>Edema. | Pull out the nematocysts that can be pulled out.<br>Pour alcohol over the wound (this fixes the nematocysts and prevents further stinging.<br>Sprinkle area with Adolfs unseasoned meat tenderizer (this prevents further poisoning). Dust area with flour or baking powder.<br>Scrape off with knife.<br>Wash with salt water.<br>Do not use fresh water.<br>Do not rub with sand. | Secondary infection<br>Respiratory arrest<br>Shock<br>Allergic reaction |
| Punctures | Coneshells<br>Stingrays<br>Sea urchins<br>Sculpins | Intense pain, nausea, vomiting, weakness, syncope (sin′ko-pe). | Immerse injured part in hot water (110°–114°) for 30–60 minutes to inactivate venom.<br>Elevate injured part<br>Cover with a sterile dressing. | Shock<br>Secondary infection<br>Allergic reaction<br>Tetanus |
| Bites | Sea snake<br>Octopus | Two fang marks | Basic life support | Respiratory arrest<br>Secondary infection |

EMTs who serve the coastal areas of the United States should be familiar with the more venomous marine life that inhabits local waters.

Most injuries due to venomous marine life occur to those who step on them, pick them up, or swim into them, especially scuba and snorkling enthusiasts. The EMT should also be familiar with local treatments and specific antivenins. Local treatments vary. It is best to seek the most current treatment regimen from the local emergency medical service advisor. Certain medical supplies should be added to the medical supply kit for marine injuries. These medical supplies often include agents which neutralize marine animal venom such as isopropyl alcohol, meat tenderizer, flour, ammonia, lemon juice, and equipment used to heat fresh water where the injured parts need to be immersed.

All persons stung or bitten by venomous marine life should have follow-up care by a physician. Although there are many species of venomous marine life, Table 31-4 lists only those that can produce a bite or sting that can cause medical concern.

*References*

Arnold, R. E. *What To Do About Bites and Stings of Venomous Animals.* New York: Macmillan Publishing Company, 1974.

Barber, J. M., and Budassi, S. A. *Mosby's Manual of Emergency Care: Practices and Procedures*, pp. 272–284. St. Louis, MO: The C. V. Mosby Company, 1979.

Biery, T. I. USAFR, BSC, "Venomous Arthropod Handbook: Envenomation Symptoms/Treatment Identification Biology and Control," Supt. of Documents, U.S. Government Printing Office, Washington, D.C., Stock No. 008-070-00397.

Frazier, C. A. "Diagnosis and Treatment of Insect Bites," *Clinical Symposium*, 20:74–100, July/August/September 1968. Summit, N. J.: CIBA Pharmaceutical Comp.

Frazier, Charles, *Insect Allergy: Allergic Reactions to Bites of Insects and Other Arthropods.* St. Louis, MO: Warren H. Green, Inc., 1969.

Harwood, R. F., and James, M. T. *Entomology in Human and Animal Health*, 7th ed. New York: Macmillan Publishing Company, 1979.

Parrish, H. M. "Analysis of 460 Fatalities From Venomous Animals in the United States," *Am. J. Med. Sci.*, 245:129–141, 1963.

Parrish, H. M. "Deaths From Bites and Stings of Venomous Animals and Insects in the United States," *Archives of Internal Medicine*, 104:198–207, 1959.

Russell, F. E. "Injuries by Venomous Animals," *American Journal of Nursing*, pp. 1322–1326, June 1966.

Russell, F. E. "Jaws That Bite, Things That Sting," *Emergency Medicine*, pp. 25–59, July 1978.

Shields, T. L., and Walsh, E. N. "'Kissing Bug' Bite," *Archives of Dermatology*, 74:14–21, 1956.

Smith. F. D., *et. al* "Insect Bite by Arilus Cristatus, A North American Reduvied," *Archives of Dermatology*, 77:324–330, 1958.

Smith, J. D., and Smith, E. B. "Multiple Fire Ant Stings: A Complication of Alcoholism," *Archives of Dermatology*, 103: 438–441, April 1971.

U.S. Department of Health and Human Services. "The Brown Recluse," Supt. of Documents, U.S. Gov't Printing Office, Washington, D.C., Publication No. 2062, 1970.

U.S. Department of Health and Human Services, Public Health Services. "Insects That Carry Disease," DHEW Pub. No. (CDC) 77-8281, Atlanta, GA: Center for Disease Control, Aug. 1977.

# Chapter 32

# Snakebites

Depending on geographical location the EMT may have occasion to treat a victim from the bite of a venomous snake. The importance of proper treatment in the prehospital setting will reduce the chance of permanent limb disability and perhaps death, depending on the initial steps taken.

There are about 120 species of snakes in the United States, of which approximately thirty are poisonous and, therefore, have the potential to harm man. Only Maine, Alaska, and Hawaii are free from current ranges of poisonous snakes. Snakes that are dangerous to man in the United States, and therefore concern the EMT, are divided into two families and four major species:

1. Family Viperidae—The Pit Vipers

   Species: a. Rattlesnakes—Crotalus

   b. Moccasins (Cottonmouths)—Agkistrodon piscivorus

   c. Copperheads—Agkistrodon contortrix

2. Family Elapidae—The Coral Snake

   a. Eastern Coral—Micrurus fulvius

   b. Texas Coral—Micrurus tenere

   c. Arizona Coral—Micrurus euryxanthus

There are about 45,000 reported snakebites in the United States every year. Of this number, about 8000 are inflicted by venomous snakes. Fewer than fifteen deaths, however, have occurred from snakebites each year for the last eight years. Of these deaths each year, most occur in Texas, Georgia, Florida, Alabama, and South Carolina.

# RANKING THE DANGER OF VENOMOUS SNAKES IN THE UNITED STATES

## Extremely Dangerous

This group of extremely dangerous snakes includes the Eastern and Western Diamondback rattlesnake (See Fig. 32-1), Coral snake, and the Mojave rattlesnake.

The Eastern and Western Diamondback rattlesnakes account for 95 percent of all deaths incurred by venomous snakes in the United States. However, they account for only 10 percent of all snakebites. Their aggressiveness and size contribute to the largest amount of venom deposited in their victims when bitten (the major reason for the high percentage of deaths incurred by this species). Their venom is more potent than any snake in the United States, except for the Coral snake.

Coral snakes are a top contender, too, but they are scarce and their bite is usually not complete because their short mouth interferes with getting a firm grasp on their victim. Their short erect fangs also make penetration of clothing difficult. Because of these physical deficiencies and their general lifestyle, they account for only 1-2 percent of the total deaths each year. The Mojave rattlesnake also has a deadly bite, but they too are quite shy and reclusive and attack on a very infrequent basis.

## Moderately Dangerous

This group includes the Moccasin (Cottonmouth, Water Moccasin) (See Fig. 32-2) and most other rattlesnakes, other than the ones mentioned above.

## Minimally Dangerous

This group includes the Copperhead (See Fig. 32-3), Massasauga, and Pygmy rattlesnake. These snakes are not aggressive, but will attack when overly provoked. These snakes also adapt well close to human habitat, where other pit vipers seldom venture.

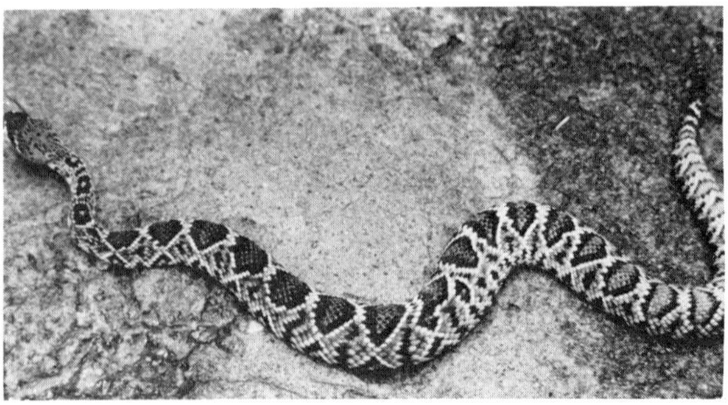

**Figure 32-1.** The Eastern diamondback rattlesnake.

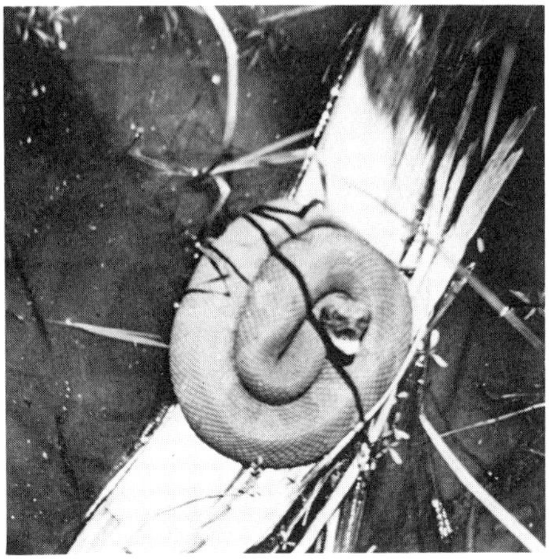

**Figure 32–2.** The cottonmouth or water moccasin. Note the cottony white mouth from which the name is derived. (Courtesy of Tony Wilson, Department of Natural Resources, Indianapolis, IN)

## IDENTIFYING CHARACTERISTICS OF VENOMOUS SNAKES

### Pit Vipers

Pit vipers have such a name because of a facial pit located between the eye and nostril. This pit serves as a heat-sensing organ, allowing the reptile to locate warm-blooded prey. Also characteristic to pit vipers are (See Fig. 32–4):

1. A triangular head.

2. Movable hollow upper jaw fangs. The fangs of pit vipers are about one-half inch long, but can attain lengths of one inch. At rest the fangs are

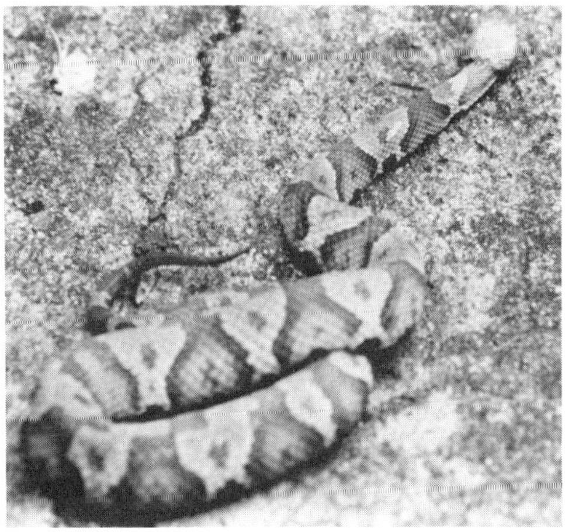

**Figure 32–3.** The copperhead.

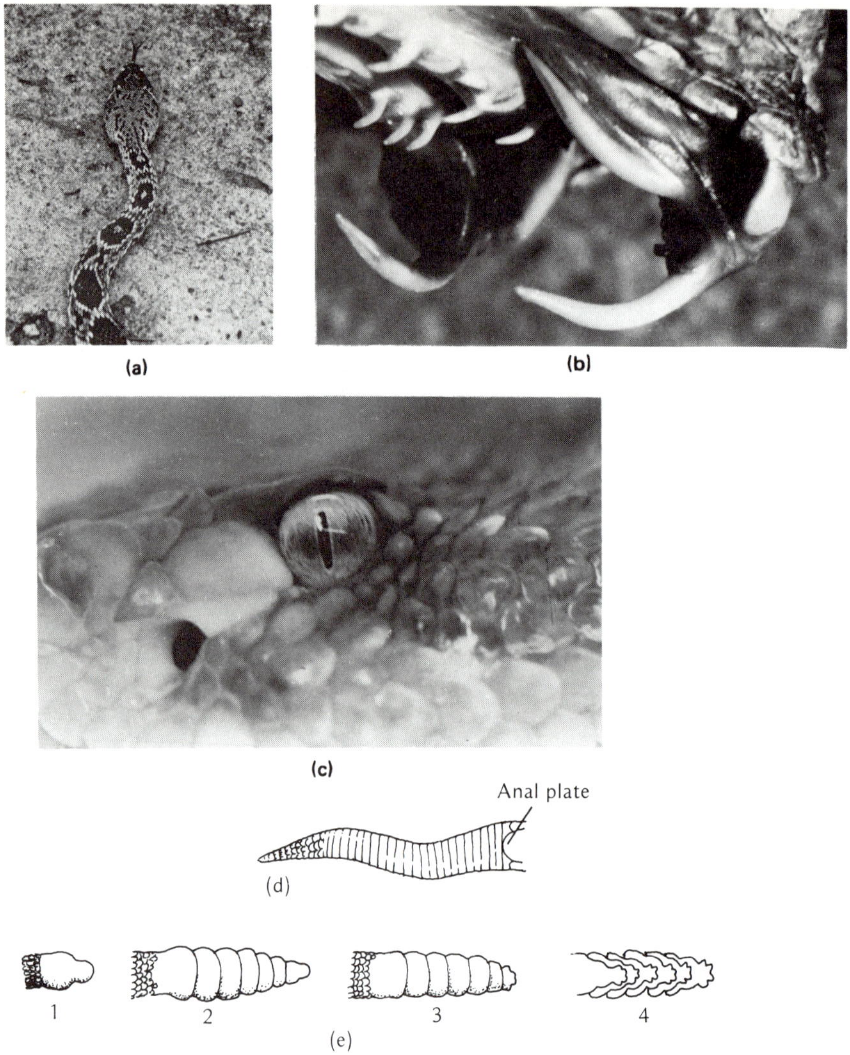


**Figure 32–4.** (a) Characteristic triangular head of most pit vipers. This snake is an Eastern diamondback. (b) Fang arrangement in pit vipers. Note the reserve fangs folded back ready to drop into place when the main fangs have been broken or dropped. (Courtesy of Tony Wilson, Department of Natural Resources, Indianapolis, IN) (c) This close view shows the characteristic pit found between the nose and eye of the pit viper and the elliptical pupil of the viper. (d) The characteristic single row of scales with a single anal plate of most poisonous snakes. (e) Rattle arrangements of the rattlesnake: (1) a button; (2) immature rattle with button still retained; (3) mature rattle with terminal joints broken off; (4) cross-section displays how rattles are interlinked.

folded back up against the roof of the mouth. Because of the fang curvature, the jaw must be opened about 180° in order to provide a perpendicular angle to the striking surface to achieve effective penetration.

3. Elliptical pupils (cat's eyes). Extremely difficult to tell when encountered, even at close range.

4. A single row of scales on the undersurface of the tail.

5. Rattles. Any snake that has rattles is poisonous. The Moccasin and Copperhead do not have this organ.

## Coral Snakes

Coral snakes belong to the same family of snakes that include Cobras, Mambas, and Kraits. There are three species found in the United States (See Fig. 32-5).

1. Eastern Coral—Micrurus fulvius
2. Texas Coral—Micrurus tenere
3. Arizona Coral—Micrurus euryxanthus

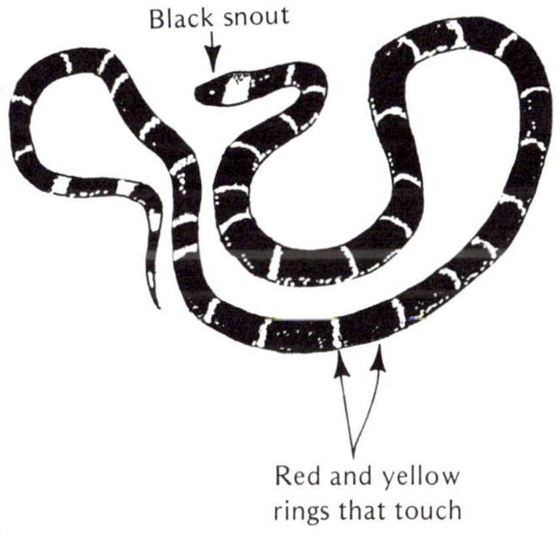


**Figure 32-5.** The Eastern coral snake.

Coral snakes have the following characteristics:

1. Relatively short fangs. The fangs of coral snakes are not hinged and do not fold back up against the roof of their mouth as do pit vipers. Instead, they always stand erect toward the front of the mouth. They are not hollow, but solid and sharply grooved where the venom slides down and into the puncture or scratch wound.

2. A black snout with a yellow or yellowish-white head ring and colored rings of red and yellow that touch. (Coral snakes are very colorful and vary considerably in color patterns. [See Fig. 32-6.] One should never rely on color markings alone to rule out whether or not these snakes are poisonous).

3. Round pupils.

**Figure 32–6.** Color pattern arrangement of the coral snake.

## IDENTIFYING CHARACTERISTICS OF NONVENOMOUS SNAKES

1. Round pupils
2. No facial pit
3. Double row of scales on the undersurface of the tail. (See Fig. 32–7.)

Because of a lack of knowledge and general fear associated with snakes, many people associate nonpoisonous snakes and their behaviors and habitat with poisonous species. Nonpoisonous snakes which are often mistaken for poisonous species include the Hognose, Scarlet, King, Mexican Milk, and Banded Water snakes.

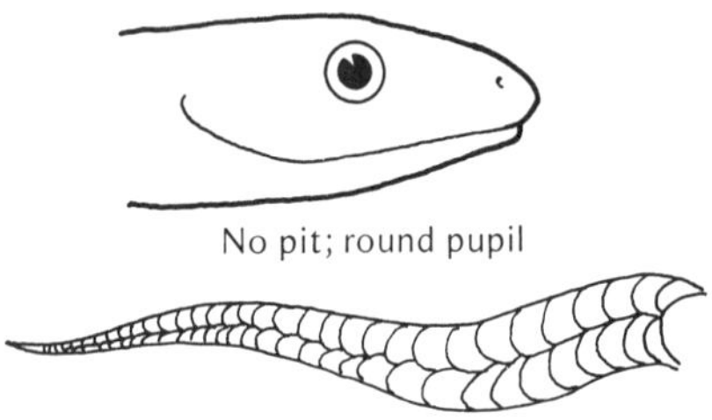


**Figure 32–7.** Characteristics of non-poisonous snakes.

## SIGNS AND SYMPTOMS—ENVENOMATION

Signs and symptoms of envenomation and the rapidity at which they appear are dependent upon several factors:

1. The size and species of the snake. (As previously mentioned, the Eastern and Western Diamondback rattlesnake, Coral snake, and Mojave rattlesnake are extremely dangerous.)

2. The location, depth, and number of bites. Although rare, the injection of venom directly into a vein can cause death within several minutes.

3. The amount of venom injected into the victim.

4. The age and weight of the victim. Children and elderly victims are more prone to the lethal effects of venom because of the smaller size of children and the general health of the elderly patient.

5. General health of the victim. The victim with cardiovascular, respiratory or nervous system diseases are more prone to the lethal effects of venom.

6. Individual sensitivity to venom.

7. Micro-organisms (type and number) in the oral cavity of the snake.

Envenomation by a poisonous snake may or may not have taken place, so be skeptical and check quickly, but thoroughly. Some 20–30 percent of all pit viper bites result in no significant venom injection. Another 25–30 percent of the victims bitten receive only small to moderate amounts of venom. Although it may seem logical to inspect for two fang marks, there may be only scratches, just one puncture wound or more than two puncture wounds. The reasons for this vary. If the snake does not get a firm grasp on the victim, there may be only scratch wounds. The Coral snake often has an incomplete bite, leaving scratch marks. One puncture wound may indicate that the other fang had been broken off in previous attack encounters. It is also possible that the snake may have more than two fangs. This is because several times a year the snake sheds its skin and when it does, it adds new fangs to replace old or broken ones. Therefore, the snake could be sporting one, two, or more fangs, depending on the given situation. (See Fig. 32–8.)

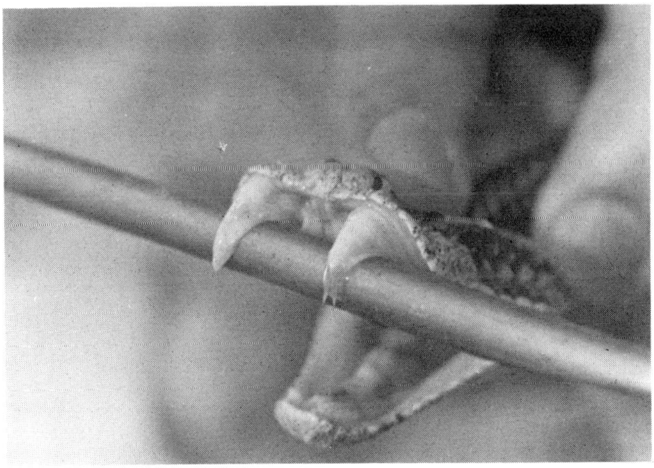

**Figure 32–8.** Some pit vipers may be sporting more than two fangs, as noted in this photo. A muscular sheath covers the left fang.

Early emergency assessment of any snake bite should be focused on the inflicted wound and condition of the patient. The immediate signs and symptoms of snakebites' envenomation should be assessed before invasive management steps take place. The bite from the pit viper may be minimal, moderate or severe.

A minimal bite may show:

1. Scratch or slight puncture wounds
2. Slight pain
3. Minimal swelling after thirty to sixty minutes

A moderate bite may show:

1. Puncture wounds
2. Intense burning pain
3. Swelling within ten minutes

A severe bite may show:

1. Puncture wounds from which capillary blood and fluid is oozing
2. Numbness around the wound
3. Muscle fasciculation (especially from the bite of the Eastern Diamondback)
4. Tingling sensation around the mouth associated with a rubbery or metallic taste (especially from severe bites of the Eastern and Western Diamondback)
5. Early shock state

The Coral snake bite may only show scratches or rarely puncture wounds. Envenomation from a Coral snake is less painful than that of pit vipers, and may not manifest symptoms for up to eighteen hours.

### *Pit Vipers*

#### *Immediate and Early Responses*

Signs and symptoms associated with envenomation beside scratch or puncture wounds include the following local tissue reactions:

1. Swelling within five to ten minutes
2. Burning pain
3. Numbness and paresthesias
4. Hypotension
5. Discoloration
6. Paralysis of the injured limb

*Delayed Systemic Responses*

1. Ecchymosis
2. Nausea
3. Vomiting
4. Bleb and blister formation
5. Bleeding
6. Sweating
7. Weakness
8. Syncope
9. Tachycardia or bradycardia
10. Shock

Weakness, sweating, nausea, and syncope are all common but may arise from the fear of being bitten.

*Coral Snakes*

*Immediate and Early Responses*

1. Minimal or no swelling
2. Discoloration
3. Paresthesia
4. Fasciculations around the wound.
5. Transitory pain or none at all

*Delayed Systemic Responses*

1. Blurred vision
2. Ptosis (to′sis) of the eyelids
3. Slurred speech
4. Dyspnea (disp′ne-ah)
5. Hypersalivation (hi″per-sal″ĭ-va′shun)
6. Euphoria (u-fo′re-ah)
7. Paralysis
8. Respiratory failure

The EMT must remember that with Coral snake bites, signs may be minimal, and symptoms may be delayed for as long as eighteen hours. The reason for this is that the main fraction of Coral snake venom is neurotoxic, and therefore, has less effect on the envenomated tissues. On the other hand, pit vipers' venom contains more hemotoxic properties causing local tissue reactions, except the Mojave rattlesnake, which is more neurotoxic. However, it is important to realize that the venom of all poisonous snakes is a complex mixture of enzymes and nonenzymatic proteins which include three main fractions that affect the human body's systems. They include: neurotoxins (poison to the nervous system), hemotoxins (poison to the circulatory system), and cardiotoxins (poison to the heart). Because these poisonous components of venom are found in all poisonous snakes, it is incorrect to label certain snake species as being just neurotoxic, hemotoxic, or cardiotoxic in nature.

## PREHOSPITAL MANAGEMENT OF SNAKEBITE

### Pit Vipers

In most situations, only general supportive care will be necessary.

1. Perform a primary survey. Institute CPR if necessary.

2. Reassure and quiet the victim. Have him lie down. The general confusion associated with this type of emergency call can be challenging. Some patients are convinced that all bites from venomous snakes are fatal. Continual reassurance of the patient will help in the general treatment. Once the patient realizes that he is not going to die, some symptoms may disappear.

3. Look for early signs and symptoms of envenomation.

4. Apply a constricting band to the injured extremity (98 percent of all bites are incurred to the hands and lower legs), about three to four inches above the bite. If the bite is to the fingers or toes, apply the constricting band just above the wrist or ankle joint. (See Fig. 32-9.) The purpose of the constricting band is to obstruct lymphatic and venous flow only, so as to prevent system absorption of the venom. Therefore, arterial and deep venous blood flow should not be occluded and the arterial pulse should be palpable. It may be difficult to palpate the distal pulse depending on the rapidity of tissue swelling.

5. Immobilize the extremity and keep it at or below the level of the heart.

6. Remove all jewelry to avoid vascular occlusion, should tissue swelling occur.

7. Do not allow the victim to perform any work. The patient should be considered a litter case, and should be carried by stretcher or Stokes Basket to the emergency vehicle.

8. Administer oxygen at 4–6 *l*/min. by face mask.

9. Transport the patient in a semi-Fowler's position if normotensive. If hypotensive, place in a shock position.

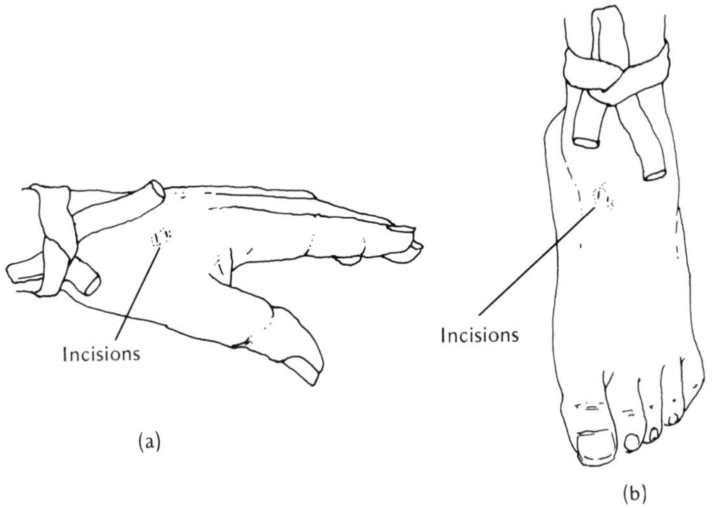


**Figure 32-9.** Linear incisions should be made on the patient only when indicated. Note the venous lymphatic tourniquet applied above the ankle and wrist.

10. Obtain baseline vital signs and monitor every five to ten minutes.

11. Record the time that progressive signs and symptoms developed and when treatment was instituted.

12. Do not allow the victim to consume alcohol, smoke, or eat.

13. Do not apply ice or any other coolant to the injured area. (Controversy exists concerning the cooling of the injured area. The EMT should consult local treatment protocol concerning cold treatment in snakebites. Under *no* circumstances should the EMT ever pack the extremity in ice or immerse the extremity in a cold water solution.)

14. Identification of the snake is important. If possible, bring the snake along with the patient, preferably dead. The EMT should not go out of his way to kill or capture the snake.

15. Alert the emergency department as to what kind of patient you are about to deliver to them. Include in your report the age of the patient, vital signs, and species of snake, if possible, that attacked the patient.

If the victim can be reached within thirty minutes, if the victim has moderate or severe signs of envenomation, and if a treatment protocol has been established by the medical director, incision and suction treatment should be instituted. If instituted promptly this technique can remove 20–25 percent of the injected venom. It has been estimated that as much as 22–50 percent of the venom can be removed if this technique is done within three minutes. Steps in incision and suction include:

1. With the constricting band in place, wash or wipe around the bite with an antiseptic solution or soap and water.

2. With a sterile scalpel or knife, make a linear incision (not cross marks "× ×") through each fang mark. They should be about one-fourth inch long and no more than one-eighth inch deep. (See Fig. 32–9.)

3. Using a suction cup from the snakebite kit (you can also use a breast pump, empty syringe, ECG suction cup, etc.), apply suction for about twenty to thirty minutes. Although not recommended, the mouth can be used to apply suction if no other device is available. The extracted wound fluid from mouth suction should be discarded (spit out) regularly. However, if swallowed, the venom will be inactivated in the stomach. The mouth should be free from lesions if the mouth suction technique is used. Otherwise, the venom will enter the rescuer's bloodstream. The mouth harbors much bacteria. Therefore, the possibility of secondary infection to the wound is a consideration. If more than thirty minutes has elapsed since the bite, this technique is of little value and could merely further traumatize the surrounding tissue.

## Coral Snakes

With Coral snake bites, the following treatment should be instituted:

1. Perform a primary survey. Institute CPR if necessary.

2. Reassure and quiet the victim. Have him lie down.

3. Wash the bitten area to prevent spreading, diffusion, and absorption of the venom into the wound. Since Coral snakes have to chew their victim so that venom enters the inflicted wound, residual venom may still be left on the skin surface. Therefore, the skin should be washed or wiped with an antiseptic solution.

4. Look for early signs and symptoms of envenomation.

5. Apply a constricting band above the wound. Remember that it should be tight enough to obstruct lymphatic and superficial venous flow only.

6. Immobilize the extremity and keep it at or below the level of the heart.

7. Remove all jewelry to avoid vascular occlusion should swelling occur.

8. Do not allow the victim to perform any work. He should be carried by stretcher or Stokes Basket to the emergency vehicle.

9. Apply oxygen at 4–6 *l*/min. by face mask.

10. Transport the patient in a semi Fowler's position if normotensive. If hypotensive, place in a shock position.

11. Obtain baseline vital signs and monitor every five to ten minutes.

12. Do not allow the victim to consume alcohol, smoke, or eat.

13. Record the time that progressive signs and symptoms developed and when treatment was instituted.

14. Do not apply ice or any other coolant to the injured area.

15. Positive identification of the snake is important. Specific antivenin is available for both pit vipers and Coral snakes. Valuable time can be saved if one knows whether the bite was inflicted by a pit viper or Coral snake, so that the correct antivenin can be given at the medical facility.

16. Alert the medical facility as to what kind of patient you are about to deliver to them. It is helpful if you can report the type of snake that bit the patient.

Incision and suction should not be performed on the patient who has been bitten by a Coral snake. This technique is useless because the effects are not to local tissue but to the central nervous system.

About 30 percent of the snakebites in the United States are bites from captive snakes. Zookeepers, hobbyists, and amateur herpetologists are usually the victims. Many of these bites are incurred by exotic snakes species not native to the United States, and require specific antivenin. To provide assistance for specific exotic snake bites, the EMT should consult the local medical expert who has experience in dealing with venomous snakes.

## PREVENTION

The EMT should be familiar with identification of poisonous snakes indigenous to his geographical location. Proper identification will aid in the treatment of the bitten patient once at the hospital, and may prevent him from being bitten if he knows the snake is poisonous. Other measures that will lessen the chance of being a victim of a snake bite include:

1. Wearing footgear that comes above the ankle when afield in snake country.

2. Never reaching for anything where you cannot see.

3. Never handle a freshly killed snake with bare hands. Reflex striking activity may persist an hour or more after death.

4. Never step over a log if the other side is not visible. Step on the log and look first.

5. Never gather firewood or wander afield after dark. Snakes are nocturnal and many seek their prey at night.

6. Never go out of the way to disturb or kill a snake.

*References*

Arnold, Robert E. *What To Do About Bites and Stings of Venomous Animals.* New York: Collier, 1973.

Barber, Janet M., and Budassi, Susan A. *Mosby's Manual of Emergency Care: Practice and Procedures.* St. Louis, MO: The C. V. Mosby Co., 1979.

Ellis, M. D. *Dangerous Plants, Snakes, Arthropods and Marine Life Toxicity and Treatment.* Hamilton, ILL: Drug Intelligence Publications.

Glass, T. G., Jr. "Early Debridement in Pit Viper Bites," *JAMA,* 235: 2513–16, June 7, 1976.

McCullough, N. C., and Gennaro, J. F., Jr. "Evolution of Venomous Snakebite in the Southern U.S.," *Journal of Florida Medicine Association,* 40:959–967, 1963.

"Patient Care: Snakebite? Get the Facts, Then Hurry," *American Journal of Nursing,* June 1, 1976.

Russell, Finley E. "Jaws That Bite, Things That Sting," *Emergency Medicine,* pp. 25–41, July 1978.

Russell, Finley E., and Puffer, H. W. "Pharmacology of Snake Venoms," *Clinical Toxicology* 3(3): 433–444, September 1970.

Watt, C. H. "Poisonous Snakebite Treatment in the U.S.," *JAMA,* 240: 654–656, August 18, 1978.

# Chapter 33

# Water-Related Accidents

## DROWNING AND NEAR-DROWNING

Drowning may be defined as suffocation by submersion in water or other liquid medium. Near-drowning denotes a recovery that has occurred after initially being submerged in water or other liquid medium.

More than 8000 deaths each year in the United States are attributed to drowning. This figure would be much higher if cases of near-drowning were included, since victims do not become fatality statistics. Over 50 percent of the drowning victims die in private swimming pools.

It is the second leading cause of accidental death in the United States, and the fourth leading cause of death in children. It accounts for 10 percent of all accidental deaths, with close to 50 percent of those deaths in children under four years of age. The highest incidence of drowning and near-drowning occurs in the fifteen- to nineteen-year-old age group, and it is five times higher in men than women. Statistics also show that 35 percent of the drownings occur with people who were good swimmers and 65 percent occur in healthy people under the age of thirty.

### Causes

Drowning and near-drowning events are attributed to numerous causes:

1. *Trauma.* Diving into shallow water and injuring the cervical spine occurs frequently. The diver is then paralyzed and cannot swim. Striking an object also occurs, which renders the person unconscious and he drowns. (See Fig. 33–1.) It must be pointed out that in all cases of drowning and near-drowning, the EMT should always suspect a cervical spine injury, especially when a history is unknown, there is facial trauma, or if a history of diving was reported.

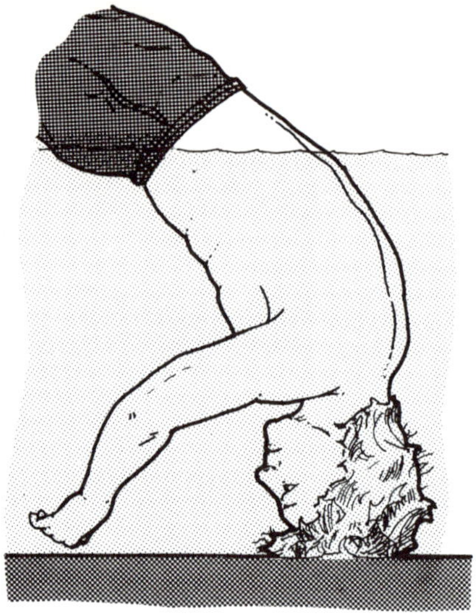

**Figure 33–1.** A common cause of drowning is diving in shallow water, injuring the cervical spine.

2. *Drug or Alcohol Intoxication.* A person who is or has taken depressant drugs or who has been drinking inordinate amounts of alcohol has a decreased ability to swim. The person is not acting in a rational manner, and tries to overextend his ability to swim.

3. *Exhaustion.* When the person becomes overly exhausted, he realizes that he cannot make it to safety, panic begins to develop, and he drowns.

4. *Hypothermia.* Exposure to cold water for any length of time tires the patient quickly. His ability to swim decreases and he loses consciousness.

Other causes that the EMT should not overlook may include: suicide attempts, heart attack, battered child syndrome, seizure disorders, and hyperventilation syndrome. (Many good swimmers hyperventilate to blow off carbon dioxide, and enrich their body with oxygen so they can stay under the water longer. Since carbon dioxide is the normal stimulus that causes us to breathe, and since it has been blown off by hyperventilating, the breathing drive is lowered. The swimmer becomes hypoxic and finally loses consciousness.)

## The Drowning Process

Drowning may occur from any of the above mentioned causes. The process the victim may follow when he is drowning can take place in one of two ways.

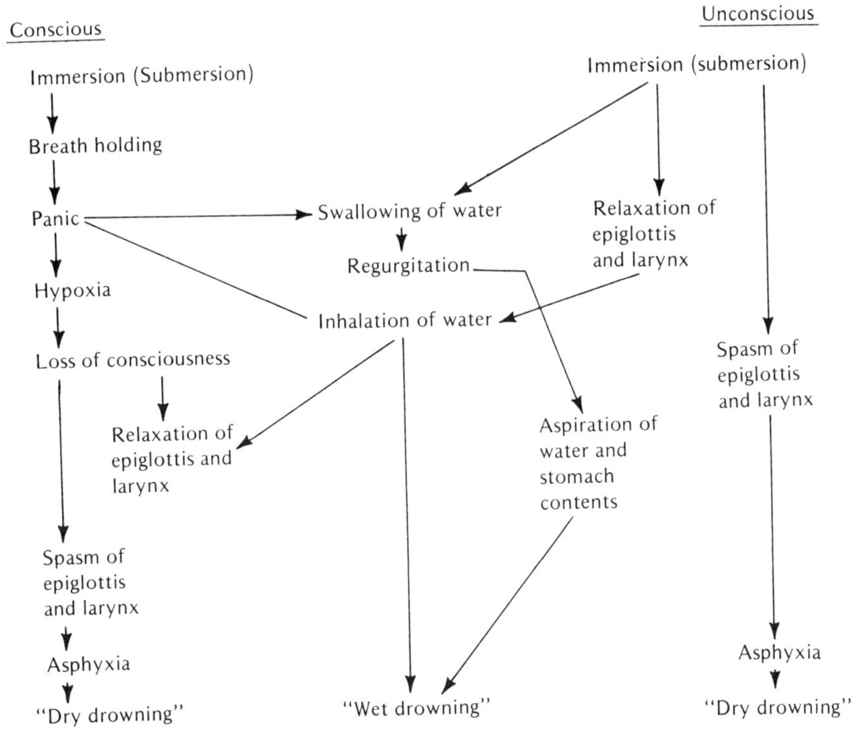


**Figure 33-2.** The process of drowning. (Reprinted with permission from "Drowning: An Overview," John E. Spoor, M.D., *Emergency Medical Services*, March–April, 1980.)

When a person in the water realizes that he cannot make it to safety, he begins to struggle and fight the water to stay afloat and breathe. As the struggle for treading the water and breathing continues, the person begins to tire; at this stage panic is the major opponent.

The drowning victim then does one of two things at this point. (See Fig. 33-2.) He may swallow lots of water while bobbing up and down in the process of his struggle, and then aspirate the water and stomach contents into the lungs. This is called a *wet drowning*. Or, he may inhale a small amount of water (< 20 cc) into the trachea. This irritating water passes by the epiglottis (ep'ĭ-glot'is), vocal cords, and trachea. This causes the vocal cords to spasm and seal off the airway. Since the person can no longer breathe due to the laryngospasm (lah-ring'go-spazm), he becomes hypoxic and becomes unconscious. This, of course, leads to suffocation and the patient becomes a drowning statistic. The laryngospasm prevents any further entry of air and water into the lungs and stomach because the person cannot inhale any longer. This is called a *dry drowning*.

Wet drownings occur in about 80–90 percent of all cases. Obviously, the victim of a dry drowning has a better chance of survival because pulmonary injury is not as severe. If the person is unconscious when he is submerged in the water, he is subjected to the same paths of a wet or dry drowning; it will depend on whether or not laryngospasm occurs.

Fresh $H_2O$ aspiration

- Transient hypervolemia
- Hemolysis
- Pulmonary edema
- Hypoxia

Sea $H_2O$ aspiration

- Hypovolemia
- Mild ↑ in hematocrit
- Pulmonary edema
- Hypoxia

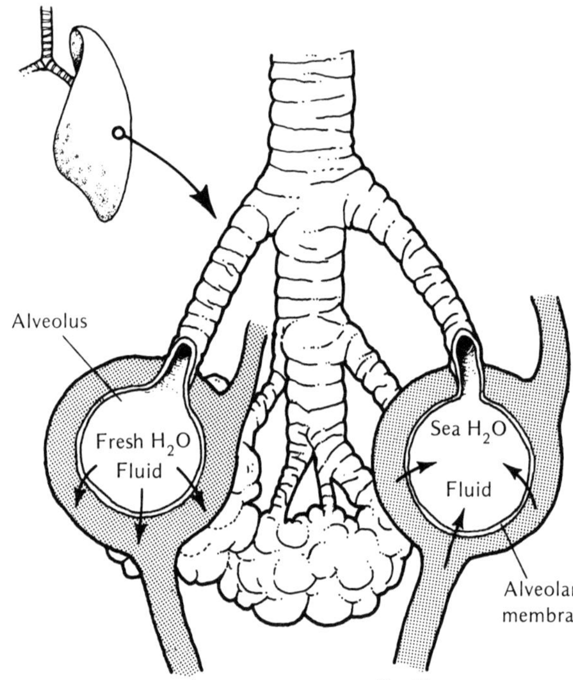


**Figure 33-3.** The body responds differently to fresh water aspiration than to salt water aspiration. Fresh water is shunted across the alveolar membrane to the capillary system, while salt water causes plasma from the capillaries to be shunted into the alveoli.

## Pathophysiology—Pulmonary

Physiological differences exist in the victim who has been submerged in fresh water versus sea water. (See Fig. 33-3.)

### *Fresh Water Submersion*

Because fresh water is less concentrated than normal body fluids, it is rapidly absorbed into the patient's blood stream once it has entered the lungs. This process of water transfer through the alveoli to the capillary system takes only about three to four minutes after aspiration (as″pĭ-ra′shun) occurs. Although this may seem to be good, fresh water decreases a necessary protein mixture called *surfactant* (sur-fak′tant), which coats the alveoli to enable them to expand when breathing. Since surfactant is decreased, there is an increase in airway resistance.

*Sea Water Submersion*

Sea water contains 3–4 percent more salt than the body's normal fluids (the body's fluid concentration is isotonic or 0.9 percent normal saline). Therefore, when sea water enters the lungs, plasma in the capillaries shunts across the alveoli and into the lung to attempt dilution of the hypertonic (more than 0.9 percent saline) solution. The alveoli eventually clog and the victim develops pulmonary edema. This patient will have very wet lungs. Rales (rahlz) can easily be heard.

## Treatment

Once the victim has been removed from the water, the EMT must rapidly evaluate the patient and institute a treatment protocol at once. A treatment protocol for the near-drowning victim should include:

1. Stabilize the cervical spine before maneuvering the patient in different positions.
2. Perform a quick primary survey. Provide a patent airway and check the circulatory status. Be aware during your survey that the patient may have other injuries if the victim was subjected to a shallow dive or if the victim has tried to commit suicide.
3. Institute CPR if no pulse and respirations are detected.
4. Give oxygen at 100 percent. If the victim responds to ventilation, which they often do, put a nonrebreathing mask on the patient to give the highest percentage of oxygen.
5. If intravenous fluids are available, advanced EMTs should start an IV of 0.9 percent saline at a keep-open rate.
6. If a heart monitor is available, run a ECG strip to establish a rhythm. Most cardiac dysrhythmias (dis-rith″me-ahz) are due to hypoxia in the near-drowning victim.
7. Monitor the patient en route to the medical facility, taking vital signs at least every five minutes.
8. Transport the victim in a left-lateral recumbent position if unconscious.
9. Report your situation to the medical facility. Let the medical personnel know:
    a. Whether the patient was submerged in fresh or sea water
    b. Present condition of patient
    c. Treatment given
    d. Position of the patient during transport
    e. Estimated time of arrival

In the United States, more than three million SCUBA (self-contained underwater breathing apparatus) diving enthusiasts take to the water to enjoy what they may see and find in the lower depths. Because the sport of scuba diving is increasing each year, more and more people will encounter diving problems.

Ideally, every scuba diver should be certified in the sport before diving. In this way every person becomes acquainted with the hazards related to diving, and his scuba diving knowledge and skills are attested to by passing an examination before certification is approved.

Basically, the physiological problems encountered with diving are related to one of the cardinal physical laws concerned with scuba diving: Boyle's Law. Boyle's Law states that at a constant temperature, the volume of a gas is inversely proportional to the pressure. In other words, as a diver descends (increasing pressure on the body), the gas volume (air mixture) in the lungs decreases. On the other hand, as a diver ascends from lower depths (decreasing pressure on the body), the gas volume (air mixture) in the lungs increases. As one can see from Boyle's Law, most problems occur with descension and ascension in the water.

## Problems of Descent

The most common problem that accompanies descent in diving is that of compression, so-called squeeze injuries. (See Fig. 33-4.) When a person dives and descends in water, the body is exposed to greater atmospheric pressure than what he is normally accustomed to. At sea level we live under the constant pressure influence of one atmosphere. When a diver reaches a depth of thirty-three feet, the body experiences a pressure of two atmospheres. At sixty-six feet the pressure is three atmospheres. Normal air cavities in the body, such as the nasal sinuses, middle ear, and lungs, cannot equalize increasing atmospheric pressure as the diver descends if the passages connecting the nose and mouth are blocked; in such situations as nasal congestion or ear infections.

As the diver descends and external pressure increases, pain will be experienced. This pain usually prevents the diver from going deeper and is a natural safeguard.

If the diver descends with pausing intervals, the pressure will equalize in the body air cavities and pain will not be experienced. This sort of descent problem is usually not seen by the EMT because, for the most part, it is self-limited. The pain caused by the external pressure is lessened by the application of cold packs to the affected area.

Complications of external pressure may exist when the diver's eardrum is ruptured. In this case, there is an increased risk of middle ear infection if the victim is not seen and treated by a physician. The EMT should suspect a ruptured eardrum if a history of quick descent is given, the pa-

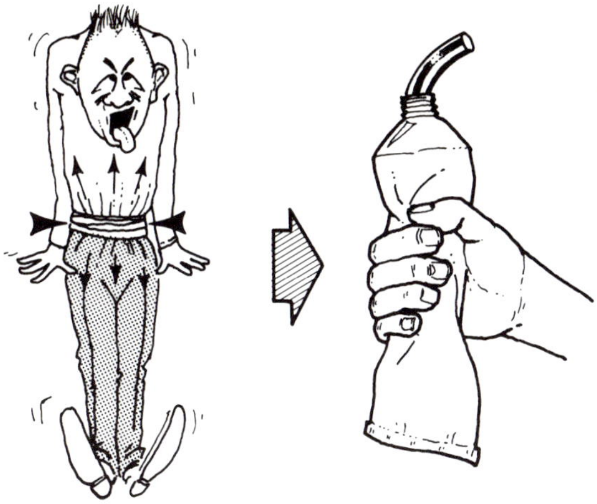

**Figure 33-4.** The squeeze injury.

tient complains of ear pain, or blood is seen oozing from the ear canal. If the EMT suspects a ruptured eardrum, the patient should be transported to a medical facility.

Compression problems can be avoided by the diver if he pushes air into the eustachian tube, thereby equalizing the external pressure. This is accomplished by performing a Valsalva maneuver, a process by which the diver holds his nose and attempts to exhale forcibly through his nose.

Accompanying a ruptured eardrum may be cold water that enters the middle ear. When this happens, the diver may lose his equilibrium or sense of balance and panic, ascending rapidly to the surface with a lung full of air, thereby increasing the chance of air embolism (em'bo-lizm). Air embolism is discussed later in the chapter.

*Nitrogen Narcosis*

A problem that may arise when the diver has descended too deeply is called *nitrogen narcosis.* The mixture of air that we breathe contains oxygen, nitrogen, and carbon dioxide. Approximately four-fifths of the air that we breathe is nitrogen. As the diver remains at certain depths for a certain period of time (see Table 33-1), the increased external pressure

TABLE 33-1. NITROGEN NARCOSIS

| *Depth of Water at Which Signs/Symptoms Appear* | *Symptoms* |
|---|---|
| 130–150 feet | Joviality, carefree attitude |
| 150–200 feet | Drowsiness |
| 200–250 feet | Fatigue drowsiness |
| 250–300 feet | Listless and feeling of uselessness |
| 300–400 feet | Unconsciousness, death |

dissolves the nitrogen gas in the nervous system tissues of the body, thereby reducing nerve excitability. This produces an effect on the body much like alcohol intoxication. For this reason, nitrogen narcosis has been called "raptures of the depths." At sea level, of course, this does not happen because there is no increased external pressure to "force" the nitrogen gas to dissolve.

The skin diver usually has to be subjected to these certain depths and pressures for at least one hour or more before nitrogen gas dissolves in the body to cause its effects. This condition is easily reversible by ascending to shallower water, thereby decreasing external pressure. Treatment for nitrogen narcosis includes basic life support and prompt rescue.

## Problems of Ascent

The two most common and dangerous problems of ascension in water are air embolism and decompression sickness.

### *Air Embolism*

Air embolism is the most frequent problem of scuba diving. It occurs from the overexpansion of air in the lung, causing the lung to rupture, creating a spontaneous pneumothorax (nu″mo-tho′raks) or pneumomediastinum (nu″mo-me″de-as-ti′num). Because of the expanding internal pressure (Boyle's Law at work here), air is forced from the alveoli into the capillaries, where air emboli (air bubbles) may pass to the heart, brain, spinal cord, or brain, blocking the circulating blood to those areas.

In severe cases, large air bubbles may accumulate in the heart, causing it to beat improperly. Fatal dysrhythmias may develop and the diver may die. The mechanism of injury in air embolism is that the diver holds his breath during the ascent process. Air embolism can be prevented if the diver exhales during the ascent. In this way, the increasing pressure is equalized and decreased during the surface ascent.

#### *Signs and Symptoms*

1. Tightness in the chest
2. Shortness of breath
3. Mottling (blotching) or itching of the skin
4. Frothy pink sputum from the nose and mouth
5. Chest pain
6. Nausea and vomiting
7. Dizziness
8. Seizures
9. Speaking difficulty
10. Possible paralysis and unconsciousness

*Treatment:* The EMT should have a strong suspicion that the diver has an air embolism with any of the above signs or symptoms, especially with a history of breath holding during the surface ascent.

The patient should be kept quiet and calm. Oxygenation is important. Give the victim 100 percent oxygen by mask, and maintain a patent airway. Rule out a pneumothorax. Auscultate (aws'kul-tāt) both lung fields for air exchange. The patient should be placed in a left-lateral Trendelenburg position to reduce the chance of air embolization to the brain. Provide basic life support during transportation and monitor vital signs. Call the designated medical facility and inform them of your situation and the type of patient being transported.

This type of patient may require immediate recompression in a pressure chamber. It is important that the EMT know which medical facility in the region has pressure chamber capabilities so that the patient can receive appropriate care.

### *Decompression Sickness*

Decompression sickness (also called the bends, caisson disease, diver's paralysis, and dysbarism) occurs when the diver has been at a depth long enough for nitrogen to be dissolved. Therefore, when the diver ascends rapidly, nitrogen is not absorbed quickly enough by the body, and nitrogen gas bubbles form, blocking small blood vessels.

If the diver ascends at appropriate water levels and pauses for specific time intervals, the nitrogen gas will be permitted to be reabsorbed by the body. Dive tables exist which give the rate of ascent and the number and length of pauses that should be made for divers of a given duration at a given depth. If the diver follows these tables, decompression sickness will not ordinarily occur. (See Appendix 9.)

*Signs and Symptoms:* A wide variety of signs and symptoms may accompany decompression sickness. Some of them may include:

1. Skin rash
2. Joint pain
3. Loss of strength and fatigue
4. Dizziness
5. Crepitus (krep'ı-tus)
6. Seizures
7. Paralysis
8. Visual loss
9. Shortness of breath
10. Unconsciousness

Unlike the immediate effects of air embolism, the signs and symptoms of decompression sickness may not occur until several hours after the dive.

*Treatment:* Recompression in a pressure chamber is the appropriate definitive treatment. Once in the pressure chamber, the diver is subjected to high pressure as he would be under water at his original depths. Because of this high external pressure, nitrogen bubbles will be reduced, forcing them back into the tissues of the body. The diver is gradually recompressed so that the remaining nitrogen can be exhaled gradually.

Enroute to the designated hospital, the EMT should provide basic life support, giving the patient 10 *l*/min. of oxygen by mask. The patient should be transported in a left lateral Trendelenburg position to decrease the chance of air embolization.

*References*

American Academy of Orthopedic Surgeons, Committee on Allied Health. *Emergency Care of the Sick and Injured.* 2nd ed. Chicago: American Academy of Orthopedic Surgeons, 1977.

Baldwin and Pierce, eds. *Mobile Intensive Care,* St. Louis: The C. V. Mosby Co., 1978.

Barber, Janet M., and Budassi, Susan A. *Mosby's Manual of Emergency Care: Practices and Procedures.* St.Louis, MO: The C. V. Mosby Company, 1979.

Erven, Lawrence W. *Handbook of Emergency Care and Rescue.* Beverly Hills, CA: Glencoe Press, 1976.

Gresham, Bayne, LCdr. C. "Acute Decompression Sickness: 50 Cases," *Journal of American College of Emergency Physicians,* 7:10, October 1978, pp. 351–354.

Guyton, A. C. *Textbook of Medical Physiology,* 4th ed. Philadelphia, PA: W. B. Saunders Co., 1971.

Hooper, Allen, H. "Near Drowning," *Emergency,* May 1980, pp. 75–77.

Knudsen, R. O. "Practical Guides to Resuscitation After Submersion," *Hospital Medicine,* May 1975.

Moser, R. "Drowning: A Seasonal Disease," *JAMA* 229:563–566, 1974.

Orlowski, J. "Prognostic Factors in Pediatric Cases of Drowning and Near Drowning," *JACEP* 8(5), May 1979.

Patton, John. "Seamergencies: The Lower Depths," *Emergency Medicine,* June 1976, pp. 155–166.

Spoor, J. E.: "Drowning: An Overview," *Emergency Medical Services,* March/April, 1980.

# Chapter 34

# Extrication, Patient Transfer, and Hazardous Materials

Emergency Medical Technicians are among the first to arrive on the scene of vehicular accidents or emergency situations requiring specialized rescue, to reach and care for the patient. Ideally, the ambulance and rescue unit should be separate and respond together when accidents are reported. This type of system will allow the EMTs and/or paramedics to attend to the patient and will allow the specialized rescue team to provide the needed extrication (eks″trĭ-ka′shun) procedures. Unfortunately, this dual response of services is usually not available, especially in rural areas. Therefore, where this system does not exist, the EMT must have a sufficient knowledge base to deal with rescue procedures. Because extrication training requires extensive "hands-on" experience (complete courses exist on the subject of extrication), it is not within the scope of this chapter to deal with all facets of rescue and extrication. The EMT should take an additional training course in extrication and specialized rescue. This training varies depending on the geographic location of the service area. The emergency service that employs the EMT will sometimes regulate the type of extrication training required to work within its system. However, the EMT should have a basic knowledge of the principles of gaining access to wrecked vehicles and stabilizing and removing patients from places of entrapment.

Rescue operations may be divided into three levels of complexity: light, medium, and heavy. Light rescue generally requires only the use of small tools such as crowbars and screwdrivers to gain access to the patient. Medium rescue necessitates the use of larger extrication tools such as hydraulically operated equipment. Heavy rescue necessitates the use of trained specialists to handle problems such as mine entrapment, high-rise building rescue, cave-ins, and the like.

The EMT's roles at the accident scene where extrication procedures are necessary are:

1. To stabilize the accident scene and create a safe working environment

2. To reach, provide immediate life-saving measures, and extricate entrapped persons from vehicles and other enclosures without causing additional injuries

3. Provide additional medical care

4. Transport injured persons to an appropriate medical facility

## EXTRICATION AND PATIENT HANDLING

*Websters New Collegiate Dictionary* defines extrication as a means to "remove from an entanglement or difficulty" or "to free from what binds or holds back." Such would be the case if a person were trapped in a building, automobile, or piece of heavy machinery. As the EMT becomes involved in extrication procedures, he must not lose sight of the care and protection of the patient, self and fellow rescuers. This is best accomplished by:

1. A quick but thorough survey of the scene
2. A common sense approach
3. An understanding of the safe procedures for quick access to the patient

### Survey of the Scene

One of the most important responsibilities of the EMT is, of course, to prevent further harm to the patient and to treat injury and illness properly. There are many hazards that accompany vehicular accidents which must be recognized and neutralized before care of the patient begins. Those hazards most frequently encountered are:

1. Traffic congestion
2. Gasoline spills
3. Downed electrical lines
4. Unstable vehicles
5. Submerged vehicles

#### *Traffic Congestion*

Proper parking of the rescue vehicle is essential. This is best accomplished by looking at the topography and the type of accident. Park the vehicle in such a manner that it does not needlessly block the normal flow of traffic. Park along the roadside or shoulder if at all possible, allowing at least one lane of traffic around the accident scene. However, if it is recognized that patients are lying on the road, it may be necessary to use the rescue vehicle as protection for the patient from other automobiles. If this is the case, the rescue vehicle must be positioned in such a way as to keep the exhaust fumes as far away from the patient as possible.

Other problems to consider are hills and curves. One must realize that an unsuspecting motorist may not be aware of an accident which lies just over the hill or just around the bend. A warning to the approaching motorists may prevent an additional accident from occurring. Flares or persons with flashlights should be used until law enforcement officials arrive.

It is also good practice not to park an emergency vehicle downhill from a traffic accident. In the event that flammable liquids or gases are present on the scene the positioning of the rescue vehicle downhill or downwind may prove disastrous if these materials are ignited.

### *Gasoline Spills*

Gasoline tanks are frequently ruptured during impact, creating fire or the possibility of fire. If a gas spill is suspected, the EMTs should call for assistance from the nearest fire department. An excellent piece of equipment which can be easily carried on all ambulances and rescue vehicles, is a twenty-pound light-water fire extinguisher. Light water has different properties from dry chemical-and/or water-type extinguishers in that it is probably the most effective substance for putting out or preventing petroleum fires. A quick spray under the vehicle and once around the perimeter will decrease the possibility of fire. A washdown with water is satisfactory if there is enough of it available; otherwise, because gas and water do not mix, the washdown will only spread the flammable liquid into a larger area.

### *Downed Electrical Wires*

Electrical hazards may be among the most frustrating and deadly problems EMTs are faced with at the accident scene. A quick and careful survey of the vehicles involved and the immediate area surrounding the accident scene may save the patient's life and those of the rescue personnel.

If when arriving at the scene of an accident, EMTs notice a downed power line is in the area or is making contact with the wrecked vehicles, their first course of action should be to keep people and themselves away from the area. A call to the local electric company should then be made. EMTs not trained in the proper removal of electrical power lines should stand by until the authorized personnel arrive.

The intense flashing of certain power lines can cause eye injury and can easily start fires, as well as electrocute untrained and unsuspecting persons.

## *Unstable Vehicles*

An unstable vehicle can be defined as any vehicle not on all four wheels, or in a position that may allow it to roll. Before entry into the vehicle is made, stabilization of that vehicle must occur. Items that are frequently used to stabilize a vehicle are:

1. Ropes
2. Wood cribbing (4 × 4s and/or 2 × 4s eighteen-inches long made from Douglas fir or straight pine)
3. Wood wedges (Douglas fir or straight pine)
4. Other vehicles

If an EMT in his enthusiasm to help jumps onto a car which is on its side, before it is stabilized, his weight may be just enough to flip the car back over. This action may injure other rescue personnel and may cause more harm to the patient than the original accident. Placing wooden cribbing and wedges in various locations around the auto will give the vehicle a greater ground contact area, thus making it more stable. For an auto on its side, the placement of cribbing or wedges should be under the tires. Additional wood (see Fig. 34-1) should be forced under the side supports of the roof, on the other side of the car. Vehicles may be tied off by use of ropes also. Ropes should be strong enough to handle the heavy load. They will be discussed later in this chapter. It also may be necessary to use your rescue vehicle or another vehicle to help stabilize an unstable auto. One must remember, however, that once a vehicle is used to stabilize another, it becomes immobile and unable to be used elsewhere.

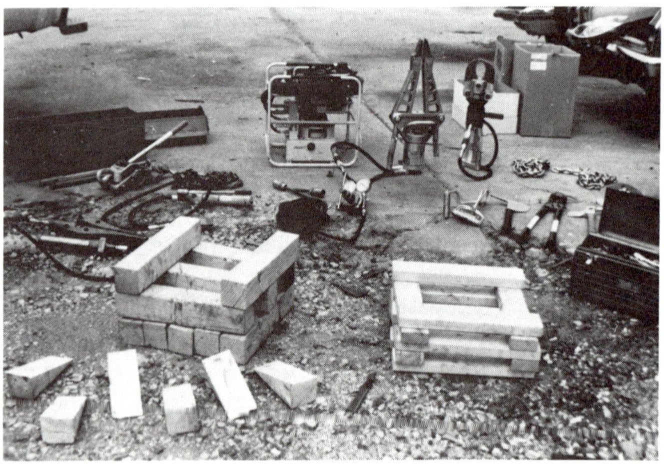

**Figure 34-1.** Wood cribbing and wedges are used to stabilize unstable vehicles.

### *Submerged Vehicles*

If an ambulance service or rescue squad has bodies of water within its service area, it is recommended that they have the basic equipment available to handle those situations in which an auto becomes submerged. Water rescue is very involved and should be left for those trained, but certain basic procedures may be used to buy more time for the patient, until removal is made possible. An eight-inch flathead screwdriver, or spring-loaded punch, along with a tank of fresh compressed air and a long air hose can give the rescuer additional time to effect a total rescue.

Placing the air hose inside the submerged auto and pumping air into it creates an air bubble which may sustain the patient until trained water rescue personnel arrive.

If the windows are closed it will be necessary to break a side or back window in order to insert the air hose. Techniques for window removal will be discussed later.

## GAINING ACCESS TO THE PATIENT

Upon completion of the initial survey of the situation, two important questions need to be answered before advancing:

1. Are all potential hazards neutralized?
2. Is there enough of the proper rescue personnel and equipment available to assure a safe and efficient extrication operation?

Ambulance and rescue organizations should be aware of the many resources available to them if the need arises for assistance. Dispatch centers should have a list of the following resources that can be called upon when requested:

1. Additional ambulances
2. Light and heavy rescue squads
3. Helicopters
4. Wreckers
5. Water rescue teams
6. Hazardous material teams
7. Construction equipment (cranes, lifts, etc.)
8. Farm equipment
9. Railways

In the event of a major disaster, all available resources may be pressed into action, so cooperation must be established *before* the need arises.

## Forcible Entry

Forcible entry refers to a quick forceful method of entering an automobile, and is used in what appears to be a life or death situation. Time in this instance is critical. Situations requiring forceful entry include:

1. Vehicle on fire with patient inside
2. Trapped patient with respiratory inadequacy
3. Patient with severe bleeding
4. Situations in which the EMT is in fear of loosing patient's life

The purpose behind forceful entry is to get emergency medical personnel to the patient as quickly as possible for the initiation of life saving emergency care. Once this has been accomplished, plans to remove the patient safely can be made if the situation allows.

One of the simplest ways of entering an auto is by grabbing the door handle and operating the latch. It's surprising the number of doors that will still open after a severe collision. Walk around the wrecked auto and try to open all doors before proceeding. If the doors are inaccessible, entry through a window should be considered. It is unlikely that following a collision all of the windows are intact, but there are those medical situations in which a patient may have collapsed inside a locked auto.

Before discussing how to break windows, it must be recognized that automobiles contain two different types of glass. For safety purposes, windshields are comprised of laminated glass. The technique for the manufacturing of this glass involves molding two sheets of glass around a thin but tough layer of plastic. This gives the window strength, thus preventing easy ejection through a windshield upon front end impacts. It also keeps pieces of broken glass together, not allowing them to explode into the auto upon breaking or collision. The glass will break, but the fractures and pieces hold together and must be cut or torn out. (See Fig. 34–2.) The other type of glass is used for side and rear windows. This type of window is known as tempered or hurculite glass. When this glass is broken, the entire window shatters into thousands of tiny pieces. (See Fig. 34–3.) This glass has been heat treated and does not contain the plastic layer as in the case of the windshield.

It is recommended that entry into an auto by breaking windows only be used when necessary. If it is necessary, however, to reach a critically ill or injured patient, it is recommended that the back window be used. This will more than likely keep glass bits away from the patient and allow ample room to enter. If a person is locked inside an undamaged vehicle, it may be preferable to break a small vent window in order to open the door from the inside, and prevent a large repair bill. However, the quickest, most efficient method will be at the discretion of the rescuer and is determined by the condition of the patient and the accident scene itself.

If entry is to be made through the windshield, which may be necessary but not recommended, a hole must be physically cut into the

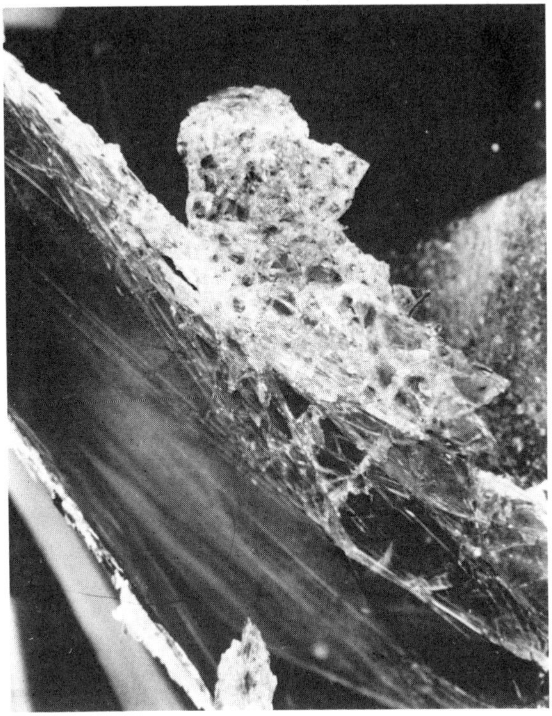

**Figure 34-2.** Laminated glass is bonded to a sheet of plastic, which is sandwiched between two layers of glass. Because of this construction, laminated glass in windshields of vehicles does not shatter into tiny pieces.

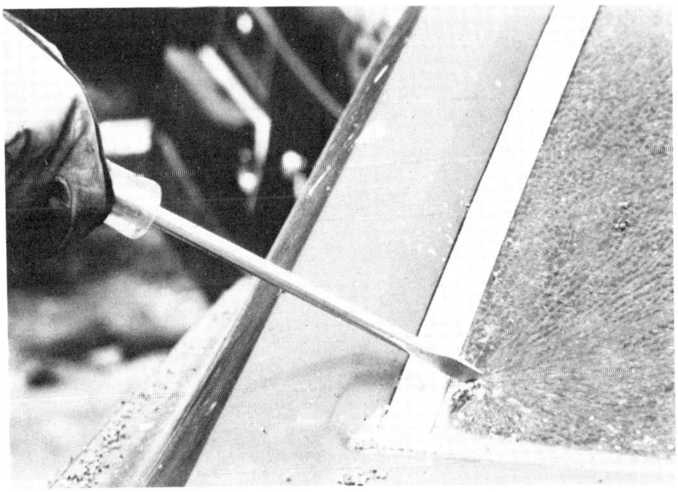

**Figure 34-3.** Tempered glass contained in side and back windows will shatter into thousands of pieces upon impact.

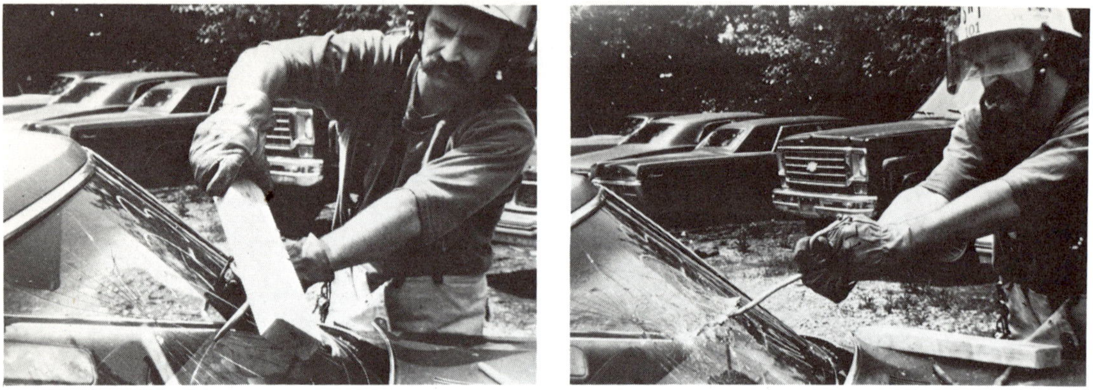

**Figure 34-4.** Technique for gaining access through a windshield using a bailing hook and cribbing. (a) The bailing hook tip is placed where the hole is to be made and driven through with cribbing. (b) An upward and outward pull of the bailing hook allows the tip to break new glass.

window. This is best accomplished with either a bailing hook or a crash-axe. (See Fig. 34-4.)

If a bailing hook is to be used, place the tip of the hook in the area the hole is to be made. Deliver a sharp blow to the back of the hook, driving the point through the window. Protecting yourself by using goggles and gloves, begin an upward and outward pull of the bailing hook, as to allow the pointed tip to break new glass. A three-sided cut should be all that's necessary, across the top and then down both sides. The flap can then be folded down, out of the way.

A crash axe is also acceptable for cutting a windshield. The axe face is serrated, as to give the tool some grip, which makes it more difficult to go completely through the window. A hole can be made by either chopping a section out or by using a sawing action with the serrated edge of the axe. (See Fig. 34-5.)

Entry through the side or rear windows, if possible, is recommended. Simple hand tools are the most effective for side or rear window removal. Some of these tools include:

1. Flathead screwdriver (good condition)
2. Springloaded punch
3. Pick-head axe
4. Crash-axe

The actual procedure for breaking the window should remain the same for all tools. First stand next to the auto on one side or the other of the window. Select a lower corner of the window closest to you. If a flathead screwdriver is to be used, the point of the flathead should be

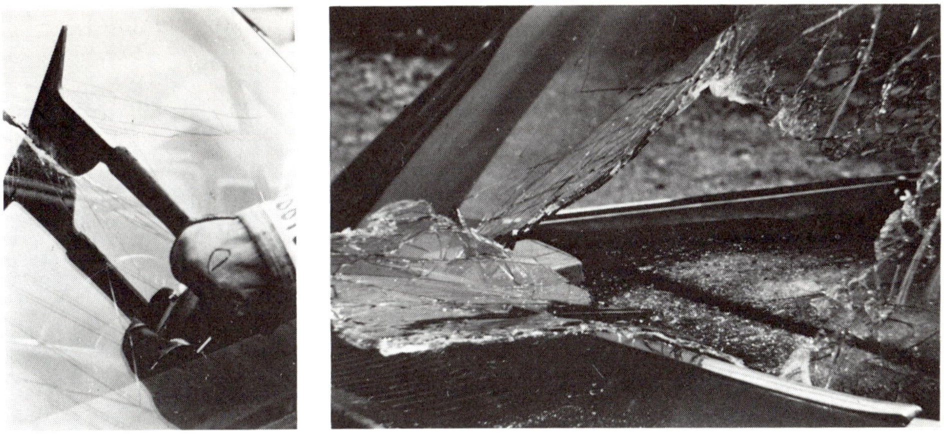

**Figure 34-5.** Technique for gaining access through the windshield using a crash axe.

"whipped" into the window. (See Fig. 34-6a.) This does not take much force. If heavier tools are to be used, beware of driving the tool through the window, and possibly harming the patient. By properly positioning yourself alongside the auto and striking the lower corner closest to you, the door or window supports will prevent the axe from entering the interior of the vehicle. The glass may then be pulled out or pushed in, depending on the situation. (See Fig. 34-6b.)

*Reminders*

A few important facts must be reviewed and considered when dealing with forceful entry. They are:

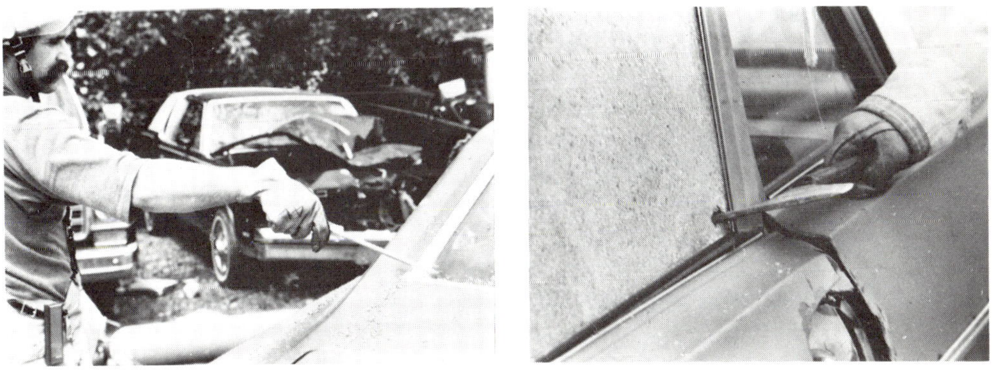

**Figure 34-6.** (a) Technique for breaking a rear window using a flathead screwdriver. (b) Technique for breaking a side window using a crash axe.

1. Use forceful entry only in life-threatening situations.
2. Before glass is broken, quickly try all doors.
3. The purpose of quick forceful entry is to get emergency care personnel into the auto as soon as possible to tend to the patient's apparent severe condition.
4. Be aware of the fact that broken glass will enter the auto, which may prove to be an additional hazard for the patients and rescuers. For this reason, it is recommended that side or rear windows be the first choice if windows need breaking.
5. Once emergency care personnel have entered and begin treating the patient, the actual extrication procedures can begin.

## REMOVAL OF THE PATIENT

The detailed knowledge needed for the safe operation and removal of patients from places of entrapment will not be covered in this chapter. The major responsibilities of the EMT at the scene of injury or illness include:

1. Protection of self and fellow rescuers
2. Protection of the patient as to prevent further harm
3. Proper handling and emergency care procedures

The old concept of auto extrication was to remove the patient from the car. The updated theory is to remove the car from around the patient. The key to an effective extrication is to make ample room for rescue workers to move and to allow enough space so proper manipulating of the patient can occur without the risk of further damage or injury. It is vitally important that those individuals responsible for the actual extrication be totally knowledgeable with all the tools they will be using. This promotes efficiency and allows fast proper handling of the patient. It is important to have a general knowledge regarding the various tools available because it may be necessary to assist rescue personnel at times. As mentioned earlier, a major responsibility of the EMT is to prevent further harm to the patient. This can be accomplished by staying with the trapped patient at all times. Metal, steel, and more, will often have to be displaced to free a patient. The EMT should constantly moniter all movement of the metals, as it is occurring by placing your hand in between the patient and the area of the car being displaced. If it is felt by the EMT that the parts of the auto are further encasing the patient, extrication procedures should be stopped and reevaluated. Communication between the EMT and the tool operator is important. The EMT should also explain to the patient a little about the procedures taking place around him. The sounds of bending metal and power tools may be frightening to the unsuspecting patients. Care must be taken to protect patients from broken glass and flying pieces of debris. This is best accomplished by covering the patient with a blanket, tarp, or fire resistant rescue blanket. Steps should be taken to ensure that the patient has adequate ventilation while being covered. It is good practice to get under the tarp with the patient, in case complications were to develop which need immediate attention.

Protection of the cervical spine is commonly required for patients involved in motor vehicle accidents.

Prior to moving the conscious patient from the auto, the EMT should ask the following questions:

1. "Do you have pain in your neck?"
2. "Do you feel any numbness anywhere?"

If the patient answers yes to either of these two questions, the EMT should check to see if the patient can:

1. Flex and extend his hands and arms
2. Move his legs

The EMT should *NOT:*

1. Ask the patient to move his neck
2. Move the patient's neck passively to check for pain

The neck should be stabilized in the position found and a cervical collar applied.

If the patient is unconscious due to a head injury or from intoxication, the EMT should treat the patient as if he has a cervical spine injury. It has been estimated that nearly 10 percent of all head injuries involve cervical fractures.

The EMT should be alert to the person who is walking around in a "daze" after being in an automobile accident. Often these types of people have injuries and do not even realize it due to the psychological trauma of being involved in the accident, especially if other persons are injured and he does not know quite what to do. These persons should be instructed to sit or lie down until you have assessed possible injuries.

Spinal injuries are best managed by immobilizing the patient on a spine board. Spine boards are available in two different sizes, long and short. (See Fig. 34–7.)

## Long Boards

Long spine boards measure approximately eighteen inches wide and seventy-two inches in length. They are commercially available in both wood and aluminum type construction. The advantage of the aluminum spine board is that most fold in the middle, making for easy storage, and because it is aluminum, its life is extremely long. However, the aluminum board does not float in water, should rescue and spinal immobilization be employed. It also absorbs heat and cold when exposed to extreme temperatures; therefore, if this type of spine board is to be utilized, a

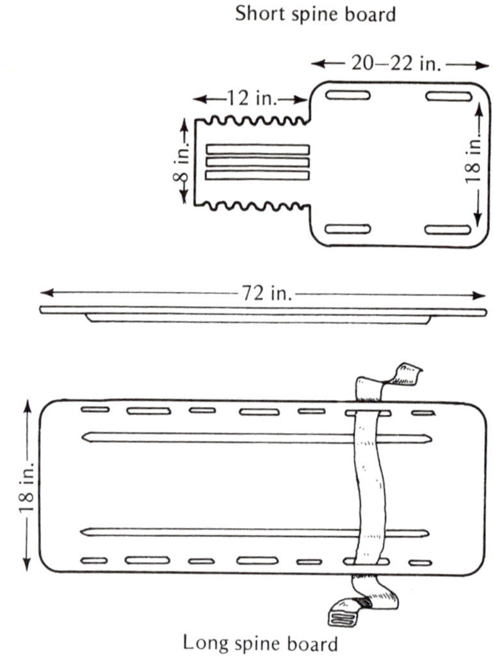


**Figure 34–7.** Long and short spine boards.

blanket or sheet should be placed on the board for patient comfort. The EMT should remember, too, that in cold weather regions where a victim has been placed on the board, body heat will be absorbed to the cold aluminum, perhaps potentiating hypothermia. Again, remember to place a blanket or sheet on the board before placing the patient onto it.

Wooden spine boards, on the other hand, do float and provide support for stabilization should they be needed in water rescue. However, over time and with use, they have the potential to splinter, thereby creating a possible hazard to both the patient and the EMT.

Regardless of construction, the long spine board is a versatile piece of equipment that can be used in stabilization of not only spinal fractures, but fractures of the hip and pelvis as well.

*Application of Long Spine Boards*

The patient with a suspected spinal or lower extremity fracture in a supine position is best placed on the long spine board by either the log-rolling method (see Fig. 34–8), or by the straddle-slide method. (See Fig. 34–9.)

## Short Spine Boards

The short spine board measures eighteen inches in width and thirty-two inches in length. Construction is generally of either wood or aluminum although space-age plastic boards are being utilized. Short spine boards are generally used to immobilize the cervical spine of patients involved in auto accidents because of their size and ability to fit in tighter working spaces. The short spine board is also useful in spinal, pelvic, or hip fractures of the pediatric patient. The short spine board can also be used as a cardiac press board if improvision is called for.

The effectiveness of the short spine board depends on the space in which the EMT must work. In some situations, the EMT will not be able to effectively apply the short spine board because of the patient's position in the wrecked vehicle. This is often the case with patients trapped in small foreign vehicles. However, the EMT usually can ensure cervical spine immobilization by placing a cervical collar on the patient and guarding against further neck movement. All too often, valuable time is spent mak-

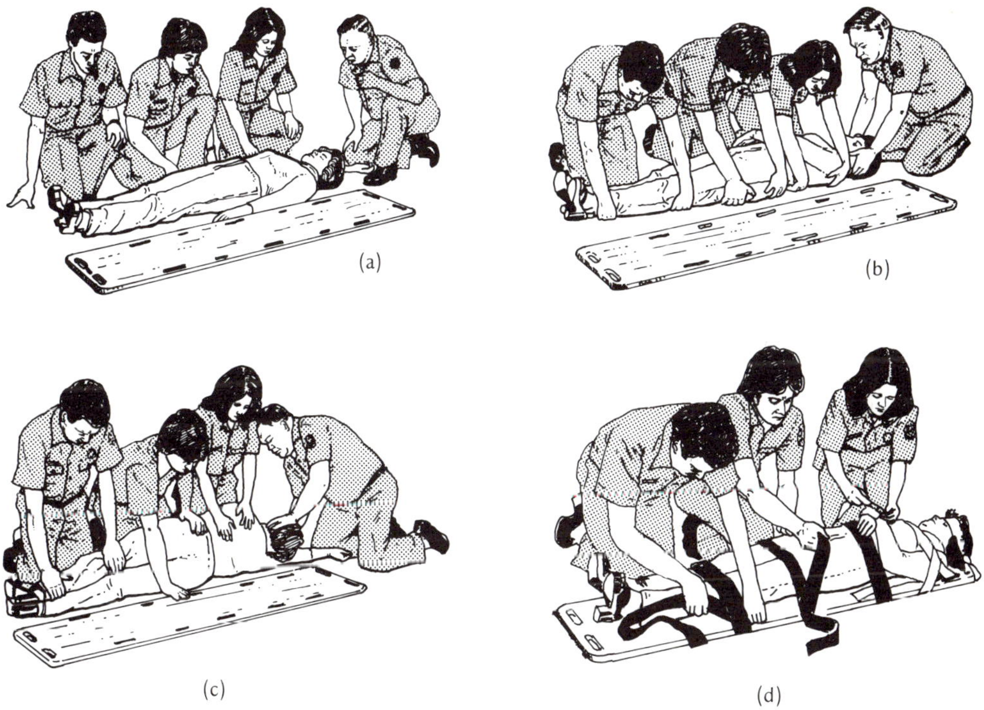


**Figure 34–8.** Positioning the injured patient on a long spine board using the log-rolling method. (a) EMT-As are in proper position to roll the patient. (b) The EMT-A at the head of the patient stabilizes the neck while the other EMT-As grasp the patient for turning. (c) As the patient is rolled as a unit toward the EMT-As, the neck is stabilized with the roll. The spine board is pulled as close to the patient as possible. (d) The patient is carefully rolled as a unit back onto the spine board and stabilized. Note: It is extremely important to stabilize all injuries prior to moving the patient onto the spine board.

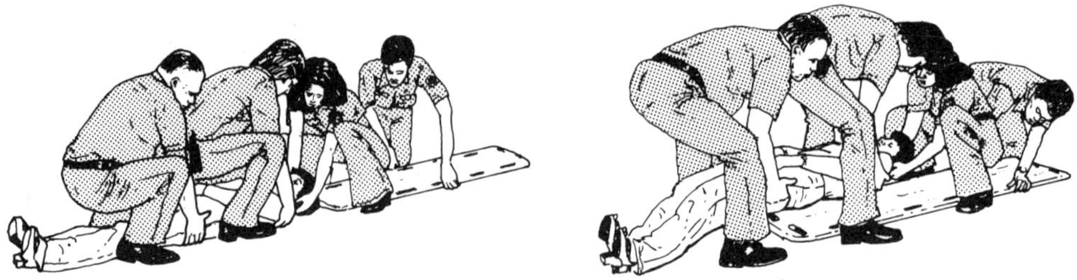

**Figure 34–9.** Positioning the patient on a long spine board using the straddle-slide method. Again, all injuries should be stabilized before moving the patient onto the spine board.

ing sure that, whatever it takes, the patient will come out of the vehicle with a spine board applied.

Many spinal injuries occur because of improper handling of the patient during spine board application. It is often more medically prudent to have one EMT stabilize the head and neck of the patient while efforts are being made to adjust the spine board at a right angle to the sitting patient's seat and carefully sliding the patient onto it. The short spine board is ideally used on those patients who are sitting in an upright position with plenty of room to their front and rear. In actual practice, the patient will rarely be in an upright position, and the EMT's working space never seems large enough, especially in high-impact vehicle collisions.

Spine board application requires many hours of practice under simulated emergency situations. The EMT should become thoroughly acquainted with all spinal immobilization equipment that might be used before it must actually be applied on a patient.

### *Positioning*

Positioning of the patient on the spine board is important. With all victims of trauma, there is the possibility of vomiting, especially if blood has entered the stomach from an injured nose or mouth. Suction equipment should always be at hand. It is recommended that the patient be placed, if necessary, in a left-lateral position to avoid aspiration of vomitus. Since the head cannot be turned with a suspected cervical spine injury, the patient's whole body must be turned. Therefore, it is imperative that the patient be firmly immobilized to the spine board, especially the cervical spine.

Regardless of what piece of equipment is used to affect proper immobilization of the spine, the patient will still need to be moved out of the car sooner or later. Tools are available which can dismantle an auto, giving rescuers the needed room to treat and move the patient correctly. Doors can be pulled out of the way or removed altogether. Seats can be moved back, steering columns and dashboards may be lifted, and roofs can be either folded back or taken completely off. With the proper equipment two-door cars can be converted to three doors, thus allowing more room to work and care for the patient.

It must be reemphasized that extrication involving powerful tools should be left up to those thoroughly trained in that field. A little knowledge may be just enough to injure yourself or others.

## COMMON TOOLS AND EQUIPMENT USED IN EXTRICATION

Equipment used for extrication can range from a simple screwdriver to a sophisticated piece of hydraulic machinery. What must be emphasized is that equipment and tools do not make a good extrication team. Total knowledge of what tools are available, what they can do, what they cannot do, and the hazards associated with particular tools are the necessary ingredients for an effective extrication team. A combination of many tools is the answer to a totally successful rescue. Tools commonly used in extrication can be broadly classified into four categories. They are:

1. Basic hand tools
2. Gasoline powered tools
3. Air powered tools
4. Hydraulically powered tools

### Basic Hand Tools

With the advent of new ultra-powerful equipment on the market for extrication, it becomes easy to forget the small hand tools. However, no rescue squad should be without certain basic hand tools. (See Fig. 34-10.) Basic hand tools, by being small, can be used in places where bigger tools

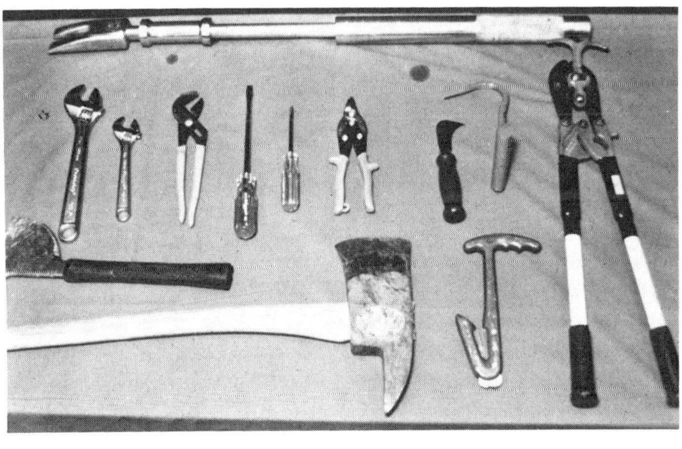

**Figure 34-10.** Common basic hand tools used in extrication.

cannot fit. Those hand tools which should be available on a rescue squad include, but are not limited to:

1. Flathead screwdrivers (various sizes)
2. Phillips head screwdrivers (various sizes)
3. Channel-lock pliers
4. Short handle sledgehammer (7½ lb.)
5. Linoleum knives
6. Vice-grip pliers
7. Aircraft snips
8. Needle nose pliers
9. Hacksaw
10. Adjustable wrenches (various sizes)
11. Pipe wrench (various sizes)
12. Socket wrench (various sizes)
13. Pick-head axe
14. Crash axe
15. Pry axe
16. 36 inch bolt cutters
17. Wrecking bar

## Gasoline-Powered Tools

The gasoline-powered disc saws are slowly being phased out of vehicle rescue because of their potential hazard if used improperly. The blades of such tools turn approximately 6000 times per minute, allowing them to cut quickly through all types of material. A charged water line must be available to shower the cutting area with a spray of water because of the tremendous amount of sparks thrown off while cutting. (See Fig. 34–11.) The tool when used improperly can set autos and clothing on fire.On the other hand, if a trained operator is available, safe and efficient usage of the tool is possible.

## Air-Powered Tools

Air-powered tools in use today include chisels for cutting metal of various thicknesses, bolts, and supports. (See Fig. 34–12.) Also included is the gun in which the chisels are secured and a regulator which tells the operator how many pounds per square inch (psi) the tool is operating off of, plus how much air is left in the supply tank. Air chisels work most effectively if they operate at 300 psi. Any more pressure than 300 psi wastes air and anything less takes more time, thus using more air. Air chisels are

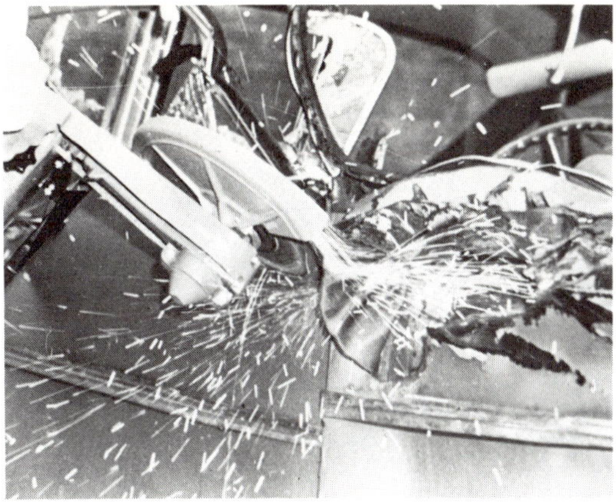

**Figure 34-11.** A gasoline powered saw. Note the sparks being emitted. When using this tool, a fine spray of water should be showered on the cutting area to decrease spark throw-off. A fire extinguisher should be available when the saw is in use.

frequently used for removing a car top for proper extrication of patients inside automobiles that are resting on their sides. Air chisels are also very affective for totally removing a roof by cutting the front window posts and the rear supports.

## Hydraulically-Powered Tools

Hydraulically-powered tools range from the manually operated porta-power tools up to the motor driven Hurst and Lucas tools. The manually-powered tools take a minimum of two operators. The tools

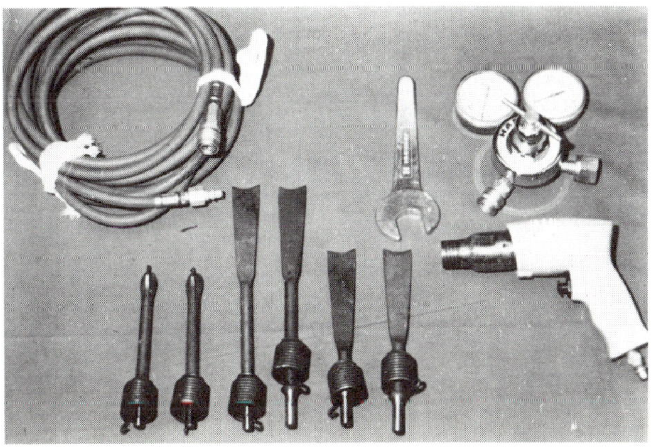

**Figure 34-12.** Air-powered chisel and blades.

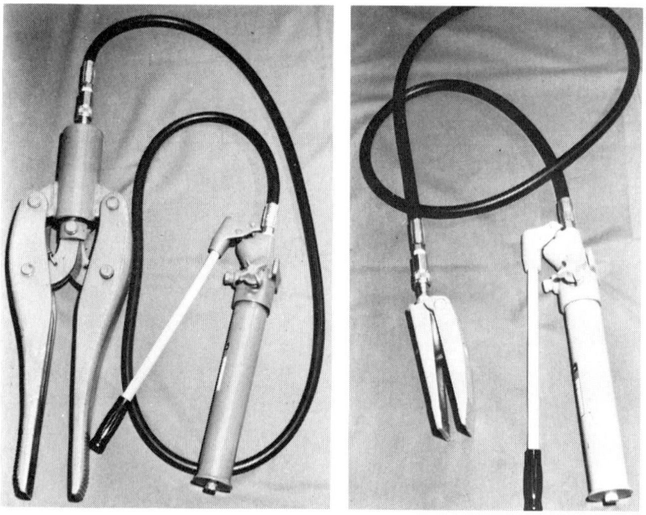

(a) (b)

**Figure 34–13.** Hydraulically-powered spreading devices: (a) This tool is known as a "spreader." (b) This tool is smaller and is called a "wedgie."

themselves are designed as small spreading devices capable of delivering anywhere from two to twenty tons of spreading and lifting power. (See Fig. 34–13.) The two-ton capacity units are most frequently used by rescue squads and serve to open jammed doors, lift or move brake and clutch pedals, and displace light metal.

The power source of the Hurst and Lucas tools come from a two-stroke engine which pumps fluid to the spreading and cutting devices of the tool. (See Fig. 34–14.) The Hurst tool is capable of exerting a force of approximately 10,000 psi at the tips of its spreader arms or jaws. The Lucas generates approximately 9000 psi at its tips. Both tools can be adapted with chains for the pulling of steering columns and cutting devices for roof removal. Hydraulic jacks are also widely used in rescue. These jacks come in an assortment of capacities from two-ton to twenty-ton units. (See Fig. 34–15.)

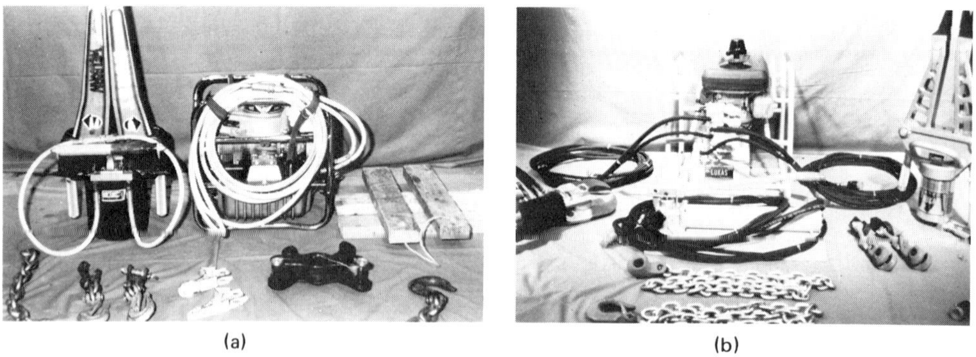

(a) (b)

**Figure 34–14.** (a) The Hurst tool; (b) the Lucas tool.

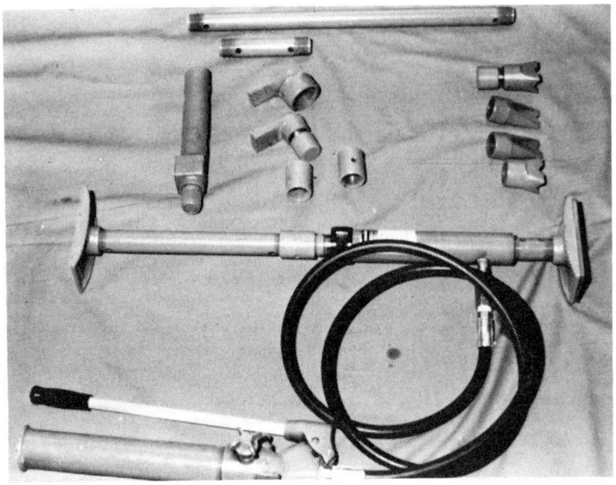

**Figure 34-15.** A hydraulically-powered jack (ram) with extension tubing.

## Pulling Devices

The come-a-long is the most widely used manually operated pulling device used in extrication. (See Fig. 34-16.) Most units are rated at one and one-half ton capacities. However, through the proper use of pulleys, cables and blocks, the pulling strength can far exceed the one and one-half ton limits. The come-a-long is frequently used to pull steering columns out of the way, as well as doors. It also can be used to pull seats back, lift break and clutch pedals, and pull back roofs. A set of chains are used with the come-a-long. One is five feet in length and the other is twelve feet long. One chain is always used as an anchor, while the other attaches to the object being moved. While the come-a-long is often used, it must be stressed that proper rigging of the chains is critical for safe operation. Improper hook-ups may snap a steering column, possibly causing injury to the patient or others. Detailed training by qualified personnel in the proper use of the come-a-long as well as all other pieces of equipment is mandatory.

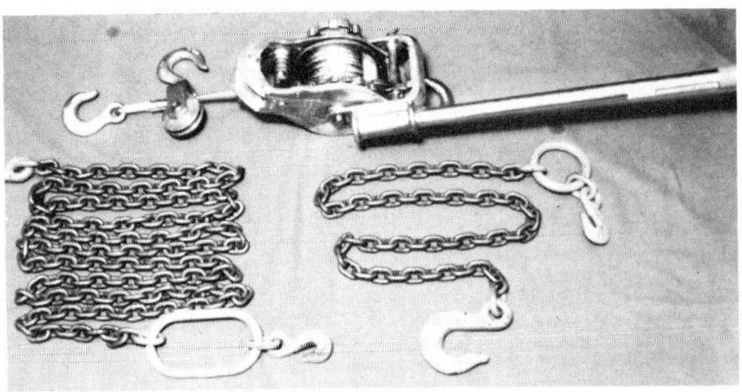

**Figure 34-16.** The come-a-long pulling device.

It must be emphasized as with extrication, the use of ropes for patient evacuation should be left to those thoroughly trained in that area. However, EMTs should have general knowledge concerning; (1) why ropes are needed in EMS, (2) types of ropes available, and (3) hardware used in conjunction with rope rescue.

People must realize that the use of special ropes, hardware, and riggings are not used solely for the evacuation of people from high-rise structures. There are countless situations which call for the use of ropes for the safe transfer of people from one area to another. Tall buildings and high structures really have little influence when determining whether a rescue squad should develop skills in rope work or not. Even though ropes may be a squad's only method available for the rescue of people from extreme heights, there are many other situations in which ropes are needed. Some of these situations are:

1. Transfer of patients over rough, dangerous terrain
2. Removal of patients from inaccessible places such as attics, roofs, ledges, and cliffs
3. Bringing patients up from mine shafts and wells
4. Transference of people from one area to another by transferring over swollen rivers, etc.
5. Securing of machinery, car, etc.

The use of ropes is largely influenced by geographical location and terrain. However, once a squad becomes proficient in rope rescue through formal training programs, it is then that the true value of line rescue can be appreciated. Fire department ladders and shackle units have the capability of reaching seventy to one-hundred feet and should be used whenever possible. But what about those cases in which the fire apparatus is tied up somewhere else, or ladders cannot be extended because of trees or lines, or because buildings and alleys won't allow entry of large trucks?

EMS personnel are concerned with delivering the best emergency care available to the patient. That includes proper patient handling, and to protect from further injury, it may be necessary to immobilize and remove patients from windows instead of narrow, curving stairwells.

## General Information About Rescue Ropes

There are dozens of ropes marketed today, but only a few are suitable for rescue work involving people. The characteristics that qualify a rope for rescue are:

1. Strength
2. Resistance to rot

3. Resists abrasion well
4. Elongation properties
5. Absorbs shock loads

Some of the first ropes used for climbing or rescue work were natural fiber ropes. These ropes were frequently made from cotton that contained fibers of only one-half to two inches long. The disadvantages of natural fiber ropes are:

1. Subject to rot
2. Easily abrased
3. Contain short fibers causing them to break easily
4. Fall of more than sixteen to twenty feet would break rope

Hemp and Manila ropes were introduced in the Nineteenth Century. These ropes had a few advantages over the cotton fiber ropes in that the fibers were longer within the rope, giving it more strength. Manila ropes are also treated with an oily substance during manufacturing for more stability and ease of handling. As this oily substance is lost, so is some of the strength of the rope. It is the opinion of this author that natural fiber ropes should not be used when handling people. Manila ropes may be used to secure machinery or automobiles or as salvage lines.

The first synthetic ropes were introduced during World War II. These ropes were made of nylon fibers which were twisted around each other. This property gave the rope stretch. Nylon ropes used in rescue are either laid (fibers twisted around each other) or of the kernmantle design. Kernmantle rope is made up of a center core of long nylon fibers, surrounded by a tightly woven sheath. Kernmantle ropes are further divided into stretch and nonstretch categories. There are advantages to both, depending on the rescue situation. The overall advantages of nylon laid and kernmantle ropes are:

1. Tremendous strength
2. Good elongation ability
3. Absorbs great shock loads
4. Can be inspected easily
5. Resists abrasion

Ropes used in rescue must be maintained as any other life-saving piece of equipment. You and your patient's life are literally "on the line." Care must be taken to keep the rope clean. Nylon ropes can be washed and dried at medium temperatures. They should be stored in dry areas, out of prolonged contact with direct sunlight, and should be wrapped in big loops when stored. A visual inch-by-inch inspection should occur after each use. Records indicating time used and whether the rope had been subjected to shock loading should be kept. It should also be mentioned that rescue ropes

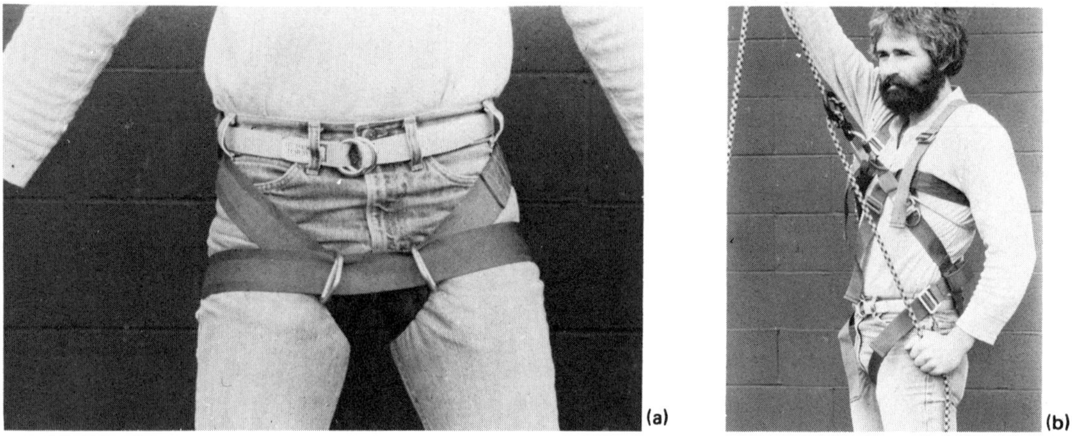

Figure 34-17. (a) A body harness; (b) a Texas seat harness.

should not be used for towing or pulling vehicles. If this occurs, the rope must be retired because of the possibility of severe internal damage, making it unsafe for the rescue of people.

## Common Hardware Used With Rescue Ropes

### *Harnesses*

There are numerous harnesses available for use by rescue personnel. However, there are two major categories into which harnesses fall: the full body harness and the seat-type device. (See Fig. 34-17.) When removing untrained personnel from heights or depths, it is recommended that the full body harness be used because it assures rescuers that the patient will always be in an upright position. It is a matter of personal preference whether a seat type or full body harness is used by the rescuer.

### *Carabiners*

Also known as D-rings, carabiners (kah-rob'in-erz) are made of either steel or aluminum and resemble an oval or D. They are designed with a gate, which opens to different sizes depending on the type, and some are equipped with a locking device that prevents the gate from opening unexpectedly. (See Fig. 34-18.) Carabiners are used to attach other pieces of hardware together or to the rescuer's harness. Strengths of the carabiners range from approximately 3000 to 10,000 pounds before damage can occur.

### *Braking Devices*

In order to descend a rope, it is necessary to use a friction device through which the rope is fed. These devices range from a simple D-Ring to items such as racks, bank/plates, descending rings, and figure 8s. All brak-

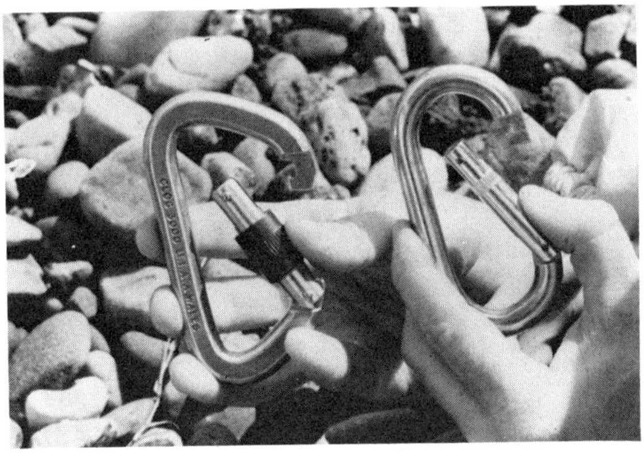

**Figure 34-18.** Carabiners.

ing devices have different properties, some allowing for a more controlled descent or friction adjustment while in operation. (See Fig. 34-19.)

*Ascending Devices*

It may be necessary at times to ascend back up a rope. This can be accomplished through the use of ascenders. Ascenders grip the rope when downward pressure is exerted against them. (See Fig. 34-20.)

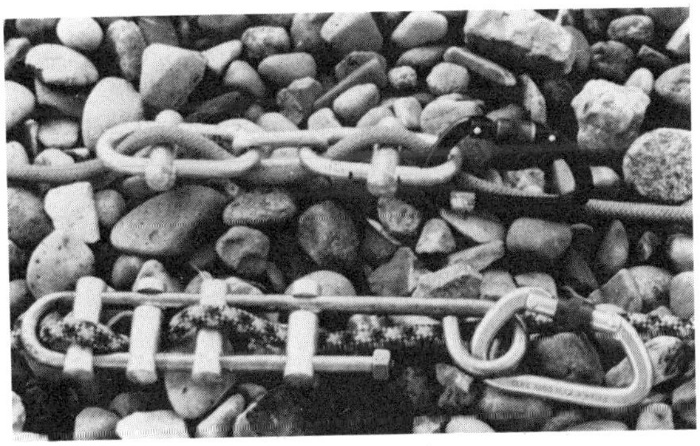

**Figure 34-19.** Descent control devices.

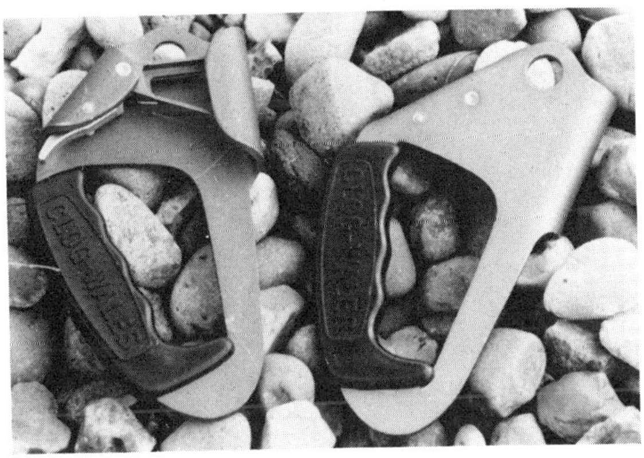

**Figure 34-20.** Ascending devices.

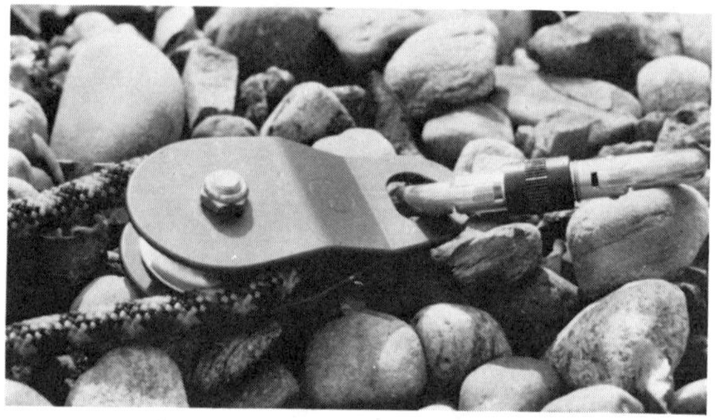

**Figure 34-21.** A rescue pulley.

*Pulleys*

It is frequently necessary to lift or move patients from one area to another. This task can be made less strenuous by using pulleys, which cut friction and give rescuers greater pulling capacity. (See Fig. 34-21.)

# PATIENT TRANSFER TECHNIQUES

## Mechanical Patient Transfer

Some emergency situations will dictate transfer of the patient onto a wheeled stretcher and then into the ambulance. Equipment used to facilitate difficult transfer may include a stair chair, scoop stretcher, or Stokes Basket.

*Stair Chair*

The stair chair is constructed of lightweight aluminum. It has rear wheels and folds easily for storage. (See Fig. 34-22.) The stair chair is used when other conventional types of stretchers cannot be utilized. It is usually needed when carrying a patient from an upstairs or downstairs location to a larger area for complete stabilization. The patient can be easily transfered up or down narrow stairways or through hallways, but must be securely strapped into the chair. (See Fig. 34-23.) The patient should be instructed

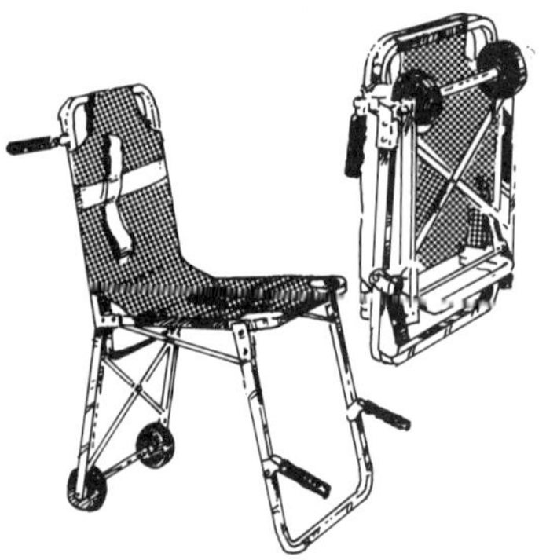

**Figure 34-22.** The stair chair.

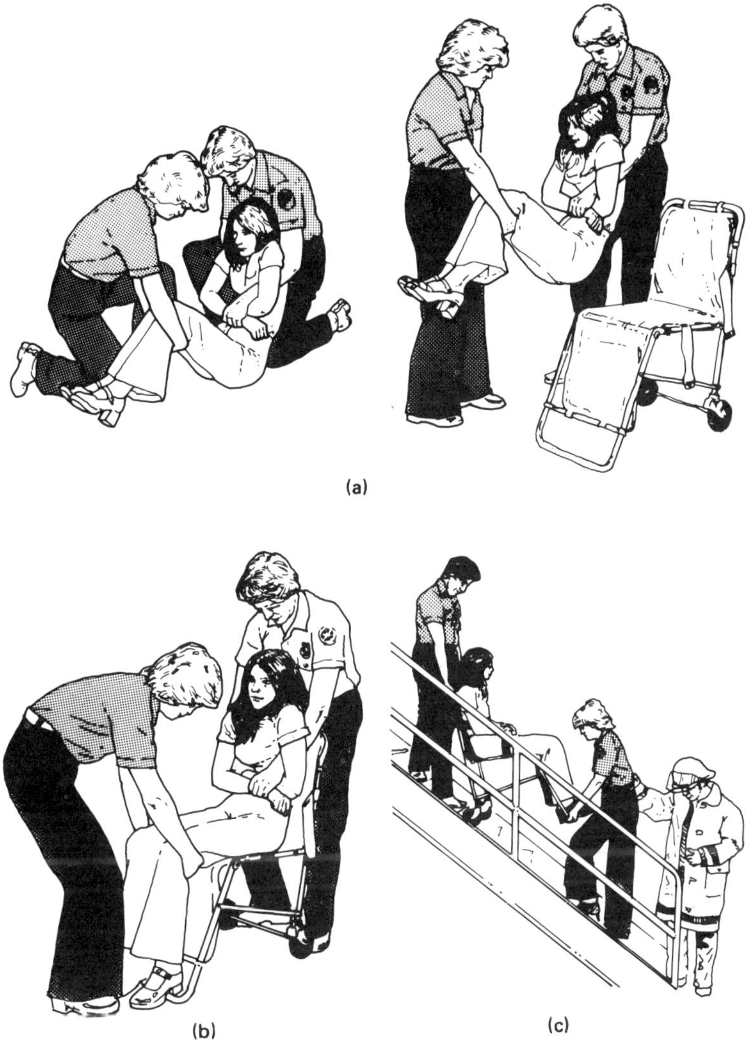


**Figure 34–23.** Procedure for transporting a patient in a stair chair. (a) The patient is moved from the injury site to the stair chair. (b) All patient injuries are stabilized. (c) The patient is instructed to keep arms and legs immobile to facilitate the transport.

(if conscious) to keep arms crossed over the abdomen and legs together while being transported. (These instructions are contingent upon patient injury). The unwheeled stair chair legs should be taken down the stairs first so that the patient's head rests in the EMT-A's body at the back of the chair. When transporting upstairs, the procedure is reversed.

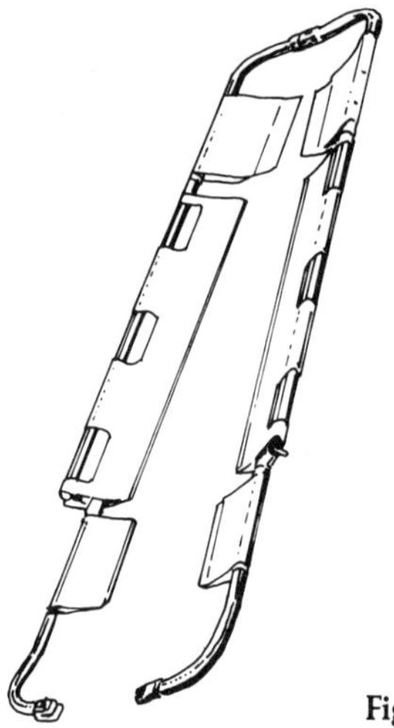

**Figure 34–24.** The scoop stretcher.

*Scoop Stretcher*

The scoop stretcher is so named because it can actually "scoop" the patient from his position. However, both sides of the patient must be accessible. The stretcher is constructed of a durable lightweight aluminum that is divided longitudinally in half. (See Fig. 34–24.) When the locking mechanisms at both ends of the stretcher are released, the stretcher breaks

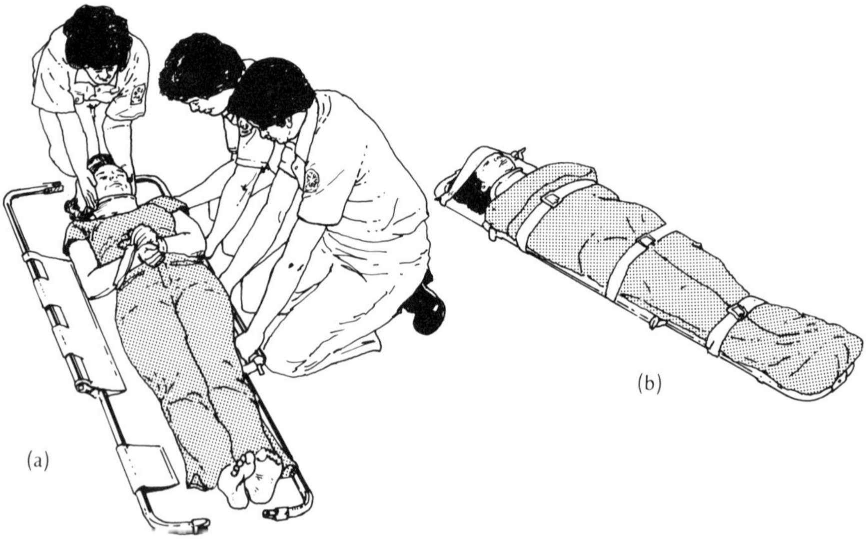


**Figure 34–25.** Procedure for positioning the patient on the scoop stretcher. (a) All injuries should be stabilized before moving the patient. Note that cervical collar placement has been established. (b) The patient is now stabilized and ready for transport.

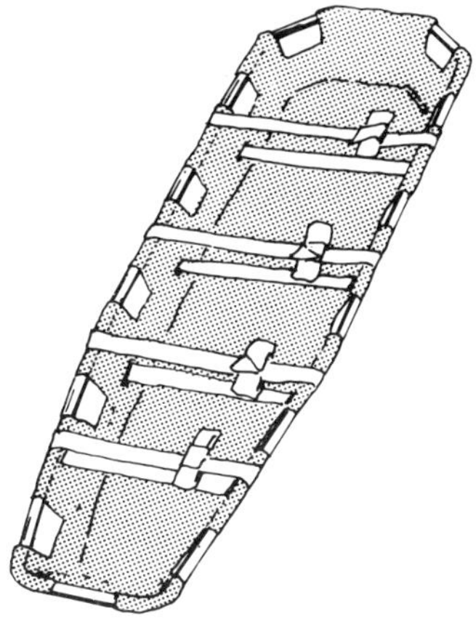

**Figure 34-26.** The Stokes Basket.

apart, allowing the patient to be scooped into the device. To avoid pinching, the patient must be log rolled or slightly lifted as the stretcher slides under the patient. At this point, all patient injuries must be stabilized, especially suspected cervical spine injury. Once on the stretcher, the patient is secured by straps. The patient can then be moved from the scene. (See Fig. 34-25.)

*Stokes Basket*

The stokes basket is made from high-impact plastic or lightweight aluminum and is oblong in design. (See Fig. 34-26.) It is primarily used for specialized rescue. The patient is encased in the basket once rescue straps are secured into place. This facilitates safe transport should the basket be raised or lowered vertically. (See Fig. 34-27.) Once the patient is placed into the basket, it is difficult to remove him. For this reason, a sheet or blanket should first be fitted as a liner into the basket onto which the patient is placed. When the patient has to be removed, the rescuers grip the sides of the liner and lift him out of the basket.

## Manual Patient Transfer

When transporting the patient from the scene to the stretcher, it may be necessary to employ certain rescue carrying techniques, especially if the routine types of transfer are not possible. This may be the case with patients who cannot walk and must be evacuated quickly. Three rescue carrying techniques that should only be employed when the life of the patient is endangered and must be quickly evacuated from the emergency area are the blanket drag, clothes drag, and fireman's drag. (See Fig. 34-28). Each rescue carry should be practiced to insure proper technique and patient safety.

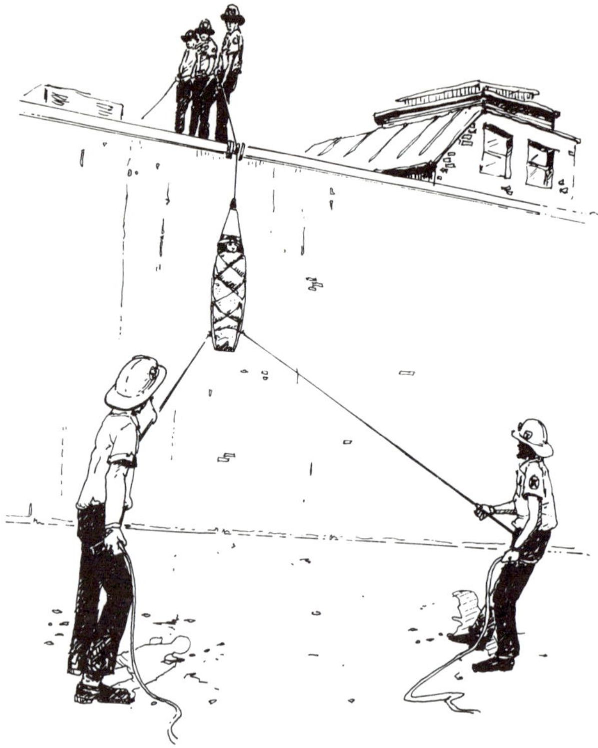

**Figure 34–27.** The patient is thoroughly secured for vertical rescue operation.

*Summary* Emergency Medical Services has within its structure many components. Job responsibilities vary from one organization to another. As EMTs, the care of patients comes first. While special rescue procedures are best left to those specifically trained to handle the job, EMTs, being a part of the entire rescue effort, must have a general knowledge of what is going on around them. If the organization employing EMTs has not only patient care responsibilities, but rescue responsibilities as well, additional formal training in extrication and/or rope rescue is suggested.

## HAZARDOUS MATERIALS

A new phenomenon that accompanies growing technology and complicated industrial processes is transportation accidents involving hazardous materials. A hazardous material may be defined as a substance or material which has been determined to be capable of posing an unreasonable risk to health, safety, and property when transported in commerce. Because of our vast transportation network, including interstate

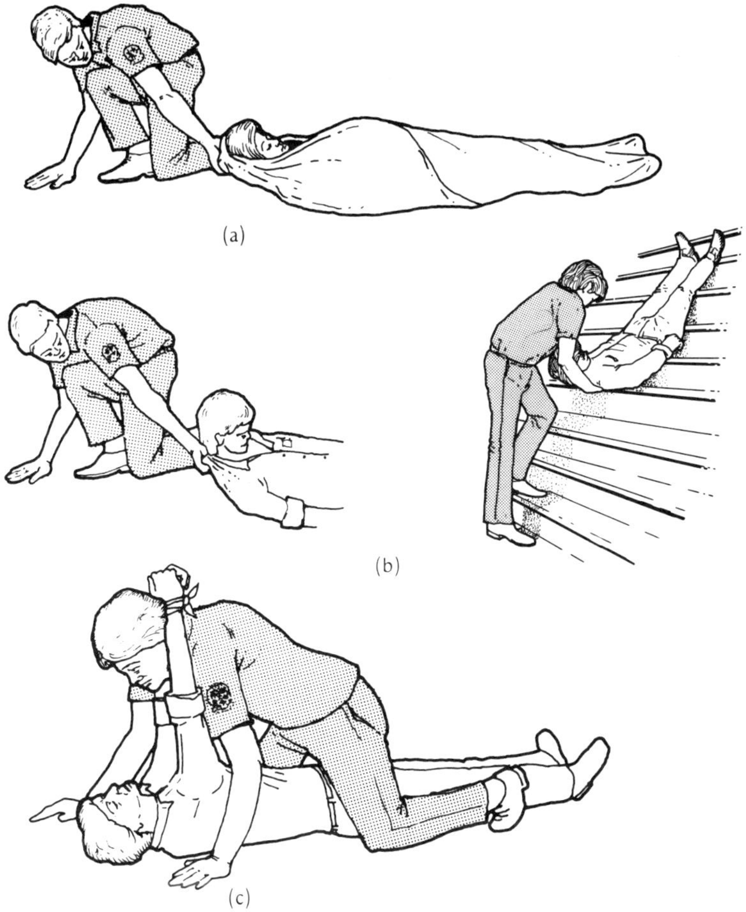


**Figure 34–28.** (a) The blanket drag; (b) clothes drag; (c) fireman's drag.

highways, railways, and air routes, there is increasing danger of catastrophic consequences from transportation accidents.

In 1980, an estimated 16,000 hazardous material incidents occurred. Daily, more than 2300 hazardous materials traverse the United States via rail, truck, air, and water. It has been estimated that ten percent of all interstate trucks and one rail car in twenty-three carry hazardous materials.

The EMT and other emergency service personnel have no control over the cause or circumstances of a hazardous material incident. Thrown into action on only minutes notice, responding emergency service personnel arrive on the scene and must make immediate decisions based on available information, experience, and training. The goals are always the same:

1. To prevent loss of life and minimize the risk of bodily injury

2. To prevent or minimize property damage to the surrounding community

3. To provide maximum safety for all emergency service personnel

To achieve these goals, the emergency planning process must have been completed as well as training on possible situations and knowledge of available technical assistance in incidents involving hazardous materials.

## Hazardous Material Readiness Factors

There are three major readiness factors in handling hazardous material incidents:

1. *Planning* that incorporates teamwork, command, and control during an incident, and includes a written control plan that involves all the emergency agencies and possible technical assistance.

2. *Training* for first-time responders with an emphasis on identification of hazardous materials, life safety considerations, and actions to be taken.

3. *Knowledge* of the characteristics, locations, transportation routes, and storage areas.

### *Planning*

Planning is essential for all emergency service organizations and personnel. It is important that all involved agencies in the local community be included in a written plan, and that the plan be tested at least twice a year using different situations and locations. It is important that a command post be set up in each situation, with a repesentative of each service involved at the command to answer any questions or lend technical assistance. With these things in mind, teamwork between emergency service agencies becomes easier as time goes by. Again, the most important things are good communication, a written plan, a command post, and testing the system and the plan.

### *Training*

Training is the most important part of any good emergency services planning program. Specialized teams are usually chosen to interact with others involved in a hazardous material incident. Specialized training is required to identify, understand, and protect the safety of others when such accidents occur.

### *Knowledge*

It is necessary in the planning stage to identify agencies in the local community which deal with hazardous materials. Even though it is impossible to identify all of them, businesses should be informed of certain agencies to call for this type of information.

The EMT should know how to cope with chemical hazards if called to the scene of such an accident. The National Highway Traffic Safety Administration (NHTSA) has prepared a small handout to aid the EMT in cases involving hazardous materials. The book should be stocked in every emergency vehicle for reference. The handbook is entitled, "Hazardous Materials—Emergency Action Guide," and copies are available from:

National Highway Traffic Safety Administration
General Service Division (NAD-42)
400 7th Street, S.W.
Washington, D.C. 20590

Chemical information that is not listed in the handbook can be obtained from CHEMTREC (Chemical Transportation Emergency Center). CHEMTREC is a non-profit organization established by the Manufacturing Chemists Association. The EMT should have the following information ready to relay to the communication center so the communications operator can call CHEMTREC:

1. Name of transport company or service
2. Vehicle numbers
3. License number of transport vehicle

CHEMTREC monitors the shipments of hazardous materials and can advise the communication center of what action should be taken. CHEMTREC may be reached by calling toll-free: (800) 424-9300. In the District of Columbia, the Virgin Islands, Guam, Samoa, Puerto Rico, and Alaska, call: (202) 483-7616 for information and advice.

## *References*

American Academy of Orthopedic Surgeons, Committee on Allied Health. *Emergency Care of the Sick and Injured,* 2nd ed. Chicago, IL: American Academy of Orthopedic Surgeons, 1977.

American Red Cross For the Instruction of First Aid Classes. *Standard First Aid and Personal Safety.* Garden City, NY: Doubleday and Co., Inc. 1975.

"CHEMTREC: Chemical Transportation Emergency Center." Washington, D.C.: Manufacturing Chemists Association, 1979.

Cloward, Ralph B. "Acute Cervical Spine Injuries," *Clinical Symposium,* 32:15, 1980.

*Crash Victim Extrication Training Course,* EMT Students Manual. U.S. D.O.T., National Highway Traffic Safety Administration, Emergency Medical Services.

Grant, H. D., and Murray, R. H. Jr. *Emergency Care,* 2nd ed. Bowie, MD: Robert J. Brady Co., 1978.

*Hazardous Materials: Emergency Action Guide.* U.S. Dept. of Transportation, National Highway Traffic Safety Administration, 1976.

Meyer, Eugene. *Chemistry of Hazardous Materials.* Englewood Cliffs, NJ: Prentice Hall, Inc., 1978.

# Chapter 35

# Aeromedical Transportation

The usefulness of aircraft in rescuing and transporting the sick and injured has long been recognized in both military and civilian operations. In the early 1900s, the military experimented with fixed wing aircraft to transport patients from remote areas to distant medical installations. Military aeromedical (a″er-o-med′ĭ-kal) transportation proved successful and over the years has been refined and expanded into a total system. In the last few years the civilian health care team's ability to sustain life for the critically ill and injured patient has increased exponentially. Unfortunately, emergency medical services cannot reach its ultimate effectiveness unless the patient is able to reach the appropriate facility or the community has instituted a plan whereby emergency care can be rendered at the scene. Aeromedical transportation has the capacity to help achieve this goal.

Aeromedical transportation systems consist of a medically managed transport operation which functions primarily to provide a comprehensive program employing educated emergency medical personnel who have been trained to function in a unique aviation environment. All associated personnel must possess efficient knowledge in order to oversee the physiological and psychological factors that may influence the patient's condition. Aeromedical systems are designed to save time while transporting the patient to the medical facility, and to provide life-sustaining measures, both pre- and intra-flight. Stabilization of the patient is the primary goal, with transporting secondary. (See Fig. 35–1.)

## ADVANTAGES OF AEROMEDICAL TRANSPORTATION

Transporting patients quickly by air from remote sites to the appropriate medical treatment facility has long been recognized as a major advantage. Today, the range and speed of present day fixed wing aircraft make it possible to transport patients by air over relatively long distances in short periods of time. Helicopters can be used to transport patients

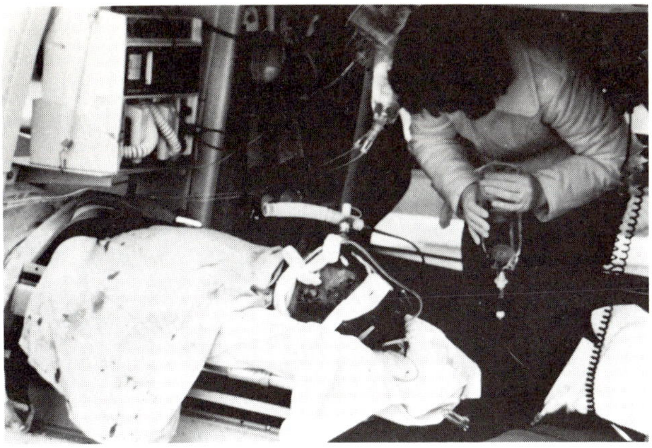

**Figure 35–1.** Patient stabilization should be completed before air transportation. (*Courtesy of Methodist Hospital, Indianapolis, Indiana*)

quickly over terrain where evacuation by other means, even four-wheel-drive vehicles, would be difficult and perhaps impossible to accomplish. Combining the speed, range, flexibility, and versatility of both types of air transportation, patients can be stabilized, then moved directly to medical treatment facilities best equipped to handle their particular injury or illness.

An often overlooked advantage is the management of patient flow through establishment of aeromedical transportation systems. Patients en route to an overloaded facility can oftentimes be diverted to other facilities with fewer patients, thus minimizing patient waiting time from hospital arrival to treatment. Selectivity in the use of appropriate medical treatment facilities made possible by aeromedical transportation can help stimulate cost effectiveness in health care. Fewer specialty treatment centers are required geographically because of the increasing capability of moving patients to care facilities with established medical specialities. This can help control the present-day perceived need for placing costly specialty care teams in every hospital in order for that hospital to treat the entire range of patient illnesses and injuries that could occur in that area.

Finally, comfort and cost of movement by air transportation in many cases can reduce patient discomfort and shock that might otherwise be suffered by more handling or rougher modes of transportation. This can be of significant importance to the patient both physically and psychologically when long-distance transportation is indicated.

## PROBLEMS ASSOCIATED WITH AEROMEDICAL TRANSPORTATION

Probably the foremost recognized problem in both civilian and military operations is the tendency to overevacuate patients. The capabilities of modern aircraft to transport patients great distances in short time spans may create a tendency to move patients farther than required or a tendency to overfly intramediate facilities along the way. This can be particularly true if the request for aeromedical transportation is not processed properly through communications centers responsible for and familiar with the role of aeromedical operations.

Through these channels trained personnel, based upon a number of medical and situational factors, determine if transport by air is indicated and appropriate. Weather factors such as fog, snow, low ceilings, freezing percipitation, sand storms, strong gusty winds (over forty knots), and turbulence can restrict aeromedical operation. In many operations aircraft are equipped with avionic instrumentation that allows flights into marginal weather and instrument conditions provided that appropriate instrument ground facilities are available in the area. Night transports are accomplished routinely; however, this depends on related weather conditions, type of aircraft to be used, qualifications of the pilot, and the patient's condition.

Rescue, mountain, and over-water operations differ greatly from normal land operations in that they pose restrictions due to the lack of suitable landing areas. Few aircraft in aeromedical operations today have all the special equipment and skilled personnel necessary to function with a high degree of safety in these environments. The capabilities and limitations of aeromedical transportation systems operating in your area must be known by all personnel who have the authority to request such aircraft. The degree of risk involved in the use of aircraft in these situations is great; therefore, it should be utilized only when no other options are found to be available. At the initial request for rescue, mountain, and overwater flights, the pilot and/or communications operator will need specific information concerning possible landing sites, terrain, weather conditions, altitudes, and alternative means of transportation. Based on that information and the patient's condition, a decision is made as to the risk involved and if the circumstances warrant such risk.

## AIRCRAFT

Aircraft used today can be divided into two categories: fixed and rotor wing. (See Fig. 35–2.) These aircraft must be specifically designed and equipped for aeromedical transportation. The type of aircraft selected will depend primarily on the type of service needed and the distance the patient is to be transported. Aircraft available for emergency, and elective air transport include light unpressurized single engine, unpressurized and pressurized multiengine and pressurized jet models.

### *Fixed Wing Aircraft*

Since there is such a wide variety of fixed wing aircraft applicable for use as an air ambulance, only general guidelines will be provided. Fixed wing aircraft are more useful when a distance of greater than 150 miles is

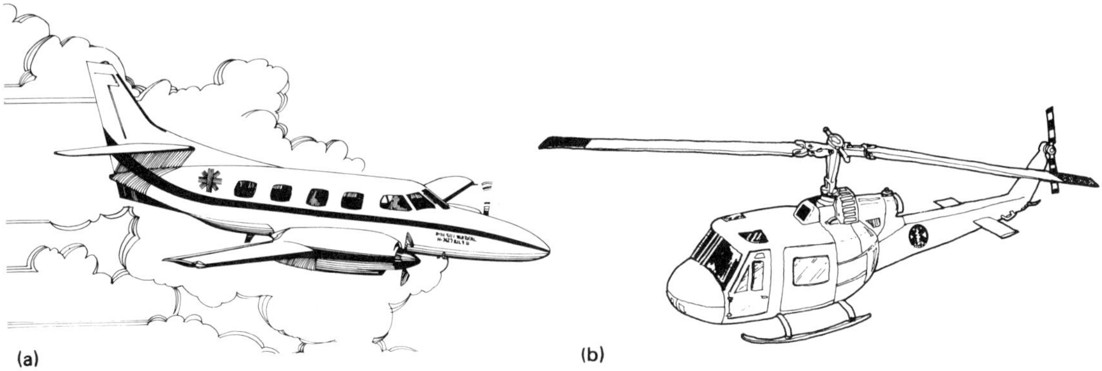

(a) (b)

**Figure 35-2.** (a) A fixed-wing aircraft; (b) a rotor wing aircraft.

involved, but they do require airport runway facilities or air strips plus the support of a ground ambulance for transportation. All fixed wing aircraft used and equipment installed must be in compliance with prevailing federal aviation regulations (FARs) for the type of aircraft in question and flying conditions under which the aircraft will be operated. Any fixed wing aircraft used for air transport of emergency patients should provide for basic emergency care equipment, advanced life support equipment, and communications equipment similar to that used in ground ambulances.

The aircraft selected must be capable of carrying a minimum of one patient on a stretcher in the horizontal position, located so as not to obstruct the pilot's vision or interfere with the performance of any member of the flight crew or required medical personnel. There must be a means of securing the stretcher to either the floor (deck), walls (bulkheads), seats, or specific stretcher racks and attaching the patient securely to the stretcher. If the aircraft provides for carrying of more than one stretcher patient at a time, there should be a minimum vertical spacing of not less than thirty inches between stretchers with the upper service of any stretcher not closer than thirty inches from the ceiling of the aircraft. The head, thorax, and abdomen of the patient should be accessible by at least two medical personnel at the same time from at least one side of the stretcher without obstructions. Patient compartments must have adequate lighting available for patient observation; however, this lighting should not in any way interfere with or restrict the pilot's vision. The patient compartment likewise should have adequate fresh air ventilation and temperature regulation to assure patient and attendant comfort at all altitudes in all conditions. The aircraft should provide at least one door large enough for ease of stretcher patient loading and unloading. Electrical systems of the aircraft must be capable of supporting all necessary equipment without the threat of overloading and causing system failures. Medical communications equipment of voice and telemetry can be either installed or portable, but must be capable of accessing ground medical communications systems at all points during the flight.

### *Rotor Wing Aircraft*

The helicopter in the early days of its military and civilian applications might have been classified as a luxury rather than a necessity; a luxury not in the sense that it provided an overwhelming degree of comfort, but rather in the sense of being highly desirable, yet not readily affordable or available. Helicopters are capable of operating from unprepared takeoff and landing areas and in some cases through instrument conditions in day or night operations. Capable of flying forward, backward, sideways, hovering, and performing completely vertical takeoffs or landings, these aircraft are ideal for maneuvering into otherwise inaccessible areas and flying into and out of heavily congested locations such as those encountered in most large urban centers. Due to the versatility of today's turbine-powered helicopters, they are becoming the aircraft of choice for intrastate aeromedical transportation and rescue operations.

Even though the helicopter is capable of vertical takeoffs and landings, these are the least desirable flight conditions. Cold weather has little to no adverse effects on helicopter operations. Adverse conditions that can occur year around and do affect operations are air turbulence, thunderstorms, heavy rains that accompany thunderstorms and ice. These four conditions should be avoided at all times for the safety of everyone involved.

## Medical Equipment

Both fixed and rotor wing aircraft must carry basic life support equipment and should carry critical care equipment, which includes electrocardiographic monitors, defibrillators, endotracheal intubation equipment, intravenous fluids in plastic containers, emergency medications, and transport isolettes (i″so-letz′), making the aircraft an airborne emergency room. (See Fig. 35–3.)

## Landing Sites

Since fixed-wing aircraft normally confine operations to improved (paved) landing areas, discussion in this section is directed to landing site preparation primarily for rotor wing aircraft; however, many items are applicable in fixed wing operations.

Even with sophisticated instrumentation, pilots rely heavily on ground personnel for assistance during the approach in landing phases. Generally, a pilot feels most safe when he can see the ground. In marginal weather or night operations, trees, wires, antennas, and other obstructions near the landing area are difficult, if not impossible, to see.

Approach zones to the landing area should be free of all obstructions, thus permitting the aircraft to land and takeoff into prevailing winds. A normal approach to landing with an unobstructed path is the safest and most desirable. Sufficient space must be provided for aircraft maneuvering while on the ground. (See Fig. 35–4.) Definite measurements for landing

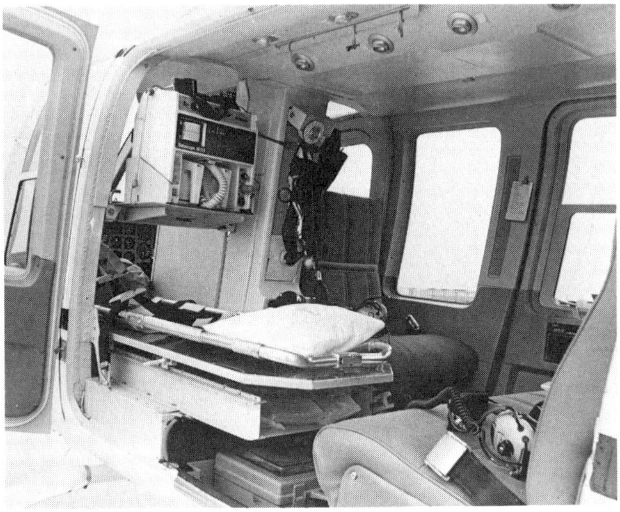

**Figure 35–3.** Appropriately placed medical equipment on board a rotor-wing aircraft. Note that the airway equipment is situated near the head of the patient and monitoring equipment is located for easy access. (*Courtesy of Methodist Hospital, Indianapolis, Indiana*)

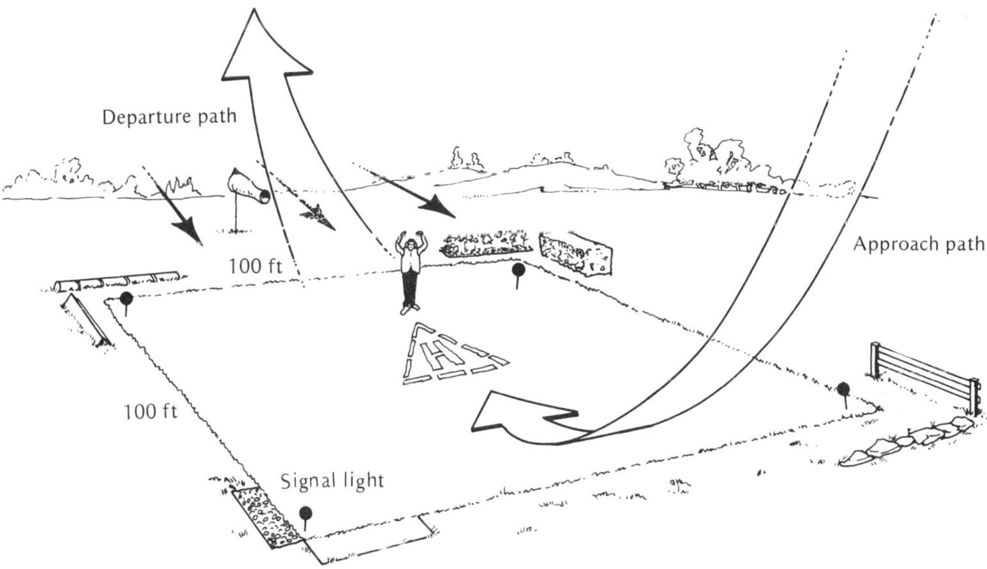


**Figure 35–4.** A typical approach and departure zone for rotor-wing aircraft.

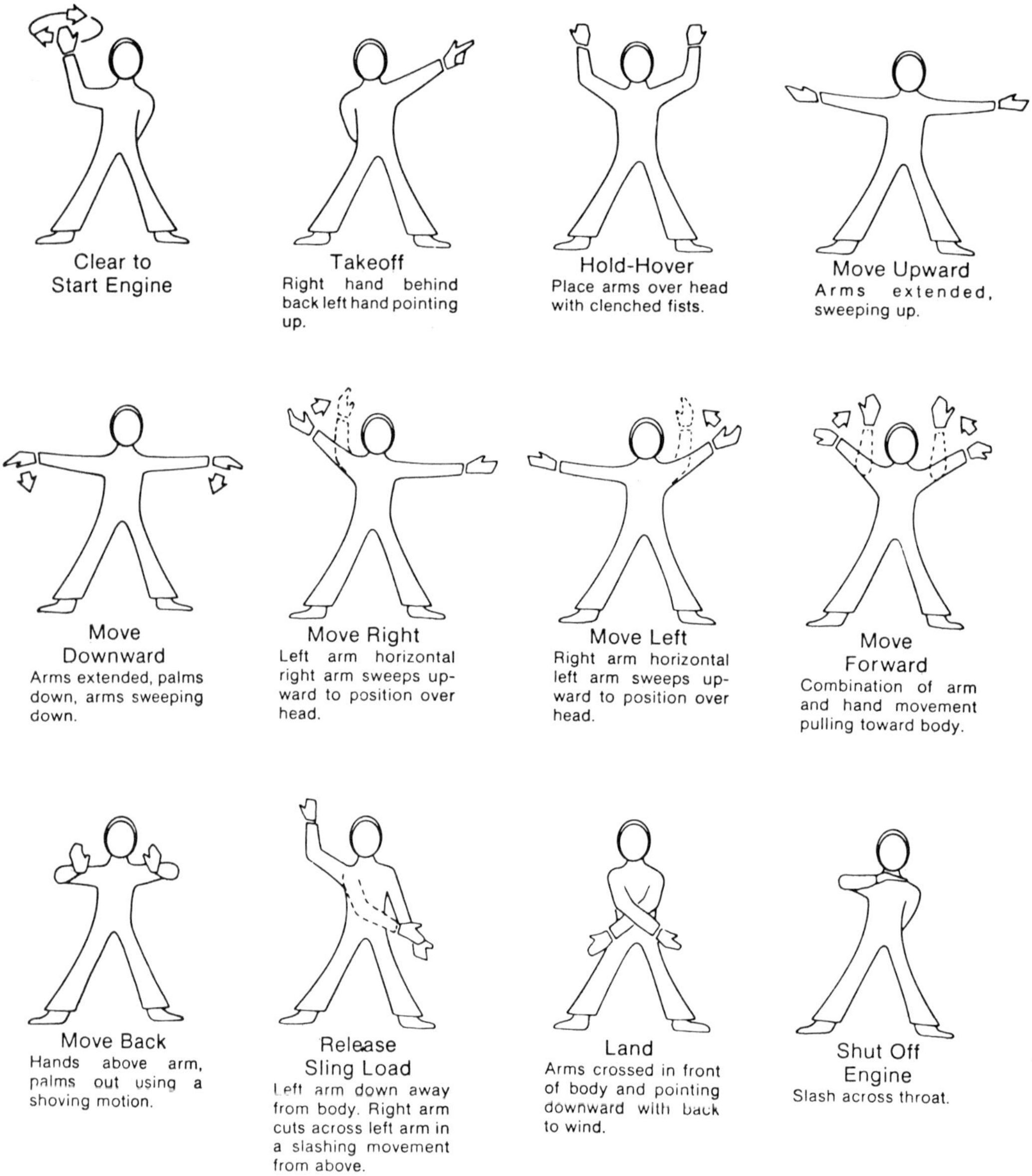
Clear to Start Engine
Takeoff
Right hand behind back left hand pointing up.
Hold-Hover
Place arms over head with clenched fists.
Move Upward
Arms extended, sweeping up.
Move Downward
Arms extended, palms down, arms sweeping down.
Move Right
Left arm horizontal right arm sweeps upward to position over head.
Move Left
Right arm horizontal left arm sweeps upward to position over head.
Move Forward
Combination of arm and hand movement pulling toward body.
Move Back
Hands above arm, palms out using a shoving motion.
Release Sling Load
Left arm down away from body. Right arm cuts across left arm in a slashing movement from above.
Land
Arms crossed in front of body and pointing downward with back to wind.
Shut Off Engine
Slash across throat.

**Figure 35–5.** Helicopter hand signals.

sites cannot be given since they must vary with temperature, altitude, wind, terrain, loading conditions, and individual aircraft characteristics. For light helicopters, clear areas one-hundred feet in diameter, with an approach and departure zone clear of obstructions, is most desirable, although an unobstructed 60 × 60 landing site can be used if necessary. Objects that are likely to be blown around by downwash (wind) from the rotors should be removed from the landing area. Obstacles such as cables, wires, and poles that cannot be removed must be clearly marked. Daytime marking can be accomplished by securing bright red cloth or plastic streamers to obstructions. During night operations hazards should be identified by the use of lights or reflective devices. One of the best ways to mark a landing site is to place stick-mounted flags or lights at each of the four corners of the usable landing area. The top of these markers should not extend more than twenty-four inches in height above the ground. When using lights, each should be colored in order to distinguish them from other lights in the vicinity. A particular color may also serve as one element of identifying the landing site. Flares or other types of open lights should not be used. They are usually blown out by rotor downwash and often create a glare on the aircraft windshield, possibly blinding the pilot. The site can be further identified by the use of strobe lights, flashlights, or vehicle lights.

The individual responsible for hand signaling the aircraft should take a position on the upwind side of the landing site with his or her back toward the wind. (See Fig. 35–5.) By directing a beam of light or extending hand and arms downward along the ground, the landing area is bisected. The pilot is kept advised of the direction of ground winds. Usually the pilot will make his approach for landing down the imaginary line, or the line of the beam of light and towards its source, landing at the center of the marked area. Care should be taken so as to prevent lights from being shined on the aircraft windshield which could temporarily blind the incoming pilot. Pocket-sized red or white strobes are an excellent means for aiding pilots and recognizing landing sites.

Wind direction and speed are of vital importance to the pilot and may be indicated by using a small hand-held windsock or streamer attached to the end of a stick. The windsock or streamer, like the person directing the aircraft, should be located on the upwind side of the field.

Orange colored smoke bombs are very useful in helping to identify the field, indicating wind direction, and marking snow-covered landing areas. The smoke devices should be ignited only when the aircraft is seen by the ground personnel or when radio communication has established that the aircraft is approximately one minute from landing. It is important, especially in helicopter operations, that smoke devices in the immediate landing area be extinguished prior to the aircraft making contact with the ground. Rotor and propellor wash winds in excess of fifty miles per hour can be expected and could cause burning smoke devices to be flung about, thus endangering personnel on the ground (See Fig. 35–6.)

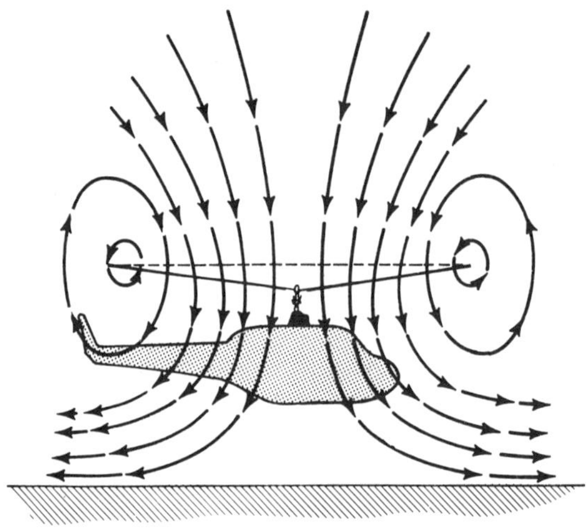

**Figure 35-6.** Wash winds produced by rotor wing aircraft.

Ground personnel, if in radio contact with the pilot, can further assist by informing him of where he is in relationship to the landing zone and guiding the aircraft toward that area. While the aircraft is maneuvering towards the landing site, the pilot can be briefed on landing details along with light or signals being displayed. If the landing area is not relatively flat, it is important for the pilot to be made aware of the direction and if possible, the degree of slope prior to his landing. Usually a slope of more than eight degrees will prevent a helicopter from landing. For this reason, it is preferred that a relatively flat landing area be located and utilized. Usually the pilot will be able to take off without the assistance of light. During takeoff, only those lights requested by the pilot should be displayed. In many cases, it is as difficult for a pilot to locate a hospital facility as it is for him to locate a remote accident scene. Strobe lights affixed to the top of the hospital, which could be turned on when it is known that an aircraft is enroute to that facility, are inexpensive and very effective. When this device is displayed it can save time, as pilots are able to go directly to the correct hospital rather than wasting valuable minutes searching for its location. If multiple hospitals in the area are using this technique, care should be taken to ensure that the strobe lights are of various colors and that the pilot is well informed as to which color strobe he will be looking for.

Should a hospital have a designated landing area, it can be identified by installing a wind cone (lighted or unlighted) adjacent to the takeoff and landing area, at a point magnetically north of this area. However, it should not be installed as to be hazardous to helicopter flight or taxiing operations, nor should it be shielded from giving a true indication of wind direction. This device, in addition to marking the area, serves as a valuable aid to the pilot during takeoff and landing.

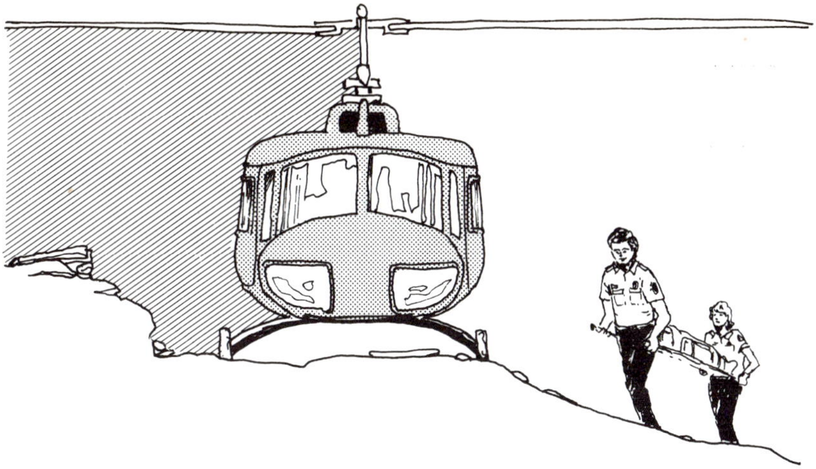

**Figure 35–7.** The proper loading approach to a rotor wing aircraft on a hill is from the downhill side.

Prior to the aircraft's arrival it is helpful for dust to be held to a minimum around the landing area by lightly sprinkling the area (but not to the point that it is muddied). This can prevent the pilot from losing visual contact with the ground during landing, which could result in the aircraft striking the ground or obstacles in the area.

## PATIENT LOADING AND SAFETY

All aircraft are engineered with crew and passenger safety in mind. The pilot of any aircraft is responsible for insuring that all patients are loaded in the prescribed manner for safe operation of the aircraft and, therefore, have the final decision as to how many patients can be safely transported. When loading and unloading the aircraft, certain precautionary measures must be observed. The aircraft must not be approached until signaled to do so by the pilot or flight crew member, and should then be approached slowly. Helicopters are usually approached from a forty-five degree angle from the front of the aircraft. If the helicopter is on a slope and conditions permit, personnel should approach the aircraft from the downhill side. (See Fig. 35–7.) Under no circumstances should anyone approach the tail of a helicopter. The tail rotor is difficult to see and may not be noticed in the surrounding noise and flashing lights. (See Fig. 35–8.) Immediately after landing, one or more persons should be stationed near the rear of the helicopter to warn others to remain clear. Personnel involved in the loading and unloading must keep as low a silhouette as possible and remain clear of the rotor blades at all times. Bystanders should be kept at a minimum of one-hundred feet from the aircraft.

Directions given by the crew must always be followed. Lay-down patients usually are positioned in the aircraft according to the nature of their

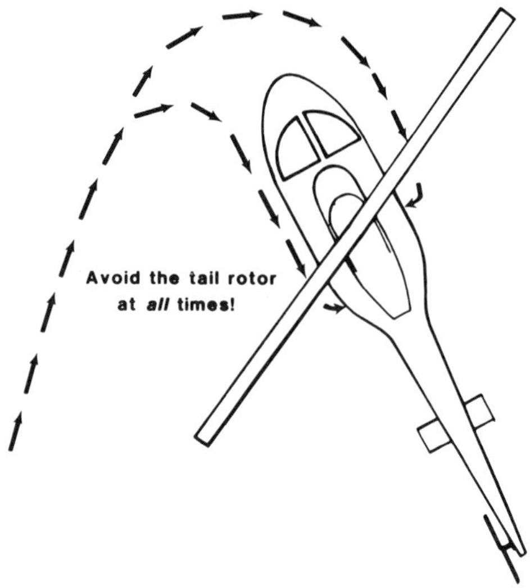


**Figure 35–8.** The correct approach for all rotor wing aircraft. (Courtesy of Methodist Hospital, Indianapolis, IN)

injuries or their condition. Personnel on board the aircraft supervise the loading and positioning of patients. The most seriously injured patients must be placed in a position that will freely permit on-board medical personnel to provide the necessary flight care. Patients receiving intravenous fluids should not be positioned on the top row or tier, but should be placed as low as possible in order to promote fluid infusion. Patients in traction, leg splints, or similar devices that have support or foot rests are usually loaded last.

Smoking is usually not permitted within fifty feet of any aircraft because aircraft fuel can be highly volatile, and ground personnel should be prepared in the event fire does erupt. At emergency landing sites and hospital landing sites, fire extinguishers provide a reasonable degree of fire rescue protection.

At permanent landing sites, large, dry chemical extinguishers are recommended by the National Fire Protection Association Fire Code Standards. If portable fire extinguishers are to be installed permanently at the sites, they should be in weatherproof boxes painted red and adequately labeled. These boxes should permit ready access in an emergency, but should not interfere with aircraft approaches or ground maneuvering.

If fire apparatus is used, it should have the capacity of discharging foam at a rate of 200 gallons per minute through the nozzle for fifteen minutes.

The primary mission of the military aeromedical component is to provide aeromedical evacuation for the sick and wounded within combat zones and theaters of operation. This includes battlefield pick-up of patients, their air transportation to initial points of treatment, and subsequent moves to other hospital facilities. The armed forces have authorized aircraft which are specifically designed for aeromedical evacuation and transportation. Most utility and transport aircraft used by the military can be equipped for air transportation of patients. Fixed wing aircraft routinely used range in size from the Army U21AUTE to the Air Force C141 Starlifter. General size of rotor craft range from the six patient utility to the thirty-one patient cargo models.

## MAST

Military Assistance to Safety and Traffic (MAST), a cooperative program of The Department of Defense, The Department of Transportation, and the Department of Health and Human Services, provides military helicopter ambulances for transporting civilian medical emergencies. The MAST program supplements existing emergency medical service systems by providing helicopters configured as air ambulances staffed with crew members, medical equipment, and supplies, all of which are maintained in a constant state of readiness to respond efficiently and effectively to serious medical emergencies. The military defines serious medical emergencies as those situations where an individual's condition is such that he should be air evacuated to a medical facility as soon as possible to prevent his/her death or further aggravation of his illness or injury.

MAST came into existence in September 1970, and was successfully evaluated at five test sites in the western United States. On November 16, 1973, a public law was enacted which allowed the expansion of MAST services to additional sites. This act limited the individual liability of military units participating and stipulated several limitations. These included: (1) assistance is limited to those areas where military units able to provide such assistance are regularly assigned (transfer of units from one location to another for MAST support is prohibited); (2) assistance is authorized only to the extent that it does not interfere with the military mission; and (3) emergency medical service assistance cannot cause any increase in funds required for the operation of the Department of Defense. Compliance with the latter limitation is possible because military units can substitute MAST missions for specific training requirements. Aeromedical and rescue units must devote a set number of flight hours to maintain proficiency in flight and aeromedical evacuation skills. Actual missions provide better training for the military than could be realized from simulated exercises. The result is that valuable services are provided to the taxpayers at little or no additional expense.

At the community level, MAST is usually organized, operated, and administered by a local MAST coordinating committee. This committee functions in accordance with the general policies developed at the federal level by the MAST interagency executive group. After a MAST site is established, federal involvement is minimal and consists only of guidance when requested and resolution of problems. The coordinating committee is generally composed of individuals representing a variety of disciplines that provide emergency medical services in that geographic area. The military project officer and civilian coordinator work hand in hand as the local administrative staff reporting collectively to their committee and individually to their respective command and civilian organizations.

At present, there are twenty-three MAST installations throughout the United States: three in Texas; two in Georgia, Kentucky, and Washington; and one in Alabama, California, Colorado, Florida, Hawaii, Idaho, Kansas, Louisiana, Michigan, New York, North Carolina, South Carolina, Oklahoma, and Wyoming, respectively. Sixteen army and seven air force units are presently involved in a MAST program.

Requests for MAST missions can originate from local or state law enforcement agencies, public safety personnel, doctors, and also from various federal groups such as the national park and forest rangers. Once determined a MAST or civilian mission is necessary, and the receiving hospital and physician have been contacted to arrange admissions, the following information is generally required:

1. Name, title, organization, and phone number of person requesting
2. Type of request (field pick-up, hospital transfer, blood or organ transfer, etc.)
3. Pick-up sites:
   (a) City,
   (b) Direction and distance from prominent land marks in area,
   (c) Type of landing area,
   (d) Destination of patient(s),
   (e) Number of patients (stretcher and/or ambulatory,)
   (f) Nature of injury or illness,
   (g) Special equipment or medical care needed en route, brief medical history,
   (h) Radio frequencies, call sign of personnel at pick-up site,
   (i) Other agencies notified and assistance they are to provide,
   (j) If interhospital transfer, time patient(s) will be ready for transfer

Weather conditions obviously are a prime consideration of an aircraft commander deciding to approve or disapprove a mission. However, circumstances surrounding the incident and the condition of the injured are factors that are always considered.

The MAST project is clearly an outgrowth of many traditional activities of the armed forces and the intense interest of the civilian sector to improve their emergency medical services. Its proven success can have great impact on community programs in the future. It is difficult to properly express what MAST projects have meant to the citizens of the United States. It has been said, "MAST is a beautiful marriage between the military and civilian sectors."

## THE AEROMEDICAL TEAM

Aeromedical crew members responsible for in-flight patient care must possess both basic and advanced patient care and life support skills in order to provide proper management of all patients encountered, both on the ground as well as airborne. These skills must include basic and advanced cardiac life support training.

Basic and advanced life support skill levels are essential, but proper patient management and care en route requires a host of additional skills. Each aeromedical team member must be able to assess flight-related medical problems and must be skilled in instituting the necessary therapy and supportive measures. Necessary technical skills include: history taking, physical assessment, positioning, treatment, insertion of peripheral IVs, arterial puncture, endotracheal intubation, and pneumothorax relief techniques. If newborn transports are conducted, the team member must possess additional skills in neonatal assessment and support, insertion of umbilical catheters, thermal regulation, and interpretation of routine chest x-rays.

Aeromedical teams have traditionally been composed of physicians and RNs; however, the expense and availability of this team has posed problems for many organizations. In many areas, the use of specially trained nurses and/or paramedics are replacing the physicians on many flights. Even though the physician has been released from actual flights, the need for communications between the aeromedical crew and the physician must remain constant.

Prior to each flight, a preflight conference between pilots and aeromedical personnel must take place. During this session, information on weather forecast, cruising altitudes, and patient conditions is discussed and a plan for patient care is developed. Additionally, it is necessary for the aeromedical team to consider alternatives for situations such as emergencies en route, extended flights due to severe weather, etc. Planning, organizing, and patient management are three of the most important factors in providing excellent patient care enroute.

## MEDICAL CONSIDERATIONS

In addition to normal medical problems, several other areas deserve special attention in aeromedical transportation, including hypoxia, dysbarism, and motion sickness.

## Hypoxia

As altitude increases, barometric air pressure decreases. This pressure drop translates from about thirty inches mercury at sea level to around eight inches at thirty-five thousand feet. Even though the atmospheric pressure decreases with altitude, the composition of air (20 percent oxygen and 80 percent nitrogen) remains constant. The amount of oxygen that can be picked up by the blood is dependent on the pressure oxygen exerts on the blood as it passes through the alveoli. As the partial pressure of oxygen decreases with altitude, the amount of blood oxygen likewise decreases. At sea level, normal blood oxygen saturation should be 100 percent. At altitudes of 5000 feet, most individuals will retain approximately 95 percent saturation. As the altitude is increased to 10,000 feet, saturation will decrease to around 85 percent, and at 14,000 feet to approximately 80 percent. At the 80 percent level, the average, healthy person will begin to display noticeable signs of hypoxia (hi-pok′se-ah)—headaches, loss of concentration, and increased breathing rate. Individuals whose health has been compromised by certain illnesses or disease may have extreme problems at these altitudes.

Persons who have recently suffered myocardial infarctions or who have heart disease, congenital defects, or severe anemia are aggravated severely by hypoxia.

Respiratory diseases such as asthma, pneumonia (nu-mo′ne-ah), and emphysema (em″fĭ-se′mah), may cause increased respiratory distress which at high altitutes may result in respiratory failure. Patients transported with any of the above problems will usually do better if given supplemental oxygen via a rebreathing mask while en route.

## Dysbarism

As pressure decreases with altitude, gas trapped in cavities of the body can cause problems. At 10,000 feet a gas bubble increases to one and one-half times its sea level volume; at 18,000 feet, twice its volume; and at 25,000 feet, three times its volume. Gas trapped in sinuses, inner ears, intestines, lungs, and teeth may cause discomfort and pain to the patient. During air transit, medical personnel must keep in mind some specific problem areas which may be aggravated due to decreased atmospheric pressure: (1) peptic ulcers and their possible perforation; (2) bowel obstructions due to adhesions or tumors which may become aggravated; (3) hernias, which could become incarcerated (in-kar′ser-āt″ed); and (4) bronchial (brong′ke-al) and lung tumors, which may cause airway obstruction.

## Motion Sickness

Turbulence and temperature extremes can aggravate any patient condition as can noise. Motion sickness may occur even in perfect flight conditions. Persons who have traveled by air previously without ill effects may experience motion sickness when transported in a recumbent position. Patients transported with immobilized jaws, pregnant women who are high-risk mothers, diabetics, and epileptics may cause some special problems for the aeromedical team.

Patients whose jaws have been immobilized due to fractures present dangerous situations if vomiting is produced. Under these circumstances, the wires or rubber bands used for immobilization must be cut immediately to prevent blockage of the airway. Diabetics who may vomit could go into diabetic coma. Pregnant women who miscarry easily can begin delivery as a result of rough air turbulence and vomit.

With all patients, a light diet prior to transport is indicated, and in some cases light sedation will be needed. Useful medications include diazepam (valium) 5 to 10 mg for anxiety; prochlorperazine (compazine) 10 mg for nausea; and diphenhydramine (dramamine) 50 mg for motion sickness.

Patients with IVs will require constant monitoring during transport, especially during descent. All IVs should (when possible) be in plastic bag containers. This allows pressure cuffs to be wrapped around them and inflated as needed for control of flow rates during flight. For those solutions that are packaged only in glass bottles, each bottle should be wrapped with a continuous strip of tape (two-inch tape is preferable.) A narrow space between wraps should be allowed so that the content level of the bottle can be monitored. This tape provides an additional margin of safety should the bottle break.

## *References*

Brown, H. N. *Pilots Aeromedical Guide.* Lombard, IL: 1969.

"Evacuation of the Sick and Wounded." Washington, D.C.: Headquarters, Dept. of the Army, FM 8-35, January 1977.

"Heliport Design Guide." DOT/FAA No. 150/5390-1B, August 1977.

Mayer, G. "Helicopter Safety During Emergency Rescue," *Journal of Emergency Nursing,* July-August 1978, p. 13.

McCombs, C. M. "Air Ambulance Services: New Horizons for Emergency Nursing," *Journal of Emergency Nursing,* July-August 1978, pp. 21-23.

O'Rourke, B. "EMS Med-A-Vac: Do it Yourself," *Emergency,* July 1978, pp. 67-68.

Simmons, P. K. "Medicopters in Ohio," *ECHO,* February 1978, p. 13.

# Chapter 36

# Stabilization and Care of the Patient During Extended Transport

The basic EMT may be involved in caring for a patient during an extended transport, and may be expected to cope with equipment and procedures outside the usual realm of training or experience. The purpose of this chapter is to provide a brief orientation to caring for patients during such transports and to familiarize the EMT with fundamental equipment commonly employed.

## AIRWAY DEVICES

Although a discussion of the airways was presented in Chapter 10, the endotracheal tube was not discussed since its use is considered outside the practice area of the basic EMT. However, since the EMT may be caring for a patient who has had such a tube placed prior to transport to another facility, its use will be reviewed briefly.

The endotracheal tube is positioned in the trachea by using a laryngoscope, an instrument that permits direct visualization of the larynx through which the tube is passed. This tube permits direct access to the respiratory tract for ventilation and suctioning. The patient can be ventilated directly using a standard adaptor and the bag-valve-mask. There is no problem with gastric distention, since air enters directly into the trachea. It is advantageous for CPR, too, since it permits a certain ease of interfacing ventilation and compressions. Although the tube is passed into the trachea and its placement is secured with an inflated cuff, the tube may migrate into a mainstem bronchus and deprive the opposite lung of air. In order to check tube location after placement, an x-ray is taken. Prior to transport, the tube is checked and anchored securely with tape or a commercial device that fixes its position. However, since lifting or moving the patient could alter the tube's position, the EMT should listen with a stethoscope periodically to ensure bilateral breath sounds which are equal over both sides of the thorax. If only one side of the chest is being ventilated, a slight adjustment of the tube (pulling it *back* 1/4" or so) may restore its proper location, permitting air delivery to both mainstem bronchi.

The endotracheal tube may require suctioning, particularly if the patient has incurred chest trauma. Follow guidelines discussed in Chapter 10, being careful not to induce hypoxia by prolonged suctioning. If the patient vomits, emesis should be removed from the mouth and pharynx *using a different catheter* than the one used to suction endotracheally to prevent introduction of contaminants and irritants into the trachea. Although the cuff of the endotracheal tube should prevent emesis from threatening the airway directly, the presence of gastric contents in the upper respiratory tract linings could create an inflammatory response, and thus they should be promptly removed by suctioning. (See Fig. 36-1.)

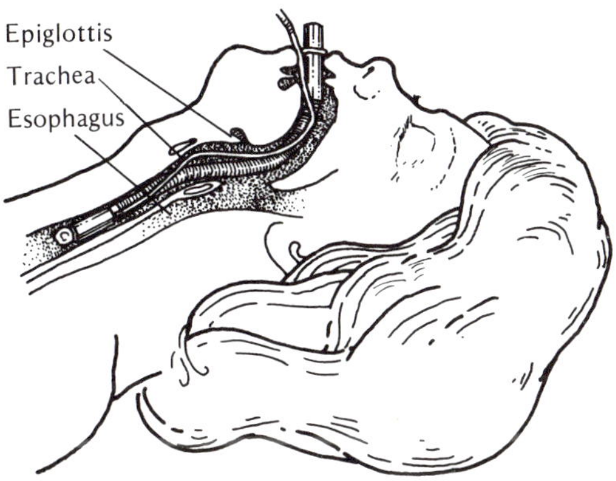


**Figure 36-1.** Endotracheal tube in place.

## CHEST TUBES

If a patient suffers a pneumothorax or chest trauma, it is probable that chest tubes will be placed prior to transport. The purpose of such devices is to drain the chest cavity, thus permitting re-expansion of the lungs.

Chest drainage can involve a closed-system disposable unit, a series of glass bottles, or a single collection receptacle. Regardless of the type of system, the EMT's major responsibility is to ensure that the tubing is patent and to maintain the continuity and integrity of the drainage network. Great care should be exercised to prevent traction on the tubes. The tubes are usually well secured by sutures, tapes, or dressings, but dislodgement could occur under extreme stress. Drainage bottles should always be kept lower than the thorax. Under no circumstances should they be placed on the cot for patient transfer!

If a receptacle for drainage is broken or if the tubes are inadvertently disconnected, they should ordinarily *not* be clamped, since such action could contribute to a tension pneumothorax. The EMT should obtain specific instructions about care and observations related to chest drainage before embarking on transport, and should be thoroughly familiar with procedures to be followed in the event of problems.

Patient care should include frequent listening for breath sounds and periodic monitoring of vital signs.

## MONITORING LEADS

It may be desirable to monitor heart activity en route to a secondary facility, and to transmit a continuous heart tracing to the hospital. This is ordinarily accomplished by a series of electrodes (called monitoring leads) which are placed on the chest wall. The leads are interfaced with a modulator that converts the ECG signals to an FM tone, which is sent on a predetermined radio frequency to a hospital for interpretation. Some units can also be "patched" to a telephone if the radio signal is of poor quality.

The EMT's basic responsibility in monitoring leads is to ensure that they remain well secured to the skin throughout transport and that wires remain disentangled and free in order to minimize interference.

Remember that no electronic monitoring system is a substitute for clinical observations and the regular monitoring of vital signs.

## INTRAVENOUS INFUSIONS

Most patients will have one or more intravenous infusions in progress before transport begins. Such infusions may be used for replacing fluid volume and for delivery of medications. The EMT who accompanies a patient should be prepared to "troubleshoot" a dysfunctional IV and to regulate flow throughout the trip.

Although IVs are generally well secured, the stresses of transport may interrupt steady flow. If the flow rate ordered before the transport cannot be maintained merely by adjusting the flow clamp screw, the EMT should attempt the following maneuvers. Inspect the bottle and tubing and clear any kinks in the line. Gently manipulate the needle or catheter at the skin entry site, since it may simply be obstructed by tissue of the vessel wall. Merely raising the height of the bottle or squeezing the drip chamber may restore a sluggish flow to a normal rate. Check the arm or leg. Occasionally, straightening the elbow, turning the arm slightly, or realigning the wrist and hand may help.

Infusions at times accidentally flow into subcutaneous tissue (rather than into the vein lumen) as a result of needle movement and its lodging in the vessel wall or the tissue surrounding the site. This complication, called *infiltration*, can be confirmed by lowering the IV bottle or flask below the level of the cot. If the IV is patent, blood will "flash back" into the line and be visible proof of patency. If infiltration has occurred, lowering the receptacle will have no effect.

Infiltration of fluids into tissue can be dangerous, particularly when the solution contains drugs or electrolytes that are irritating to tissue. Besides injuring the tissue, the patient is, of course, not receiving the drug or electrolyte as planned by the IV route. Infiltration may produce considerable local edema, which can impair circulation. If this occurs, the IV should be clamped off and the extremity elevated for the remainder of the transport. (Remember to assess extremity circulation by palpating the peripheral pulse.)

A "runaway" IV can be even more dangerous than one that is dripping poorly. For example, if a control clamp is accidentally opened, a great quantity of fluid could be given within a few minutes, overwhelming the heart's ability to handle it. Guard against this by periodically checking the drip rate and ensuring that it is within normal limits. (Taping fluid levels according to clock-time intervals on the bottle's calibration system will serve as a guide to flow rate maintenance.)

The EMT may be required to change a bottle en route and should be familiar with the method. Ordinarily the change only requires disconnecting one unit and connecting the second via a stopper system. Prior practice accomplishing this is recommended even though it is a simple procedure. Improper procedure could lead to air entering the line or excessive loss of fluid reserved for IV administration. Of course, care should always be exercised to prevent contamination of the line system during the changing of bottles.

## NASOGASTRIC TUBES

A patient may have a tube in place for decompression of the stomach. Ordinarily the tube will be connected to a receptacle, but it could be merely clamped off en route. If the tube is clamped, periodic aspiration (using a syringe) may be required to maintain patency and to ensure that the stomach does not become distended.

An EMT who is charged with transporting a patient with such a tube should understand its intended use and the care to be given en route.

## URINARY CATHETER

A Foley catheter is placed in most ill or injured patients before transport to a secondary facility. The catheter ensures that the bladder is decompressed and provides a method to assess output of urine.

The EMT should note the characteristics of the urine (clear? bloody?) and the amount eliminated at least every thirty minutes during transport.

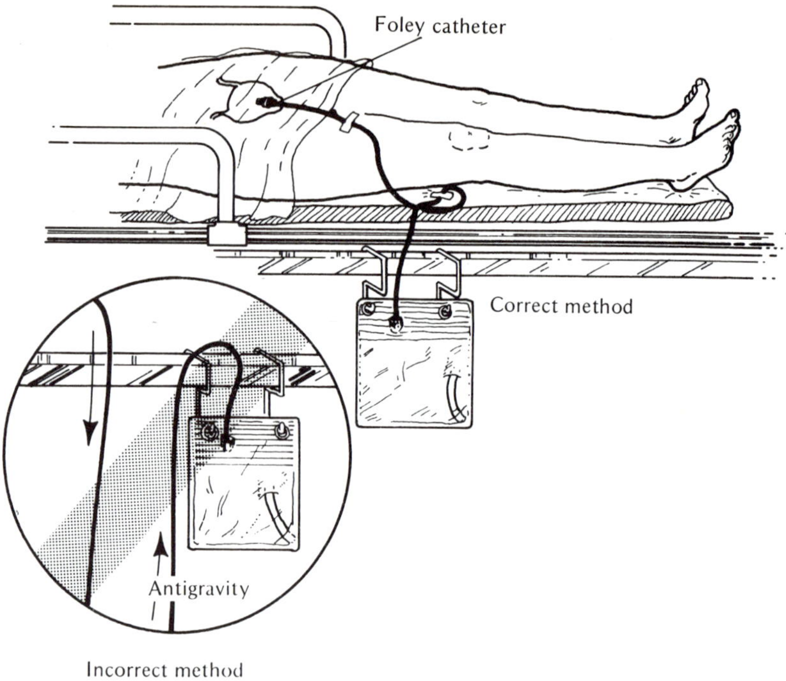


**Figure 36–2.** Urinary drainage tubing should be coiled on the cot and not permitted to loop below the cot.

The collection receptacle must always be kept below the level of the cot; should it be permitted to reach cot level, backflow of urine into the bladder would result, inviting infection. Tubing should not be permitted to loop below the level of the cot either. (See Fig. 36–2.)

The transporting hospital staff should ensure that the catheter is draining freely before transport to the secondary facility is initiated.

## OTHER CARE

A long-distance or prolonged transport is difficult for a critically ill patient, despite stabilization procedures. The EMT who cares for this individual en route should be sensitive and supportive in communications.

Comfort measures are indeed important. Changing the patient's position, even slightly, adjusting a pillow, or straightening the linens conveys concern.

Airway, breathing, and circulation must be assessed and reassessed. Periodic recordings should be made regarding their status. Changes in the patient's condition (either improvements or deterioration) must be noted, along with contributing factors.

It is important for the EMT who cares for a patient during transport to a secondary treatment facility to have a checklist of observations to be made at various times. Vital signs, IV fluid flow, urinary output, and so forth should be noted according to a specific timetable which has been predetermined.

A careful documentation of care throughout the transport is mandatory, and this should be transferred to the receiving hospital team along with a verbal report.

If circumstances permit, take time to add a personal touch for your patient. Express concern for his outcome and indicate that you are pleased to have had the opportunity to care for him during this critical time. Remember, touch conveys caring and warmth, and this brief contact upon your leaving will prove mutually rewarding!

*References*

Barber, Janet S., and Budassi, Susan A. *Mosby's Manual of Emergency Care: Practices and Procedures.* St. Louis, MO: The C. V. Mosby Co., 1979.

Barber, Janet S.; Stokes, Lillian S.; and Billings, Diane M. *Adult and Child Care, A Client-Approach to Nursing,* 2nd ed. St. Louis, MO: The C. V. Mosby Co., 1977.

# Appendix 1

# Weight Equivalencies

| *Lb.* | *Kg.* |
|---|---|
| 1 | 0.45 |
| 2 | 0.9 |
| 3 | 1.4 |
| 4 | 1.8 |
| 5 | 2.3 |
| 6 | 2.7 |
| 7 | 3.2 |
| 8 | 3.6 |
| 9 | 4.1 |
| 10 | 4.5 |
| 20 | 9.0 |
| 30 | 13.6 |
| 40 | 18.2 |
| 50 | 22.7 |
| 60 | 27.2 |
| 70 | 31.8 |
| 80 | 36.3 |
| 90 | 40.9 |
| 100 | 45.4 |
| 110 | 50.0 |

| *Lb.* | *Kg.* |
|---|---|
| 120 | 54.5 |
| 130 | 59.0 |
| 140 | 63.6 |
| 150 | 68.1 |
| 160 | 72.6 |
| 170 | 77.2 |
| 180 | 81.7 |
| 190 | 86.3 |
| 200 | 90.8 |
| 210 | 95.3 |
| 220 | 100.0 |
| 230 | 104.4 |
| 240 | 109.0 |
| 250 | 113.5 |
| 260 | 118.0 |
| 270 | 122.6 |
| 280 | 127.1 |
| 290 | 131.7 |
| 300 | 136.2 |

# Appendix 2

# Cardiopulmonary Resuscitation Standards

AMERICAN HEART ASSOCIATION
CARDIOPULMONARY RESUSCITATION AND EMERGENCY CARDIAC CARE
PERFORMANCE TEST FOR ONE RESCUER CPR (HEARTSAVER)

NAME: ______________________ DATE: ______________

| ELAPSED TIME (Seconds) Min. | Max. | ACTIVITY AND TIME (Seconds) | CRITICAL PERFORMANCE | PASS | FAIL |
|---|---|---|---|---|---|
| 4 | 10 | Establish unresponsiveness and call out for help. Allow 4 - 10 sec. if face down and turning is required. | Tap, gently shake and shout "Are you OK?" Call out - "Help!" Turn if necessary. | | |
| | | | Adequate time | | |
| 7 | 15 | Open airway. Establish breathlessness. (Look, Listen, and Feel) (3 - 5 sec.) | Kneels properly | | |
| | | | Head tilt with one hand on forehead and neck lift or chin lift with other hand. | | |
| | | | Ear over mouth, observe chest. | | |
| 10 | 20 | Four ventilations (3 - 5 sec.) | Ventilate properly 4 times and observe chest rise. | | |
| 15 | 30 | Establish pulse and simulate activation of EMS system (5 - 10 sec.) | Fingers palpate for carotid pulse on near side (other hand on forehead maintains head tilt) Know local EMS number. | | |
| | | | Adequate time | | |
| 69 | 96 | Four cycles of 15 compressions 2 ventilations (54 - 66 sec.) | Proper body position | | |
| | | | Landmark check each time | | |
| | | | Position of hands | | |
| | | | Vertical compression | | |
| | | | Says mnemonic | | |
| | | | Proper rate | | |
| | | | Proper ratio | | |
| | | | No bouncing | | |
| | | | Ventilates properly | | |
| 72 | 101 | Check for return of pulse and spontaneous breathing. (Pupil check optional) (3 - 5 sec.) | Check pulse and breathing. (Pupil check optional) If no pulse, resume one cycle of ventilations and compressions | | |

Number of compressions 60 Number of ventilations 12

INSTRUCTOR: ______________________ (Check) PASS ___ FAIL ___

Reprinted with permission of the American Heart Association.

AMERICAN HEART ASSOCIATION
CARDIOPULMONARY RESUSCITATION AND EMERGENCY CARDIAC CARE
RATIONALE FOR ONE RESCUER CPR (HEARTSAVER)

| ELAPSED TIME (Seconds) Min. | Max. | ACTIVITY AND TIME (Seconds) | CRITICAL PERFORMANCE | RATIONALE |
|---|---|---|---|---|
| 4 | 10 | Establish unresponsiveness and call out for help. Allow 4 - 10 sec. if face down and turning is required. | Tap, gently shake and shout "Are you OK?" Call out - "Help!" Turn if necessary. | Frequently victim will be face down. Effective closed chest heart compression can only be provided with victim flat on back on hard surface. |
| | | | Adequate time | Accurate diagnosis is important. 4 to 10 seconds gives time to do that and to review mentally the sequence of CPR. |
| 7 | 15 | Open airway. Establish breathlessness. (Look, Listen, and Feel) (3 - 5 sec.) | Kneels properly | |
| | | | Head tilt with one hand on forehead and neck lift or chin lift with other hand. | Airway must be opened to establish breathlessness. Many victims may be making respiratory efforts that are ineffective because of obstruction. |
| | | | Ear over mouth, observe chest. | |
| | 20 | Four ventilations. (3 - 5 sec.) | Ventilate properly 4 times and observe chest rise. | |
| 15 | 30 | Establish pulse and simulate activation of EMS system (5 - 10 sec.) | Fingers palpate for carotid pulse on near side (other hand on forehead maintains head tilt) | This activity should take 5 to 10 seconds, because not only does it take time to find the right place, but the pulse may be very slow or very weak and rapid. |
| | | | Know local EMS number | |
| | | | Adequate time | |
| 69 | 96 | Four cycles of 15 compressions 2 ventilations (54 - 66 sec.) | Proper body position | |
| | | | Landmark check each time | |
| | | | Position of hands | Precision in hand placement is essential to avoid serious injury. |
| | | | Vertical compression | |
| | | | Says mnemonic | Necessary to establish rhythm |
| | | | Proper rate | Should attempt to accomplish 60 compressions and 8 ventilations per minute |
| | | | Proper ratio | |
| | | | No bouncing | |
| | | | Ventilates properly | |
| 72 | 101 | Check for return of pulse and spontaneous breathing. (Pupil check optional) (3 - 5 sec.) | Check pulse and breathing (Pupil check optional) | Pupil size helps to monitor changes in the patient. |

Revised
8/20/80

AMERICAN HEART ASSOCIATION
CARDIOPULMONARY RESUSCITATION AND EMERGENCY CARDIAC CARE
PERFORMANCE TEST FOR ONE AND TWO RESCUER CPR

NAME: ____________________ DATE: ____________

| | ELAPSED TIME (Seconds) Min. | Max. | ACTIVITY AND TIME (Seconds) | CRITICAL PERFORMANCE | PASS | FAIL |
|---|---|---|---|---|---|---|
| SINGLE RESCUER | 4 | 10 | Establish unresponsiveness and call out for help. Allow 4 - 10 sec. if face down and turning is required. | Tap, gently shake shoulder and shout - "Are you OK?" Call out "Help!" Turn if necessary. | | |
| | | | | Adequate time | | |
| | 7 | 15 | Open Airway. Establish breathlessness. (Look, Listen, and Feel) (3 - 5 sec.) | Kneels properly. Head tilt with one hand on forehead and neck lift or chin lift with other hand. | | |
| | | | | Ear over mouth, observe chest. | | |
| | 10 | 20 | Four ventilations. (3 - 5 sec.) | Ventilate properly 4 times and observe chest rise. | | |
| | 15 | 30 | Establish pulselessness and simulate activation of the EMS System. (5 - 10 seconds) | Fingers palpate for carotid pulse on near side (other hand on forehead maintains head tilt) Know local EMS number | | |
| | | | | Adequate time. | | |
| | 69 | 96 | Four cycles of 15 compressions and 2 ventilations (54 - 66 sec.) | Proper body position. | | |
| | | | | Landmark check each time. | | |
| | | | | Position of hands. | | |
| | | | | Vertical compression/no bouncing. | | |
| | | | | Says mnemonic. | | |
| | | | | Proper rate and ratio. | | |
| | | | | Ventilates properly. | | |
| | 72 | 101 | Check for return of pulse and spontaneous breathing (3 - 5 sec.) | Check pulse and breathing | | |
| TWO RESCUER | | | 1st rescuer resumes CPR. 2nd rescuer identifies himself and checks pulse for effective compressions. | Technique for single rescuer. 2nd rescuer says, "I know how to do CPR." Fingers palpate for carotid pulse. | | |
| | | | 2nd rescuer calls out "Stop compressions" and checks for spontaneous pulse and breathing. (5 sec.) | Five second pause to check for spontaneous pulse and breathing. 2nd rescuer should inform the 1st rescuer of the status of the victim and the need for either ventilations, compressions or both. Says "No pulse, continue CPR" | | |
| | | | Second rescuer ventilates once. | Ventilates properly and observes chest rise. | | |
| | | | First rescuer resumes compressions. | Two-rescuer rate and ratio. | | |
| | | | Minimum of two cycles of 5 compressions and 1 ventilation. (8 - 10 sec.) Switch and repeat until examiner is satisfied. | Correct rate of compression. | | |
| | | | | Says mnemonic. | | |
| | | | | Interposes breath. | | |
| | | | | No pause for ventilations. | | |
| | | | | Calls for switch. | | |
| | | | | Switches. | | |
| | | | | Switches back. | | |
| | | | | Checks pulse (ventilator). | | |
| | | | | | | |
| | | | | Technique as above. | | |

For single rescuer - Number of compressions 60 Number of ventilations 12

INSTRUCTOR: ____________________

Single Rescuer technique (check) PASS___ FAIL___
Two Rescuer technique (check) PASS___ FAIL___

Revised
8/20/80

AMERICAN HEART ASSOCIATION
CARDIOPULMONARY RESUSCITATION AND EMERGENCY CARDIAC CARE
RATIONALE FOR ONE AND TWO RESCUER CPR

SINGLE RESC

| ELAPSED TIME (Seconds) Min. | Max. | ACTIVITY AND TIME (Seconds) | CRITICAL PERFORMANCE | RATIONALE |
|---|---|---|---|---|
| 4 | 10 | Establish unresponsiveness and call out for help. Allow 4-10 sec. if face down and turning is required. | Tap, gently shake shoulder and shout - "Are you OK?" Call out - "Help!" Turn if necessary. | Frequently victim will be face down. Effective closed chest heart compression can only be provided with victim flat on back on hard surface. |
| | | | Adequate time. | Accurate diagnosis is important. 4 to 10 seconds gives time to do that and to review mentally the sequence of CPR. |
| 7 | 15 | Open airway. Establish breathlessness. (Look, Listen, and Feel) (3 - 5 sec.) | Kneels properly | |
| | | | Head tilt with one hand on forehead and neck lift or chin lift with other hand. | Airway must be opened to establish breathlessness. Many victims may be making respiratory efforts that are ineffective because of obstruction. |
| | | | Ear over mouth, observe chest. | |
| 10 | 20 | Four Ventilations. (3 - 5 sec.) | Ventilate properly 4 times and observe chest rise. | |
| 15 | 30 | Establish pulse and simulate activation of EMS system (5 - 10 sec.) | Fingers palpate for carotid pulse on near side (other hand on forehead maintains head tilt) | This activity should take 5 to 10 seconds, because not only does it take time to find the right place, but the pulse may be very slow or very weak and rapid. |
| | | | Know local EMS number. | EMS is activated at this time so information on breathing and pulse can be given to dispatcher. |
| | | | Adequate time. | |
| 69 | 96 | Four cycles of 15 compressions, 2 ventilations (54-66 sec.) | Proper body position | |
| | | | Landmark check each time. | |
| | | | Position of hands | Precision in hand placement is essential to avoid serious injury. |
| | | | Vertical compression | |
| | | | Says mnemonic | Necessary to establish rhythm |
| | | | Proper rate | Should attempt to accomplish 60 compressions and 8 ventilations per minute |
| | | | Proper ratio | |
| | | | No bouncing | |
| | | | Ventilates properly | |
| 72 | 101 | Check for return of pulse and spontaneous breathing. (3 - 5 sec.) | Check pulse and breathing | |

Revised
8/20/80

-over-

TWO RESCUERS

| ELAPSED TIME (Seconds) Min. Max. | ACTIVITY AND TIME (Seconds) | CRITICAL PERFORMANCE | RATIONALE |
|---|---|---|---|
| | 1st rescuer resumes CPR. 2nd rescuer identifies himself and checks pulse for effective compressions. | Technique for single rescuer. 2nd rescuer says, "I know how to do CPR" Fingers palpate for carotid pulse. | To locate the carotid pulse. |
| | 2nd rescuer calls out "Stop compressions" and checks for spontaneous pulse and breathing. (5 sec.) | Five second pause to check for spontaneous pulse and breathing. 2nd rescuer should inform the 1st rescuer of the status of the victim and the need for either ventilations, compressions or both. Says "No pulse, continue CPR." | Provides a second assessment of pulse and breathing and the need for CPR. |
| | 2nd rescuer ventilates once. | Ventilates properly and observes chest rise. | |
| | 1st rescuer resumes compressions. | Two-rescuer rate and ratio. | 2nd Rescuer ventilation triggers change of rate and ratio. |
| | Minimum of two cycles of 5 compressions & 1 ventilation. 8 - 10 seconds Switch and repeat until examiner is satisfied. | Correct rate of compressions. | |
| | | Says mnemonic. | Necessary to establish rhythm. |
| | | Interposes breath. | |
| | | No pause for ventilation. | |
| | | Calls for switch. | Signal for change must be clear. |
| | | Switches. | |
| | | Switches back. | |
| | | Checks pulse (by ventilator). | |
| | | | |
| | | Technique as above. | |

Revised
8/20/80

AMERICAN HEART ASSOCIATION
CARDIOPULMONARY RESUSCITATION AND EMERGENCY CARDIAC CARE
PERFORMANCE TEST FOR INFANT RESUSCITATION

NAME:______________________________ DATE:______________

| ELAPSED TIME (Seconds) Min. | Max. | ACTIVITY AND TIME (Seconds) | CRITICAL PERFORMANCE | PASS | FAIL |
|---|---|---|---|---|---|
| 3 | 5 | Establish unresponsiveness and call out for help (including turning) (3 - 5 sec.) | Tap, gently shake shoulder, and see if infant responds. Call out - "Help!" Turn if necessary | | |
| | | | Infant horizontal | | |
| | | | Adequate time | | |
| 6 | 10 | Open airway. Establish breathlessness. Look at chest. Listen with ear over mouth. Feel for breathing. (3 - 5 sec.) | Tip head back. Do not hyperextend. | | |
| | | | Put ear over mouth and look toward chest to look, listen and feel for breathing. | | |
| 9 | 15 | Four ventilations (3 - 5 sec.) | Use breath large enough to make chest rise. | | |
| 14 | 25 | Establish pulse and simulate activation of EMS system (5-10 sec.) | Fingers palpate for brachial pulse in infant. | | |
| | | | Know local EMS number. | | |
| 44 | 55 | 10 cycles of 5 compressions and 1 ventilation Continue uninterrupted (30 sec.) | Two fingers on mid-sternum for compressions at rate of 100 compressions per minute. | | |

Number of Compressions 100 per minute

Number of Ventilations 20 per minute

INSTRUCTOR______________________________(Check) PASS______ FAIL______

Revised
8/20/80

AMERICAN HEART ASSOCIATION
CARDIOPULMONARY RESUSCITATION AND EMERGENCY CARDIAC CARE
RATIONALE FOR INFANT RESUSCITATION

| ELAPSED TIME (Seconds) Min. | Max. | ACTIVITY AND TIME (Seconds) | CRITICAL PERFORMANCE | RATIONALE |
|---|---|---|---|---|
| 3 | 5 | Establish unresponsiveness and call out for help (including (3 - 5 sec.) | Tap, gently shake shoulder, and see if infant responds. Call out - "Help!" Turn if necessary.<br>Infant horizontal.<br>Adequate time. | Diagnosis must be equally accurate in children and infants. With this emotionally charged situation, time must be taken to establish the diagnosis of cardiac arrest. Horizontal position aids effective circulation. |
| 6 | 10 | Open airway. Establish breathlessness. (3 - 5 sec.) Look-Listen-Feel | Tip head back. Do not hyperextend.<br>Put ear over mouth and look toward chest to look, listen and feel for breathing. | Hyperextension can collapse trachea or cause cervical spine injury. |
| 9 | 15 | Four ventilations (3 - 5 sec.) | Use small breaths to ventilate. | Lung capacity of infant smaller than adult. Avoid gastric distention. |
| 14 | 25 | Establish pulse and simulate activation of EMS system (5 - 10 sec.) | Fingers palpate for brachial pulse in infant.<br>Know local EMS number. | Brachial pulse easier to feel in infant than carotid. |
| 44 | 55 | 10 cycles of 5 compressions and 1 ventilation Continue uninterrupted (30 sec.) | Two fingers on mid-sternum in infant for compressions at rate of 100 compressions per minute. | Infants (100/min) need a more rapid cardiac compression rate with breaths interposed every 5 compressions. |

Revised
8/20/80

AMERICAN HEART ASSOCIATION
CARDIOPULMONARY RESUSCIATION AND EMERGENCY CARDIAC CARE
PERFORMANCE TEST FOR OBSTRUCTED AIRWAY

CONSCIOUS VICTIM, SITTING OR STANDING; COMPLETE AIRWAY OBSTRUCTION

NAME:______________________________ DATE:______________

| ELAPSED TIME (Seconds) Min. | Max. | ACTIVITY AND TIME (Seconds) | CRITICAL PERFORMANCE | PASS | FAIL |
|---|---|---|---|---|---|
| 2 | 3 | Rescuer asks: "Can you speak?" (2 - 3 sec.) | Rescuer must identify complete airway obstruction by asking victim if he is able to speak. | | |
| 5 | 8 | 4 Back Blows * (3 - 5 sec.) | Deliver 4 sharp blows rapidly and forcefully to the back between the shoulder blades; support the victim's chest with other hand | | |
| 9 | 13 | 4 Abdominal Thrusts (4 - 5 sec.) | Stand behind victim and wrap your arms around his waist. Grasp one fist with your other hand and place thumb side of your fist in the midline between the waist and ribcage. Press fist into abdomen with quick inward and upward thrusts. | | |
| | | OR | | | |
| | | 4 Chest Thrusts (4 - 5 sec.) | Stand behind victim and place your arms under victim's armpits to encircle the chest. Grasp one fist with other hand and place thumb side of fist on breastbone. Press with quick backward thrusts. | | |
| | | Verbally indicate repeat of above sequence until effective. | Verbalize alternating the above maneuvers in rapid sequence.. | | |

* NOTE: Although the above sequence of back blows followed by manual thrusts is preferred, the reverse sequence of manual thrusts followed by back blows is acceptable.

INSTRUCTOR:______________________________(Check) PASS_____ FAIL_____

Revised
8/20/80

AMERICAN HEART ASSOCIATION
CARDIOPULMONARY RESUSCITATION AND EMERGENCY CARDIAC CARE
RATIONALE FOR OBSTRUCTED AIRWAY

CONSCIOUS VICTIM, SITTING OR STANDING; COMPLETE AIRWAY OBSTRUCTION

| ELAPSED TIME (Seconds) Min. | Max. | ACTIVITY AND TIME (Seconds) | CRITICAL PERFORMANCE | RATIONALE |
|---|---|---|---|---|
| 2 | 3 | Rescuer asks: Can you speak?" (2 - 3 sec.) | Rescuer must identify complete airway obstruction by asking victim if he is able to speak. | |
| 5 | 8 | 4 Back Blows * (3 - 5 sec.) | Deliver 4 sharp blows rapidly and forcefully to the back between the shoulder blades; support the victim's chest with other hand. | Continually check for success. |
| 9 | 13 | 4 Abdominal Thrusts (4 - 5 sec.) | Stand behind victim and wrap your arms around his waist. Grasp one fist with your other hand and place thumb side of your fist in the midline between the waist and ribcage. Press fist into abdomen with quick inward and upward thrusts. | The sequence of back blows and abdominal or chest thrusts is more effective than either maneuver used alone. Each back blow or manual thrust should be delivered with the intent of relieving the obstruction. |
| | | OR | | |
| | | 4 Chest Thrusts (4 - 5 sec.) | Stand behind victim and place your arms under victim's armpits to encircle the chest. Grasp one fist with other hand and place thumb side of fist on breastbone. Press with quick backward thrusts. | Chest thrusts are more easily delivered than are abdominal thrusts when the abdominal girth is large, as in gross obesity or in advanced pregnancy. |
| | | Verbally indicate repeat of above sequence until effective. | Verbalize alternating the above maneuvers in rapid sequence. | Time is of the essence: the two techniques are rapidly repeated alternatively until obstruction is relieved or unconsciousness occurs. |

* NOTE: Although the above sequence of back blows followed by manual thrusts is preferred, the reverse sequence of manual thrusts followed by back blows is acceptable.

AMERICAN HEART ASSOCIATION
CARDIOPULMONARY RESUSCITATION AND EMERGENCY CARDIAC CARE
PERFORMANCE TEST FOR OBSTRUCTED AIRWAY

CHOKING VICTIM WHO BECOMES UNCONSCIOUS

NAME: ______________________ DATE: ______________________

| ELAPSED TIME (Seconds) Min. | Max. | ACTIVITY AND TIME (Seconds) | CRITICAL PERFORMANCE | PASS | FAIL |
|---|---|---|---|---|---|
| 4 | 10 | Position the victim and call for help. Allow 4 - 10 sec. if face down and turning is required. | Turn victim supine if neces- sary, call out for help. Adequate time. | | |
| 7 | 15 | Open airway and attempt to ventilate (3 - 5 sec.) | Kneel properly, utilize head tilt-neck lift or head tilt-chin lift. Attempt ventilation. Airway remains obstructed. | | |
| 9 | 17 | Activate EMS System (2 sec.) | If second rescuer is present, he should activate EMS system. Know local EMS number. | | |
| 13 | 23 | 4 Back Blows* (4 - 6 sec.) | Roll victim toward you, using your thigh for support. Give 4 forceful and rapidly delivered blows to back between shoulder blades. | | |
| 18 | 29 | 4 Abdominal Thrusts (5 - 6 sec.) | Position yourself with your knees close to victim's hips. Place heel of one hand in the midline between the waist and the ribcage and second hand on top. Press into abdomen with quick inward & upward thrusts. This maneuver may be done astride the victim. | | |
| | | OR 4 Chest Thrusts (5 - 6 sec.) | Same hand position as for applying closed chest cardiac compression. Exert quick downward thrusts. | | |
| 24 | 37 | Check for foreign body using finger sweep. (6 - 8 sec.) | Turn head up, open mouth with jaw-lift technique and sweep deeply into mouth with hooked finger. May need to remove dentures. | | |
| 27 | 42 | Attempt to ventilate. (3 - 5 sec.) | Reposition head. Airway remains obstructed. | | |
| | | Verbally indicate repeat of above sequence until effective. | Verbalize alternating the above maneuvers in rapid sequence. | | |

* NOTE: Although the above sequence of back blows followed by manual thrusts is preferred, the reverse sequence of manual thrusts followed by back blows is acceptable.

INSTRUCTOR: ______________________ (Check) PASS _____ FAIL _____

Revised
8/20/80

AMERICAN HEART ASSOCIATION
CARDIOPULMONARY RESUSCITATION AND EMERGENCY CARDIAC CARE
RATIONALE FOR OBSTRUCTED AIRWAY

CHOKING VICTIM WHO BECOMES UNCONSCIOUS

| ELAPSED TIME (Seconds) Min. | Max. | ACTIVITY AND TIME (Seconds) | CRITICAL PERFORMANCE | RATIONALE |
|---|---|---|---|---|
| 4 | 10 | Position the victim and call for help. 4 - 10 sec. if face down and turning is required. | Turn victim supine if necessary. Call out for help. Adequate time. | Initial call is to alert bystanders, collapsed victim will need to be properly positioned. |
| 7 | 15 | Open airway and attempt to ventilate (3 - 5 sec.) | Kneel properly - utilize head tilt-neck lift or head tilt-chin lift. Attempt ventilation. Airway still obstructed. | Lack of oxygen or falling and jarring motion may loosen foreign body enough to permit ventilation. |
| 9 | 17 | Activate EMS System (2 sec.) | Second person present activate EMSS. Know local EMS number. | Advanced life support capability may be required. |
| 13 | 23 | 4 Back Blows * (4 - 6 sec.) | Roll victim toward you, using your thigh for support. Give 4 forceful and rapidly delivered blows to back between shoulder blades. | Continually check for success. Each back blow or manual thrust should be delivered with the intent of relieving the obstruction. |
| 18 | 29 | 4 Abdominal Thrusts (5 - 6 sec.) | Position yourself with your knees close to victim's hips. Place heel of one hand in the midline between the waist and ribcage and second hand on top. Press into abdomen with quick inward & upward thrusts. This maneuver may be done astride the victim. | Kneeling at victim's side gives the rescuer greater mobility and access to the airway. The sequence of back blows and abdominal thrusts is more effective than either method when used alone. |
| | | OR 4 Chest Thrusts (5 - 6 sec.) | Same hand position as that for applying closed chest cardiac compression. Exert quick downward thrusts. | Chest thrusts are preferred in the presence of large abdominal girth (advanced pregnancy & obesity). Downward thrusts generate effective airway pressures. |
| 24 | 37 | Check for foreign body using finger sweep. (6 - 8 sec.) | Turn head up, open mouth with jaw-lift technique and sweep deeply into mouth along cheek with hooked finger. May need to remove dentures. | A dislodged foreign body may now be manually accessible if it has not been expelled. Dentures may need to be removed to improve fingersweep. |
| 27 | 42 | Attempt to ventilate (3 - 5 sec.) | Reposition head. Airway remains obstructed. | By this time another attempt must be made to get some air into the lungs. |
| | | Verbally indicate repeat of above sequence until effective. | Verbalize alternating the above maneuvers in rapid sequence. | Persistent attempts are rapidly made in sequence in order to relieve the obstruction. |

* NOTE: Although the above sequence of back blows followed by manual thrusts is preferred, the reverse sequence of manual thrusts followed by back blows is acceptable.

Revised 8/20/80

AMERICAN HEART ASSOCIATION
CARDIOPULMONARY RESUSCITATION AND EMERGENCY CARDIAC CARE
PERFORMANCE TEST FOR OBSTRUCTED AIRWAY

UNCONSCIOUS VICTIM, SUPINE

NAME:______________________ DATE:______________

| ELAPSED TIME (Seconds) Min. | Max. | ACTIVITY AND TIME (Seconds) | CRITICAL PERFORMANCE | PASS | FAIL |
|---|---|---|---|---|---|
| 4 | 10 | Establish unresponsiveness and call out for help. Allow 4 - 10 sec. if face down and turning is required. | Tap, gently shake shoulder and shout - "Are you OK?" Call out - "Help!" Turn if necessary. | | |
| | | | Adequate time. | | |
| 7 | 15 | Open airway. Establish breathlessness. (Look, Listen, and Feel) (3 - 5 sec.) | Kneels properly. | | |
| | | | Head tilt with one hand on forehead and neck lift or chin lift with other hand. | | |
| | | | Ear over mouth, observe chest. | | |
| 10 | 20 | Attempt to ventilate (3 - 5 sec.) | Attempt ventilation. Airway remains obstructed. | | |
| 13 | 25 | Reattempt ventilation (3-5 sec.) | Reposition head, airway remains obstructed | | |
| 15 | 27 | Activate EMS System (2 sec) | If a second rescuer is present he should activate the EMS System. Know local EMS number. | | |
| 19 | 33 | 4 Back Blows * (4 - 6 sec.) | Roll victim toward you, using your thigh for support. Give 4 forceful and rapidly delivered blows to back between shoulder blades. | | |
| 24 | 39 | 4 Abdominal Thrusts (5 - 6 sec.) OR | Position yourself with your knees close to victim's hips. Place heel of one hand in the midline between the waist and ribcage with second hand on top. Press into abdomen with quick inward & upward thrusts. This maneuver may be done astride victim. | | |
| | | 4 Chest Thrusts (5 - 6 sec.) | Same hand position as for applying closed chest cardiac compression. Exert quick downward thrusts. | | |
| 30 | 47 | Check for foreign body using finger sweep (6 - 8 sec.) | Turn head up, open mouth with jaw-lift technique and sweep deeply into mouth with hooked finger. May need to remove dentures. | | |
| 33 | 52 | Attempt to ventilate. (3 - 5 sec.) | Reposition head. Airway remains obstructed. | | |
| | | Verbally indicate repeat of above sequence until effective. | Verbalize alternating the above maneuvers in rapid sequence. | | |

*NOTE: Although the above sequence of back blows followed by manual thrusts is preferred, the reverse sequence of manual thrusts followed by back blows is acceptable.

Revised 8/20/80 INSTRUCTOR______________________ (Check) PASS_____ FAIL_____

AMERICAN HEART ASSOCIATION
CARDIOPULMONARY RESUSCITATION AND EMERGENCY CARDIAC CARE
RATIONALE FOR OBSTRUCTED AIRWAY

UNCONSCIOUS VICTIM, SUPINE

| ELAPSED TIME (Seconds) Min. | Max. | ACTIVITY AND TIME (Seconds) | CRITICAL PERFORMANCE | RATIONALE |
|---|---|---|---|---|
| 4 | 10 | Establish unresponsiveness and call out for help. Allow 4 - 10 sec. if face down and turning is required. | Tap, gently shake shoulder and shout - "Are you OK?" Call out "Help!" Turn if necessary. | This initial call for help is to alert bystanders. |
| | | | Adequate time | |
| 7 | 15 | Open airway. Establish breathlessness. (Look, Listen, and Feel) (3 - 5 sec.) | Kneels properly | |
| | | | Head tilt with one hand on forehead and neck lift or chin lift with other hand | |
| | | | Ear over mouth, observe chest | |
| 10 | 20 | Attempt to ventilate (3 - 5 sec.) | Attempt ventilation. Airway remains obstructed. | Complete airway obstruction by a foreign body is assumed present, but at this point an attempt must be made to get some air into the lungs. |
| 13 | 25 | Reattempt ventilation (3-5 sec.) | Reposition head, airway remains obstructed | Improper head tilt is most common cause of airway obstruction |
| 15 | 27 | Activate EMS System (2 sec) | If a second rescuer is present he should activate the EMSS. Know local EMS number. | Advanced life support capability may be required. |
| 19 | 33 | 4 Back Blows * (4 - 6 sec.) | Roll victim toward you, using your thigh for support. Give 4 forceful and rapidly delivered blows to back between shoulder blades. | Continually check for success. Each back blow or manual thrust should be delivered with the intent of relieving the obstruction. |
| 24 | 39 | 4 Abdominal Thrusts (5 - 6 sec.) | Position yourself with your knees close to victim's hips. Place heel of one hand in the midline between the waist and ribcage and second hand on top. Press into abdomen with quick inward & upward thrusts. Maneuver may be done astride victim. | Kneeling at victim's side gives the rescuer greater mobility and access to the airway. The sequence of back blows and manual thrusts is more effective than either technique when used alone. |
| | | OR 4 Chest Thrusts (5 - 6 sec.) | Same hand position as that for applying closed chest cardiac compression. Exert quick downward thrusts. | Chest thrusts are preferred in the presence of large abdominal girth (advanced pregnancy & obesity). Downward thrusts generate effective airway pressures. |
| 30 | 47 | Check for foreign body using finger sweep. (6 - 8 sec.) | Turn head up, open mouth with jaw-lift technique and sweep deeply into mouth along cheek with hooked finger. May need to remove dentures. | A dislodged foreign body may now be manually accessible if it has not been expelled. Dentures may need to be removed to improve finger sweep. |
| 33 | 52 | Attempt to ventilate (3 - 5 sec.) | Reposition head. Airway remains obstructed. | By this time another attempt must be made to get some air into the lungs. |
| | | Verbally indicate repeat of above sequence until effective. | Verbalize alternating the above maneuvers in rapid sequence. | Persistent attempts are rapidly made in sequence in order to relieve the obstruction. |

* NOTE: Although the above sequence of back blows followed by manual thrusts is preferred, the reverse sequence of manual thrusts followed by back blows is acceptable.

Revised 8/20/80

AMERICAN HEART ASSOCIATION
CARDIOPULMONARY RESUSCITATION AND EMERGENCY CARDIAC CARE
PERFORMANCE TEST FOR COMPLETE OBSTRUCTION
CONSCIOUS CHOKING INFANT

NAME:______________________________ DATE:______________________

| ELAPSED TIME (Seconds) Min. | Max. | ACTIVITY AND TIME (Seconds) | CRITICAL PERFORMANCE | PASS | FAIL |
|---|---|---|---|---|---|
| 2 | 3 | Rescuer checks for airway obstruction (2 - 3 sec.) | Rescuer must identify complete obstruction by looking, listening and feeling for ventilation, for blueness of the lips. | | |
| 5 | 8 | 4 Back Blows (3 - 5 sec.) | The infant is straddled over the rescuer's arm with the head lower than the trunk. The 4 back blows are delivered rapidly and forcefully between the shoulder blades. | | |
| 9 | 13 | 4 Chest Thrusts (4 - 5 sec.) | The infant is supported between 2 hands, turned onto the back, and the thrusts are delivered in the mid sternal region in the same manner as external chest compression. The head is lower than the trunk. | | |
| | | Verbally indicate repeat of above sequence until effective. | Verbalize alternating the above maneuvers in rapid sequence. | | |

INSTRUCTOR______________________________ (Check) PASS_____ FAIL_____

Revised
8/20/80

AMERICAN HEART ASSOCIATION
CARDIOPULMONARY RESUSCITATION AND EMERGENCY CARDIAC CARE
RATIONALE FOR COMPLETE OBSTRUCTION
CONSCIOUS CHOKING INFANT

| ELAPSED TIME (Seconds) Min. | Max. | ACTIVITY AND TIME (Seconds) | CRITICAL PERFORMANCE | RATIONALE |
|---|---|---|---|---|
| 2 | 3 | Rescuer checks for airway obstruction (2 - 3 sec.) | Rescuer must identify complete obstruction by looking, listening and feeling for ventilation, for blueness of the lips. | The presence of complete airway obstruction must be properly diagnosed before proceeding with treatment. |
| 5 | 8 | 4 Back Blows (3 - 5 sec.) | The infant is straddled over the rescuer's arm with the head lower than the trunk. The 4 back blows are delivered rapidly and forcefully between the shoulder blades. | Back blows when used alone may relieve the obstruction. |
| | 13 | 4 Chest Thrusts (4 - 5 sec) | The infant is supported between 2 hands, turned onto the back, and the thrusts are delivered in the mid sternal region in the same manner as external chest compression. The head is lower than the trunk. | The combination of back blows and chest thrusts is superior to one technique when used alone. Abdominal thrusts are not recommended in infants because of the potential injury to the abdominal organs. |
| | | Verbally indicate repeat of above sequence until effective. | Verbalize alternating the above maneuvers in rapid sequence. | Time is of the essence: The two techniques are rapidly repeated alternatively until obstruction is relieved or unconsciousness occurs. |

AMERICAN HEART ASSOCIATION
CARDIOPULMONARY RESUSCITATION AND EMERGENCY CARDIAC CARE
PERFORMANCE TEST FOR INFANT OBSTRUCTED AIRWAY
CHOKING INFANT WHO BECOMES UNCONSCIOUS OR IS FOUND UNCONSCIOUS

NAME:______________________________ DATE:____________________

| ELAPSED TIME (Seconds) Min. | Max. | ACTIVITY AND TIME (Seconds) | CRITICAL PERFORMANCE | PASS | FAIL |
|---|---|---|---|---|---|
| 4 | 10 | Establish unresponsiveness. Call for help. Turn victim. (4 - 10 sec.) | Gently shake, tap, call out for help. Turn infant horizontal and supine. | | |
| 7 | 15 | Open airway, Establish breathlessness. Look, listen, feel. (3 - 5 sec) | Tip head back, do not hyperextend. Rescuer looks toward chest with ear over mouth to look listen and feel for breathing. Utilize head tilt-neck lift or, if needed, head tilt-chin lift. | | |
| 10 | 20 | Attempt to ventilate (3 - 5 sec.) | Ventilate - airway remains obstructed | | |
| 13 | 25 | Reattempt to ventilate. (3 - 5 sec.) | Reposition the head. Airway remains obstructed. | | |
| 15 | 27 | Activate EMS system (2) sec.) | If a second rescuer is present he should activate the EMS system. Know local EMS number. | | |
| 19 | 33 | 4 Back Blows (4 - 6 sec.) | Same as for conscious infant. | | |
| 24 | 39 | 4 Chest Thrusts (5 - 6 sec.) | Same as for conscious infant. | | |
| 30 | 47 | Tongue-Jaw Lift (6 - 8 sec.) | Thumb in victim's mouth over tongue. Lift tongue and jaw forward with fingers wrapped around lower jaw. Remove foreign body if visualized. | | |
| | | Verbally indicate repeat of above sequence until effective. | Verbalize alternating the above maneuvers in rapid succession. | | |

INSTRUCTOR ______________________________(Check) PASS_____ FAIL_____

Revised
8/20/80

AMERICAN HEART ASSOCIATION
CARDIOPULMONARY RESUSCITATION AND EMERGENCY CARDIAC CARE
RATIONALE FOR INFANT OBSTRUCTED AIRWAY
CHOKING INFANT WHO BECOMES UNCONSCIOUS OR IS FOUND UNCONSCIOUS

| ELAPSED TIME (Seconds) Min. | Max. | ACTIVITY AND TIME (Seconds) | CRITICAL PERFORMANCE | RATIONALE |
|---|---|---|---|---|
| 4 | 10 | Establish unresponsiveness. Call for help. Turn victim. (4 - 10 sec.) | Gently shake, tap, call out for help. Turn infant horizontal and supine. | An accurate diagnosis of unresponsiveness must be made before resuscitation begins or continues. |
| 7 | 15 | Open airway, Establish breathlessness. Look, listen, feel. (3 - 5 sec.) | Tip head back, do not hyperextend. Rescuer looks toward chest with ear over mouth to look, listen and feel for breathing. Utilize head tilt-neck lift or, if needed, head tilt-chin lift. | Hyperextension of the head can collapse the trachea or cause cervical spine injury in the infant. An accurate diagnosis must be made to establish the presence of cardiopulmonary arrest or airway obstruction. |
| 10 | 20 | Attempt to ventilate (3 - 5 sec.) | Ventilate - airway remains obstructed | Complete airway obstruction or a foreign body is assumed. |
| 13 | 25 | Reattempt to ventilate. (3 - 5 sec.) | Reposition the head. Airway remains obstructed. | Improper head tilt is the most common cause of airway obstruction. Airway obstruction is confirmed. |
| 15 | 27 | Activate EMS system (2 sec.) | If a second rescuer is present he should activate the EMSS. Know local EMS number! | ALS Capability will be needed. |
| 19 | 33 | 4 Back Blows (4 - 6 sec.) | Same as for conscious infant. | |
| 24 | 39 | 4 Chest Thrusts (5 - 6 sec.) | Same as for conscious infant. | |
| 30 | 47 | Tongue-Jaw Lift (6 - 8 sec.) | Thumb in victim's mouth over tongue. Lift tongue and jaw forward with fingers wrapped around lower jaw. Remove foreign body if visualized. | Blind finger sweeps are to be avoided in the infant since the foreign body can easily be pushed back and cause further obstruction. |
| | | Verbally indicate repeat of above sequence until effective. | Verbalize alternating the above maneuvers in rapid succession. | Persistent attempts are rapidly made in sequence in order to relieve the obstruction. |

# Appendix 3

# ''Head To Toe'' Assessment of Multiple Trauma

*Step 1 *Primary survey: diagnose and treat

a. Inadequate ventilation
b. Circulatory insufficiency
c. Hemorrhage

*Remember always to suspect C-spine injuries

*Step 2 Obtain and record pertinent injury history

*Step 3 Identify injured areas: perform systematic review

a. Head
   1. Calculate *Glasgow Coma Scale*
   2. Inspect *head* and *scalp*
   3. Explore *nasal* and *auditory* canals for blood, CSF
   4. Inspect *eyes* (movement, pupils, visual acuity)
   5. Search the *mouth* (malocclusion, lacerations, missing teeth)
   6. Inspect *face* for fractures (nose, zygoma, mandible)
b. Neck
   1. Inspect for tracheal deviation, vein distention, ecchymosis
   2. Palpate for subcutaneous emphysema, bony abnormalities, tenderness
c. Chest
   1. Inspect for wounds, symmetry in breath excursions, rate and rhythm of breathing
   2. Listen for breath sounds, heart sounds
   3. Palpate stability of thoracic cage for masses and tenderness
d. Abdomen
   1. Inspect for wounds, ecchymosis, old surgical scars
   2. Listen for bowel sounds, bruits
   3. Palpate for masses, tenderness, pelvic stability, subcutaneous emphysema

e. Musculoskeletal system
   1. Inspect for pathological posturing, spastic hemiplegia, appearance and function of extremities.
   2. Palpate for pulses, sensation, tenderness, deformities, muscle strength

f. Perineum and genitalia
   1. Inspect for blood at meatus, ecchymosis of scrotum and perineum, open wounds.
   2. Note any urinary incontinence or unusual urge to void

g. Back and buttocks
   1. *Logroll patient* and
      Inspect for ecchymosis, hematoma, wounds
   2. Palpate vertebrae, ribs, and pelvis for deformities, fractures, swelling, tenderness.

# Appendix 4

# Oxygen Administration Devices, Flow, and Oxygen Concentrations

| *Oxygen Device* | *Flow Rate* | *Concentration* |
|---|---|---|
| Nasal prongs or cannula | 2–6 *l*/min | 25–40% |
| Simple mask | 10 *l*/min | 50–60% |
| Reservoir mask | 10–12 *l*/min | 90% |
| Venturi | Fixed concentration determined by settings. | |
| Pocket mask | 10 *l*/min | 50% |
| Bag-valve mask | 12 *l*/min | 40–90% |
| | room air | 21% |
| Oxygen-powered unit | 100 *l*/min | 100% |

# Appendix 5

# Selected Medical Abbreviations For The EMT

| | |
|---|---|
| abd | abdomen |
| AE | above elbow |
| AK | above knee |
| AMA | against medical advice |
| ant | anterior |
| ASA | aspirin |
| A & P | auscultation and percussion |
| ASAP | as soon as possible |
| AX | axillary |
| B/F | black female |
| BID | bring in dead |
| bil | bilateral |
| BK | below knee |
| B/M | black male |
| BM | bowel movement |
| B/P | blood pressure |
| BOW | bag of waters |
| CC | chief complaint |
| CHF | congestive heart failure |
| CNS | central nervous system |
| C/O | complains of |
| CO | carbon monoxide |
| $CO_2$ | carbon dioxide |
| COLD | chronic obstructive lung disease |
| COPD | chronic obstructive pulmonary disease |
| CP | cerebral palsy |
| CPR | cardiopulmonary resuscitation |
| CSF | cerebrospinal fluid |
| CVA | cerebrovascular accident (stroke) |

| | |
|---|---|
| DC | discontinue |
| DOA | dead on arrival |
| DOE | dyspnea on exertion |
| DT | delirium tremens |
| Dx | diagnosis |
| | |
| ECG | electrocardiogram |
| ED | emergency department |
| EENT | eye, ear, nose and throat |
| e.g. | for example |
| EKG | electrocardiogram |
| EOA | esophageal obturator airway |
| ER | emergency room |
| Et tube | endotracheal tube |
| ETOH | ethyl alcohol |
| ext | external |
| epi | epinephrine |
| | |
| FB | foreign body |
| FHT | fetal heart tones |
| FUO | fever of undetermined origin |
| Fx | fracture |
| | |
| GC | gonorrhea |
| GI | gastrointestinal |
| GSW | gunshot wound |
| GU | genitourinary system |
| Gyn | gynecology |
| | |
| H & L | heart and lungs |
| H & P | history and physical |
| HR | heart rate |
| $H_2O$ | water |
| Hx | history |
| | |
| IC | intracardiac |
| ICS | intercostal space |
| ICU | intensive care unit |
| IM | intramuscular |
| inf | inferior |
| IUD | intrauterine device |
| IV | intravenous |
| IVC | inferior vena cava |
| | |
| KUB | kidney, ureter, bladder |
| | |
| LLL | left lower lobe |
| LLQ | left lower quadrant |

| | |
|---|---|
| LMP | last menstrual period |
| LOM | limitation of motion (movement) |
| LOS | length of stay |
| LRQ | lower right quadrant |
| LSB | left sternal border |
| LUL | left upper lobe |
| LUQ | left upper quadrant |
| | |
| MCL | mid-clavicular line |
| mg | milligram |
| MI | myocardial infarction |
| ml | milliliter |
| ML | midline |
| mm | millimeter |
| Mod | moderate |
| MVA | motor vehicle accident |
| | |
| Na | sodium |
| $NaHCO_3$ | sodium bicarbonate |
| NaCl | sodium chloride |
| NG | nasogastric |
| $N_2O$ | nitrous oxide |
| NS | normal saline |
| NSR | normal sinus rhythm |
| NT | nasotracheal |
| N/A | not applicable |
| NVD | nausea, vomiting, diarrhea |
| | |
| OB | obstetrics |
| OD | overdose |
| OR | operating room |
| $O_2$ | oxygen |
| O & E | observation and examination |
| | |
| P & A | percussion and auscultation |
| PE | physical examination |
| per os | by mouth |
| PERL | pupils equal, react to light |
| PI | personal injury |
| PND | paroxysmal nocturnal dyspnea |
| P.O. | by mouth |
| PRN | when necessary |
| Pt | patient |
| | |
| q | every |
| qd | every day |
| qh | every hour |
| qid | four times a day |

| | |
|---|---|
| RCM | right costal margin |
| RDS | respiratory distress syndrome |
| RHC | respirations have ceased |
| RLL | right lower lobe |
| RLQ | right lower quadrant |
| R/O | rule out |
| ROM | range of motion |
| R | respiration |
| RUL | right upper lobe |
| RUQ | right upper quadrant |
| Rx | treatment, prescription |
| SIDS | sudden infant death syndrome |
| sol | solution |
| stat | at once, immediately |
| SVC | superior vena cava |
| sx | signs, symptoms |
| TB | tuberculosis |
| T & C | type and cross match |
| TID | three times a day |
| TKO | to keep open |
| TPR | temperature, pulse, respiration |
| UA | urinalysis |
| ung | ointment |
| URI | upper respiratory infection |
| UTI | urinary tract infection |
| VD | venereal disease |
| V/S | vital signs |
| WD WN | well developed, well nourished |
| WF | white female |
| WNL | within normal limits |
| WM | white male |
| y.o. | year old |

## MISCELLANEOUS SYMBOLS

| | |
|---|---|
| @ | at |
| ≠ | does not equal |
| + | plus, positive |
| # | number, pounds |
| – | minus, negative |
| ′ | foot |

| | |
|---|---|
| ″ | inch |
| Ⓛ | Left |
| Ⓡ | Right |
| > | greater than |
| < | less than |
| ♀ | female |
| ♂ | male |
| = | equals |
| → | causes |
| ← | due to |
| ↓ | decreased |
| ↑ | increased |
| ° | degree |
| ✓'d | checked |
| ~ | approximately |
| s̄ | without |
| c̄ | with |
| c̄/ | which |
| % | percent |
| s̄s̄ | half |

# Appendix 6

# Communication with the Deaf

"May I help you?"

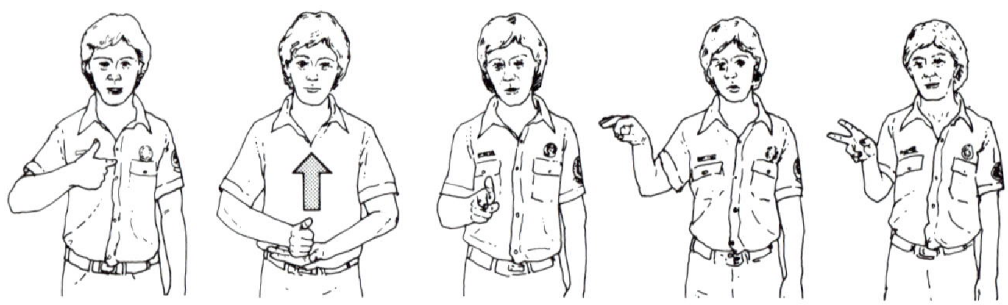

ME HELP YOU O K

"I'll ask questions that you can answer with a 'yes' or 'no.' O.K?"

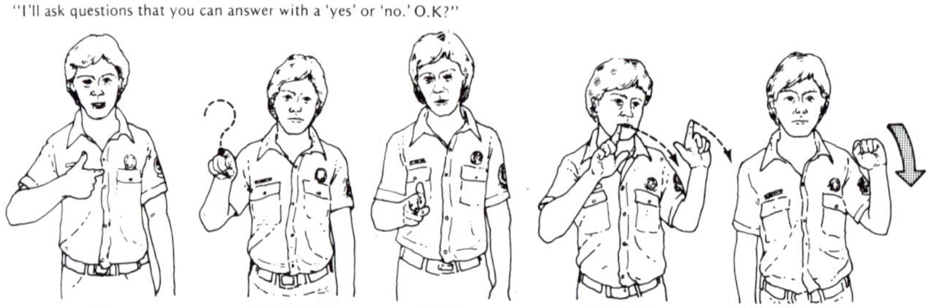

ME QUESTION YOU ANSWER YES

"Are you sick?"

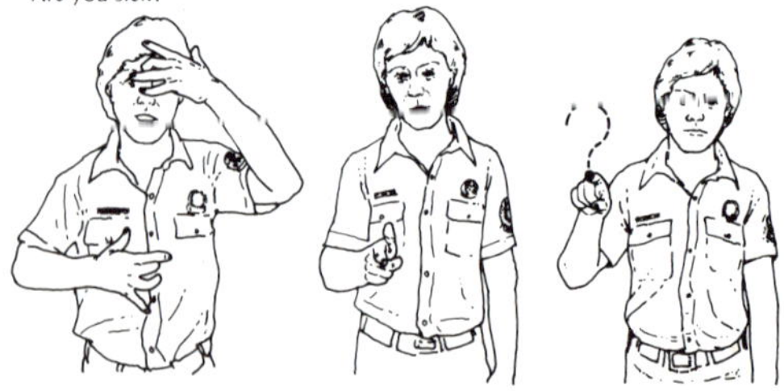

SICK YOU ?

"I'm an emergency medical technician."

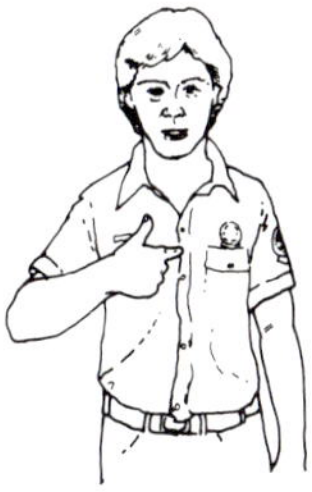

ME

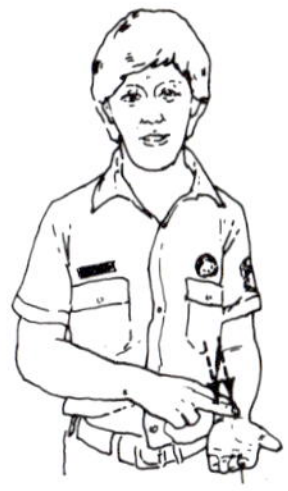

MEDICAL

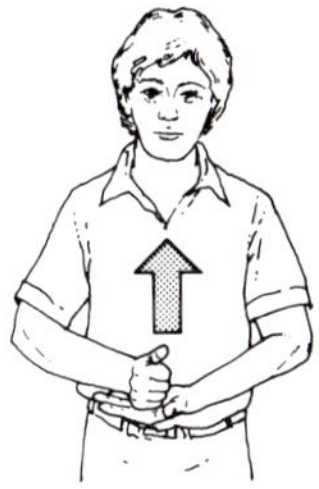

HELP

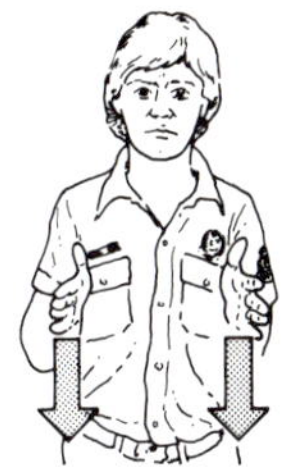

-ER

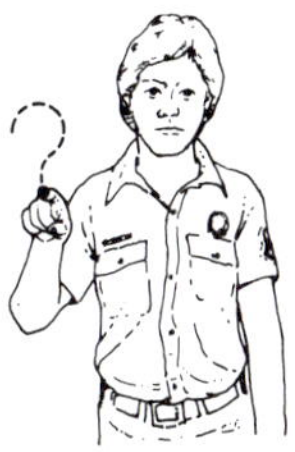

?

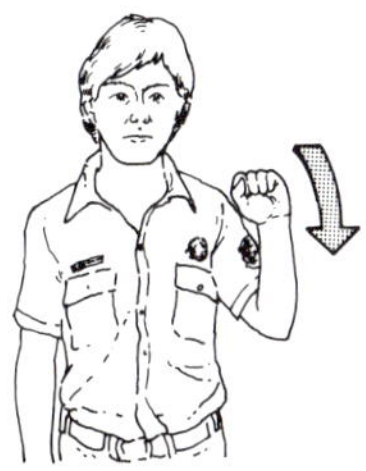

YES

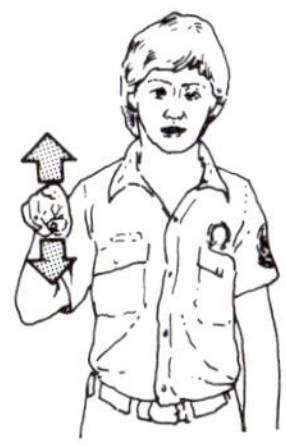

NO

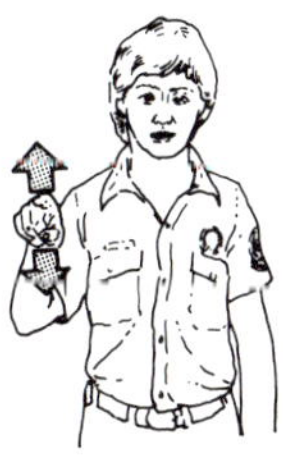

NO

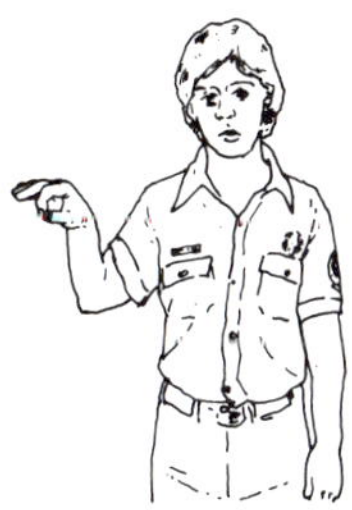

O

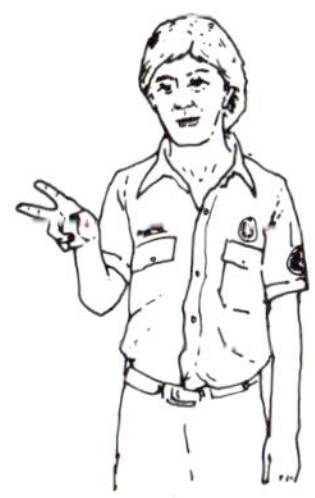

K

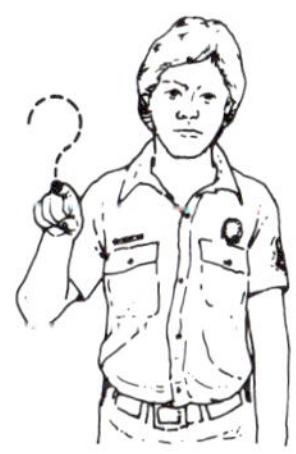

?

"Are you hurt?"

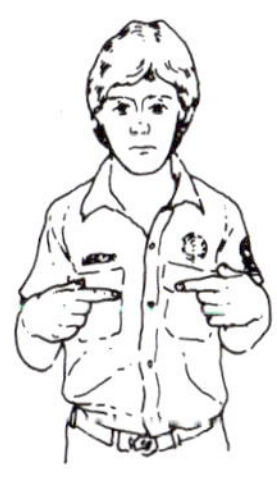

HURT

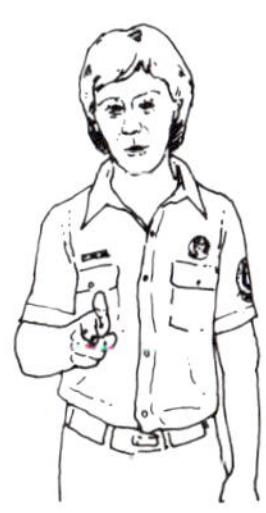

YOU

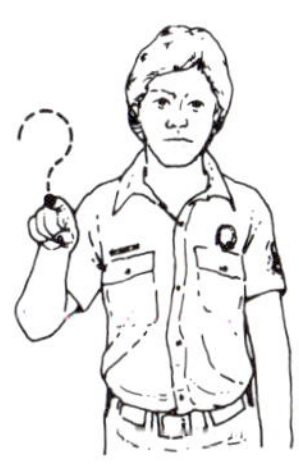

?

"May I check you for injuries (pain)?"

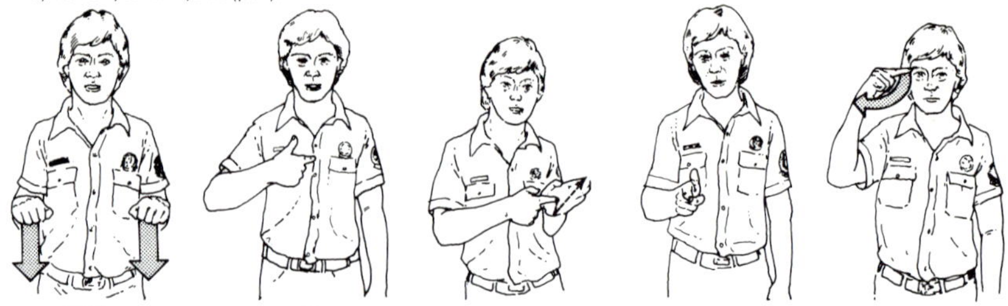

MAY ME CHECK YOU FOR

"May I check your blood pressure?"

Hold the B/P cuff in front of you so the patient can see it. Convey the idea of using it on him.

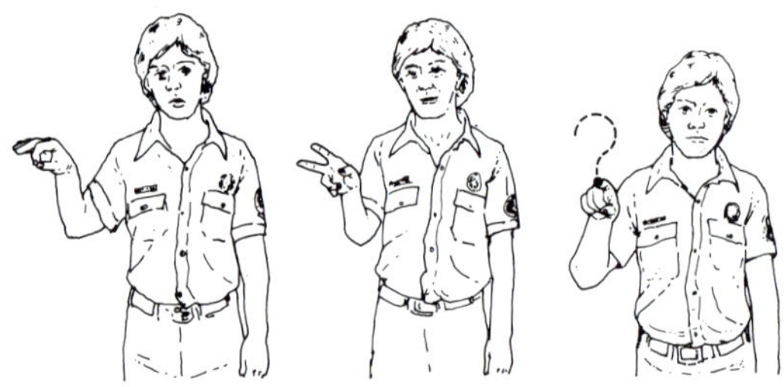

O K ?

"I'm going to touch a possible injury site. It may hurt. O.K?"

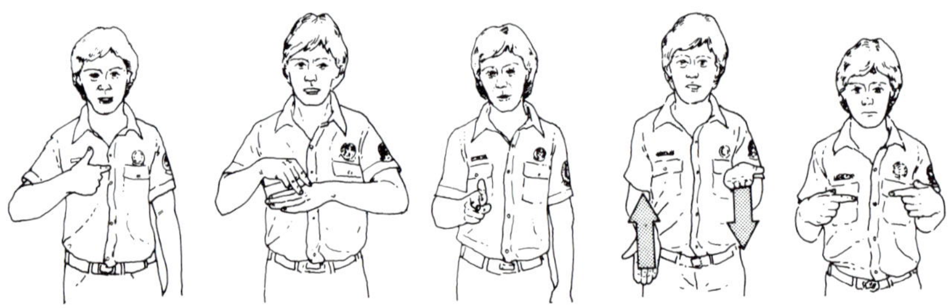

ME TOUCH YOU MAY HURT

"I'm finished with the examination."

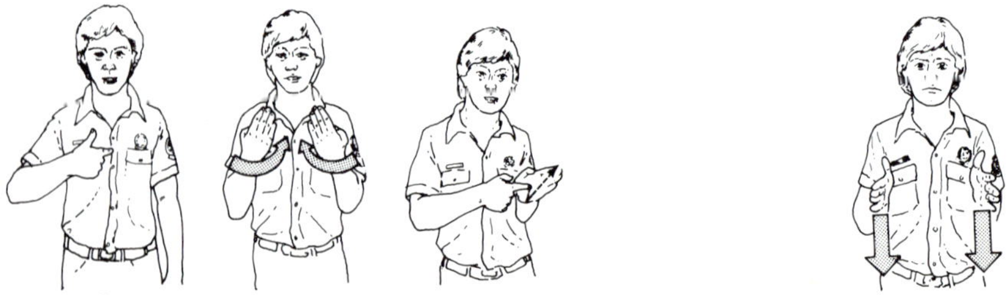

ME FINISH CHECK MAY

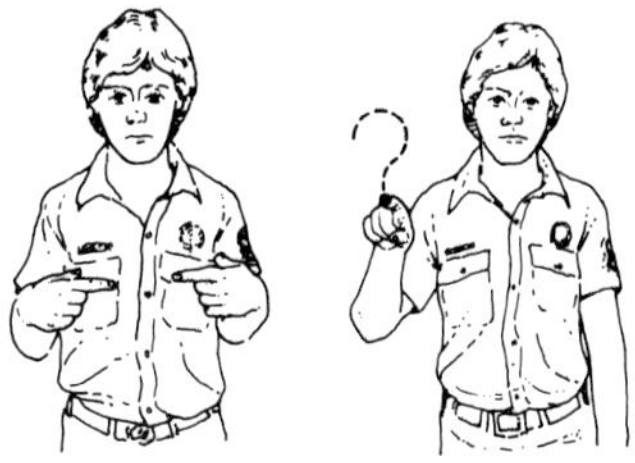

HURT ?

"May I adjust (remove) your (article of clothing)?"

Open your shirt or roll up your sleeve to convey the idea that you must do the same with your patient.

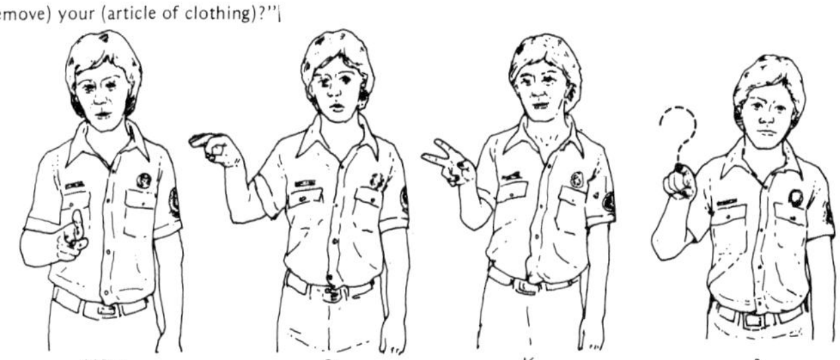

YOU O K ?

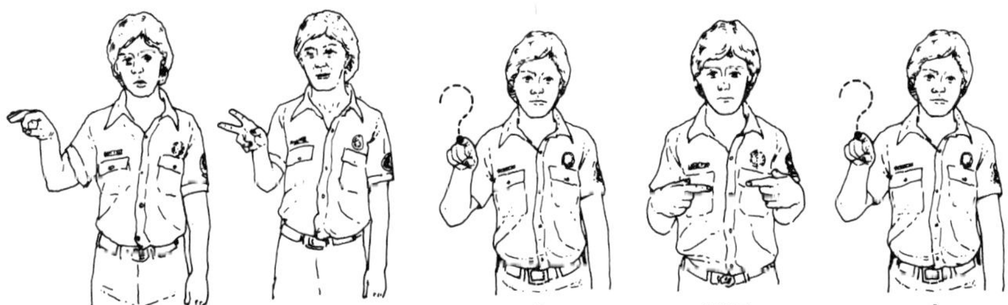

O K ? HURT ?

"May I go on with the emergency care procedure?"

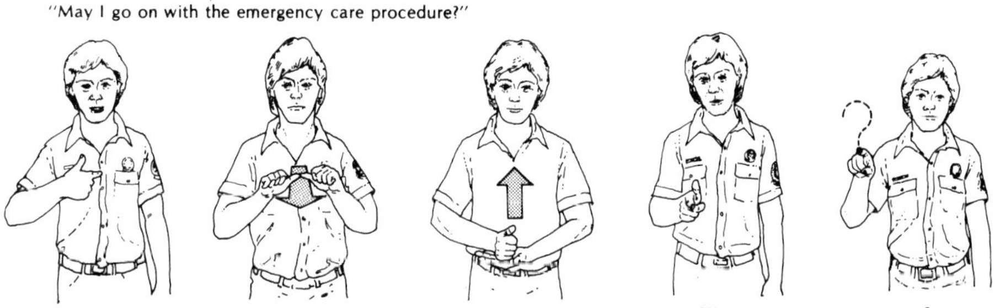

ME CONTINUE HELP YOU ?

# Appendix 7

## Poisonous Plants, Trees, Shrubs, and Vines

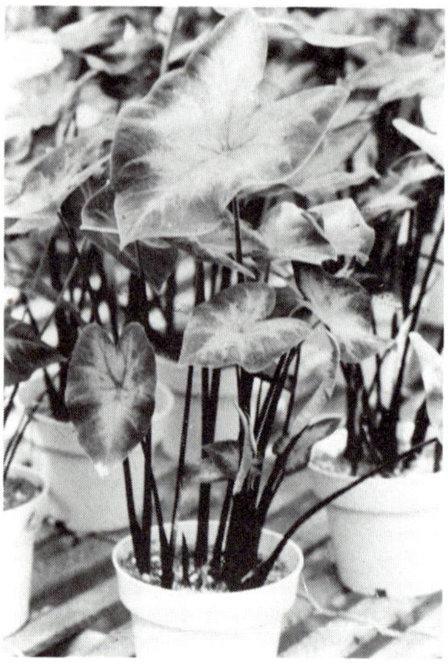

**Figure A-1.** Caladium.

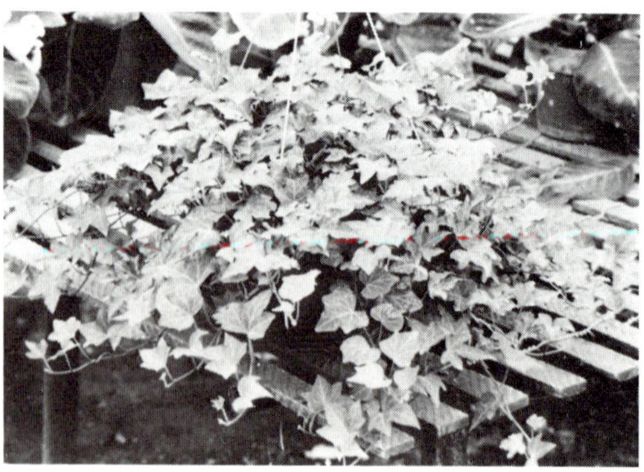

**Figure A-2.** English ivy.

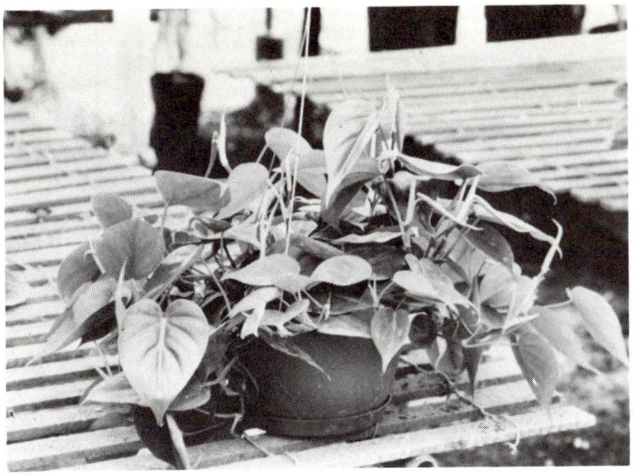

**Figure A-3.** Philodendron.

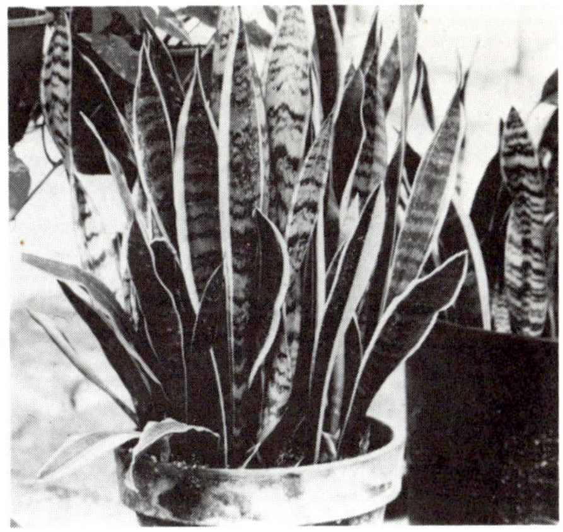

**Figure A-4.** Mother-in-law tongue.

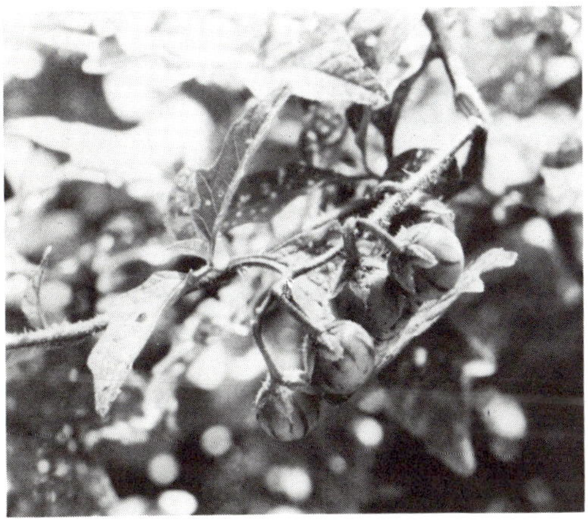

**Figure A-5.** Horsenettle plant and berries.

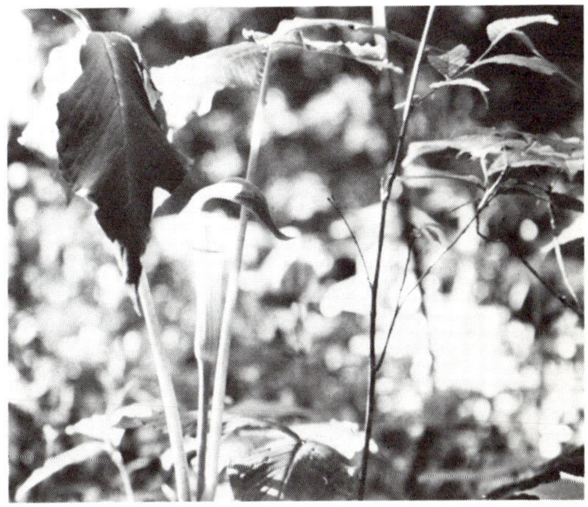

**Figure A-6.** Jack-in-the-pulpit.

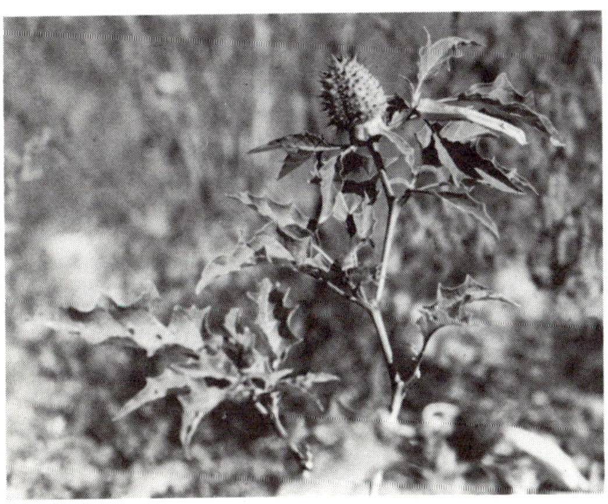

**Figure A-7.** Jimson weed, flower, and seed pod.

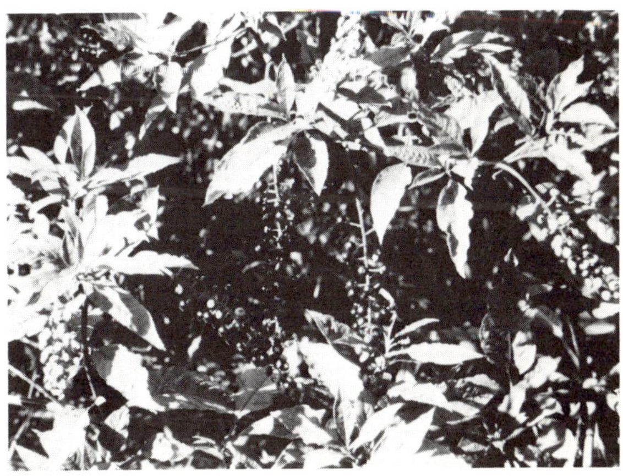

**Figure A-8.** Pokeweed and berries.

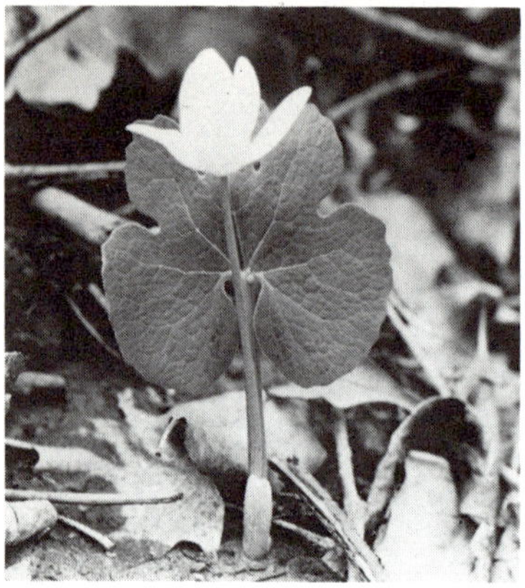

**Figure A–9.** Bloodroot and its flower.

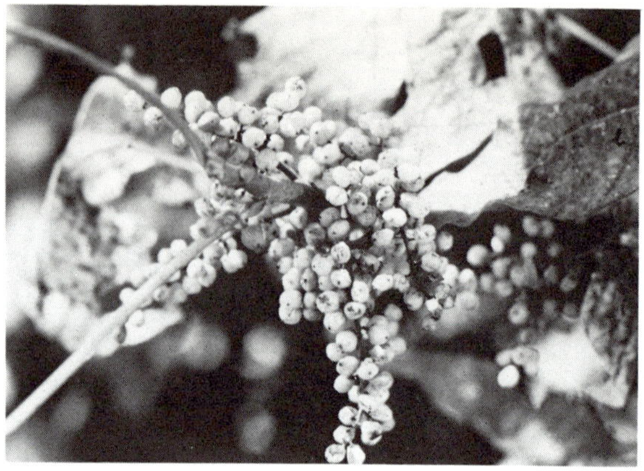

**Figure A–10.** Poison ivy and its winter berries.

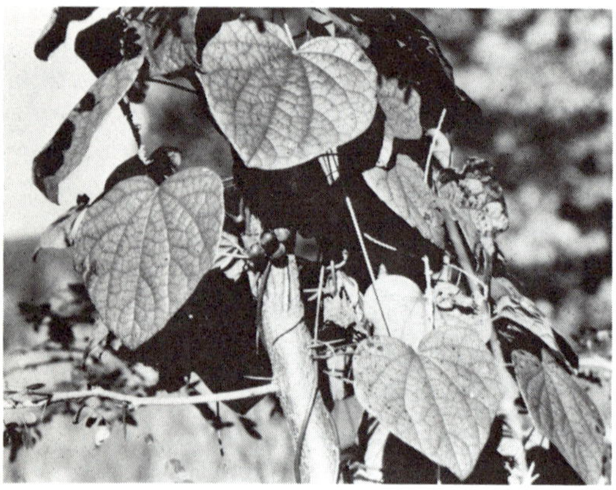

**Figure A–11.** Canada moonseed vine and fall berries.

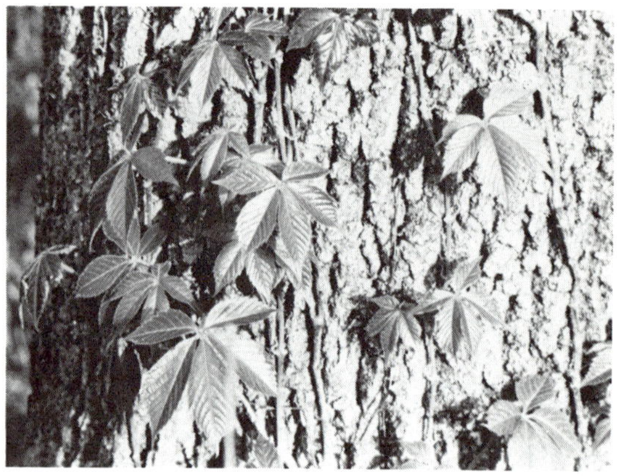

**Figure A–12.** Virginia creeper.

*References*

Ellis, M. D. *Dangerous Plants, Snakes, Arthropods, and Marine Life: Toxicity and Treatment.* Hamilton, IL: Drug Intelligence Publications, 1978.

Hardin, J. W., and Arena, J. M. *Human Poisoning From Native and Cultivated Plants,* 2nd ed. Durham, NC: Duke University Press, 1977.

Lee, Cheryl, and Little, D. "Update Your Poison Plant List" (pamphlet). Indianapolis, IN: Indiana State Board of Health, 1980.

Muenscher, W. C. *Poisonous Plants of the United States.* New York: Collin Books, 1975.

Tampion, J. *Dangerous Plants.* New York: Universe Books, 1977.

| House Plants Name | Scientific Name | Distribution | Poisonous Part(s) | Poisonous Principle | Signs/Symptoms | Treatment |
|---|---|---|---|---|---|---|
| 1. Asparagus fern | Asparagus plumosus | Throughout the U.S., except in hot areas. Commercially available as a potted plant. | Berries, uncooked young shoots. Sap | Glycoside hederagenin | Dermatitis of the mouth, lips and tongue. Nausea and vomiting. | Symptomatic and supportive care. |
| 2. Caladium (Fig. 1) | Caladium | Throughout the U.S. Commercially available as a potted plant | Entire plant | Calcium oxalate | Intense burning sensation of mouth, lips and tongue. Possible pharyngeal and laryngeal edema. Respiratory difficulties. | Administration of demulcents (milk, aluminum-magnesium hydroxide. Pain may persist for days. |
| 3. Castor bean | Ricinus communis | Southern U.S., Hawaii. Commercially available as a potted plant. | All parts, mainly seeds | Phytotoxin ricitin | Burning sensation of mouth, tongue & lips. Nausea, vomiting, & bloody diarrhea. Seed coat must be broken for poisoning. Intact seeds will pass harmlessly through G.I. tract. 2–4 seeds—serious poisoning 8 seeds—considered lethal | Gastric lavage. Basic life support. |
| 4. Dieffenbachia (Dumbcane) | Dieffenbachia sequine or picta | Throughout U.S. & Canada as potted plant. Native to South America. | All parts | Calcium oxalate. Toxic protein | Same as Caladium | Same as Caladium. |
| 5. English ivy (Fig. 2) | Araliaceae | Throughout U.S. & Canada Commercially available as potted plant. | Leaves & berries | Glycoside hederagenin | Restlessness, anxiety, excitement, dyspnea, respiratory arrest | Gastric lavage. Basic life support. |

| *House Plants (cont'd.)* *Name* | *Scientific Name* | *Distribution* | *Poisonous Part(s)* | *Poisonous Principle* | *Signs/Symptoms* | *Treatment* |
|---|---|---|---|---|---|---|
| 6. Philodendrcn (Fig. 3) | Philodendron | Throughout U.S. as a potted plant. | All parts | Calcium oxalate, toxic protein | Same as Caladium | Same as Caladium. |
| 7. Jeruselum cherry | Solanum pseudocapsicum | Throughout U.S. as a potted plant. | Leaves unripened berry | Solanine (Cardio-active substance) | Abdominal cramps, vomiting, diarrhea, circulatory & respiratory depression, paralysis, shock, coma & death. | Symptomatic and supportive care. Basic life support. |
| 8. Lantana | Lantana camara | Throughout U.S. & Canada as a potted plant. Common southern coastal plant. | Entire plant, berries | Alkaloid | Central nervous system depression, profuse sweating, convulsions, respiratory arrest | Gastric lavage. Basic life support. |
| 9. Mother-in-law tongue (Fig. 4 | Sansevieria trifasciata | Throughout U.S. & Canada as a potted plant. | All parts Sap | Calcium oxalate | Same as Caladium. Permanent corneal opacification may occur if sap is rubbed in eyes. | Same as caladium. |
| 10. Poinsettia | Euphorbia pulcherrima | Throughout U.S. & Canada as a potted plant. Native to tropical Mexico & Central America. | Leaves, flowers, fruit, sap | Various poisons in milky sap. | Nausea & vomiting, blistering of lips and tongue, dermatitis | Induce vomiting. Administer demulcents |
| 11. Rosary pea | Abrus precatorius | Central & Southern Florida Commercially available as a potted plant. | Seeds | Phytotoxin abrin and the tetanic glycoside abric acid | Extremely toxic—one chewed seed is said to be fatal. Nausea, vomiting, diarrhea, weakness, drowsiness, circulatory collapse, coma | Induce vomiting or gastric lavage. Basic life support. |

| Garden Plants Name | Scientific Name | Distribution | Toxic Part(s) | Toxin(s) Involved | Signs/Symptoms | Treatment |
|---|---|---|---|---|---|---|
| 1. Potato | Solanum tuberosum | Throughout North America, Britain & Europe. Originally from South America. | Green "sunburned" spots. Green stems, leaves | Alkaloids | Vomiting, diarrhea, cold clammy skin, nausea, mental confusion. Respiratory & cardiac depression. | Symptomatic and supportive care. Basic life support. |
| 2. Rhubarb | Rheum rhaponticum | Cultivated in North America, Britain & Europe | Leaf blades, roots | Calcium oxalate | Intermittent abdominal pain, muscle cramps, & tatany due to hypocalcemia. Large amounts of raw, uncooked leaves can cause convulsions & coma, followed by death. | Administer milk or lime water. Induce vomiting or gastric lavage with lime water. |
| 3. Tomato | Lycopersicon esculentum | Throughout U.S. & Canada | Leaves, vine | Alkaloids | Vomiting, diarrhea, nausea, cold clammy skin, decrease in temperature, dilated pupils, paralysis, shock, circulatory & respiratory depression, Confusion & death. | Induce vomiting or gastric lavage with activated charcoal. Basic life support. |
| 4. Narcissus (Daffodil) | Narcissus | Cultivated in North America, Britian & Europe | Bulb | Alkaloids | Nausea, vomiting, abdominal pain, diarrhea | Induce vomiting. Symptomatic and supportive care. |
| 5. Iris | Iris versicolor | Eastern U.S. & Canada | Leaves, root, stalks | Resinous substance, irisin | Nausea, vomiting, dermatitis | Symptomatic and supportive care. |

| *Garden Plants (cont'd) Name* | *Scientific Name* | *Distribution* | *Toxic Part(s)* | *Toxin(s) Involved* | *Signs/Symptoms* | *Treatment* |
|---|---|---|---|---|---|---|
| 6. Oleander | Nerium oleander | Southern U.S. & Hawaii. Native to tropical America. | Stems, flowers, leaves | Cardiac glycosides | Begins several hrs after ingestion. Local irritation of mouth. Nausea, vomiting, irregular heart rate, dilated pupils, discoloration of mouth, bloody diarrhea, respiratory paralysis. *One leaf has been known to kill an adult.* Bees can make poisoned honey from nectar of flowers. | Symptomatic and supportive care. Basic life support. |
| 7. Morning glory | Ipomoea violacea | Cultivated in North America, Britain & Europe | Seeds | Several alkaloids related to L.S.D. | 50–200 seeds are capable of inducing hallucinationlike states. Nausea. Death has occured from ingestion. | Symptomatic and supportive care. *Chlorpromazine effective as antidote* |
| 8. Sweet pea | Lathyrus odoratus | Cultivated in North America | Seeds or peas | Beta-amino-propionitrile | Slow & weak pulse, depressed respirations, convulsions | Symptomatic and supportive care. |
| 9. Foxglove | Digitalis purpurea | Throughout U.S. & Hawaii. Native to Britain & Europe. | All parts | Cardiac glycosides | Stimulates heart, irregular heartbeat, gastrointestinal upset, mental confusion. May be fatal. | Induce vomiting or gastric lavage. Basic life support. |
| 10. Hyacinth | Hyacinthius crientalis | Throughout U.S. & Canada as cultivated plant | Bulb | Unidentified | Intense digestive upset, dermatitis. | Induce vomiting or gastric lavage. Symptomatic and supportive care. |

|  |  |  |  |  |  |  |
|---|---|---|---|---|---|---|
| 11. Daphne | Daphne mezereum | Cultivated in North America, Britain, & Europe. | Berries, bark, leaves | Bitter glycosides | Very pungent odor. Burning of oral cavity. Vomiting, diarrhea with blood & mucus. Stupor, convulsions, death. | Induce vomiting or gastric lavage. Symptomatic and supportive care. |
| 12. Autumn crocus | Colchicum autumnale | Throughout U.S. & Canada. Native to Britain & Europe. | All parts, bulbs, seeds | Alkaloid colchicine | Mental depression, nausea, vomiting, circulatory collapse | Administer activated charcoal. Gastric lavage. |
| 13. Nightshade | Solanum nigram & dulcamara | Throughout U.S. & Canada. Native to Britain & Europe. | Leaves, unripe fruit | Glycoalkaloid | Burning of oral cavity. Nausea, dizziness, dilated pupils, convulsions, death | Induce vomiting. Basic life support. |
| 14. Lilly-of-the-Valley | Convallaria majalis | Cultivated in North America. Native to Britain & Europe. | Leaves, flowers, roots | Cardiac glycosides | Heart stimulant, dizziness & vomiting within 1–2 hrs after ingestion, heart irregularities | Induce vomiting or gastric lavage. Basic life support. |
| 15. Larkspur | Delphinium | Throughout U.S. & Canada | All parts, especially the seeds | Alkaloids | Gastrointestinal upset, excitement & depression. May be fatal. | Gastric lavage. Basic life support. |
| 16. Hydrangea | Hydrangea macrophylla | Cultivated in North America, Britain, & Europe. Native to Japan. | Leaves, buds | Cyanogenic glycoside (cyanide poisoning) | Nausea, vomiting, abdominal pain, diarrhea, dyspnea, weakness, stupor, coma, convulsions. Death is rapid. | Induce vomiting or administer activated charcoal. Perform gastric lavage. Basic life support. |
| 17. Horsenettle (Fig. 5) | Solanum carolinese eleagnifolium & americanum | Eastern U.S. & Canada | All parts, especially the green berries. | Glycoalkaloid | Appears several hours after ingestion. Nausea, vomiting, abdominal pain & diarrhea, dizziness, pupil dilation, salivation may be present. Headache is common. Convulsions, stupor, respiratory arrest, death. | Induce vomiting and administer activated charcoal. Gastric lavage. Administer demulcents. |

| *Wild Plants Name* | *Scientific Name* | *Distribution* | *Toxic Part(s)* | *Toxin(s) Involved* | *Signs/Symptoms* | *Treatment* |
|---|---|---|---|---|---|---|
| 1. Baneberry (Doll's Eyes) | Aceta rubra, alba, and spicta | Canada south to Georgia, Alabama, Louisiana, Oklahoma. Britain & Europe, temparate Asia. Rich woods & thickets. | All parts, especially the berries. | Essential oil | Abdominal pain, nausea, vomiting, diarrhea, tachycardia, coma. Six berries can cause symptoms, death has occurred in children. | Induce vomiting or gastric lavage. Basic life support. |
| 2. Dogbane | Apocynum cannabunum | Throughout U.S. Dry woods, fields, roadsides. | All parts | Glycosides | Elevated temperature, heartrate & blood pressure. Sweating, anorexia (an"o-rek'se-ah), nausea, vomiting. Death has been reported. | Induce vomiting. *Tannic Acid is reported as specific antidote.* |
| 3. Dutchmans breeches | Dicentra cucullaria & canadensis | Eastern U.S., Southern Canada. Rich woods. | All parts | Alkaloids | Nausea, vomiting, abdominal pain | Induce vomiting. Symptomatic and supportive care. |
| 4. Jack-in-The-Pulpit (Fig. 6) | Arisaema triphyllum | Northeastern & Central U.S. & Southern Canada. Damp woods & swamps. | All parts, especially leaves, roots | Calcium oxalate | Intense burning of mouth, lips & tongue. Possible swelling of pharynx, dyspnea. Nausea, vomiting, abdominal pain. | Rinse mouth with water. Administer milk or aluminum-magnesium hydroxide. |
| 5. Jimson weed (Fig. 7) | Datura strammonium | Throughout U.S. & Canada, Britain extending in Europe | All parts, especially the seeds | Alkaloids atropine scopalamine | Increased thirst, vomiting, dry-mouth, rapid-weak pulse, dilation of pupils, delirium, decreased respirations. | Cholinergic drugs (Physostigmine). Basic life support. |
| 6. Mayapple | Fodophyllum peltatam | Throughout U.S. & Southern Canada. Rich woods. | Greenfruit, leaves, roots | Resinoid podophyllin | Severe vomiting, abdominal pain. Deaths have been reported. | Induce vomiting. Symptomatic & supportive care. Basic life support. |

| | | | | | | |
|---|---|---|---|---|---|---|
| 7. Pokeweed (Fig 8) | Phytolacca americana | Eastern U.S. & Southern Canada open woods | Roots, leaves fruit | Alkaloid | Burning of mouth, abdominal cramps, vomiting, diarrhea, perspiration, salivation, weak pulse & respiration, coma | Induce vomiting. Activated charcoal. Basic life support. |
| 8. Skunk cabbage | Symplocarpus foetidus | Southern Canada Northeastern U.S. rich woods | Leaves, roots | Calcium oxylate | Burning of mouth, lips & tongue, possible swelling | Rinse mouth with water. Administer demulcents. |
| 9. Water hemlock | Cicuta maculata | Eastern U.S. & Canada. Wet marshy areas. | All parts, especially roots | Cicutoxin | Symptoms usually appear in 15–20 minutes. Severe abdominal pain, vomiting, violent convulsions, hypersalivation, dilated pupils, coma. Death may occur within 15 minutes after lethal dose. | Induce vomiting or gastric lavage. Basic life support. |
| 10. Marsh marigold (Cowslip) | Calatha palustris | Across Canada south to North Carolina, west to Tennessee, Iowa & Nebraska. Swamps, marshes, wet meadows, along streams. | Top leaves & stems | Protoanemonin | Sap causes increased salivation. Vomiting, abdominal pain. Large quantity may cause convulsions. | Induce vomiting. Administer demulcents. |
| 11. Death camus | Zygadenus nuttalli | Northeastern & Southern U.S. Along coastal plains, sandy pinelands, bogs. | Flowers, leaves, roots | Alkaloids | Intense burning of mouth, lips & tongue, may occur. Vomiting, diarrhea headache, weakness, hypotension, coma | Induce vomiting or gastric lavage. Administer activated charcoal. Basic life support. |
| 12. Blood root (Fig. 9) | Sanguinaria canadensis | Canada to Florida, Texas. Rich woods and along streams. | Underground stems, roots, red juice | Alkaloid | Intense burning of oral cavity. Nausea, vomiting; C.N.S., depression, coma | Induce vomiting, followed with milk. Basic life support. |

| Wild Plants (cont'd) Name | Scientific Name | Distribution | Toxic Part(s) | Toxin(s) Involved | Signs/Symptoms | Treatment |
|---|---|---|---|---|---|---|
| 13. Green or false hellebore (Indian Poke) | Veratrum viride | Eastern Canada to Minnesota. Mountains of South Carolina, Georgia, & Tennessee. Swamps, wet woods. | Roots, leaves, seeds | Alkaloid | Increased salivation, diaphoresis (di″ah-fo-re′sis), hypotension, dyspnea, convulsions. Death due to asphyxia. | Induce vomiting or gastric lavage. Basic life support. **Epinephrine is contraindicated.* |
| 14. Poison hemlock | Conium maculatum | Eastern U.S. & Southern Canada. Wet meadows, thickets, freshwater swamps. | All parts | Lambdaconicene coniine | Nausea, vomiting, respiratory distress, weakness, convulsions. | Induce vomiting or gastric lavage. |
| 15. Poison ivy (Fig. 10) | Toxicodendron radicans | Throughout U.S. & Canada | All parts, even the smoke from burning it. | Urushiol | Severe allergic response, causing dermatitis upon contact, resulting in inflammation, blistering & vesicles, as skin breaks a liquid flows out & scabs over. | Lotions & creams for symptomatic relief. **Do not use alcohol as it spreads urushiol.* |
| 16. Poison oak | Toxicodendron quercifolium | Maryland to Texas | All parts | Urushiol | See Poison Ivy | See Poison Ivy. |
| 17. Poison sumac | Toxicodendron vernix | Maine to Ontario southward. Common in swamps. | All parts | Urushiol | See Poison Ivy | See Poison Ivy. |
| 18. Mushrooms | Thousands of species | Across Canada & U.S. | Many species are edible, but many more are poisonous. The best rule to follow is never eat a mushroom that one cannot identify. Many deaths have been reported from their ingestion. | | | |

| Trees Name | Scientific Name | Distribution | Toxic Part(s) | Toxin(s) Involved | Signs/Symptoms | Treatment |
|---|---|---|---|---|---|---|
| 1. Apple | Pyrus sylvestris | Throughout the U.S. and Canada | Seeds | Cyanogenic glycoside | Nausea, vomiting, abdominal pain, diarrhea, dyspnea, weakness, stupor, coma, convulsions | Induce vomiting. Administer activated charcoal. Gastric lavage. Basic life support. |
| 2. Apricot | Prunus armeniaca | Throughout the U.S. and Canada | Leaves, stems. Bark and seed pits. | Cyanogenic glycoside | Same as apple. seed ingestion. | Same as Apple. *Ingestion of 3–5 seed pits in children is considered serious poisoning.* |
| 3. Black locust | Robinia pseudoacacia | Northcentral & Southeastern U.S. Southern Canada | Young leaves. Inner bark. Seeds. | Glycoside | Nausea, vomiting, weakness, dilated pupils, irregular heart rate. | Administer demulcents. Basic life support. |
| 4. Cherry (wild) | Prunus serotina and virginiana | Eastern U.S. & Southern Canada | Leaves, stems. Bark & seed pits. | Cyanogenic glycoside | Same as apple seed ingestion | Same as apple seed ingestion. |
| 5. Chinaberry tree | Melia Azedarach | Southern U.S. | Berries, leaves | Saponin<br>Toxic alkaloid | Onset of symptoms often delayed. Nausea, vomiting, bloody diarrhea, dyspnea, syncope, sweating, dilated pupils & dyspnea may occur. | Induce vomiting. Administer activated charcoal. Gastric lavage. Basic life support. |

| *Trees (cont'd) Name* | *Scientific Name* | *Distribution* | *Toxic Part(s)* | *Toxin(s) Involved* | *Signs/Symptoms* | *Treatment* |
|---|---|---|---|---|---|---|
| 6. Holly | Llex cornuta and opaca | | Berries | Ilicin | Rapid onset of nausea, abdominal pain, vomiting & diarrhea | Induce vomiting. Administer demulcents. |
| 7. Osage orange | Maclura pomifera | Northeastern & Southern U.S. | Milky sap | Unidentified | Dermatitis | Wash with soap and water. |
| 8. Peach | Prunus persica | Commercially available throughout the U.S. & Canada | Seed kernels (pits) | Cyanogenic glycoside | See Apple | See Apple. |
| 9. Plum | Prunus americana | Commercially available throughout the U.S. & Canada | Seed kernels (pits) | Cyanogenic glycoside | See Apple | See Apple. |
| 10. Red buckeye | Aesculus pavia | Southeastern U.S. | Leaves, flowers, young sprouts and seeds | Glycosidic saponin aesculin | Salivation, nausea, vomiting, abdominal pain, severe diarrhea, weakness, incoordination, paralysis, respiratory arrest | Induce vomiting. Administer activated charcoal. Gastric lavage. Administer demulcents. Basic life support. |

| *Shrubs Name* | *Scientific Name* | *Distribution* | *Toxic Part(s)* | *Toxin(s) Involved* | *Signs & Symptoms* | *Treatment* |
|---|---|---|---|---|---|---|
| 1. Japanese yew | Podocarpus macrophylla | Throughut U.S. as ornamental shrub. | Leaves, seeds | Alkaloid toxins | Nausea, vomiting, diarrhea, cardiac disturbances | Induce vomiting. Basic life support. |
| 2. Mountain laurel (mescal bean) | Kalamia Latifolia | Native to Eastern U.S. | Entire plant, especially the seeds. | Cytisine (alkaloid with nicitine-like action). | One chewed seed is considered lethal. Symptoms within 1 hour. Nausea, vomiting, diarrhea, abdominal pain, headache, confusion, convulsions, paralysis, coma, respitory failure, death. | Gastric lavage. Basic life support. |
| 3. Golden chain | Laburnum anagyroids | Northern U.S. | Beanlike capsules | Alkaloids | Excitement, incoordination, vomiting, convulsions, coma, respiratory arrest. | Induce vomiting or gastric lavage with glucose saline solution—5 percent. Basic life support. |
| 4. Boxwood | Boxus sempervirens | Southern U.S. | Leaves, stems | Alkaloids | Same as above | Same as above. |
| 5. Rhododendron | Rhododendron albiflorum | Canada south to Appalacians | All parts | Same as Mountain Laurel | Same as Mountain Laurel | See Mountain Laurel. |
| 6. Snowberry | Symphoricarpus albus | Northern U.S. & Canada | Berries | Saponins, tannins, coumarins | Nausea, vomiting, Stupor | Induce vomiting, Symptomatic & supportive care. |
| 7. Privet | Ligustrum vulgare | Cultivated in North America & Europe as a hedge plant. Native to Britain & Europe. | Berries | Unidentified | Rapid onset of nausea, vomiting, diarrhea. Death has occurred in children. | Induce vomiting. Administer demulcents before gastric lavage. Activated charcoal. |

| Shrubs Name | Scientific Name | Distribution | Toxic Part(s) | Toxin(s) Involved | Signs & Symptoms | Treatment |
|---|---|---|---|---|---|---|
| 8. Jessamine (yellow) | Gelesemium sempervirens | Southern U.S., Hawaii. | Entire plant berries | Alkaloids | Sweating, weakness, convulsions, paralysis, respiratory arrest | Induce vomiting or gastric lavage. Basic life support. **Morphine said to be specific antidote* |
| 9. Yaupon | Llex vomitoria | Southern U.S. | Berries | Unidentified | See Privet | See Privet. |
| 10. Poinciana (Bird-of-Paradise) | Poinciana Gilliesii | Southern U.S. Commercially available as a potted plant. | Green seed, pods | Unidentified | See Privet | See Privet. |
| 11. Wisteria | Wisteria | Cultivated throughout U.S. & Canada. Native to Japan. | Seeds, pods | Unidentified | See Privet | See Privet. |
| 12. Senna-bean | Sesbania drummondii | Southern U.S. | Seeds, entire plant | Saponins (irritating & corrosive) | Nausea, vomiting, abdominal pain, diarrhea, depression, weakness, dyspnea, cardiac irregularities | Induce vomiting or gastric lavage. Administer activated charcoal. Basic life support. |
| 13. Purple rattlebox | Sesbania punicea | Southern U.S. | Seeds, entire plant | Saponins | See Senna-Bean | See Senna-Bean. |

| *Vines* *Name* | *Scientific Name* | *Distribution* | *Toxic Part(s)* | *Toxin(s) Involved* | *Signs/Symptoms* | *Treatment* |
|---|---|---|---|---|---|---|
| 1. Mistletoe | Phoradendron flavescens | Southern U.S. Commercially available as ornamental decoration. | Berries | Beta-phenylethylamine and tryamine | Abdominal pain, bracycardia, cardiovascular collapse. Death has occurred in children, approximately 10 hours after ingestion of berries. | Induce vomiting or gastric lavage. Basic life support. |
| 2. Bittersweet | Solanum dulcamara | Eastern U.S. | Leaves, fruit | Glycoalkaloid | Nausea, dizziness, muscle weakness, vomiting, diarrhea, dilated pupils, convulsions, paralysis, coma | Induce vomiting. Basic life support. |
| 3. English ivy | Hedera helix | Throughout U.S. & Canada. Native to Britain & Europe. | Leaves, berries | Glycoside hederagenin | Excitement, dyspnea coma | Induce vomiting or gastric lavage. Basic life support. |
| 4. Canada moonseed (Fig. 11) | Menispermum canadense | Southern Canada to Georgia & Oklahoma. Resembles grape vine. Berries contain a single seed. Grapes have several. | Roots, berries | Alkaloids | Fruit seeds can cause mechanical injury to intestines. Deaths have been reported. | Symptomatic and supportive care. Basic life support. |
| 5. Virginia creeper (American ivy) (Fig. 12) | Parthenocissus quinquefolia | Southern Canada, Eastern U.S. Cultivated in Britain & Europe. | Leaves, berries | Calcium oxylate (corrosive action) | Symptoms appear about 24 hours after ingestion. Nausea, vomiting, diarrhea (may contain blood), headache, stupor, muscle cramping. | Induce vomiting or gastric lavage with milk, calcium hydroxide (lime water), calcium gluconate or calcium lactate. Administer activated charcoal. |

# Appendix 8

# Diving Tables

## U. S. NAVY STANDARD AIR DECOMPRESSION TABLE

| Depth (feet) | Bottom time (min) | Time first stop (min:sec) | Decompression stops (feet) | | | | | Total ascent (min:sec) | Repetitive group |
|---|---|---|---|---|---|---|---|---|---|
| | | | 50 | 40 | 30 | 20 | 10 | | |
| 40 | 200 | | | | | | 0 | 0:40 | * |
| | 210 | 0:30 | | | | | 2 | 2:40 | N |
| | 230 | 0:30 | | | | | 7 | 7:40 | N |
| | 250 | 0:30 | | | | | 11 | 11:40 | O |
| | 270 | 0:30 | | | | | 15 | 15:40 | O |
| | 300 | 0:30 | | | | | 19 | 19:40 | Z |
| | 360 | 0:30 | | | | | 23 | 23:40 | ** |
| | 480 | 0:30 | | | | | 41 | 41:40 | ** |
| | 720 | 0:30 | | | | | 69 | 69:40 | ** |
| 50 | 100 | | | | | | 0 | 0:50 | * |
| | 110 | 0:40 | | | | | 3 | 3:50 | L |
| | 120 | 0:40 | | | | | 5 | 5:50 | M |
| | 140 | 0:40 | | | | | 10 | 10:50 | M |
| | 160 | 0:40 | | | | | 21 | 21:50 | N |
| | 180 | 0:40 | | | | | 29 | 29:50 | O |
| | 200 | 0:40 | | | | | 35 | 35:50 | O |
| | 220 | 0:40 | | | | | 40 | 40:50 | Z |
| | 240 | 0:40 | | | | | 47 | 47:50 | Z |
| 60 | 60 | | | | | | 0 | 1:00 | * |
| | 70 | 0:50 | | | | | 2 | 3:00 | K |
| | 80 | 0:50 | | | | | 7 | 8:00 | L |
| | 100 | 0:50 | | | | | 14 | 15:00 | M |
| | 120 | 0:50 | | | | | 26 | 27:00 | N |
| | 140 | 0:50 | | | | | 39 | 40:00 | O |
| | 160 | 0:50 | | | | | 48 | 49:00 | Z |
| | 180 | 0:50 | | | | | 56 | 57:00 | Z |
| | 200 | 0:40 | | | | 1 | 69 | 71:00 | Z |
| | 240 | 0:40 | | | | 2 | 79 | 82:00 | ** |
| | 360 | 0:40 | | | | 20 | 119 | 140:00 | ** |
| | 480 | 0:40 | | | | 44 | 148 | 193:00 | ** |
| | 720 | 0:40 | | | | 78 | 187 | 266:00 | ** |
| 70 | 50 | | | | | | 0 | 1:10 | * |
| | 60 | 1:00 | | | | | 8 | 9:10 | K |
| | 70 | 1:00 | | | | | 14 | 15:10 | L |
| | 80 | 1:00 | | | | | 18 | 19:10 | M |
| | 90 | 1:00 | | | | | 23 | 24:10 | N |
| | 100 | 1:00 | | | | | 33 | 34:10 | N |
| | 110 | 0:50 | | | | 2 | 41 | 44:10 | O |
| | 120 | 0:50 | | | | 4 | 47 | 52:10 | O |
| | 130 | 0:50 | | | | 6 | 52 | 59:10 | O |
| | 140 | 0:50 | | | | 8 | 56 | 65:10 | Z |
| | 150 | 0:50 | | | | 9 | 61 | 71:10 | Z |
| | 160 | 0:50 | | | | 13 | 72 | 86:10 | Z |
| | 170 | 0:50 | | | | 19 | 79 | 99:10 | Z |

* See No Decompression Table for repetitive groups

**Repetitive dives may not follow exceptional exposure dives

| Depth (feet) | Bottom time (min) | Time first stop (min:sec) | 70 | 60 | 50 | 40 | 30 | 20 | 10 | Total ascent (min:sec) | Repetitive group |
|---|---|---|---|---|---|---|---|---|---|---|---|
| | | | Decompression stops (feet) | | | | | | | | |
| 80 | 40 | | | | | | | | 0 | 1:20 | * |
| | 50 | 1:10 | | | | | | | 10 | 11:20 | K |
| | 60 | 1:10 | | | | | | | 17 | 18:20 | L |
| | 70 | 1:10 | | | | | | | 23 | 24:20 | M |
| | 80 | 1:00 | | | | | | 2 | 31 | 34:20 | N |
| | 90 | 1:00 | | | | | | 7 | 39 | 47:20 | N |
| | 100 | 1:00 | | | | | | 11 | 46 | 58:20 | O |
| | 110 | 1:00 | | | | | | 13 | 53 | 67:20 | O |
| | 120 | 1:00 | | | | | | 17 | 56 | 74:20 | Z |
| | 130 | 1:00 | | | | | | 19 | 63 | 83:20 | Z |
| | 140 | 1:00 | | | | | | 26 | 69 | 96:20 | Z |
| | 150 | 1:00 | | | | | | 32 | 77 | 110:20 | Z |
| | 180 | 1:00 | | | | | | 35 | 85 | 121:20 | ** |
| | 240 | 0:50 | | | | | 6 | 52 | 120 | 179:20 | ** |
| | 360 | 0:50 | | | | | 29 | 90 | 160 | 280:20 | ** |
| | 480 | 0:50 | | | | | 59 | 107 | 187 | 354:20 | ** |
| | 720 | 0:40 | | | | 17 | 108 | 142 | 187 | 455:20 | ** |
| 90 | 30 | | | | | | | | 0 | 1:30 | * |
| | 40 | 1:20 | | | | | | | 7 | 8:30 | J |
| | 50 | 1:20 | | | | | | | 18 | 19:30 | L |
| | 60 | 1:20 | | | | | | | 25 | 26:30 | M |
| | 70 | 1:10 | | | | | | 7 | 30 | 38:30 | N |
| | 80 | 1:10 | | | | | | 13 | 40 | 54:30 | N |
| | 90 | 1:10 | | | | | | 18 | 48 | 67:30 | O |
| | 100 | 1:10 | | | | | | 21 | 54 | 76:30 | Z |
| | 110 | 1:10 | | | | | | 24 | 61 | 86:30 | Z |
| | 120 | 1:10 | | | | | | 32 | 68 | 101:30 | Z |
| | 130 | 1:00 | | | | | 5 | 36 | 74 | 116:30 | Z |
| 100 | 25 | | | | | | | | 0 | 1:40 | * |
| | 30 | 1:30 | | | | | | | 3 | 4:40 | I |
| | 40 | 1:30 | | | | | | | 15 | 16:40 | K |
| | 50 | 1:20 | | | | | | 2 | 24 | 27:40 | L |
| | 60 | 1:20 | | | | | | 9 | 28 | 38:40 | N |
| | 70 | 1:20 | | | | | | 17 | 39 | 57:40 | O |
| | 80 | 1:20 | | | | | | 23 | 48 | 72:40 | O |
| | 90 | 1:10 | | | | | 3 | 23 | 57 | 84:40 | Z |
| | 100 | 1:10 | | | | | 7 | 23 | 66 | 97:40 | Z |
| | 110 | 1:10 | | | | | 10 | 34 | 72 | 117:40 | Z |
| | 120 | 1:10 | | | | | 12 | 41 | 78 | 132:40 | Z |
| | 180 | 1:00 | | | | 1 | 29 | 53 | 118 | 202:40 | ** |
| | 240 | 1:00 | | | | 14 | 42 | 84 | 142 | 283:40 | ** |
| | 360 | 0:50 | | | 2 | 42 | 73 | 111 | 187 | 416:40 | ** |
| | 480 | 0:50 | | | 21 | 61 | 91 | 142 | 187 | 503:40 | ** |
| | 720 | 0:50 | | | 55 | 106 | 122 | 142 | 187 | 613:40 | ** |
| 110 | 20 | | | | | | | | 0 | 1:50 | * |
| | 25 | 1:40 | | | | | | | 3 | 4:50 | H |
| | 30 | 1:40 | | | | | | | 7 | 8:50 | J |
| | 40 | 1:30 | | | | | | 2 | 21 | 24:50 | L |
| | 50 | 1:30 | | | | | | 8 | 26 | 35:50 | M |
| | 60 | 1:30 | | | | | | 18 | 36 | 55:50 | N |
| | 70 | 1:20 | | | | | 1 | 23 | 48 | 73:50 | O |
| | 80 | 1:20 | | | | | 7 | 23 | 57 | 88:50 | Z |
| | 90 | 1:20 | | | | | 12 | 30 | 64 | 107:50 | Z |
| | 100 | 1:20 | | | | | 15 | 37 | 72 | 125:50 | Z |
| 120 | 15 | | | | | | | | 0 | 2:00 | * |
| | 20 | 1:50 | | | | | | | 2 | 4:00 | H |
| | 25 | 1:50 | | | | | | | 6 | 8:00 | I |
| | 30 | 1:50 | | | | | | | 14 | 16:00 | J |
| | 40 | 1:40 | | | | | | 5 | 25 | 32:00 | L |
| | 50 | 1:40 | | | | | | 15 | 31 | 48:00 | N |
| | 60 | 1:30 | | | | | 2 | 22 | 45 | 71:00 | O |
| | 70 | 1:30 | | | | | 9 | 23 | 55 | 89:00 | O |
| | 80 | 1:30 | | | | | 15 | 27 | 63 | 107:00 | Z |
| | 90 | 1:30 | | | | | 19 | 37 | 74 | 132:00 | Z |
| | 100 | 1:30 | | | | | 23 | 45 | 80 | 150:00 | Z |
| | 120 | 1:20 | | | | 10 | 19 | 47 | 98 | 176:00 | ** |
| | 180 | 1:10 | | | 5 | 27 | 37 | 76 | 137 | 284:00 | ** |
| | 240 | 1:10 | | | 23 | 35 | 60 | 97 | 179 | 396:00 | ** |
| | 360 | 1:00 | | 18 | 45 | 64 | 93 | 142 | 187 | 551:00 | ** |
| | 480 | 0:50 | 3 | 41 | 64 | 93 | 122 | 142 | 187 | 654:00 | ** |
| | 720 | 0:50 | 32 | 74 | 100 | 114 | 122 | 142 | 187 | 773:00 | ** |
| 130 | 10 | | | | | | | | 0 | 2:10 | * |
| | 15 | 2:00 | | | | | | | 1 | 3:10 | F |
| | 20 | 2:00 | | | | | | | 4 | 6:10 | H |
| | 25 | 2:00 | | | | | | | 10 | 12:10 | J |
| | 30 | 1:50 | | | | | | 3 | 18 | 23:10 | M |
| | 40 | 1:50 | | | | | | 10 | 25 | 37:10 | N |
| | 50 | 1:40 | | | | | 3 | 21 | 37 | 63:10 | O |
| | 60 | 1:40 | | | | | 9 | 23 | 52 | 86:10 | Z |
| | 70 | 1:40 | | | | | 16 | 24 | 61 | 103:10 | Z |
| | 80 | 1:30 | | | | 3 | 19 | 35 | 72 | 131:10 | Z |
| | 90 | 1:30 | | | | 8 | 19 | 45 | 80 | 154:10 | Z |

| Depth | Bottom time (min) | Time to first stop (min:sec) | 90 | 80 | 70 | 60 | 50 | 40 | 30 | 20 | 10 | Total ascent (min:sec) | Repetitive group |
|---|---|---|---|---|---|---|---|---|---|---|---|---|---|
| | | | | | | Decompression stops (feet) | | | | | | | |
| **140** | 10 | | | | | | | | | | 0 | 2:20 | * |
| | 15 | 2:10 | | | | | | | | | 2 | 4:20 | G |
| | 20 | 2:10 | | | | | | | | | 6 | 8:20 | I |
| | 25 | 2:00 | | | | | | | | 2 | 14 | 18:20 | J |
| | 30 | 2:00 | | | | | | | | 5 | 21 | 28:20 | K |
| | 40 | 1:50 | | | | | | | 2 | 16 | 26 | 46:20 | N |
| | 50 | 1:50 | | | | | | | 6 | 24 | 44 | 76:20 | O |
| | 60 | 1:50 | | | | | | | 16 | 23 | 56 | 97:20 | Z |
| | 70 | 1:40 | | | | | | 4 | 19 | 32 | 68 | 125:20 | Z |
| | 80 | 1:40 | | | | | | 10 | 23 | 41 | 79 | 155:20 | Z |
| | 90 | 1:30 | | | | | 2 | 14 | 18 | 42 | 88 | 166:20 | ** |
| | 120 | 1:30 | | | | | 12 | 14 | 36 | 56 | 120 | 240:20 | ** |
| | 180 | 1:20 | | | | 10 | 26 | 32 | 54 | 94 | 168 | 386:20 | ** |
| | 240 | 1:10 | | | 8 | 28 | 34 | 50 | 78 | 124 | 187 | 511:20 | ** |
| | 360 | 1:00 | | 9 | 32 | 42 | 64 | 84 | 122 | 142 | 187 | 684:20 | ** |
| | 480 | 1:00 | | 31 | 44 | 59 | 100 | 114 | 122 | 142 | 187 | 801:20 | ** |
| | 720 | 0:50 | 16 | 56 | 88 | 97 | 100 | 114 | 122 | 142 | 187 | 924:20 | ** |
| **150** | 5 | | | | | | | | | | 0 | 2:30 | C |
| | 10 | 2:20 | | | | | | | | | 1 | 3:30 | E |
| | 15 | 2:20 | | | | | | | | | 3 | 5:30 | G |
| | 20 | 2:10 | | | | | | | | 2 | 7 | 11:30 | H |
| | 25 | 2:10 | | | | | | | | 4 | 17 | 23:30 | K |
| | 30 | 2:10 | | | | | | | | 8 | 24 | 34:30 | L |
| | 40 | 2:00 | | | | | | | 5 | 19 | 33 | 59:30 | N |
| | 50 | 2:00 | | | | | | | 12 | 23 | 51 | 88:30 | O |
| | 60 | 1:50 | | | | | | 3 | 19 | 26 | 62 | 112:30 | Z |
| | 70 | 1:50 | | | | | | 11 | 19 | 39 | 75 | 146:30 | Z |
| | 80 | 1:40 | | | | | 1 | 17 | 19 | 50 | 84 | 173:30 | Z |
| **160** | 5 | | | | | | | | | | 0 | 2:40 | D |
| | 10 | 2:30 | | | | | | | | | 1 | 3:40 | F |
| | 15 | 2:20 | | | | | | | | 1 | 4 | 7:40 | H |
| | 20 | 2:20 | | | | | | | | 3 | 11 | 16:40 | J |
| | 25 | 2:20 | | | | | | | | 7 | 20 | 29:40 | K |
| | 30 | 2:10 | | | | | | | 2 | 11 | 25 | 40:40 | M |
| | 40 | 2:10 | | | | | | | 7 | 23 | 39 | 71:40 | N |
| | 50 | 2:00 | | | | | | 2 | 16 | 23 | 55 | 98:40 | Z |
| | 60 | 2:00 | | | | | | 9 | 19 | 33 | 69 | 132:40 | Z |
| | 70 | 1:50 | | | | | 1 | 17 | 22 | 44 | 80 | 166:40 | Z |

| Depth | Bottom time (min) | Time to first stop (min: sec) | 110 | 100 | 90 | 80 | 70 | 60 | 50 | 40 | 30 | 20 | 10 | Total ascent (min: sec) | Repetitive group |
|---|---|---|---|---|---|---|---|---|---|---|---|---|---|---|---|
| | | | | | | | Decompression stops (feet) | | | | | | | | |
| **170** | 5 | | | | | | | | | | | | 0 | 2:50 | D |
| | 10 | 2:40 | | | | | | | | | | | 2 | 4:50 | F |
| | 15 | 2:30 | | | | | | | | | | 2 | 5 | 9:50 | H |
| | 20 | 2:30 | | | | | | | | | | 4 | 15 | 21:50 | J |
| | 25 | 2:20 | | | | | | | | | 2 | 7 | 23 | 34:50 | L |
| | 30 | 2:20 | | | | | | | | | 4 | 13 | 26 | 45:50 | M |
| | 40 | 2:10 | | | | | | | | 1 | 10 | 23 | 45 | 81:50 | O |
| | 50 | 2:10 | | | | | | | | 5 | 18 | 23 | 61 | 109:50 | Z |
| | 60 | 2:00 | | | | | | | 2 | 15 | 22 | 37 | 74 | 152:50 | Z |
| | 70 | 2:00 | | | | | | | 8 | 17 | 19 | 51 | 86 | 183:50 | Z |
| | 90 | 1:50 | | | | | | 12 | 12 | 14 | 34 | 52 | 120 | 246:50 | ** |
| | 120 | 1:30 | | | | 2 | 10 | 12 | 18 | 32 | 42 | 82 | 156 | 356:50 | ** |
| | 180 | 1:20 | | | 4 | 10 | 22 | 28 | 34 | 50 | 78 | 120 | 187 | 535:50 | ** |
| | 240 | 1:20 | | | 18 | 24 | 30 | 42 | 50 | 70 | 116 | 142 | 187 | 681:50 | ** |
| | 360 | 1:10 | | 22 | 34 | 40 | 52 | 60 | 98 | 114 | 122 | 142 | 187 | 873:50 | ** |
| | 480 | 1:00 | 14 | 40 | 42 | 56 | 91 | 97 | 100 | 114 | 122 | 142 | 187 | 1007:50 | ** |
| **180** | 5 | | | | | | | | | | | | 0 | 3:00 | D |
| | 10 | 2:50 | | | | | | | | | | | 3 | 6:00 | F |
| | 15 | 2:40 | | | | | | | | | | 3 | 6 | 12:00 | I |
| | 20 | 2:30 | | | | | | | | | 1 | 5 | 17 | 26:00 | K |
| | 25 | 2:30 | | | | | | | | | 3 | 10 | 24 | 40:00 | L |
| | 30 | 2:30 | | | | | | | | | 6 | 17 | 27 | 53:00 | N |
| | 40 | 2:20 | | | | | | | | 3 | 14 | 23 | 50 | 93:00 | O |
| | 50 | 2:10 | | | | | | | 2 | 9 | 19 | 30 | 65 | 128:00 | Z |
| | 60 | 2:10 | | | | | | | 5 | 16 | 19 | 44 | 81 | 168:00 | Z |
| **190** | 5 | | | | | | | | | | | | 0 | 3:10 | D |
| | 10 | 2:50 | | | | | | | | | | 1 | 3 | 7:10 | G |
| | 15 | 2:50 | | | | | | | | | | 4 | 7 | 14:10 | I |
| | 20 | 2:40 | | | | | | | | | 2 | 6 | 20 | 31:10 | K |
| | 25 | 2:40 | | | | | | | | | 5 | 11 | 25 | 44:10 | M |
| | 30 | 2:30 | | | | | | | | 1 | 8 | 19 | 32 | 63:10 | N |
| | 40 | 2:30 | | | | | | | | 8 | 14 | 23 | 55 | 103:10 | O |
| | 50 | 2:20 | | | | | | | 4 | 13 | 22 | 33 | 72 | 147:10 | Z |
| | 60 | 2:20 | | | | | | | 10 | 17 | 19 | 50 | 84 | 183:10 | Z |

| Depth (feet) | Bottom time (min) | Time to first stop (min:sec) | 130 | 120 | 110 | 100 | 90 | 80 | 70 | 60 | 50 | 40 | 30 | 20 | 10 | Total ascent (min:sec) |
|---|---|---|---|---|---|---|---|---|---|---|---|---|---|---|---|---|
| | | | Decompression stops (feet) | | | | | | | | | | | | | |
| 200 | 5 | 3:10 | | | | | | | | | | | | | 1 | 4:20 |
| | 10 | 3:00 | | | | | | | | | | | | 1 | 4 | 8:20 |
| | 15 | 2:50 | | | | | | | | | | | 1 | 4 | 10 | 18:20 |
| | 20 | 2:50 | | | | | | | | | | | 3 | 7 | 27 | 40:20 |
| | 25 | 2:50 | | | | | | | | | | | 7 | 14 | 25 | 49:20 |
| | 30 | 2:40 | | | | | | | | | | 2 | 9 | 22 | 37 | 73:20 |
| | 40 | 2:30 | | | | | | | | | 2 | 8 | 17 | 23 | 59 | 112:20 |
| | 50 | 2:30 | | | | | | | | | 6 | 16 | 22 | 39 | 75 | 161:20 |
| | 60 | 2:20 | | | | | | | | 2 | 13 | 17 | 24 | 51 | 89 | 199:20 |
| | 90 | 1:50 | | | | | 1 | 10 | 10 | 12 | 12 | 30 | 38 | 74 | 134 | 324:20 |
| | 120 | 1:40 | | | | 6 | 10 | 10 | 10 | 24 | 28 | 40 | 64 | 98 | 180 | 473:20 |
| | 180 | 1:20 | | 1 | 10 | 10 | 18 | 24 | 24 | 42 | 48 | 70 | 106 | 142 | 187 | 685:20 |
| | 240 | 1:20 | | 6 | 20 | 24 | 24 | 36 | 42 | 54 | 68 | 114 | 122 | 142 | 187 | 842:20 |
| | 360 | 1:10 | 12 | 22 | 36 | 40 | 44 | 56 | 82 | 98 | 100 | 114 | 122 | 142 | 187 | 1058:20 |
| 210 | 5 | 3:20 | | | | | | | | | | | | | 1 | 4:30 |
| | 10 | 3:10 | | | | | | | | | | | | 2 | 4 | 9:30 |
| | 15 | 3:00 | | | | | | | | | | | 1 | 5 | 13 | 22:30 |
| | 20 | 3:00 | | | | | | | | | | | 4 | 10 | 23 | 40:30 |
| | 25 | 2:50 | | | | | | | | | | 2 | 7 | 17 | 27 | 56:30 |
| | 30 | 2:50 | | | | | | | | | | 4 | 9 | 24 | 41 | 81:30 |
| | 40 | 2:40 | | | | | | | | | 4 | 9 | 19 | 26 | 63 | 124:30 |
| | 50 | 2:30 | | | | | | | | 1 | 9 | 17 | 19 | 45 | 80 | 174:30 |
| 220 | 5 | 3:30 | | | | | | | | | | | | | 2 | 5:40 |
| | 10 | 3:20 | | | | | | | | | | | | 2 | 5 | 10:40 |
| | 15 | 3:10 | | | | | | | | | | | 2 | 5 | 16 | 26:40 |
| | 20 | 3:00 | | | | | | | | | | 1 | 3 | 11 | 24 | 42:40 |
| | 25 | 3:00 | | | | | | | | | | 3 | 8 | 19 | 33 | 66:40 |
| | 30 | 2:50 | | | | | | | | | 1 | 7 | 10 | 23 | 47 | 91:40 |
| | 40 | 2:50 | | | | | | | | | 6 | 12 | 22 | 29 | 68 | 140:40 |
| | 50 | 2:40 | | | | | | | | 3 | 12 | 17 | 18 | 51 | 86 | 190:40 |
| 230 | 5 | 3:40 | | | | | | | | | | | | | 2 | 5:50 |
| | 10 | 3:20 | | | | | | | | | | | 1 | 2 | 6 | 12:50 |
| | 15 | 3:20 | | | | | | | | | | | 3 | 6 | 18 | 30:50 |
| | 20 | 3:10 | | | | | | | | | | 2 | 5 | 12 | 26 | 48:50 |
| | 25 | 3:10 | | | | | | | | | | 4 | 8 | 22 | 37 | 74:50 |
| | 30 | 3:00 | | | | | | | | | 2 | 8 | 12 | 23 | 51 | 99:50 |
| | 40 | 2:50 | | | | | | | | 1 | 7 | 15 | 22 | 34 | 74 | 156:50 |
| | 50 | 2:50 | | | | | | | | 5 | 14 | 16 | 24 | 51 | 89 | 202:50 |
| 240 | 5 | 3:50 | | | | | | | | | | | | | 2 | 6:00 |
| | 10 | 3:30 | | | | | | | | | | | 1 | 3 | 6 | 14:00 |
| | 15 | 3:30 | | | | | | | | | | | 4 | 6 | 21 | 35:00 |
| | 20 | 3:20 | | | | | | | | | | 3 | 6 | 15 | 25 | 53:00 |
| | 25 | 3:10 | | | | | | | | | 1 | 4 | 9 | 24 | 40 | 82:00 |
| | 30 | 3:10 | | | | | | | | | 4 | 8 | 15 | 22 | 56 | 109:00 |
| | 40 | 3:00 | | | | | | | | 3 | 7 | 17 | 22 | 39 | 75 | 167:00 |
| | 50 | 2:50 | | | | | | | 1 | 8 | 15 | 16 | 29 | 51 | 94 | 218:00 |
| 250 | 5 | 3:50 | | | | | | | | | | | | 1 | 2 | 7:10 |
| | 10 | 3:40 | | | | | | | | | | | 1 | 4 | 7 | 16:10 |
| | 15 | 3:30 | | | | | | | | | | 1 | 4 | 7 | 22 | 38:10 |
| | 20 | 3:30 | | | | | | | | | | 4 | 7 | 17 | 27 | 59:10 |
| | 25 | 3:20 | | | | | | | | | 2 | 7 | 10 | 24 | 45 | 92:10 |
| | 30 | 3:20 | | | | | | | | | 6 | 7 | 17 | 23 | 59 | 116:10 |
| | 40 | 3:10 | | | | | | | | 5 | 9 | 17 | 19 | 45 | 79 | 178:10 |
| | 60 | 2:40 | | | | | 4 | 10 | 10 | 10 | 12 | 22 | 36 | 64 | 126 | 298:10 |
| | 90 | 2:10 | | 8 | 10 | 10 | 10 | 10 | 10 | 28 | 28 | 44 | 68 | 98 | 186 | 514:10 |
| 260 | 5 | 4:00 | | | | | | | | | | | | 1 | 2 | 7:20 |
| | 10 | 3:50 | | | | | | | | | | | 2 | 4 | 9 | 19:20 |
| | 15 | 3:40 | | | | | | | | | | 2 | 4 | 10 | 22 | 42:20 |
| | 20 | 3:30 | | | | | | | | | 1 | 4 | 7 | 20 | 31 | 67:20 |
| | 25 | 3:30 | | | | | | | | | 3 | 8 | 11 | 23 | 50 | 99:20 |
| | 30 | 3:20 | | | | | | | | 2 | 6 | 8 | 19 | 26 | 61 | 126:20 |
| | 40 | 3:10 | | | | | | | 1 | 6 | 11 | 16 | 19 | 49 | 84 | 190:20 |
| 270 | 5 | 4:10 | | | | | | | | | | | | 1 | 3 | 8:30 |
| | 10 | 4:00 | | | | | | | | | | | 2 | 5 | 11 | 22:30 |
| | 15 | 3:50 | | | | | | | | | | 3 | 4 | 11 | 24 | 46:30 |
| | 20 | 3:40 | | | | | | | | | 2 | 3 | 9 | 21 | 35 | 74:30 |
| | 25 | 3:30 | | | | | | | | 2 | 3 | 8 | 13 | 23 | 53 | 106:30 |
| | 30 | 3:30 | | | | | | | | 3 | 6 | 12 | 22 | 27 | 64 | 138:30 |
| | 40 | 3:20 | | | | | | | 5 | 6 | 11 | 17 | 22 | 51 | 88 | 204:30 |

| Depth (feet) | Bottom time (min) | Time to first stop (min:sec) | 130 | 120 | 110 | 100 | 90 | 80 | 70 | 60 | 50 | 40 | 30 | 20 | 10 | Total ascent time (min:sec) |
|---|---|---|---|---|---|---|---|---|---|---|---|---|---|---|---|---|
| | | | Decompression stops (feet) | | | | | | | | | | | | | |
| 280 | 5 | 4:20 | | | | | | | | | | | | 2 | 2 | 8:40 |
| | 10 | 4:00 | | | | | | | | | | 1 | 2 | 5 | 13 | 25:40 |
| | 15 | 3:50 | | | | | | | | | 1 | 3 | 4 | 11 | 26 | 49:40 |
| | 20 | 3:50 | | | | | | | | | 3 | 4 | 8 | 23 | 39 | 81:40 |
| | 25 | 3:40 | | | | | | | | 2 | 5 | 7 | 16 | 23 | 56 | 113:40 |
| | 30 | 3:30 | | | | | | | 1 | 3 | 7 | 13 | 22 | 30 | 70 | 150:40 |
| | 40 | 3:20 | | | | | | 1 | 6 | 6 | 13 | 17 | 27 | 51 | 93 | 218:40 |
| 290 | 5 | 4:30 | | | | | | | | | | | | 2 | 3 | 9:50 |
| | 10 | 4:10 | | | | | | | | | | 1 | 3 | 5 | 16 | 29:50 |
| | 15 | 4:00 | | | | | | | | | 1 | 3 | 6 | 12 | 26 | 52:50 |
| | 20 | 4:00 | | | | | | | | | 3 | 7 | 9 | 23 | 43 | 89:50 |
| | 25 | 3:50 | | | | | | | | 3 | 5 | 8 | 17 | 23 | 60 | 120:50 |
| | 30 | 3:40 | | | | | | | 1 | 5 | 6 | 16 | 22 | 36 | 72 | 162:50 |
| | 40 | 3:30 | | | | | | 3 | 5 | 7 | 15 | 16 | 32 | 51 | 95 | 228:50 |
| 300 | 5 | 4:40 | | | | | | | | | | | | 3 | 3 | 11:00 |
| | 10 | 4:20 | | | | | | | | | | 1 | 3 | 6 | 17 | 32:00 |
| | 15 | 4:10 | | | | | | | | | 2 | 3 | 6 | 15 | 26 | 57:00 |
| | 20 | 4:00 | | | | | | | | 2 | 3 | 7 | 10 | 23 | 47 | 97:00 |
| | 25 | 3:50 | | | | | | | 1 | 3 | 6 | 8 | 19 | 26 | 61 | 129:00 |
| | 30 | 3:50 | | | | | | | 2 | 5 | 7 | 17 | 22 | 39 | 75 | 172:00 |
| | 40 | 3:40 | | | | | | 4 | 6 | 9 | 15 | 17 | 34 | 51 | 90 | 231:00 |
| | 60 | 3:00 | | 4 | 10 | 10 | 10 | 10 | 10 | 14 | 28 | 32 | 50 | 90 | 187 | 460:00 |

### Extreme exposures—250 and 300 ft

| Depth (ft) | Bottom time (min) | Time to first stop (min:sec) | 200 | 190 | 180 | 170 | 160 | 150 | 140 | 130 | 120 | 110 | 100 | 90 | 80 | 70 | 60 | 50 | 40 | 30 | 20 | 10 | Total ascent time (min:sec) |
|---|---|---|---|---|---|---|---|---|---|---|---|---|---|---|---|---|---|---|---|---|---|---|---|
| | | | Decompression stops (feet) | | | | | | | | | | | | | | | | | | | | |
| 250 | 120 | 1:50 | | | | | | | 5 | 10 | 10 | 10 | 10 | 16 | 24 | 24 | 36 | 48 | 64 | 94 | 142 | 187 | 684:10 |
| | 180 | 1:30 | | | | | 4 | 8 | 8 | 10 | 22 | 24 | 24 | 32 | 42 | 44 | 60 | 84 | 114 | 122 | 142 | 187 | 931:10 |
| | 240 | 1:30 | | | | | 9 | 14 | 21 | 22 | 22 | 40 | 40 | 42 | 56 | 76 | 98 | 100 | 114 | 122 | 142 | 187 | 1109:10 |
| 300 | 90 | 2:20 | | | | | 3 | 8 | 8 | 10 | 10 | 10 | 10 | 16 | 24 | 24 | 34 | 48 | 64 | 90 | 142 | 187 | 693:00 |
| | 120 | 2:00 | | | 4 | 8 | 8 | 8 | 8 | 10 | 14 | 24 | 24 | 24 | 34 | 42 | 58 | 66 | 102 | 122 | 142 | 187 | 890:00 |
| | 180 | 1:40 | 6 | 8 | 8 | 8 | 14 | 20 | 21 | 21 | 28 | 40 | 40 | 48 | 56 | 82 | 98 | 100 | 114 | 122 | 142 | 187 | 1168:00 |

## NO-DECOMPRESSION LIMITS AND REPETITIVE GROUP DESIGNATION TABLE FOR NO-DECOMPRESSION AIR DIVES

| Depth (feet) | No-decompression limits (min) | A | B | C | D | E | F | G | H | I | J | K | L | M | N | O |
|---|---|---|---|---|---|---|---|---|---|---|---|---|---|---|---|---|
| | | Group Designation | | | | | | | | | | | | | | |
| 10 | | 60 | 120 | 210 | 300 | | | | | | | | | | | |
| 15 | | 35 | 70 | 110 | 160 | 225 | 350 | | | | | | | | | |
| 20 | | 25 | 50 | 75 | 100 | 135 | 180 | 240 | 325 | | | | | | | |
| 25 | | 20 | 35 | 55 | 75 | 100 | 125 | 160 | 195 | 245 | 315 | | | | | |
| 30 | | 15 | 30 | 45 | 60 | 75 | 95 | 120 | 145 | 170 | 205 | 250 | 310 | | | |
| 35 | 310 | 5 | 15 | 25 | 40 | 50 | 60 | 80 | 100 | 120 | 140 | 160 | 190 | 220 | 270 | 310 |
| 40 | 200 | 5 | 15 | 25 | 30 | 40 | 50 | 70 | 80 | 100 | 110 | 130 | 150 | 170 | 200 | |
| 50 | 100 | | 10 | 15 | 25 | 30 | 40 | 50 | 60 | 70 | 80 | 90 | 100 | | | |
| 60 | 60 | | 10 | 15 | 20 | 25 | 30 | 40 | 50 | 55 | 60 | | | | | |
| 70 | 50 | | 5 | 10 | 15 | 20 | 30 | 35 | 40 | 45 | 50 | | | | | |
| 80 | 40 | | 5 | 10 | 15 | 20 | 25 | 30 | 35 | 40 | | | | | | |
| 90 | 30 | | 5 | 10 | 12 | 15 | 20 | 25 | 30 | | | | | | | |
| 100 | 25 | | 6 | 7 | 10 | 15 | 20 | 22 | 25 | | | | | | | |
| 110 | 20 | | | 5 | 10 | 13 | 15 | 20 | | | | | | | | |
| 120 | 15 | | | 5 | 10 | 12 | 15 | | | | | | | | | |
| 130 | 10 | | | 5 | 8 | 10 | | | | | | | | | | |
| 140 | 10 | | | 5 | 7 | 10 | | | | | | | | | | |
| 150 | 5 | | | 5 | | | | | | | | | | | | |
| 160 | 5 | | | | 5 | | | | | | | | | | | |
| 170 | 5 | | | | 5 | | | | | | | | | | | |
| 180 | 5 | | | | 5 | | | | | | | | | | | |
| 190 | 5 | | | | 5 | | | | | | | | | | | |

# RESIDUAL NITROGEN TIMETABLE FOR REPETITIVE AIR DIVES

*Dives following surface intervals of more than 12 hours are not repetitive dives. Use actual bottom times in the Standard Air Decompression Tables to compute decompression for such dives.

Repetitive group at the beginning of the surface interval

| Repetitive group | Z | O | N | M | L | K | J | I | H | G | F | E | D | C | B | A |
|---|---|---|---|---|---|---|---|---|---|---|---|---|---|---|---|---|
| A | | | | | | | | | | | | | | | | 0:10<br>12:00* |
| B | | | | | | | | | | | | | | | 0:10<br>2:10 | 2:11<br>12:00* |
| C | | | | | | | | | | | | | | 0:10<br>1:39 | 1:40<br>2:49 | 2:50<br>12:00* |
| D | | | | | | | | | | | | | 0:10<br>1:09 | 1:10<br>2:38 | 2:39<br>5:48 | 5:49<br>12:00* |
| E | | | | | | | | | | | | 0:10<br>0:54 | 0:55<br>1:57 | 1:58<br>3:22 | 3:23<br>6:32 | 6:33<br>12:00* |
| F | | | | | | | | | | | 0:10<br>0:45 | 0:46<br>1:29 | 1:30<br>2:28 | 2:29<br>3:57 | 3:58<br>7:05 | 7:06<br>12:00* |
| G | | | | | | | | | | 0:10<br>0:40 | 0:41<br>1:15 | 1:16<br>1:59 | 2:00<br>2:58 | 2:59<br>4:25 | 4:26<br>7:35 | 7:36<br>12:00* |
| H | | | | | | | | | 0:10<br>0:36 | 0:37<br>1:06 | 1:07<br>1:41 | 1:42<br>2:23 | 2:24<br>3:20 | 3:21<br>4:49 | 4:50<br>7:59 | 8:00<br>12:00* |
| I | | | | | | | | 0:10<br>0:33 | 0:34<br>0:59 | 1:00<br>1:29 | 1:30<br>2:02 | 2:03<br>2:44 | 2:45<br>3:43 | 3:44<br>5:12 | 5:13<br>8:21 | 8:22<br>12:00* |
| J | | | | | | | 0:10<br>0:31 | 0:32<br>0:54 | 0:55<br>1:19 | 1:20<br>1:47 | 1:48<br>2:20 | 2:21<br>3:04 | 3:05<br>4:02 | 4:03<br>5:40 | 5:41<br>8:40 | 8:41<br>12:00* |
| K | | | | | | 0:10<br>0:28 | 0:29<br>0:49 | 0:50<br>1:11 | 1:12<br>1:35 | 1:36<br>2:03 | 2:04<br>2:38 | 2:39<br>3:21 | 3:22<br>4:19 | 4:20<br>5:48 | 5:49<br>8:58 | 8:59<br>12:00* |
| L | | | | | 0:10<br>0:26 | 0:27<br>0:45 | 0:46<br>1:04 | 1:05<br>1:25 | 1:26<br>1:49 | 1:50<br>2:19 | 2:20<br>2:53 | 2:54<br>3:36 | 3:37<br>4:35 | 4:36<br>6:02 | 6:03<br>9:12 | 9:13<br>12:00* |
| M | | | | 0:10<br>0:25 | 0:26<br>0:42 | 0:43<br>0:59 | 1:00<br>1:18 | 1:19<br>1:39 | 1:40<br>2:05 | 2:06<br>2:34 | 2:35<br>3:08 | 3:09<br>3:52 | 3:53<br>4:49 | 4:50<br>6:18 | 6:19<br>9:28 | 9:29<br>12:00* |
| N | | | 0:10<br>0:24 | 0:25<br>0:39 | 0:40<br>0:54 | 0:55<br>1:11 | 1:12<br>1:30 | 1:31<br>1:53 | 1:54<br>2:18 | 2:19<br>2:47 | 2:48<br>3:22 | 3:23<br>4:04 | 4:05<br>5:03 | 5:04<br>6:32 | 6:33<br>9:43 | 9:44<br>12:00* |
| O | | 0:10<br>0:23 | 0:24<br>0:36 | 0:37<br>0:51 | 0:52<br>1:07 | 1:08<br>1:24 | 1:25<br>1:43 | 1:44<br>2:04 | 2:05<br>2:29 | 2:30<br>2:59 | 3:00<br>3:33 | 3:34<br>4:17 | 4:18<br>5:16 | 5:17<br>6:44 | 6:45<br>9:54 | 9:55<br>12:00* |
| | 0:10<br>0:22 | 0:23<br>0:34 | 0:35<br>0:48 | 0:49<br>1:02 | 1:03<br>1:18 | 1:19<br>1:36 | 1:37<br>1:55 | 1:56<br>2:17 | 2:18<br>2:42 | 2:43<br>3:10 | 3:11<br>3:45 | 3:46<br>4:29 | 4:30<br>5:27 | 5:28<br>6:56 | 6:57<br>10:05 | 10:06<br>12:00* |
| **NEW → GROUP DESIGNATION** | **Z** | **O** | **N** | **M** | **L** | **K** | **J** | **I** | **H** | **G** | **F** | **E** | **D** | **C** | **B** | **A** |

| REPETITIVE DIVE DEPTH | Z | O | N | M | L | K | J | I | H | G | F | E | D | C | B | A |
|---|---|---|---|---|---|---|---|---|---|---|---|---|---|---|---|---|
| 40 | 257 | 241 | 213 | 187 | 161 | 138 | 116 | 101 | 87 | 73 | 61 | 49 | 37 | 25 | 17 | 7 |
| 50 | 169 | 160 | 142 | 124 | 111 | 99 | 87 | 76 | 66 | 56 | 47 | 38 | 29 | 21 | 13 | 6 |
| 60 | 122 | 117 | 107 | 97 | 88 | 79 | 70 | 61 | 52 | 44 | 36 | 30 | 24 | 17 | 11 | 5 |
| 70 | 100 | 96 | 87 | 80 | 72 | 64 | 57 | 50 | 43 | 37 | 31 | 26 | 20 | 15 | 9 | 4 |
| 80 | 84 | 80 | 73 | 68 | 61 | 54 | 48 | 43 | 38 | 32 | 28 | 23 | 18 | 13 | 8 | 4 |
| 90 | 73 | 70 | 64 | 58 | 53 | 47 | 43 | 38 | 33 | 29 | 24 | 20 | 16 | 11 | 7 | 3 |
| 100 | 64 | 62 | 57 | 52 | 48 | 43 | 38 | 34 | 30 | 26 | 22 | 18 | 14 | 10 | 7 | 3 |
| 110 | 57 | 55 | 51 | 47 | 42 | 38 | 34 | 31 | 27 | 24 | 20 | 16 | 13 | 10 | 6 | 3 |
| 120 | 52 | 50 | 46 | 43 | 39 | 35 | 32 | 28 | 25 | 21 | 18 | 15 | 12 | 9 | 6 | 3 |
| 130 | 46 | 44 | 40 | 38 | 35 | 31 | 28 | 25 | 22 | 19 | 16 | 13 | 11 | 8 | 6 | 3 |
| 140 | 42 | 40 | 38 | 35 | 32 | 29 | 26 | 23 | 20 | 18 | 15 | 12 | 10 | 7 | 5 | 2 |
| 150 | 40 | 38 | 35 | 32 | 30 | 27 | 24 | 22 | 19 | 17 | 14 | 12 | 9 | 7 | 5 | 2 |
| 160 | 37 | 36 | 33 | 31 | 28 | 26 | 23 | 20 | 18 | 16 | 13 | 11 | 9 | 6 | 4 | 2 |
| 170 | 35 | 34 | 31 | 29 | 26 | 24 | 22 | 19 | 17 | 15 | 13 | 10 | 8 | 6 | 4 | 2 |
| 180 | 32 | 31 | 29 | 27 | 25 | 22 | 20 | 18 | 16 | 14 | 12 | 10 | 8 | 6 | 4 | 2 |
| 190 | 31 | 30 | 28 | 26 | 24 | 21 | 19 | 17 | 15 | 13 | 11 | 10 | 8 | 6 | 4 | 2 |

**RESIDUAL NITROGEN TIMES (MINUTES)**

# Informational Resources

American Diabetes Association
New York, NY
(212) 697-7760

American Lung Association
New York, NY
(212) 245-8000

Center for Disease Control
Atlanta, GA
(404) 633-3311-Weekdays
(404) 633-2176-Nights

Chemical Transportation Emergency Center—CHEMTREC
Washington, D.C.
(800) 424-9300 (toll free)
In the District of Columbia, the Virgin Islands, Guam, Samoa, Puerto Rico, and Alaska call (202) 483-7616

Civil Air Patrol
Building 714
Office of Information, Department E
Maxwell AFB, AL 36112

Department of Energy, Nuclear Accident Center
Albuquerque, NM
(505) 844-4667

Epilepsy Foundation of America
Washington, D.C.
(202) 293-2930

Intermountain Regional Poison Control Center
Salt Lake City, UT
(801) 581-2151
Advice concerning poisonous plant ingestion

International Association of Fire Chiefs
Washington, D.C.
(202) 833-3420

International Rescue and First Aid Association
Columbus, OH
(614) 444-4732

National Association of Emergency Medical Technicians
Newton Highlands, MA
(617) 894-7179

National Association for Search and Rescue
LaJolla, CA
(714) 276-7228

National Center for Prevention of Child Abuse
Rockville, MD
(301) 443-2954

National Emergency Medical Services Information Clearing House
Philadelphia, PA
(215) 243-6304

National Poison Center Network
Pittsburgh, PA
(412) 681-6669

National Registry of Emergency Medical Technicians
Columbus, OH
(614) 888-4484

National Response Center
Washington, D.C.
(800) 424-8802 (toll free)

National Safety Council
Chicago, IL
(312) 527-4800

National Ski Patrol
Denver, CO
(303) 237-2737

National Sudden Infant Death Syndrome Foundation
Chicago, IL
(312) 663-0650

U.S. Army Explosive Ordinance Disp.
Rockville, MD
(301) 677-5182

U.S. Navy Experimental Diving Unit
Panama City, FL
(904) 234-4351 (24-hour emergency hotline)
Information for the nearest hyperbaric unit

# Important Telephone Numbers

Ambulance Services ____________________

____________________

____________________

American Heart Association ____________________

American Red Cross ____________________

Blood Bank ____________________

Civil Defense Department ____________________

Coast Guard ____________________

Department of Public Works ____________________

Department of Natural Resources ____________________

Emergency Departments of Hospitals ____________________

Electric Company ____________________

Fire Department ____________________

Gas Company ____________________

Health Department, Local ____________________

Health Department, State ____________________

Helicopter Transport ____________________

National Weather Service
Information ______________________________

Poison Control Center, Local ______________________________

Poison Control Center, State ______________________________

Police Department ______________________________

Premature Infant Transport ______________________________

Water Company ______________________________

# Glossary

**Abdomen** (ab'do-men) The body cavity between the thorax and the pelvis.

**Abdominal cavity** (ab-dom'ĭ-nal kav'ĭ-te) The portion of the body bounded superiorly by the diaphragm and inferiorly by the pelvic cavity. It contains the liver, gallbladder, stomach, portions of the large and small intestines, kidneys, pancreas, spleen, and suprarenal glands.

**Abduction** (ab-duk'shun) Movement of a limb away from the midline of the body.

**Abortion** (ah-bor'shun) Expulsion of an embryo or fetus prior to the stage of viability (about 20 weeks of gestation).

**Abrasion** (ah-bra'zhun) An injury to the superficial skin layers from sliding or rubbing against a hard surface. Also called a brush, mat, or friction burn.

**Abruptio placentae** (ab-rup'she-o plah-sen'-tah) A condition occurring during the third trimester of pregnancy wherein the placenta is separated from the uterus before the baby, thereby blocking its exit. Bleeding is usually excessive.

**Abscess** (ab'ses) The collection in a cavity of pus formed by dead tissue and white blood cells.

**Absorption** (ab-sorp'shun) Movement of a substance through body membranes into the bloodstream or body tissues.

**Acetabulum** (as''ĕ-tab'u-lum) The bony socket formed by the pelvis into which the head of the femur fits.

**Acetaminophen** (as''et-am'ĭn-o-fen) Aspirin substitute.

**Acetone** (as'ĕ-tōn) A chemical compound normally eliminated in the urine. Increased amounts occur in the blood and urine of diabetic persons, who have an imbalance of insulin, which may give a fruity smell to the breath or urine.

**Acidosis** (as''ĭ-do'sis) An abnormally high acid content (carbonic, lactic, etc.) in the blood or body tissues, which may decrease the pH of body fluids.

**Acromioclavicular joint** (ah-kro''me-o-klah-vik'u-lar joint) The joint between the acromion and the clavicle.

**Acromion** (ah-kro'me-on) The lateral extension of the spine of the scapula, projecting over the shoulder joint and forming the highest point of the shoulder.

**Activated charcoal** (ak'tĭ-vā''tud char'kōl) Treated powdered charcoal that absorbs chemical compounds. Often given to overdose victims to absorb the poisonous effects of the chemical.

**Acute** (ah-kūt') Sharp or short; experiencing severe symptoms in a short period of time. Not chronic.

**Acute abdomen** (ah-kūt' ab-do'men) Any of a number of intra-abdominal medical conditions that causes pain, irritation, and inflammation of the peritoneum and tenderness of the abdomen. Appendicitis is an example.

**Adduction** (ad-duk'shun) Movement of a limb toward the midline of the body.

Phonetic spellings are reprinted with permission from *Dorland's Illustrated Medical Dictionary*, 25th ed. (Philadelphia, PA: W. B. Saunders Co., 1974).

**Adipose** (ad′ĭ-pos) Fatty tissue.

**Afebrile** (a-feb′ril) Without fever.

**Afterbirth** (af′ter-berth″) Delivery of the placenta and its contents after the birth of the baby.

**Agonal** (ag′o-nal) Pertaining to the process of dying. The term is often used in reference to dying respirations.

**Air embolism** (ār em′bo-lizm) Air bubbles that are introduced into the bloodstream and may travel to the brain, lung, or other organ, causing obstruction.

**Alkali** (al′kah-li) A basic substance. A compound substance which forms salts when combined with acids and soaps when combined with fats.

**Alkalosis** (al″kah-lo′sis) An abnormally high alkali content (bicarbonate) in the blood or body tissues which may increase the pH of body fluids. May result from hyperventilation, persistent diarrhea or vomiting, and excessive intake of sodium bicarbonate.

**Allergen** (al′er-jen) A foreign substance capable of producing an allergic reaction.

**Allergic reaction** (ah-ler′jik″ re-ak′shun) A localized or general body reaction to an allergen which produces hives, itching, difficulty in breathing, and swelling of tissues.

**Alopecia** (al″o-pe′she-ah) Loss of hair; baldness.

**Alveoli** (al-ve′o-li) Air sacs in the lungs. Location of the exchange of oxygen and carbon dioxide.

**Amnesia** (am-ne′ze-ah) Loss of memory.

**Amniotic fluid** (am″ne-ot′ik floo′id) The fluid within the amniotic sac that surrounds and protects the fetus.

**Amniotic sac** (am″ne-ot′ik sak) The transparent membranous sac that contains the fetus. Also termed the *bag of waters.*

**Amphetamine** (am-fet′ah-min) Any of a number of drugs that produce excitability of the central nervous system. Examples are benzedrine and ephedrine.

**Ampule** (am′pūl) A small sealed glass container of sterile medication.

**Amputation** (am″pu-ta′shun) The removal of a body part by cutting.

**Anaerobic** (an″a-er-o′bik) Without oxygen.

**Analgesic** (an″al-je′-zik) Any drug that relieves pain.

**Anaphylactic shock** (an″ah-fĭ-lak′tik shok) Shock due to an allergic reaction to a foreign substance.

**Anaphylaxis** (an″ah-fĭ-lak′sis) An allergic reaction. This term is often used in place of anaphylactic shock.

**Anasarca** (an″ah-sar′kah) Swelling of subcutaneous tissues caused by excessive accumulation of body fluid.

**Anatomical landmark** (an″ah-tom′e-kal land′mark) A readily recognizable anatomical structure used as a point of reference in establishing the location of another structure or area.

**Anatomy** (ah-nat′o-me) The form and structure of the body.

**Anemia** (ah-ne′me-ah) Deficiency of red blood cells or related substances in the blood.

**Anesthesia** (an″es-the′ze-ah) The loss of feeling or sensation in the body or its parts, generally induced by a drug.

**Aneurysm** (an′u-rizm) A sac-like defect in the wall of an artery.

**Angina pectoris** (an-ji′nah pek″to′ris) A condition in which the heart muscle receives an insufficient blood supply, causng pain in the chest. Commonly results when the arteries supplying the heart muscle are narrowed by atherosclerosis.

**Angulation** (ang″gu-la′shun) The formation of an angle or bend in an extremity or organ of the body. Usually used in reference to a fracture that causes an abnormal angle in an extremity or other body part.

**Anisocoria** (an″ĭ-so-ko′re-ah) Unequal pupils.

**Anomaly** (ah-nom′ah-le) Not normal; abnormal.

**Anorexia** (an″o-rek′se-ah) Loss of appetite.

**Anoxia** (ah-nok′se-ah) Without oxygen; abnormally low levels of oxygen in the body tissues.

**Antabuse** (an′tah-būs) A drug given in alcohol treatment programs which produces unpleasant effects when combined with alcohol.

**Antecubital fossa** (an″te-ku′bĭ-tal fos′ah) The hollow at the anterior bend of the elbow. Blood pressure is generally taken at this site.

**Anticoagulant** (an″tĭ-ko-ag′u-lant) A drug that prevents coagulation or clotting of blood. The drug Heparin is an anticoagulant.

**Antidote** (an′tĭ-dōt) A substance used to counteract the effects of a poison or drug.

**Antiemetic** (an″tĭ-e-met′ik) A drug that stops or decreases vomiting.

**Antipyretic** (an″tĭ-pi-ret′ik) Any drug that reduces fever.

**Antivenin** (an″tĭ-ven′in) A serum used to counter the effects of insect or animal venom.

**Anus** (a′nus) The rectal opening.

**Aorta** (a-or′tah) A large artery that receives blood from the lower chamber of the heart. It gives off other arteries that conduct blood to other parts of the body except the lungs.

**Apathy** (ap′a-the) Lack of feeling, emotion, or interest.

**Apex** (a′peks) A general term used to denote the top or point of a conical structure.

**Aphasia** (ah-fa′ze-ah) Loss of speech or comprehension caused by disease or injury to the speech center of the brain.

**Aphonia** (ah-fo′ne-ah) Loss of the voice.

**Apical** (ap′e-kal) Pertaining to the apex of the heart.

**Apneic** (ap-ne′ik) The absence of respiration.

**Appendicular skeleton** (ap″en-dik′u-lar skel′ĕ-ton) The skeleton consisting of the upper and lower extremities.

**Arachnoid membrane** (ah-rak′noid mem′brān) The middle membrane covering the brain and spinal cord.

**Arrhythmia** (ah-rith′me-ah) Irregularity of the heartbeat.

**Arteries** (ar′ter-ez) Blood vessels that carry blood away from the heart to the various parts of the body. They carry oxygenated blood, except for the pulmonary artery, which carries unoxygenated blood from the heart to the lungs.

**Arthralgia** (ar-thral′je-ah) Joint pain.

**Arthritis** (ar-thri′tis) A condition characterized by inflammation of the joints.

**Arthropod** (ar′thro-pod) An invertebrate animal such as an insect, a spider, or a crustacean.

**Articulate** (ar-tik′u-lāt) To unite by a joint; a juncture between bones.

**Ascites** (ah-si′tēz) Massive fluid accumulation in the abdomen.

**Aseptic** (a-sep′tik) Free from germs; preventing or not involving sepsis.

**Asphyxia** (as-fik′se-ah) Suffocation.

**Aspirate** (as′pĭ-rāt) To inhale foreign material into the lungs; to withdraw by suction.

**Asthma** (az′mah) An allergy condition which irritates the bronchi, causing them to constrict and triggering wheezing and dyspnea.

**Atelectasis** (at″e-lek′tah-sis) Collapse of the lungs or part of the lungs caused by failure of the alveoli to expand or by reabsorption of oxygen from the lungs into the blood.

**Atherosclerosis** (ath″er-o″skle-ro′sis) A type of artery hardening in which the inner layer of the arterial wall is thick and rough due to deposits of lipids and cholesterol. Eventually it can cause obstruction of the vessel.

**Atrium** (a′tre-um) The upper chambers of the heart.

**Atrophy** (at′ro-fe) The wasting away of the body, its organs, or its parts.

**Auditory meatus** (aw′dĭ-to″re me-a′tus) The hole of the ear.

**Aura** (aw′rah) A peculiar sensation of sound, sight, taste, or smell that may precede an epileptic seizure.

**Auscultate** (aws′kul-tāt) To listen to body sounds with a stethoscope for the purpose of physical assessment.

**Autonomic nervous system** (aw″to-nom′ik ner′vus sis′tem) Sometimes called the *involuntary nervous system;* controls tissues not under voluntary control, i.e., glands, heart, and smooth muscles.

**Avulsion** (ah-vul′zhun) An injury in which the skin, subcutaneous tissue, muscles, and/or bone is scooped out or torn away, leaving a flap.

**Axial skeleton** (ak′se-al skel′ĕ-ton) The bones of the head, neck, and trunk.

**Axilla** (ak-sil′ah) Armpit.

**Axillary** (ak′sĭ-lar″e) Pertaining to the armpit.

**Babinski Reflex** (bah-bin′skē re′fleks) A reflex response of the great toe observed in patients with brain trauma or certain brain diseases. The great toe turns upward instead of downward when the sole of the foot is stroked with a sharp object.

**Bandage** (ban′dij) The material used to hold or secure a dressing in place.

**Barbiturate** (bar-bit′u-rāt) A class of drugs that produce a sedative effect.

**Battles' sign** (bat′t′lz sīn) A sign in which the mastoid process is ecchymotic; usually indicative of a basilar skull fracture.

**Bends** (bendz) A painful disease of the limbs and joints caused by the release of nitrogen bubbles in body tissues; Caissons Disease.

**Benign** (be-nin′) Nonmalignant; an illness that is not dangerous.

**Benzoin** (ben′zoin) A solution that promotes adhesiveness.

**Bifurcation** (bi″fur-ka-shun) Division into two branches.

**Bile** (bīl) The yellowish-green fluid secreted by the liver. Its principal action in the body is dissolving cholesterol and aiding in peristalsis.

**Biliary system** (bil′e-a-re sis′tem) The network of ducts consisting of the gallbladder and bile ducts connecting the liver to the intestine.

**Biopsy** (bi′ŏp-se) The removal of tissue for diagnostic examination.

**Blanched** (blanch′d) A term used to denote skin that is white or pale.

**Bleb** (bleb) A small elevated swelling on the skin; a small blister.

**Blister** (blis′ter) A fluid-filled sac under the epidermis or within it.

**Blood pressure (B/P)** (blud presh′ur) An indirect measurement of the force exerted by blood against the wall of an artery during the contraction and relaxation of the ventricles of the heart.

**Blunt trauma** (blunt traw′mah) Forceful impact to the body from an object; soft tissue can be damaged and a closed injury results.

**Bolus** (bo′lus) A single large dose of a drug given all at once to maintain a certain therapeutic blood level. Food that is completely or incompletely chewed.

**Bone collar** (bōn kol′ler) The growth that occurs around a fracture site of a bone.

**Bony prominence** (bōn′e prom′ĭ-nens) Any bone that normally projects because of its shape and so is easily felt. The lateral and medial malleoli are examples.

**Bourdon gauge** (boor′den gāj) A type of pressure gauge used to calibrate the rate of flow of gas from a cylinder.

**Brachial artery** (bra′ke-al ar′ter-e″) One of the major arteries of the arm. This artery is auscultated in the anticubital fossa when a blood pressure is taken.

**Bradycardia** (brad″e-kar′de-ah) A slow heart rate, usually 60 beats per minute or less.

**Breech delivery** (brēch de-liv′er-e) A fetus that presents itself buttocks or feet first during delivery.

**Bronchioles** (brong′ke-ōlz) Small branching air passages extending from the bronchi.

**Bronchiolitis** (brong″ke-o-li′tis) An infection of the bronchioles caused by a virus. Generally affects children less than two years old.

**Bronchus** (brong′kus) One of two main branches of the trachea leading to the bronchioles.

**Bruit** (broo′e) An abnormal sound or murmur heard upon auscultation.

**Buccal** (buk′al) Pertaining to the cheek.

**Cachexia** (kah-kek′se-ah) Severe malnutrition; wasting away of muscle.

**Calcaneus** (kal-ka′ne-us) The heel bone.

**Cannula** (kan′u-lah) A tube inserted into the body to deliver or withdraw fluid or gas.

**Capillary** (kap′ĭ-lar″e) An extremely narrow tube forming a network between the arterioles and the venules. The walls are composed of a single layer of cells through which oxygen and nutritive materials pass out of the tissues and carbon dioxide and waste products are admitted from the tissues into the bloodstream.

**Capitate** (kap′ĭ-tāt) One of the eight carpal bones in the wrist.

**Carbon dioxide ($CO_2$)** (kar′bon di-ok′sīd) A product of cellular metabolism eliminated by the lungs.

**Carbon monoxide (CO)** (kar′bon mon-ok′-sīd) A colorless, odorless, tasteless, poisonous gas eliminated from incomplete combustion. Carbon monoxide has strong binding powers to hemoglobin.

**Carboxyhemoglobin** (kar-bok″se-he″mo-glo′bin) Substance produced when carbon monoxide passes unchanged through the lungs and combines with hemoglobin.

**Cardiac arrest** (kar′de-ak ah-rest) Heart stoppage.

**Cardiac tamponade** (kar′de-ak tam″pon-ād′) Acute compression of the heart due to effusion of fluid into the pericardium.

**Cardiogenic shock** (kar″de-o-jen′ik shok) A shock state caused by failure of the heart as a pump.

**Cardiopulmonary resuscitation (CPR)** (kar″-de-o-pul′mo-ner-e re-sus″ĭ-ta′shun) A procedure designed to artificially ventilate the lungs and externally compress the heart of a patient whose heart has stopped and whose breathing has ceased.

**Cardiotoxin** (kar″de-o-tok′sin) Poison that affects the heart.

**Cardiovascular** (kar″de-o-vas′ku-lar) Pertaining to the heart and blood vessels.

**Cardiovert** (kar′de-o-vert″) To restore the heart rhythm by synchronized electric shock.

**Caries** (ka′re-ēz) Tooth decay.

**Carina** (kah-ri′nah) The ridge at the bifurcation of the trachea where the right and left main bronchi divide.

**Carotid pulse** (kah-rot′id puls) Pulse taken at the principal artery in the neck.

**Carpals** (kar′palz) Bones that make up the wrist.

**Cartilage** (kar′tĭ-lij) Tough, resilient, living connective tissue.

**Cataract** (kat′ah-rakt) Clouding of the lens or its capsule of the eye, resulting in complete or partial blindness.

**Cathartic** (kah-thar′tik) Any medicine that causes an active bowel movement.

**Catheter** (kath′ĕ-ter) A slender tube, of metal or rubber, inserted into a body passage, vessel, or cavity for passing fluids and making examinations.

**Caudal** (kaw′dal) Directed toward the foot end of the body.

**Caustic** (kaws′tik) Corrosive.

**Cell** (sel) The smallest unit of life capable of independent function.

**Cellular hypoxia** (sel′u-lar hi-pok′se-ah) Insufficient oxygen for cellular life.

**Cellulitis** (sel″u-li′tis) Inflammation of cellular tissue.

**Centrifugal force** (sen-trif′u-gal fōrs) Force that directs an object away from the center.

**Centigrade (Celsius)** (sen′tĭ-grād) A temperature scale consisting of 100 graduations. Freezing point is 0 and boiling point is 100. Normal body temperature is 37° Centigrade.

**Cervical** (ser′vĭ-kal) Pertaining to the cervix.

**Cervix** (ser′viks) The lower part or neck of the uterus.

**Cesarean section** (se-sa′re-an sek′shun) A surgical procedure in which an incision is made through the abdomen and uterus for delivery of the fetus.

**Chemotherapy** (ke″mo-ther′ah-pe) The treatment or prevention of disease by drugs.

**Cheyne-Stokes respiration** (chān′ stōks res″pĭ-ra′shun) An abnormal breathing pattern characterized by crescendo–decrescendo respirations with regular periods of apnea.

**Chief complaint** (chēf kom-plānt′) What the patient feels is his/her main problem.

**Chilblain** (chil′blan) A lesion that occurs to bare skin surfaces when exposed to cold temperature for prolonged periods of time.

**Cholecystitis** (ko″le-sis-ti′tis) Inflammation of the gallbladder.

**Cholesterol** (ko-les″ter-ol) A chemical found in all animal fats and oil as well as other foods that is believed to contribute to the development of atherosclerosis when ingested in excess. Found in the brain, bile, blood, nerves, liver, kidneys, and adrenal glands. It is the major constituent of gallstones.

**Chronic** (kron′ik) A disease lasting a long time. Not acute.

**Circulation** (ser″ku-la′shun) The transportation of diffused gases in the blood to and from cells where oxygen is taken up and carbon dioxide is given off.

**Circumcision** (ser″kum-sizh′un) Surgical removal of the foreskin of the penis.

**Circumduction** (ser″kum-duk′shun) Circular movement of a limb.

**Circumferential (pressure)** (ser″kum-fer-en′shal) Pressure applied around the circumference of the body or its parts.

**Cirrhosis** (sir-ro′sis) A chronic liver disease in which the liver degenerates.

**Clammy** (klam′e) Denoting skin that is cool and damp from perspiration.

**Clavicle (Collarbone)** (klav′ĭ-k′l) The bone that acts as a support for the shoulder.

**Clitoris** (kli′to-ris) A small organ located at the anterior portion of the vulva; female counterpart of the penis.

**Clot** (klot) A thrombus; coagulation of blood.

**Clubbing** (klub′ing) Broadening and thickening of the tissues of the fingers and toenails; usually seen in patients with chronic lung disease.

**Coalesce** (ko″-ah-les′) To blend or mesh together.

**Coefficient of friction** (ko″ĕ-fish′ent ov frik′shun) The frictional forces that develop when two surfaces pass across one another. Used to predict the number of feet required to stop a vehicle at a given speed on a given surface under specific circumstances.

**Coffee ground vomitus** (kof′e grownd vom′ĭ-tus) Vomitus that resembles and has the consistency of coffee grounds. An indication of slow bleeding in the gastrointestinal tract.

**Colic** (kol′ik) Acute, intermittent abdominal pain.

**Colitis** (ko-li′tis) Inflammation of the colon (large intestine).

**Colles fracture** (kol′ēz frak′tūr) A type of wrist fracture in which the deformity in relation to the forearm looks like a supper fork. Also called a *silver fork fracture.*

**Colostomy** (ko-los′to-me) A surgically created opening in the abdominal wall to permit the elimination of fecal material.

**Coma** (ko′mah) A state of unconsciousness from which the patient cannot be aroused.

**Comminuted fracture** (kom′ĭ-nūt″ed frak′tūr) Fracture of a bone into three or more fragments.

**Compensated shock** (kom′pen-sa-ted″ shok) Initial stage of a shock condition, when the body's mechanisms attempt to adjust to prevent further shock.

**Compress** (kom′pres) The initial pad of material placed on the wound; to squeeze.

**Concussion** (kon-kush′un) A transient episode of unconsciousness, due to a temporary interruption of neural transmissions to the center of consciousness (the RAS).

**Conduction** (kon-duk′shun) Process whereby body heat may be lost by being directly transferred to another object.

**Condyle** (kon′dīl) A bony bump on the medial and lateral surface of the distal femur.

**Congenital** (kon-jen′ĭ-tal) Existing from birth; resulting from or developing during one's prenatal stage.

**Congestive heart failure** (kon-jes′tiv hart fāl′yer) Damaged heart muscle that is not able to contract forcefully enough to empty the chambers during the cardiac cycle, allowing blood to back up into the lungs.

**Conjugate** (kon′ju-gāt) Movement of the eyes together in unison.

**Conjunctiva** (kon″junk-ti′vah) Mucous membrane that lines the eyelids.

**Constriction** (kon-strik′shun) Narrowing.

**Contraction** (kon-trak′shun) Increased tension or shortening of a muscle.

**Contraindication** (kon″trah-in″dĭ-ka′shun) The undesirable use of a drug or procedure.

**Contusion** (kon-tu′zhun) A bruise; an injury of a part without a break in the skin.

**Convection** (kon-vek′shun) Passage of air across the skin, resulting in loss of body heat.

**Convulsion** (kon-vul′shun) A seizure. Violent involuntary contractions of voluntary muscles, causing jerky body movements.

**Copious** (kop′e-us) Abundant; very plentiful.

**Core temperature** (kōr tem′per-ah-tūr) Internal body temperature.

**Cornea** (kor′ne-ah) The transparent structure forming the anterior part of the eye.

**Coronary arteries** (kor′ŏ-na-re ar′ter-ez) Arteries that arise directly from the aorta and supply the heart with its blood supply.

**Coronary occlusion** (kor′ŏ-na-re ŏ-kloo′zhun) An obstruction (generally a blood clot) in a branch of one of the coronary arteries which hinders the flow of blood to some part of the heart muscle. Sometimes called a coronary, or simply a heart attack.

**Corrosive** (kŏ-ro′siv) Caustic.

**Cramp** (kramp) A painful muscle spasm.

**Craniad** (kra′ne-ad) Directed toward the head.

**Cranium** (kra′ne-um) Skull.

**Cravat** (krah-vat′) A bandage made by folding a triangular piece of cloth from its apex toward the base.

**Crepitus** (krep′ĭ-tus) A crackling sensation that may be felt upon palpation; due to bone fragments moving against one another.

**Cricothyrotomy** (kri″ko-thi″rot′o-me) The surgical opening of the cricothyroid membrane to establish an airway.

**Crisis** (kri′sis) A critical change during the period of an acute medical condition.

**Croup** (kro͞op) Laryngitis or spasm of the larynx in children.

**Cuboid bone** (ku′boid bōn) One of the bones of the foot.

**Cuneiform bone** (ku-ne′ĭ-form bōn) A bone of the ankle.

**CVA (Stroke)** Cerebrovascular accident. Results from an interruption in blood flow to the brain.

**Cyanosis** (si″ah-no′sis) A bluish tint to the skin caused by decreased blood flow to body tissues.

**Cyclic** (sik′lik) Occurring periodically.

**Cytotoxin** (si″to-tok′sin) A toxin that kills tissue cells.

**Debride** (da-brēd′) To remove foreign material and contaminated or devitalized tissue.

**Decerebrate posture** (de-ser′ĕ-brāt pos′tūr) Posture assumed by patients with acute brain dysfunction; characterized by extended and abducted arms, with legs stiffly extended and feet plantar flexed.

**Decontaminate** (de″kon-tam′ĭ-nāt) To rid of contagious disease or radioactivity.

**Decorticate posture** (de″kor′ti-kat pos′tūr) Posture assumed by patients with acute brain dysfunction; characterized by flexion of the arms, wrists, and fingers, with legs extended and feet plantar flexed.

**Defecate** (def″e-kāt′) To have a bowel movement.

**Defibrillation** (de-fib″rĭ-la′shun) Termination of ventricular fibrillation, usually by electric shock.

**Deformity** (de-for′mĭ-te) Abnormal shape or size; disfigurement.

**Dehydration** (de″hi-dra′shun) Loss of water.

**Delirium** (de-lir′ĭ-um) A mental disturbance marked by illusions, hallucinations, physical restlessness and incoherence.

**Delirium tremens** (de-lir′ĭ-um tre′menz) Alcoholic psychosis, characterized by trembling, excitement, sweating, anxiety, gastrointestinal complaints, precordial pain, and visual and auditory sensations of an unpleasant nature.

**Delivery** (de-liv′er-e) Childbirth.

**Demulcent** (de-mul′sent) A medicine that soothes and relieves mucous irritation.

**Depressant** (de-pres′ant) Any of a variety of drugs that decreases nervous or functional activity.

**Dermis** (der′mis) The living layer of tissue under the epidermis; contains blood vessels, nerves, sweat glands, oil glands, hair, and nails.

**Dextran** (dek′stran) A plasma or blood substitute used in intravenous therapy for hypovolemic shock.

**Dextrose** (deks′trōs) A sugar solution used for intravenous therapy.

**Dextrostix** (deks′tro-stiks″) Commercially available chemical-sensitive sugar testing strips that can be used (on scene) to determine blood sugar level.

**Diabetes mellitus** (di″ah-be′tēz mĕ-li′tus) A metabolic disorder in which the ability to oxidize carbohydrates is more or less completely lost, usually due to faulty pancreatic activity.

**Diagnosis** (di″ag-no′sis) The identification of a disease.

**Diagnostic signs** (di″ag-nos′tik sīnz) Characteristics exhibited by the patient that aid in determining the illness or injury.

**Diaphysis** (di-af′ĭ-sis) The shaft of the long bone.

**Diaphoresis** (di″ah-fo-re′sis) Profuse perspiration.

**Diaphragm** (di′ah-fram) The muscular partition between the thorax and abdomen.

**Diarrhea** (di″ah-re′ah) Frequent discharge of liquid feces.

**Diastole** (di-as′to-le) The relaxation part of the cardiac cycle, which occurs after contraction of the heart.

**Diastolic pressure** (di″ah-stol′ik presh′ur) Pressure exerted on vessels by the blood during relaxation of the heart ventricles.

**Diffusion** (dĭ-fu′zhun) Movement of gases across membranes; in the case of respiration, oxygen from the lungs into the bloodstream.

**Dilate** (di′lāt) To enlarge or relax.

**Diplopia** (dĭ-plo′pe-ah) Double vision.

**Dislocation** (dis″lo-ka′shun) Displacement of the bones from the joint.

**Disorientation** (dis-o″re-en-ta′shun) Confusion of identity, place, and time.

**Dissipate** (dis′ĭ-pāt″) To disperse.

**Distal** (dis′tal) Farther from any point of reference.

**Distention** (dis-ten′shun) State of being enlarged or distended.

**Diuresis** (di″u-re′sis) Increased secretion of urine.

**Diuretic** (di″u-ret′ik) Any of a number of drugs given to reduce the body's water content by increasing the secretion of urine.

**Dorsal** (dor′sal) Referring to a position more towards the back surface than some other object of reference.

**Dorsalis pedis artery** (dor-sa′lis ped′is ar′-ter-e) An important artery located on the dorsum (top) of the foot.

**Dorsiflexion** (dor″sĭ-flek′shun) Backward flexion or bending, as of the hand or foot.

**Dressing** (dres′ing) Material used to cover a wound.

**Drift angle** (drift ang′g'l) The angle that is formed when the steering wheel is turned and the center line of the front tires heads away from the direction in which the vehicle is traveling.

**Dura mater** (du′rah ma′ter) The outermost layer of the three membranes that cover the brain and spinal cord.

**Dysconjugate** (dis-kon′ju-gāt) Turning or movement of the eyes in different directions.

**Dysfunction** (dis-funk′shun) Abnormal function.

**Dysphagia** (dis-fa′je-ah) Difficulty in swallowing.

**Dysphasia** (dis-fa′ze-ah) Impaired speech.

**Dyspnea** (disp′ne-ah) Difficult or labored respirations.

**Dysrhythmia** (dis-rith′me-ah) Irregularity of the heartbeat.

**Ecchymosis** (ek″ĭ-mo′sis) Bruising. A blackish-blue and green discoloration of the skin caused by the breakdown of blood in the tissues.

**Eclampsia** (ĕ-klamp′se-ah) Seizures and coma occurring with pregnancy.

**Ectopic pregnancy** (ek-top′ik preg′nan-se) Pregnancy in which the fetus is growing outside the uterus.

**Edema** (ĕ-de′mah) The presence of abnormally large amounts of fluid in the intercellular tissue spaces of the body; swelling.

**Edematous** (ĕ-dem′ah-tus) Pertaining to or affected by edema.

**Effusion** (ĕ-fu′zhun) Leakage or escape of fluid from a vessel into the surrounding tissue or cavity.

**Electrocardiogram (ECG or EKG)** (e-lek″-tro-kar′de-o-gram) A graphic record of the heart's electrical activity made by an electrocardiograph.

**Electrolyte** (e-lek′tro-līt) Any compound whose molecules dissociate into charged particles (ions) when placed in water.

**Elixir** (e-lik′ser) An alcoholic syrup that has been artificially flavored.

**Embolism** (em′bo-lizm) Obstruction of a blood vessel by a solid, liquid, or gaseous material.

**Embolus** (em′bo-lus) A blood clot, air bubble, fat particle, or any other solid or gas that may pass through the circulation and occlude blood flow to tissue.

**Emesis** (em′ĕ-sis) Vomit.

**Emetic** (ĕ-met′ik) An agent that brings on or causes vomiting.

**Emphysema** (em″fĭ-se′mah) Characterized by an overdistention of the air sacs in the lungs, which do not empty upon expiration and evenutally rupture from overdistention.

**Encephalopathy** (en-sef″ah-lop′ah-the) Any disease state of the brain.

**Endocardium** (en″do-kar′de-um) The inner lining of the heart.

**Endocrine** (en′do krin) Applies to organs and structures whose function is to secrete into the blood or lymph, hormones that have a specific effect on another organ or part.

**Endosteum** (en-dos′te-um) Thin tissue lining the inside marrow cavity of bones.

**Endotoxin** (en″do-tok′sin) A poison within the bacterial cell.

**Endotracheal** (en″do-tra′ke-al) Within; through the trachea.

**Engorged** (en-gorjd′) Filled up.

**Enteritis** (en″ter-i′tis) Inflammation of the intestine.

**Enuresis** (en″u-re′sis) Bedwetting.

**Envenomate** (en-ven′o-mat″) The act of being poisoned by a bite from an arthropod.

**Enzyme** (en′zīm) A protein that has the potential to make chemical reactions occur faster.

**Epidemic** (ep″ĭ-dem′ik) A disease that attacks many persons at the same time.

**Epidermis** (ep″ĭ-der′mis) The outer layer or most superficial layer of skin tissue.

**Epidural** (ep″-ĭ-du′ral) The area above the dura mater.

**Epigastrium** (ep′ĭ-gas′tre-um) The upper middle region of the abdomen, located within the sternal angle.

**Epiglottis** (ep″ĭ-glot′is) The tissue that overlies and protects the larynx and trachea during swallowing.

**Epiglottitis** (ep″ĭ-glot-ti′tis) A potentially fatal respiratory tract infection that involves the epiglottis.

**Epinephrine** (ep″ĭ-nef′rin) A vasoconstrictor hormone substance.

**Epiphyseal plate** (ep″ĭ-fiz″e-al plāt) Growth center of a growing bone, located between the ends of the bone and the shaft of the bone.

**Epiphysis** (ĕ-pif′ĭ-sis) The end of a long bone.

**Epistaxis** (ep″ĭ-stak′sis) Nosebleed.

**Erythema** (er″ĭ-the′mah) Redness of the skin produced by blood-filled capillaries.

**Erythrocyte** (ĕ-rith′ro-sit) A red blood cell.

**Eschar** (es′kar) A crust of skin that sloughs off after a thermal burn or necrosis of the skin.

**Esophageal obturator airway** (ĕ-sof″ah-je′al ob′tu-ra″tor ār′wa) A device that provides a quick and effective means of establishing an airway while preventing vomiting and gastric aspirations.

**Esophageal sphincter** (ĕ-sof″ah-je′al sfingk′ter) A band of muscles that closes off the esophagus.

**Esophagus** (ĕ-sof′ah-gus) (Food tube) The tube leading from the mouth to the stomach.

**Etiology** (e″te-ol′o-je) The cause of disease.

**Euphoria** (u-fo′re-ah) A sense of well being.

**Eustachian tube** (u-sta′ke-an tūb) The tube extending from the back of the throat to the middle ear, which equalizes pressure in the middle ear.

**Evaporation** (e-vap″o-ra′shun) Change from a liquid state to a vapor.

**Eversion** (e-ver′zhun) A turning outward.

**Evisceration** (e-vis″er-a′shun) Extrusion of the viscera or internal organs from the abdomen; disembowelment.

**Exacerbate** (eg-zas′er-bat″) To make an illness or injury worse. To increase in severity.

**Exanthem** (ek-san′them) A rash or eruption of the skin observed with diseases such as measles or scarlet fever.

**Excision** (ek-sizh′un) The cutting out or removal of tissue.

**Expectorant** (ek-spek′to-rant) Any drug that increases mucous secretion and aids in its expulsion.

**Expiration** (eks″pĭ-ra′shun) The process of breathing out.

**Exsanguination** (eks-sang″wĭ-na′shun) The process of bleeding out or becoming bloodless.

**Extension** (ek-sten′shun) The straightening of any limb.

**Extracellular** (eks″trah-sel′u-lar) Between cells.

**Extravasation** (eks-trav″ah-sa′shun) Escape of fluid from a vessel into the surrounding tissues.

**Extrication** (eks″tri-ka′shun) Removal of something that has been trapped.

**Exudate** (eks-u-dāt) A fluid that exudes or oozes from the skin or body organs.

**Fahrenheit Scale** (fah′ren-hīt skāl) A temperature scale in which 212° is boiling and 32° is freezing.

**Faint** (fānt) A syncopal episode; the state of being very weak.

**Fallopian tube** (fal-lo′pe-an to͞ob) The tube that extends from the uterus to the ovary, where fertilization takes places.

**Fascia** (fash'e-ah) A membrane that joins the skin to underlying tissue and also covers, separates, and gives support to muscles.

**Fasciotomy** (fash"e-ot'o-me) A surgical procedure in which tissue is sliced open to decrease the fluid pressure inside, as in severe swelling.

**Febrile** (feb'ril) Characterized by fever.

**Feces** (fe'sēz) Solid waste from the intestine; stool.

**Femoral artery** (fem'or-al ar'ter-e) A major artery located in the leg; may be palpated in the upper femoral area.

**Femur** (fe'mur) Thigh bone.

**Fetus** (fe'tus) The unborn baby, from the eighth week of pregnancy to birth.

**Fever** (fe'ver) Elevation of the body temperature above 99°F.

**Fibrillation** (fi-brĭ-la'shun) Non-synchonous muscle contractions.

**Fibrosis** (fi-bro'sis) Fibrous tissue that replaces dead tissue.

**Fibrotic cartilage** (fi-brot'ik kar'tĭ-lij) A weak cartilage that may replace injured hyaline cartilage.

**Fibula** (fib'u-lah) The long bone in the lower leg which runs parallel to the tibia, on the lateral side of the leg.

**Fistula** (fis'tu-lah) An abnormal passage leading from an organ to the body surface or from one organ to another.

**Flaccid** (flas'sid) Weak, lax, or soft.

**Flail chest** (flāl chest) A condition wherein three or more ribs are fractured, allowing a segment of the chest wall to become loosened.

**Flank** (flank) The side of the body between the ribs and the pelvis.

**Flatulence** (flat'u-lens) Intestinal gas.

**Flexion** (flek'shun) Bending of any of the limbs.

**Fontanelles** (fon"tah-nelz') Soft membranous areas at the angles of the cranial bones of an infant.

**Foreskin** (fōr'skin) The skin that partially or completely covers the head of the penis.

**Fowler's position** (fow'lerz po-zish'un) A straight-up sitting position.

**Fracture** (frak'tūr) A break in a bone.

**Avulsion fracture** (ə-vul'shən) A fracture in which a piece of bone has been pulled away from its primary structure.

**Blow-out fracture** A fracture of the orbital floor in which the muscle of the eye becomes trapped, causing a paralyzed gaze.

**Closed fracture** (klōzd) A fracture in which the skin has not been penetrated or opened.

**Comminuted fracture** (käm'nut"ed) A fracture in which the bone is broken into three or more fragments.

**Compression fracture** (kom-presh'un) A fracture in which the bone has been pressed or squeezed together.

**Depressed Fracture** (di-prest') A fracture in which the bone has been displaced downward. Often seen in skull fractures.

**Greenstick fracture** (grēn'stik) A fracture in which the bone is incompletely broken.

**Impacted fracture** (im-pak'tid) A fracture in which the bones have been pressed into each other.

**Oblique fracture** (ō-blēk') A fracture in which the bone is broken in a diagonal line.

**Open fracture** (ō'p'n) A fracture in which the skin has been penetrated or opened.

**Spiral fracture** (spī'ral) A fracture that spirals around and through the bone.

**Transverse fracture** (tranz-vurs') A fracture in which the bone is broken straight across.

**Frontal plane** (frun'tal plān) A vertical plane at right angles to the mid-sagittal section, dividing the body into front and back portions.

**Frontal bone** (frun'tal bōn) The bone that forms the forehead.

**Frostbite** (frost'bīt) Freezing of tissue.

**Frostnip** (frost'nip) Superficial freezing of tissue.

**Fulminating** (ful'mĭ-nāt-ing) Running a rapid course. A fast-worsening condition.

**Fungus** (fung'gus) An organism that feeds on organic matter.

**Fused joints** (fūzd) Bones that have joined together, allowing little or no motion.

**Gait** (gāt) The way in which a person walks or runs.

**Gangrene** (gan'grēn) Necrosis of body tissue due to insufficient blood supply.

**Gastrointestinal** (gas″tro-in-tes′tĭ-nal) Pertaining to the stomach and intestines.

**Genitalia** (jen″ĭ-ta′le-ah) The genitals or organs of reproduction.

**Genitourinary** (jen″ĭ-to-u′rĭ-nar-e) Pertaining to the organs of reproduction and the urinary tract.

**Germ** (jerm) A microorganism that causes disease.

**Germicide** (jer′mĭ-sīd) A solution that destroys germs.

**Gestation** (jes-ta′shun) Hormonal changes in the uterus; pregnancy.

**Ginglymus** (jin′glĭ-mus) A hinge joint that allows only extension or flexion, such as the elbow joint.

**Gland** (gland) A secreting organ or group of cells.

**Glasgow Coma Scale** (glas′gō ko′mah skāl) A scale designed to quantitatively relate consciousness to motor responses, verbal responses, and eye opening.

**Glenohumeral joint** (gle″no-hu′mer-al joint) The connection (ball and socket) between scapula, clavicle, and humerus.

**Glenoid cavity** (gle′noid kav′ĭ-te) The cavity into which the head of the humerus fits.

**Glottis** (glot′is) The space between the vocal cords.

**Glucose** (gloo′kōs) A sugar solution used for intravenous therapy.

**Gluteal muscle** (gloo′te-al) Buttock muscle.

**Glycogen** (gli′ko-jen) Sugar released by the liver when insulin is not released in sufficient quantity.

**Gonorrhea** (gon″o-re′ah) A common social contagious disease transmitted chiefly through sexual intercourse. It is characterized by inflammation of the urethral tract, discharge of pus, and painful and frequent urination.

**Grand mal seizure** (grahn mahl se′zhur) A generalized body seizure.

**Granulation** (gran″u-la′shun) The formation of small fleshy granules as a wound heals.

**Gravid** (grav′id) Pregnant.

**Groin** (groin) The inguinal area.

**Hallucination** (hal-lu″sĭ-na′shun) Perception that is auditory, visual, or both, of something that does not exist.

**Hamate** (ham′at) One of eight carpal bones in the wrist.

**Hare Traction Splint** (hār trak′shun splint) A telescoping one-piece device used to stabilize lower extremity fractures.

**Heat cramps** (hēt krampz) Muscle cramps in the arms, legs, and abdomen due to the loss of water and salt through perspiration.

**Heat stroke** (hēt strōk) A serious medical condition in which the heat regulatory center of the brain (hypothalamus) ceases to function, thereby causing the body to overheat to 105°–106°.

**Hematemesis** (hem″ah-tem′ĕ-sis) The vomiting of blood.

**Hematochezea** (hem″ah-to-ke′ze-ah) The passage of bloody stool.

**Hematoma** (hem″ah-to′mah) A pocket of blood under a contused area.

**Hematuria** (hem″ah-tu′re-ah) Blood in the urine.

**Hemolysis** (he-mol′ĭ-sis) Red blood cell destruction.

**Hemopneumothorax** (he″mo-nu″mo-tho′raks) The collection of air and blood in the pleural cavity.

**Hemoptysis** (he-mop′tĭ-sis) Coughing up of blood.

**Hemorrhage** (hem′or-ij) Loss of blood from a blood vessel.

**Hemorrhagic shock** (hem″o-raj′ik shok) Shock caused by bleeding.

**Hemothorax** (hem″ah-tho′raks) Collection of blood in the pleural cavity.

**Hemotoxin** (he″mo-tok′sin) A toxin that destroys blood cells.

**Hernia** (her′ne-ah) Rupture of an organ through the wall that normally contains it.

**Heroin** (her′o-in) Diacetylmorphine. A drug that can cause physical and psychological addiction. Its use is prohibited by federal law in the United States.

**Histamine** (his′tah-min) A chemical in the body that, when released, causes constriction of the bronchioles, a fall in blood pressure, and vessel dilation. Histamine is released in anaphylactic shock.

**Hives** (hivz) Red or white elevated patches on the skin accompanied by itching. Usually associated with an allergic reaction.

**Host** (hōst) The organism or body on which a parasite lives.

**Humerus** (hu′mer-us) The upper arm bone.

**Humidity** (hu-mid′ĭ-te) The moisture contained in air.

**Humor** (hu′mor) Any clear fluid substance that occurs in the body.

**Hyaline cartilage** (hi′ah-līn kar′tĭ-lij) The cartilage that covers that articular ends of bones and aids in the free movement of joints.

**Hydrocephalus** (hi-dro-sef′ah-lus) Abnormal accumulation of fluid in the cranial vault, accompanied by enlargement of the head.

**Hydroplaning** (hi″dro-plan′ing) Traveling over surface water, as experienced when tires ride on a film of water instead of the road surface.

**Hydrostatic pressure** (hi″dro-stat′ik presh′-ur) Pressure created by volume and peripheral resistance, as in the arterial system, as well as the pumping action of the heart.

**Hymenoptera** (hi″men-op′ter-ah) A classification of insects that includes bees, wasps, yellow jackets, hornets, and ants.

**Hypercapnia** (hi″per-kap′ne-ah) Increased carbon dioxide in circulatory blood.

**Hypercarbia** (hi″per-kar′be-ah) Hypercapnia.

**Hyperflexion** (hi″per-flek′shun) Flexion of a limb or body part beyond its normal range.

**Hyperglycemia** (hi″per-gli-se′me-ah) Increased sugar in the bloodstream; high blood sugar.

**Hyperpnea** (hi″perp-ne′ah) Respiration that is deeper and more rapid than normal.

**Hyperpyrexia** (hi″per-pi-rek′se-ah) Elevation of the body temperature above 105°F.

**Hypertension** (hi″per-ten′shun) Unusually high blood pressure.

**Hyperthermia** (hi″per-ther′me-ah) Elevated or increased temperature.

**Hypertonic** (hi″per-ton′ik) A solution that has greater osmotic pressure than another.

**Hypertrophy** (hi-per′tro-fe) Increased size of an organ or body part.

**Hyperventilation** (hi″per-ven″tĭ-la′shun) A state in which there is an increased amount of air entering the alveoli, resulting in reduction of carbon dioxide tension.

**Hyphema** (hi-fe′mah) A hemorrhage into the anterior chamber of the eye, usually caused by direct trauma to the eye.

**Hypnotic** (hip-not′ik) Any drug that produces a sleepy state.

**Hypoallergenic** (hi″po-al″er-jen′ik) A decreased allergic response to a substance.

**Hypocapnia** (hi″po-kap′ne-ah) Decreased carbon dioxide in the circulatory blood.

**Hypoglycemia** (hi″po-gli-se′me-ah) Decreased sugar in the bloodstream; low blood sugar.

**Hypopnea** (hi″pop′ne-ah) Decreased depth of breathing, allowing less oxygen to enter the lungs.

**Hypotension** (hi″po-ten′shun) Unusually low blood pressure.

**Hypothalamus** (hi″po-thal′ah-mus) The part of the brain that controls and maintains normal body temperature by balancing heat production and heat loss.

**Hypothermia** (hi″po-ther′me-ah) General body cooling. A condition that results when the body temperature falls below 95°F.

**Hypovolemic** (hi″po-vo-le′mik) Abnormally decreased volume of circulating blood in the body.

**Hypovolemic shock** (hi″po-vo-le′mik shok) Shock caused by an abnormally decreased volume of circulating blood in the body.

**Hypoxia** (hi-pok′se-ah) Less than normal oxygen in the organs and tissues of the body.

**Icterus** (ik′ter-us) Jaundice.

**Idiopathic** (id″e-o-path′ik) Denoting a disease of unknown origin.

**Ileus** (il′e-us) Bowel obstruction resulting from paralysis. Caused by peritonitis or other inflammatory disease.

**Ilium** (il′e-um) Innominate bone. The bone of the pelvis that flares out to form the hip.

**Immunity** (ĭ-mu′nĭ-te) Bodily resistance to an infectious disease.

**Immunization** (im″u-ni-za′shun) Vaccination against a disease.

**Impaled object** (im-pāl′d) Any object that has been driven into the body or its parts and is stabilized by body tissue.

**Incision** (in-sizh′un) A cut made into the

soft tissue, usually a surgical cut made by a scalpel.

**Incontinence** (in-kon′tĭ-nens) Inability to control excretory functions.

**Incubation** (in″ku-ba′shun) The time from which disease-producing organisms enter the body until clinical signs and symptoms of the disease appear.

**Incubator** (in′ku-ba-ter) A container in which environmental conditions can be controlled. Often used for premature and newborn infants.

**Indolent** (in′do-lent) Without pain; sluggish.

**Infarction** (in-fark′shun) Muscle destruction due to obtruction of an artery.

**Infection** (in-fek′shun) The multiplication of bacteria or microorganisms within the body.

**Inferior** (in-fe′re-or) Below or in a lower position.

**Inflammation** (in″flah-ma′shun) A tissue change that takes place with disease or injury; signs include pain, redness, and swelling.

**Infusion** (in-fu′zhun) The therapeutic introduction of a fluid other than blood.

**Ingestion** (in″jest′shun) The swallowing of a solid or liquid into the stomach.

**Inguinal** (ing′gwĭ-nal) Pertaining to the groin area.

**Inhalation** (in″hah-la′shun) The act of breathing in.

**Innocuous** (ĭ-nok′u-us) Harmless.

**Insertion of muscle** (in-ser′shun of mus′el) The connection of muscle to the more movable part of the skeleton.

**Inspiration** (in″spĭ-ra′shun) The process of breathing in.

**Insulin** (in′su-lin) A hormone secreted by the pancreas that regulates how fast glucose in the body is consumed.

**Integument** (in-teg′u-ment) The skin.

**Intercostal** (in″ter-kos′tal) Between the ribs, as in intercostal muscles.

**Intermuscular Septum** (in″ter-mus′ku-lar sep′tum) A thin, transparent sheath that separates muscle groups.

**Internal Respirations** (in-ter′nal res″pĭ-ra′shunz) The gas exchange process at the cellular level.

**Intoxication** (in″tok-sĭ-kā′shun) Drunkenness; inebriation.

**Intracellular** (in″trah-sel′u-lar) Within the cell.

**Intravenous** (in″trah-ve′nus) Within a vein.

**Intubation** (in″tu-ba′shun) The insertion of a tube into any vessel, cavity, or canal.

**Inversion** (in-ver′zhun) The inward turning of the ankle.

**Ipecac** (ip′ĕ-kak) A drug used to induce vomiting.

**Iris** (i′ris) The colored portion of the eye.

**Irrigation** (ir″ĭ-ga′shun) Flushing with a fluid.

**Ischemia** (is-ke′me-ah) Deficiency of blood in a body part due to constriction or occlusion of an artery.

**Ischium** (is′ke-um) The lower posterior bone of the pelvis.

**Isordil** (i′sor-dil) A vasodilating drug prescribed for angina pectoris.

**Jaundice** (jawn′dis) A yellowish tint of the skin caused by the bile pigments that have escaped into the bloodstream, skin, and mucous membranes.

**Jejunum** (je-joo′num) The section of small intestine between the duodenum and the ileum.

**Joint** A region in the skeleton where two or more bones meet and permit body movement.

**Joint capsule** (joint kap′sūl) Tissue that encloses a joint.

**Jugular** (jug′u-lar) Pertaining to the neck.

**Jugular notch** (jug′u-lar noch) The hollow above the breastbone in the midline of the anterior neck.

**Keratin** (ker′ah-tin) The protein substance that forms the nails and hair.

**Ketoacidosis** (ke″to-ah″sĭ-do′sis) Acidosis accompanied by the accumulation of ketone bodies in the blood and tissue fluids. Associated with patients who are diabetic.

**Kinetic** (kĭ-net′ik) Pertaining to or related to motion.

**Knee jerk** (nē jerk) The patellar reflex.

**Kussmauls′ respirations** (koos′mowlz res″pĭ-ra′shunz) Characteristic respirations seen in diabetic acidotic or coma patients, in which the respiratory pattern is deep and rapid.

**Labor** (la′bor) The process by which the

baby and placenta are expelled from the uterus.

**Laceration** (las″er-a′shun) A jagged irregular cut. A break in the skin caused by a sharp object.

**Lacrimation** (lak″rĭ-ma′shun) The secretion of tears.

**Lactation** (lak-ta′shun) The secretion of milk.

**Laparotomy** (lap-ah-rot′o-me) A surgical incision into the abdomen.

**Laryngectomee** (lar″in-jek′to-me) A person who has had his larynx removed. The hole that remains is called a *stoma*.

**Laryngectomy** (lar″in-jek′to-me) The removal of the larynx.

**Laryngospasm** (lah-ring′go-spazm) Spasm of the laryngeal muscles which obstructs the airway.

**Larynx** (lar′inks) The voice box.

**Latent** (la′tent) Hidden, concealed.

**Lateral** (lat′er-al) To the outside, external.

**Lateral malleolus** (lat′er-al mal-le′o-lus) The bony protuberance on the lateral side of the ankle joint. The lateral malleolus is the distal bone of the fibula.

**Lavage** (lah-vahzh′) The washing or pumping out of ingested material from the stomach.

**Left lateral recumbent** (left lat′er-al rekum′bent) A position in which the patient is placed on the left side.

**Lesion** (le′zhun) A tissue wound or injury.

**Lethargy** (leth-ar-je) Drowsiness; a state of indifference.

**Ligament** (lig′ah-ment) Living tissue that stabilizes the skeleton by binding bone to bone.

**Liniment** (lin′ĭ-ment) An oily preparation used externally for sore muscles or skin protection.

**Livid** (liv′id) Cyanotic, ashen grey.

**Long bones** (long bōnz) Bones whose length is greater than their width.

**Lumbosacral spine** (lum″bo-sa′kral spīn) The area of the spine that contains the loin and sacrum.

**Lumen** (lu′men) The interior of a vessel.

**Lunate** (lu′nāt) One of the eight carpal bones in the wrist.

**Lund and Browder chart** (loond, brow′der) A chart with pre-calculated percentages representing body parts or skin surface; used for burn assessment.

**Lymph** (limf) A transparent fluid composed mainly of lymphocytes (white blood cells) and red blood cells which react with the body's immune system.

**Lymph nodes** (limf nōdz) Small nodules located throughout the body that act as a filtering system for the blood. These nodes are found primarily in the neck, groin, axilla.

**Macule** (mak′u-lah) A small non-elevated spot on the skin that differs in color from the surrounding skin.

**Malaise** (mal-āz′) A general feeling of body discomfort.

**Malignant** (mah-lig′nant) Cancerous, dangerous.

**Malleolus** (mal-le′o-lus) A bony prominence at the distal end of the tibia and fibula.

**Mandible** (man′dĭ-b′l) The lower jaw.

**Mania** (ma′ne-ah) A psychological disorder characterized by unstable thinking and excitement.

**Mastoid process** (mas′toid pros′es) The bony prominence located behind each ear. A part of the temporal bones.

**Maxillary sinus cavity** (mak′sĭ-ler″e si′nus kav′ĭ-te) One of the paired paranasal sinuses.

**Meatus** (me-a′tus) A hole or opening.

**Meconium** (mĕ-ko′ne-um) Fetal stool.

**Medial** (me′de-al) Pertaining to the middle; closer to the median plane or the midline of a body.

**Mediastinum** (me″de-as-ti′num) The area between the lungs containing the heart, nerves, and great vessels.

**Medulla** (mĕ-dul′ah) [brain] The lowest part of the brain; actually an enlarged extension of the spinal cord in the cranial cavity. It controls the heartbeat, blood pressure, and respiration.

**Medullary cavity** (med′u-lār″e kav′ĭte) The hollow part of the shaft of long bones occupied by red or yellow bone marrow.

**Melanoma** (mel′ah-no′mah) A dark-pigmented cancerous tumor.

**Melena** (mĕ-le′nah) Black tarry stools; indicative of a slow passage of leaking blood from the gastrointestinal tract.

**Membrane** (mem′brān) A tissue that covers or divides parts of the body.

**Meningitis** (men″in-ji′tis) Inflammation of the membranes of the brain or spinal cord.

**Menopause** (men′o-pawz) Termination of menstruation. Usually occurs between 45 and 55 years of age.

**Menstrual flow** (men′stroo-al flō) The vaginal discharge of blood.

**Menstrual period** (men′stroo-al pe′re-od) The time of menstrual flow, usually 3 to 7 days in duration.

**Mesentery** (mes′en-ter″e) Peritoneum covering the small intestine attached to the posterior wall of the abdomen.

**Metabolism** (mĕ-tab′o-lizm) Chemical tissue reactions by which food is changed into energy.

**Metacarpal** (met″ah-kar′pal) [hand] The long bones that articulate proximally with the phalanges and distally with the wrist.

**Metastasis** (mĕ-tas′tah-sis) The spread or shift of a disease throughout the body.

**Metatarsal bones** (met″ah-tar′sal bōnz) The five long bones in the foot.

**Methanol** (meth′ah-nol) Methyl alcohol.

**Middle Ear** (mid′l ēr) The tympanic cavity with its ossicles (small bones).

**Midsagittal plane** (mid″saj′ĭ-tal) A vertical plane dividing the body into right and left portions.

**Miosis** (mi-o′sis) Constriction of the pupils.

**Miscarriage** (mis-kar′ij) The delivery of a nonviable fetus, usually less than twenty weeks of gestational age.

**Modality** (mo-dal′ĭ-te) A condition under which symptoms develop, becoming better or worse. A method of application of any therapeutic agents.

**Morbidity** (mor-bid′ĭ-te) An injured or disease state. The ratio of ill to well persons.

**Mortality** (mor-tal′ĭ-te) Death from injury or illness.

**Mottled** (mot′tl′d) Refers to skin that has a mixed pattern of white and blue created by pooled venous blood and circulatory collapse.

**Mucous membrane** (mu′kus mem′brān) A thin layer of tissue that lines body cavities or passages that communicate with the outside of the body; the mouth is an example.

**Mucus** (mu′kus) Fluid secreted from mucous membranes.

**Multipara** (mul-tip′ah-rah) A woman who has given birth to two or more children.

**Muscle, Cardiac** (kar′de-ak) Muscle that is unique to the heart. Unlike other muscle, it requires a constant supply of oxygen.

**Muscle fasciculation** (mus′el fah-sik″u-la′-shun) A small local contraction of muscles visible through the skin.

**Muscle, Involuntary** (in-vol′un-ter″e) Muscle tissue that cannot be controlled at will.

**Muscle, Voluntary** (vol′un-ter″e) Muscle tissue that can be controlled at will.

**Mute** (mūt) Unable to speak.

**Mydriasis** (mĭ-dri′ah-sis) Dilation of the pupils.

**Myocardial Infarction** (mi″o-kar′de-al in-fark′shun) Complete blockage of a coronary artery, causing heart muscle damage.

**Myocardium** (mi″o-kar′de-um) The muscle wall of the heart.

**Myoglobin** (mi″o-glo′bin) A protein substance in muscle tissue that stores oxygen, much like the hemoglobin of blood.

**Myoglobinuria** (mi″o-glob″in-u′re-ah) The excretion of myoglobin in the urine.

**Narcosis** (nar-ko′sis) A sleep-like state; stupor; inability to perform any useful activity.

**Narcotic** (nar-kot′ik) A drug that produces stupor or sleep; used medically to relieve pain.

**Nares** (na′rēz) An opening into the nose; nostril.

**Nasal cannula** (na′zal kan′u-lah) Most frequently used oxygen delivery device for patients who have spontaneous breathing; consists of a catheter which is fitted into the nose.

**Nasopharynx** (na″zo-far′inks) The space between the posterior nares and above the level of the soft palate.

**Nausea** (naw′ze-ah) Discomfort in the stomach region which causes a feeling of impending vomiting.

**Navicular bone** (nah-vik′u-lar) A boat-shaped bone such as that found in the wrist or ankle.

**Nebulizer** (neb′u-lĭz″er) An atomizer or

device for misting or fine-spraying of a drug or other liquid.

**Necrosis** (nĕ-kro'sis) The death of tissue; undergoing the process of tissue death.

**Necrotic** (nĕ-krot'ik) Dead tissue; nonliving cells next to living ones.

**Neonate** (ne'o-nāt) A newborn infant.

**Neurogenic shock** (nu"ro-jen'ik) Spinal shock; a transient form of shock due to transection of the spinal cord.

**Neurological** (nu-ro-loj'ik-al) Pertaining to the nervous system.

**Neurotic** (nu-rot'ik) Possessing a tendency towards neurosis; an emotionally unstable individual.

**Neurotoxic** (nu-ro-tok'sik) An agent that acts as a poison to the nervous system; examples are snake venom and certain drugs in large doses.

**Nitrogen narcosis** (ni'tro-jen nar-ko'sis) A stupor or sleep-like state caused by dissolved nitrogen, which has an alcohol-like effect. This condition usually results from diving to great depths.

**Nitroglycerin** (ni-tro-glis'er-in) A vasodilating agent that promotes relaxation of the coronary arteries and thus improves their filling.

**Nocturia** (nok-tu're-ah) The need to void or urinate during the night; the need to urinate awakens the patient.

**Norepinephrine** (nor"ep-ĭ-nef'rin) A hormone manufactured by the body for the purpose of constricting blood vessels; a drug used as a vasoconstrictor.

**Normotensive** (nor"mo-ten'siv) Characterized by normal tone, tension or pressure; for example, a normal blood pressure.

**Noxious cutaneous stimulus** (nok'shus ku-ta'ne-us stim'u-lus) A disagreeable or painful provoking of the skin which produces a response.

**Nuchal rigidity** (nu'kal rĭ-jid'ĭ-te) Stiff neck due to irritation of the meninges or spasm of the neck muscles

**Nystagmus** (nis-tag'mus) Involuntary rotation or shifting of the eyeball, often due to severe brain insult.

**Obese** (o-bēs') Extremely fat.

**Oblique fracture** (ŏ-blēk) A bone broken in a diagonal line.

**Occipital bone** (ok-sip'ĭ-tal) The lower posterior portion of the skull.

**Occiput** (ok'sĭ-put) The lower back part of the head.

**Occlude** (ŏ-klo͞od') To close up tight; to obstruct.

**Occlusive dressing** (ŏ-kloo'siv) A dressing or wound covering that seals the area, not permitting the passage of fluid or air.

**Olecranon process** (o-lek'rah-non) The bony projection of the ulna at the elbow, referred to as the "funny bone" since it produces a vivid and painful sensation when traumatized.

**Olfactory** (ol-fak'to-re) Pertaining to the sense of smell.

**Orbit** (or'bit) Bony cavity surrounding the eyeball; space that confines rotation.

**Organism** (or'gah-nizm) A living plant or animal; a microorganism (germ).

**Orifice** (or'ĭ-fis) An opening into a body cavity.

**Origin of muscle** (or'-ĭ-jin) The end attachment of a muscle, which remains relatively fixed during muscle contraction.

**Oropharyngeal airway** (o"ro-fah-rin'jē-al ār'wa) An airway made of hard rubber or plastic that is shaped to conform to the curvature of the tongue and pharynx.

**Orthopnea** (or"thop-ne'ah) Denotes that the individual must assume an upright position to overcome difficulty in breathing.

**Osmosis** (oz-mo'sis) A pulling force which causes particles in solution to move through a membrane from a dilute to a more concentrated environment.

**Otorrhea** (o"to-re'ah) Drainage of fluid or blood from the ear.

**Ovary** (o'vah-re) A glandular organ in the female which produces eggs for reproduction of the species.

**Oxygen drive** (ok'sĭ-jen) The innate force that gives rise to the need to breathe or to obtain oxygen.

**Oxygen toxicity** (tok-sis'ĭ-te) A poisonous state induced by prolonged overuse of oxygen under certain adverse conditions.

**Pacemaker** (pās'māk-er) The node (concentration of nervous tissue) in the heart that stimulates the heart to beat; a mechanical device that mimics this node.

**Pallor** (pal'or) A whitish tint to the skin caused by blood vessels being severely constricted.

**Palmar** (pal'mar) Pertaining to the palm.

**Palpable** (pal'pah-b'l) Evident through touching or feeling.

**Palpation** (pal-pa'shun) The act of feeling in the process of examination.

**Pancreatitis** (pan"kre-ah-ti'tis) Inflammation of the pancreas.

**Papilledema** (pap"il-ĕ-de'mah) Engorgement of the optic nerve, which is visible by examination using an ophthalmoscope.

**Papule** (pap'ūl) A round, raised lesion on the skin that contains no fluid or air.

**Paradoxical** (par"ah-dok'se-kal) Movement against the usual forces or rules.

**Paralysis** (pah-ral'ĭ-sis) Loss of muscle function or sensation due to nerve injury.

**Paramount** (par'ah-mount) Ranking highest; more important than anything else.

**Paraplegia** (par"ah-ple'je-ah) Paralysis of the legs and the lower part of the body.

**Parasite** (par'ah-sīt) A plant or animal which lives in or on another living thing and thrives at the expense of the host.

**Parasympathetic** (par"ah-sim"pah-thet'ik) That portion of the nervous system which arises from the cranial and sacral nerve tracts. It is concerned with restoring equilibrium or normalcy; for example, slowing the heart rate or breathing when they have been accelerated.

**Parenteral** (pah-ren'ter-al) Outside of the intestinal tract; for example, substances introduced intravenously or intramuscularly.

**Paresis** (pah-re'sis) Slight or incomplete paralysis; weakness.

**Paresthesia** (par"es-the'ze-ah) A numbness or tingling sensation (sometimes stinging or burning) which results from irritation or disease of peripheral nerves.

**Parietal bones** (pah-ri'ĕ-tal) The lateral skull bones; bones which form the walls or sides of the cranium.

**Parturition** (par"tu-rish'un) The act of giving birth.

**Patella** (pah-tel'-ah) Bone of the kneecap.

**Patency** (pa'ten-se) The condition of being wide open; not obstructed.

**Patent** (pa'tent) Open; not obstructed.

**Pathogen** (path'o-jen) An organism (germ) that is capable of producing disease.

**Pedal** (ped'al) Pertaining to the foot or feet.

**Pediatric** (pe"de-at'rik) The branch of medicine that deals with the child.

**Pediculosis** (pe-dik"u-lo'sis) Infestation by lice.

**Pelvis** (pel'vis) The hip bone, which connects the upper torso to the lower torso and serves as a bony encasement for the abdominal organs.

**Percussion** (per-kush'un) The act of striking a part of the body in order to elicit a sound for the purpose of diagnosis.

**Perfusion** (per-fu'zhun) The passage of fluid (especially blood) through a vessel of a specific organ.

**Pericardium** (per"ĭ-kar'de-um) The membranous sac that encloses the heart.

**Perineum** (per"i-ne'um) The pelvic floor and the associated structures occupying the pelvic outlet.

**Periorally** (per"e-o'ra-le) Refers to something around the mouth.

**Periosteum** (per"e-os'te-um) Thin tissue surrounding the outside of bones.

**Periphery** (pĕ-rif'er-e) The outside or the side away from the center.

**Peristalsis** (per"ĭ-stal'sis) Rhythmic contractions of smooth muscle that facilitate the movement of fluid or solids through a hollow, tubular organ such as the bowel.

**Peritoneal dialysis** (per"ĭ-to-ne'al di-al'ĭ-sis) Use of the serous membrane of the abdominal wall as a medium of exchange in order to eliminate waste products from the blood when renal function is inadequate.

**Peritoneum** (per"i-to-ne'um) The serous lining of the abdominal cavity which envelops the abdominal organs.

**Peritonitis** (per"ĭ-to-ni'tis) Inflammation of the peritoneum caused by rupture of the bowel or similar trauma.

**Periumbilical area** (per"e-um-bil'ĭ-kal) Region around the navel or umbilicus.

**Peroneal nerve** (per"o-ne'al) The nerve located on the outer side of the lower leg which supplies the knee and anterior portions of the lower leg.

**Petechiae** (pe-tek′e-e) Tiny red or purple lesions which are sharply outlined. They accompany serious infections such as meningitis.

**Petit mal** (pĕ-te′mahl′) A minor seizure in which the individual does not lose consciousness.

**Phalanges** (fah-lan′jēz) Fingers or toes.

**Pharynx** (far′inks) A continuation of the nose and mouth which connects to the trachea and the esophagus.

**Phlebitis** (flĕ-bi′tis) Inflammation of a blood vessel.

**Pia mater** (pi′ah ma′ter) The innermost of the three covering membranes of the brain and spinal cord.

**Piloerection** (pi″lo-e-rek′shun) The "standing on end" of hair on the body surfaces.

**Pinna** (pin′nah) The external fleshy part of the ear.

**Pit viper** (pit′ vi′per) A snake that possesses a sac of venom. Pit refers to the depression between the eye and the nostril which serves as a heat-sensing organ to locate warm-blooded prey.

**Placebo** (plah-se′bo) A false or inactive drug which satisfies the patient's need for drugs when no medicinal effect is required.

**Placenta** (plah-sen′tah) The organ of pregnancy which serves to nourish the developing fetus; the "afterbirth."

**Plantar** (plan′tar) Refers to the sole of the foot.

**Plaque** (plak) Flat or patchy lesions on a body surface.

**Plasma** (plaz′mah) The fluid portion of the blood in which other constituents are suspended.

**Platelet** (plāt′let) A blood cell that plays a principal role in the coagulation of blood.

**Pleural** (ploor′al) The serous lining of the thorax or chest cavity which envelops the lungs.

**Plexus** (plek′sus) A tangled network; a complex intermixing.

**Pneumomediastinum** (nu″mo-me″de-as-ti′-num) Presence of air or gas in the central portion of the chest which may interfere with breathing or heart action; may lead to pneumothorax.

**Pneumothorax** (nu″mo-tho′-raks) Accumulation of air or gas in the pleural space which results in a collapsed lung.

**Point tenderness** (point ten′der-ness) Increased sensitivity over a highly circumscribed area which can lead to discovery of the exact site of injury.

**Polydipsia** (pol″e-dip′se-ah) Increased desire to drink; abnormal thirst.

**Polyphagia** (pol″e-fa′je-ah) Increased desire to eat; excessive appetite.

**Polyuria** (pol″e-u′re-ah) Increased urinary output; excessive urination.

**Popliteal** (pop-lit′e-al) Refers to the posterior portion of the knee joint.

**Posterior** (pos-tĕr′e-or) Behind; back of.

**Postictal** (pōst-ik′tal) The period of time following a seizure when the patient has not recovered his pre-seizure level of consciousness.

**Post-mortem** (pōst mor′tem) After death.

**Post-partum** (post par′tum) After delivery of a baby.

**Posturing** (pos′tu-ring) Pertaining to the position of the body.

**Precordial** (pre-kor′de-al) Pertaining to the area over the heart.

**Precursor** (pre′kur-sor) An event or condition which precedes or predisposes one to a later event; for example, smoking is a precursor to lung cancer.

**Predisposed** (pre″dis-pōzd) Having a tendency to something; susceptible.

**Preeclampsia** (pre″e-klamp′se-ah) A toxic condition occurring during the later part of pregnancy which is characterized by edema, hypertension, and loss of protein in the urine.

**Prenatal** (pre-na′tal) The period of time before the delivery of a baby; during pregnancy.

**Priapism** (pri′ah-pizm) A pathological or abnormal erection of the penis which is usually due to obstruction of blood flow out of the organ or a serious spinal cord injury; this erection is not associated with sexual desire.

**Primary survey** (pri′ma-re ser-vay) The first part of patient assessment, consisting of the ABCs and immediate correction of any compromise that may be found.

**Primigravida** A woman who is having her first pregnancy.

**Prognosis** (prog-no′sis) Forecast of probable outcome from a disease or other state of imbalance.

**Prolapse** (pro-laps′) Abnormal falling or sinking of an organ; in childbirth, a prolapsed cord indicates that the delivery of the cord precedes that of the infant.

**Pronation** (pro-na′shun) Assumption of a down-turned position, such as turning the palm down.

**Prone** (prōn) Positioned with the face down.

**Prosthesis** (pros-the′sis) An artificial device that takes the place of an absent body part, such as an artificial leg or dentures.

**Protocol** (pro′to-kol) A standard set of guidelines for action in a designated circumstance.

**Proximal** (prok′sĭ-mal) Nearest or closer to any point of reference.

**Pruritus** (proo-ri′tus) Itching; a condition that induces the desire to scratch.

**Ptosis** (to′sis) Drooping or downward displacement; for example, of the eyelid.

**Pubis** (pu′bis) Lower anterior bone of the pelvis.

**Pulmonary edema** (pul′mo-ner″e ĕ-de′mah) Congestion of the lungs resulting from leakage of fluid from the bloodstream.

**Pulmonary embolus** (pul′mo-ner″e em′bo-lus) A blood clot that obstructs the flow of blood in or around the lungs.

**Pulse points** (puls pointz) Points on the body where the heart rate may be counted; usually the sites are where arteries overlie superficial bony structures.

**Pulse rate** (puls rāt) A reflection of the heartbeat obtained by palpation of the artery as it expands in response to the pumping action of the heart; number of beats per minute.

**Pulsus alternans** (pul′sus awl-ter′nanz) A strong pulse beat followed by a weak beat.

**Pupil** (pu′pil) The opening in the eye that admits light.

**Quadrant** (kwod′rant) One quarter of a circle or surface area.

**Quadriceps** (kwod′rĭ-seps) Upper thigh muscles.

**Quadriceps femora** (kwod′rĭ-seps fem′o-rah) Tendon that holds the patella in place.

**Quadriplegia** (kwod″rĭ-ple′je-ah) Paralysis of all extremities (arms and legs).

**Radial artery** (ra′de-al ar′ter-e) Artery located in wrist area; the most frequently palpated artery for obtaining a pulse.

**Radial pulse** (ra′de-al puls) Pulse taken in wrist area over the radial artery.

**Radius** (ra′de-us) Long bone of lower arm.

**Rales** (rahlz) Abnormal breathing sound; a vibrating disconnected breath sound heard during inspiration. Usually indicates that air is passing by secretions in lower airways.

**Reactivity** (re″ak-tiv′ĭ-te) Response. When a light is shown in the eye, the pupil will get smaller or constrict.

**Regurgitation** (re-gur″jĭ-ta′shun) A backward flowing of undigested food from the stomach to the esophagus. Term can also be applied to other backflows, as in large blood vessels or within heart chambers.

**Reticular activating system (RAS)** (rĕ-tik′-u-lar ak′tĭ-vā-ting sis′tem) Brain's center of consciousness or wakefulness.

**Retina** (ret′ĭ-nah) The nervous tissue that receives the light image in the eye and transfers it to the brain's sight center.

**Retraction** (re-trak′shun) The pulling inward of intercostal muscles which are used to facilitate air intake during periods of obstructed airway or other compromise in breathing.

**Retroperitoneal bleeding** (re″tro-per″ĭ-to-ne′al) Bleeding that accompanies renal injury; loss of blood behind the peritoneum.

**Retrosternal** (re″tro-ster′nal) Behind the sternum or breastbone.

**Rhinorrhea** (ri″no-re′ah) Leakage of CSF fluid from the nose.

**Rhonchi** (rong′kī) Abnormal breathing sounds; a musical vibration (fine popping noises) sometimes heard during expiration. They are usually the result of narrowed larger airways.

**Rigor mortis** (rig′or mor′tis) The stiffening of a dead body.

**Rotation** (ro-ta′shun) Movement of a body part around a joint.

**Sager traction splinting** (sā′ger trak′shun splint′ing) A one-piece metal telescoping tube that is placed on the medial side of the lower extremities to stabilize fractures.

**Salicylates** (sal'ĭ-sil"ātz) Any salt of salicylic acid; aspirin and wintergreen are two examples.

**Saline** (sa'līn) Salt solution; usually refers to an isotonic mixture of sodium chloride (0.9%).

**Saliva** (sah-li'vah) Glandular secretion that moistens the mouth, softens food, and prepares it for digestion before it reaches the stomach.

**Salivation** (sal"ĭ-va'shun) The act of producing saliva.

**Scab** (skab) An encrustation that covers and protects a healing lesion.

**Scaphoid** (skaf'oid) One of eight carpal (wrist) bones located on top of the wrist.

**Scapula** (skap'u-lah) A flat triangular bone situated on the posterior thoracic rib cage; the shoulder blade.

**Sclera** (skle'rah) The white, tough outer cover of the eyeball.

**Sclerema neonatorum** (skle-re'mah ne"o-na-tor'um) A yellowing and tallow-like hardening of the subcutaneous fat in infants who have been subjected to prolonged shock states and whose body temperature is subnormal.

**Sebaceous glands** (se-ba'shus glandz) Oil glands connected directly to each hair follicle.

**Sebum** (se'bum) Oily substance secreted by sebaceous glands.

**Secondary survey** (sek'un-der"e sur'va) Consists of the examination of the level of consciousness, an interview of the patient, and a detailed examination of each body system.

**Seizure** (se'zhur) An attack of epilepsy; a convulsion.

**Sellar** (sel'ar) Saddle-like joint.

**Semi-consciousness** (sem"e-kon'shus-nes) An altered state of consciousness in which the patient will at least respond to painful stimuli.

**Semi-Fowler's position** (sem"e-fow'lerz po-zish'un) Semi-sitting position of about 45 degrees in angle.

**Senile** (se'nīl) Characteristic of the aged individual.

**Sepsis** (sep'sis) Presence of both micro-organisms and their toxins in the bloodstream or body tissue during the process of infection.

**Septic shock** (sep'tik shok) Shock characterized by circulatory collapse induced by the release of endotoxins of sepsis into the bloodstream.

**Septum** (sep'tum) A dividing wall of tissue within an organ.

**Sequela** (se-kwel'ah) The aftermath or residual consequences of an illness or injury.

**Serum** (se'rum) The clear portion of a body fluid that remains when solid particles have been eliminated.

**Shock** (shok) Inadequate utilization of oxygen by the cells, caused by low volume states, heart failure, loss of peripheral resistance, and as a complication of certain disease states.

**Shock position** (shok po-zish'un) Placement of the patient in a supine position with legs elevated 30–40 degrees.

**Short bones** (short bōnz) Bones whose length equals (or nearly equals) their width.

**Shoulder girdle** (shōl'der ger'd'l) The bony structure formed by the scapula, or shoulder blade, and the clavicle, or collarbone.

**Shunt** (shunt) To divert; to send in a different direction. A mechanical device used for patients on dialysis therapy to facilitate frequent entry into the circulation. Usually placed in the forearm.

**Sickle cell anemia** (sik'el sel ah-ne'me-ah) A blood disorder of Negroes characterized by joint pain, fever, and abdominal pain. Condition is caused by a clumping of red blood cells in small vessels, thus creating an obstruction to circulation and oxygenation.

**SIDS** Sudden infant death syndrome; crib death.

**Signs** (sīnz) Visible indications.

**Sinus** (si'nus) A cavity or portal of outflow.

**Slough** (sluf) The casting off or shedding of non-living tissue from living tissue.

**Spasm** (spazm) A sudden violent, involuntary contraction of a muscle or a group of muscles.

**Spheroidal** (sfe-roi'dal) Pertaining to a ball and socket joint; round.

**Sphygmomanometer** (sfig"mo-mah-nom'ĕ-ter) An instrument used to measure blood pressure.

**Spontaneous pneumothorax** (spon-ta′ne-us nu″mo-tho′raks) Collapse of the lung in the absence of traumatic insult.

**Sputum** (spu′tum) Matter ejected from the lungs, bronchi, and trachea through the mouth.

**Status epilepticus** (sta′tus ep″ĭ-lep′ti-kus) Two or more successive seizures in which consciousness is not regained before the onset of another seizure.

**Sterile** (ster′il) Free from living microorganisms.

**Sternoclavicular joint** (ster″no-klah-vik′u-lar) Point where the clavicle meets the sternum.

**Sternocleidomastoid muscle** (ster″no-kli″-do-mas′toid mus′el) Anterior muscle in the neck.

**Sternum** (ster′num) Breastbone.

**Stethoscope** (steth′o-skōp) Instrument used to listen to breath sounds, record blood pressure, and count heart rate.

**Stoma** (sto′mah) The external opening such as occurs with a colostomy, tracheostomy, or laryngectomy.

**Strain** (strān) Stretched or torn muscle.

**Stridor** (stri′dor) A high-pitched crowing or "seal-bark" sound classically caused by obstruction of the larynx.

**Stupor** (stu′por) A depressed level of awareness nearing an unconscious state.

**Subcapital** (sub-kap′ĭ-tal) Fracture at base of the femoral head.

**Subcutaneous emphysema** (sub″ku-ta′ne-us em″fĭ-se′mah) The presence of air or gas in the subcutaneous tissues of the body.

**Subcutaneous space** (sub″ku-ta′ne-us spās) Layer of tissue made up of adipose tissue or fat cells in addition to blood vessels, nerves, hair follicles, and sweat glands. Major role of this layer is insulation and protection.

**Subdural hematoma** (sub-du′ral hem″ah-to′mah) Pocket of blood caused by bleeding between dura and arachnoid membranes.

**Subluxation** (sub″luk-sa′shun) Partial or incomplete dislocation of bones that form a joint.

**Substernal** (sub-ster′nal) Under the sternum.

**Subtrochanteric** (sub″tro-kan-ter′ik) Fracture just below the trochanter.

**Subungual hematoma** (sub-ung′gwal hem″-ah-to′mah) Pocket of blood under a fingernail or toenail caused by a solid object impacting on the top of the nail.

**Sucking chest wound** (suk′ing chest wo͞ond) An open pneumothorax with a chest wall wound which permits air to enter or leave the chest, creating a "sucking" sound.

**Superficial arteries** (su″per-fish′al ar′ter-ez) Arteries near the body surface.

**Superior** (su-pe′re-or) Above or in a higher position.

**Supination** (su″pĭ-na′shun) Assumption of the supine position; applied to the hand, the act of turning the palm forward or upward.

**Supine** (su′pīn) A back-down position; lying on the back.

**Supracondylar** (su″prah-kon′dĭ-lar) Lower portion of the humerus.

**Supraorbital ridge** (su″prah-or′bĭ-tal rij) The bony prominence where the eyebrows are located. Part of the frontal bone.

**Surfactant** (sur-fak′tant) Protein mixture that coats the alveoli, enabling them to expand when breathing.

**Suture line** (su′chur līn) The point where two bones meet and are not yet fused, as in the skull of an infant.

**Sympathetic nervous system** (sim″pah-thet′ik ner′vus sis′tem) A part of the automatic nervous system, concerned with mediating the involuntary response to alarm by speeding the heart, increasing B.P., etc.

**Symphysis pubis** (sim′fĭ-sis pu′bis) The joint formed by the union of the pubic bones at the midline.

**Symptom** (simp′tum) A subjective indication of illness or injury which cannot be detected by external observation.

**Syncope** (sin′ko-pe) Fainting due to inadequate perfusion of the brain.

**Syndrome** (sin′drōm) A set of classic symptoms that occur together to indicate a given condition.

**Synovial fluid** (sĭ-no′ve-al floo′id) A thick gel-like substance that lubricates joints, allowing for friction-free movement.

**Synovial joints** (sĭ-no′ve-al jointz) Movable joints.

**Systemic** (sis-tem'ik) Affecting the entire body; generalized.

**Systole** (sis'to-le) The pumping or contraction part of the cardiac cycle in which blood is ejected from the heart into circulation.

**Systolic pressure** (sis-tol'ik presh'ur) Pressure that the blood exerts during the contraction of the ventricles of the heart.

**Tachycardia** (tak"e-kar'de-ah) Unusually rapid heart rate.

**Tachypnea** (tak"ip-ne'ah) Excessive rapidity of respiration; quick shallow breathing.

**Talus** (ta'lus) Ankle bone; articulates with the tibia and fibula to form the ankle joint.

**Tamponade** (tam"pon-ād') Compression of a structure resulting in obstruction of blood flow.

**Tarsal bones** (tahr'sal bonz) Ankle.

**Telemetry** (tĕ-lem'e-tre) Transmission of graphed information such as an ECG by telephone or radio signals.

**Temporal bones** (tem'po-ral bonz) Bony portion of the skull where the ears are located.

**Temporomandibular joint** (tem"po-ro-mandib'u-lar joint) Permits movement of the lower jaw. Located just in front of the hole in the ear.

**Tendon** (ten'dun) The terminal position of a muscle that crosses over joints and attaches the muscle to bone.

**Tenesmus** (te-nez'mus) The act of straining.

**Tension pneumothorax** (ten'shun nu"mo-tho'raks) Caused when air builds up in the chest cavity and collapses the injured lung, causing displacement of the mediastinum to the opposite side and compressing the uninjured lung.

**Testicular torsion** (tes-tik'u-lar tor'shun) A clinical emergency characterized by a twisting of the spermatic cord or the testicle.

**Tetanus** (tet'ah-nus) Infection characterized by severe contractures of the muscles of the face and back; "lockjaw."

**Thalamus** (thal'ah-mus) Portion of the brain that relays sensory impulses.

**Thermal** (ther'mal) Pertaining to temperature.

**Thomas half-ring splint** (tom'as) Splinting device to which leg cradles and traction mechanisms must be added for use. Used to stabilize lower extremity fractures.

**Thoracic cavity** (tho-ras'ik kav'ĭ-te) Chest; extends from the shoulders to the diaphragm.

**Thoracic spine** (tho-ras'ik spīn) That part of the spine which extends from the shoulder area to the diaphragm area.

**Thready pulse** (thre'de) Weak and rapid pulse; difficult to detect upon palpation.

**Thrombus** (throm'bus) A blood clot formed inside a blood vessel or the heart.

**Thyroxine** (thi-rok'sin) A hormone released from the thyroid gland which increases cellular metabolism.

**TIA, "mini-strokes"** Transient ischemic attack. A temporary interruption of blood supply to a localized area of the brain, causing a stroke-like condition which is short-lived and without any residual damage.

**Tibia** (tib'e-ah) The long bone in the lower leg which runs parallel to the fibula on the medial side of the leg.

**Tibiofemoral joint** (tib"e-o-fem'or-al) Knee joint.

**Tibiotalus joint** (tib"e-o-ta'lus) Ankle joint.

**Tic** (tik) A spasmodic twitch.

**Tinnitus** (tĭ-ni'tus) Ringing in the ear.

**Topographic anatomy** (top"o-graf'ik ah-nat'o-me) Anatomy of the surface area of the body.

**Toxemia** (tok-se'me-ah) Poisoning of the blood by toxins.

**Toxin** (tok'sin) Poison produced by microorganisms as they multiply within the body.

**Tracheal tug** (tra'ke-al tug) A pulling in at the neck, just above the sternum, during a struggle to take in air.

**Tracheostomy** (tra"ke-os'to-me) Creation of a surgical opening into the trachea through the neck.

**Traction** (trak'shun) Longitudinal pulling.

**Transfusion** (trans-fu'zhun) The introduction of blood, saline, or other liquid into a blood vessel.

**Transverse** (trans-vers′) A horizontal plane at the shoulders which divides the body into upper and lower portions.

**Transverse fracture** (trans-vers′ frak′tur) A bone that is broken straight across.

**Trapezium** (trah-pe′ze-um) One of eight carpal (wrist) bones, located on bottom of wrist.

**Trapezius muscle** (trah-pe′ze-us mus′el) Anterior muscle in the neck; forms the top of the shoulders.

**Trapezius pinch** (trah-pe′ze-us pinch) Pinching of the trapezius muscle as a mode of assessing for nervous system dysfunction by the application of unpleasant stimuli.

**Trapezoid** (trap′e-zoid) One of the eight carpal (wrist) bones, located on bottom of wrist.

**Trauma** (traw′mah) Presence of wounds and injuries.

**Traumatic asphyxia** (traw-mat′ik as-fik′-se-ah) Inability to breathe due to severe injury to the upper airways or chest cage.

**Trendelenburg position** (tren-del′en-berg po-zish′un) A supine position with the head down and the remainder of the body up at about a 30° angle.

**Triage** (tre-ahzh′) In multiple victim scenes, the sorting of victims into categories for care based on priorities of types of injuries.

**Triquetrum** (tri-kwe′trum) One of eight carpal (wrist) bones, located on top of wrist.

**Trochanter** (tro-kan′ter) Either of the two processes below the neck of the femur.

**Trochoid** (tro′koid) A pivot joint; allows bones to pivot on one another.

**Turgid** (tur′jid) Swollen or congested.

**Turgor** (tur′gor) Swollen or full; elasticity; suppleness.

**Tympanum** (tim′pah-num) Eardrum.

**Ulcer** (ul′ser) A local defect on the surface of body tissue due to erosion of necrotic tissue which has been inflamed.

**Ulna** (ul′nah) Long bone of lower arm.

**Umbilicus** (um-bil′ĭ-kus) Navel.

**Unconscious** (un-kon′shus) Unarousable; unresponsive; lacking any response to stimulus, even deep pain.

**Uremia** (u-re′me-ah) Retention in the bloodstream of waste products normally eliminated by the kidneys.

**Urethra** (u-re′thrah) Tube that transports urine from the bladder.

**Urticaria** (ur″tĭ-ka′re-ah) A vascular skin reaction characterized by burning and itching.

**Uterus** (u′ter-us) Womb; organ that supports a developing fetus.

**Vaccine** (vak-sēn) A mixture of dead (or disabled) microorganisms administered to prevent or modify infectious diseases which are contagious.

**Vagina** (vah-ji′nah) The hollow tube which connects the uterus to the external perineum. The female organ of intercourse; the birth canal.

**Valsalva maneuver** (val-sal′vah mah-noo′-ver) A process by which a person attempts to forcibly exhale through his nose against a closed glottis.

**Vascular** (vas′ku-lar) Pertaining to or full of vessels.

**Vasoconstriction** (vas″o-kon-strik′shun) Contraction of the vascular system or narrowing of vessels, resulting in increased resistance to blood flow. Violent contraction of a blood vessel to eliminate hemorrhage.

**Vasodilation** (vas″o-di-la′shun) Vessel relaxation; decreased resistance to blood flow.

**Vasopressor** (vas″o-pres′or) An agent that constricts or narrows blood vessels and raises peripheral resistance.

**Vasospasm** (vas′o-spazm) Clamping down of a severed blood vessel to reduce blood loss.

**Vein** (vān) Any one of a series of vessels that carries blood from various parts of the body back to the heart. All veins in the body conduct unoxygenated blood except the pulmonary veins, which conduct freshly oxygenated blood from the lungs back to the heart.

**Vena cava** (ve′nah ka′vah) Inferior: Vein returning blood from lower extremities, pelvis, and abdominal area. Superior: Vein returning blood from head, neck, upper extremities, and chest.

**Venipuncture** (ven′ĭ-punk″tūr) Needle entry into a vein.

**Venom** (ven′um) Poisonous substance secreted by a snake or insect.

**Venous congestion** (ve′nus kon-jest′yun) Abnormal accumulation of blood in veins.

**Ventilation** (ven″tĭ-la′shun) Exchange of air between the lungs and the ambient air.

**Ventral** (ven′tral) Denoting a position more toward the belly surface than some other object of reference; same as anterior.

**Ventricle** (ven′trĭ-k'l) One of the two lower chambers of the heart. Left ventricle pumps oxygenated blood through the arteries to the body. Right ventricle pumps unoxygenated blood through the pulmonary artery to the lungs.

**Ventricular contraction** (ven-trik′u-lar kon-trak′shun) Pumping action of the ventricles of the heart.

**Ventricular fibrillation** (ven-trik′u-lar fi-brĭ-la′shun) Arrhythmia characterized by rapid contractions of the ventricular muscle.

**Venule** (ven′ūl) A small vessel that collects blood from capillaries for return to the venous system.

**Vermilion border** (ver-mil′yun bor′der) The definitive color line between the lips and surrounding skin.

**Vertigo** (ver′tĭ-go) Dizziness.

**Vesicle** (ves′ĭ-k'l) A small elevation of the skin containing fluid; a blister.

**Vesication** (ves-i-ka′shun) Blistering.

**Viable** (vi′ah-b'l) Living; alive.

**Viscera** (vis′er-ah) Body organs.

**Volkmann's ischemic contracture** (fōlk′-mahnz is-kem′ik kon-trak′tūr) Condition evidenced by shrinking and hardening of muscles in limbs, leaving the patient with a stiff limb and claw-like hands or feet. It can be a complication of an untreated fracture.

**Vomitus** (vom′ĭ-tus) Emesis; expelled contents of the stomach.

**Vulva** (vul′vah) The external genital organs of a female.

**Wheal** (hwēl, wēl) A small, raised, fluid-filled lesion, usually just under the epidermis.

**Wheezing** (hwē′zing) Abnormal breathing sounds; a high-pitched or whistle-like noise usually noted on exhalation. May be caused by constriction or obstruction in the lower airways.

**White blood cell** (hwīt blud sel) A colorless cell of the blood which plays several roles in protecting the organism against infections and other disease states.

**Wind chill factor** (wind chil fak′tor) The temperature derived when the forces of wind are added to the baseline temperature; reflects total cooling force of the wind upon the exposed body.

**Womb** (wōōm) The uterus.

**Xiphoid** (zif′oid) Lower part of the sternum area.

**X-ray** (eks′ra) A diagnostic test to detect internal pathology by using electrically generated rays to produce a radiograph.

**Zygoma** (zi-go′mah) The arch formed by the zygomatic processes of the temporal bone and the maxilla, and the zygomatic bone.

**Zygomatic bone** (zi″go-mat′ik bōn) Cheek bone.

# Index